The Palgrave Handbook of Disability and Communication

"The communication discipline has incredibly valuable insights to offer on the experience and enactment of disability. The four editors collected and organized *The Palgrave Handbook of Disability and Communication*, offering tremendous breadth and depth of communication scholarship. The chapter authors span interpersonal, health, mediated, rhetorical, and critical approaches to understanding and living the experience of disability in human life. This volume represents excellence in current scholarship and practices and will be extremely valuable for scholars across academic disciplines, practitioners, and persons experiencing disability."
—Dawn O. Braithwaite, *Willa Cather Professor of Communication Emerita, University of Nebraska-Lincoln, USA*

"Always engaging and eminently readable, the handbook includes a breadth and depth of subject matter and methodologies—ideal for the disability studies classroom. The handbook provides foundational material that contextualizes contemporary, pressing issues in the field. Most importantly, contributors never lose sight of the lived experience of disability in all its variety. I am eager to enliven and update the curriculum in my disability arts and culture courses with this exceptional collection."
—Carrie Sandahl, PhD, *Director Program on Disability Art, Culture and Humanities, Disability and Human Development at University of Illinois Chicago, USA*

"This is an exciting collection of essays bringing together disability and communication, but the scope is much larger than the title suggests. Communication is expanded to include the varied uses of language, rhetoric, and media-driven content that is so crucial to our postmodern lives. There is something of great interest in every essay, and the book made me rethink many important ideas in disability studies. It is definitely a must-read book."
—Lennard J. Davis, *Distinguished Professor of Liberal Arts and Science at the University of Illinois at Chicago, USA*

"*The Palgrave Handbook of Disability and Communication* expertly explores the intersection of disability and communication and illustrates the cultural power all societies have to transmit communication frameworks that have long stigmatized the experience of disability and its representations. *The Handbook* deconstructs ableist communication of past and present, as well as showing how present-day empowered disabled people have more agency to control communicative structures. *The Handbook* interrogates many of the ways humans communicate disability concepts but with contemporary sociocultural-informed research that highlights disability identity and pride, new online communication methods, and major interactions with the ableist world. Chapters cover language, identity, intersectionality, cultural artifacts, institutional structures, activism, and social policy. Specifically, topics include: microaggressions, memes, collaborative

podcasting, artificial intelligence, masking during a pandemic, accessibility in video games, Brexit, service dogs, police brutality, TikTok, Deaf children, and much more. A variety of methods are used from autoethnography to content analysis to case studies. All in all, *The Handbook* skillfully moves forward much-needed research that interweaves Disability Studies and Communication Studies into a substantial inquiry now but with the hope that new scholars in these fields will continue this critical work into the future."
—Beth A. Haller, PhD, author, *Representing Disability in an Ableist World, Essays on Mass Media*

"The Palgrave Handbook of Disability and Communication accomplishes what all handbooks should: it positions itself as the anthology you need to guide your thinking about the intersections of the central areas of study, disability and communication; it offers groundbreaking chapters that are indispensable for further research in the fields; and it does all of this in an accessible, engaging manner. For scholars in disability studies and communication studies, this anthology will be a required resource."
—Robert McRuer, *Professor of English, George Washington University, and author of Crip Theory (2006) and Crip Time (2018)*

"This collection explores, evokes, and enmeshes the overlaps and intersections between disability and communication from a vast and impressive range of perspectives—27 chapters! Yet the book is so clearly organized, and each chapter so well-written, that the result is both encyclopedic and concise. *The Palgrave Handbook of Disability and Communication* also could not feel more timely, with every chapter connecting to contemporary issues. This is a tremendous accomplishment, and an incredibly useful resource."
—Jay Dolmage, *Professor of English, University of Waterloo, Founding Editor of the Canadian Journal of Disability Studies*

"Boasting an amazing collection of authors addressing disability from different perspectives and identities, this *Handbook* shows the importance of conceiving of disability as a complex set of professional, personal, and political relations—always meaningful and always more than we expect. Readers are provided many pathways to encounter what disability experience and representation means to communication studies and what communication means to disability studies. The array of chapters constitutes a brilliant way to nurture deeper relations to our embodied selves."
—Tanya Titchkosky, PhD, *The Ontario Institute for Studies in Education of the University of Toronto, Canada*

Michael S. Jeffress • Joy M. Cypher
Jim Ferris • Julie-Ann Scott-Pollock
Editors

The Palgrave Handbook of Disability and Communication

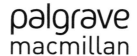

Editors
Michael S. Jeffress
Medical University of the Americas
Nevis, Saint Kitts and Nevis

Jim Ferris
Department of Disability Studies
The University of Toledo
Toledo, OH, USA

Joy M. Cypher
Department of Communication Studies
Rowan University
Glassboro, NJ, USA

Julie-Ann Scott-Pollock
Department of Communication Studies
University of North Carolina Wilmington
Wilmington, NC, USA

ISBN 978-3-031-14446-2   ISBN 978-3-031-14447-9   (eBook)
https://doi.org/10.1007/978-3-031-14447-9

© The Editor(s) (if applicable) and The Author(s), under exclusive licence to Springer Nature
Switzerland AG 2023
This work is subject to copyright. All rights are solely and exclusively licensed by the Publisher,
whether the whole or part of the material is concerned, specifically the rights of translation,
reprinting, reuse of illustrations, recitation, broadcasting, reproduction on microfilms or in any
other physical way, and transmission or information storage and retrieval, electronic adaptation,
computer software, or by similar or dissimilar methodology now known or hereafter developed.
The use of general descriptive names, registered names, trademarks, service marks, etc. in this
publication does not imply, even in the absence of a specific statement, that such names are exempt
from the relevant protective laws and regulations and therefore free for general use.
The publisher, the authors, and the editors are safe to assume that the advice and information in
this book are believed to be true and accurate at the date of publication. Neither the publisher nor
the authors or the editors give a warranty, expressed or implied, with respect to the material
contained herein or for any errors or omissions that may have been made. The publisher remains
neutral with regard to jurisdictional claims in published maps and institutional affiliations.

Cover illustration: Orkidia / Alamy Stock Vector.

This Palgrave Macmillan imprint is published by the registered company Springer Nature
Switzerland AG.
The registered company address is: Gewerbestrasse 11, 6330 Cham, Switzerland

CONTENTS

1 Introduction   1
Michael S. Jeffress, Joy M. Cypher, Jim Ferris, and
Julie-Ann Scott-Pollock

Part I   Language and Disability   15

2 Language Matters: Disability and the Power of Taboo Words   17
Joanne Arciuli and Tom Shakespeare

**3 Communicating by Accident: Dysfluency, the Non-Essential,
and the Catastrophe**   31
Joshua St. Pierre

4 Cross-Neurotype Communication Competence   45
Emily Stones

5 Microaggressions Toward People with Disabilities   67
Danielle Sparrow, Erin Sahlstein Parcell, Emily R. Gerlikovski,
and Dathan N. Simpson

**6 "When We Say That It's Private, a Lot of People Assume It
Just Doesn't Exist": Communication, Disability, and Sexuality**   81
Ameera Ali

Part II   Identity and Intersectionalities   97

7 Ableism and Intersectionality: A Rhetorical Analysis   99
James L. Cherney

vi CONTENTS

8 **Performing FitCrip in Daily Life: A Critical Autoethnographic Reflection on Embodied Vulnerability**   113
Julie-Ann Scott-Pollock

9 **On a Scale of One to Ten: A Lyric Autoethnography of Chronic Pain and Illness**   129
Shelby Swafford

10 **On Being a Diabetic Black Male: An Autoethnography of Race, Gender, and Invisible Disability**   145
Antonio L. Spikes

11 **Physical Disability in Interabled Romantic Relationships: Exploring How Women with Visible, Physical Disabilities Navigate and Internalize Conversations About Their Identity with Male Romantic Partners**   163
Lisa J. DeWeert and Aimee E. Miller-Ott

12 **Disposable Masks, Disposable Lives: Aggrievement Politics and the Weaponization of Disabled Identity**   185
Brian Grewe and Craig R. Weathers

Part III   Cultural Artifacts and Disability   203

13 **Communicating AI and Disability**   205
Gerard Goggin, Andrew Prahl, and Kuansong Victor Zhuang

14 **Thinking Inclusiveness, Diversity, and Cultural Equity Based on Game Mechanics and Accessibility Features in Popular Video Games**   221
Alexandra Dumont and Maude Bonenfant

15 **Posthuman Critical Theory and the Body on *Sports Night***   243
Peter J. Gloviczki

16 **Never Go Full Potato: Discourses of Ableism and Sexism in "I Can Count to Potato" Memes**   253
Jeff Preston

CONTENTS vii

17 #DisabilityTikTok 273
Jordan Foster and David Pettinicchio

Part IV Institutional Constructs and Constraints 293

18 Communicating Vulnerability in Disasters: Media Coverage of People with Disabilities in Hurricane Katrina and the Tōhoku Earthquake and Tsunami 295
Liz Shek-Noble

19 "Kept in a Padded Black Cell in Case He Accidently Said 'Piccaninny'": Disability as Humor in Brexit Rhetoric 317
Emmeline Burdett

20 "Oh, We Are Going to Have a Problem!": Service Dog Access Microaggressions, Hyper-Invisibility, and Advocacy Fatigue 331
Robert L. Ballard, Sarah J. Ballard, and Lauren E. Chu

21 "The Fuzzy Mouse": Unresolved Reflections on Podcasting, Public Pedagogy, and Intellectual Disability 351
Chelsea T. Jones, Jennifer Chatsick, Kimberlee Collins, and Anne Zbitnew

22 Organizational Communication and Disability: Improvising Sense-Sharing 369
Amin Makkawy and Shane T. Moreman

Part V Advocacy, Policy, and Action 383

23 Overlooked and Undercounted: Communication and Police Brutality Against People with Disabilities 385
Deion S. Hawkins

24 Critical Disability Studies in Technical Communication: A 25-Year History and the Future of Accessibility 401
Leah Heilig

25 Communication Infrastructures: Examining How Community Storytelling Facilitates or Constrains Communication Related to Medicaid Waivers for Children 417
Whittney H. Darnell

viii CONTENTS

26 Governing Deaf Children and Their Parents Through (and into) Language 441
Tracey Edelist

27 #ImMentallyIllAndIDontKill: A Case Study of Grassroots Health Advocacy Messages on Twitter Following the Dayton and El Paso Shootings 461
Sarah Smith-Frigerio

References 475

Index 545

Notes on Contributors

Ameera Ali, PhD is an educational developer specializing in equity, diversity, and inclusion at York University in Toronto, Canada. Her broad research interests include critical disability studies, equity-oriented pedagogies in higher education, and childhood studies. Her most recent disability-related publication is featured in Jeffress' latest edited volume, *Disability Representation in Film, TV, and Print Media* (2021).

Joanne Arciuli, PhD is a full professor and Dean of Research in the College of Nursing and Health Sciences at Flinders University, Australia. She has been involved in child development and disability research for several decades. Her much loved brother, Andrew, had Duchenne muscular dystrophy and taught her a lot about life. She has been continuously funded by the Australian Research Council since 2007 and has published over 100 peer-reviewed journal articles including many co-authored papers with international collaborators.

Robert L. Ballard, PhD is the former Blanche E. Seaver Professor of Communication at Pepperdine University. He is now the owner/operator of Dog Training Elite Denver, a company that specializes in service dog training and disability advocacy. He is the author of numerous publications in communication ethics, disability, and transracial adoption, identity, and family communication. He has a Bernedoodle service dog named Binh An who assists with hearing alert, anxiety, and mobility.

Sarah J. Ballard, MA is Former Professor of Practice at Pepperdine University. She is now the owner/operator of Dog Training Elite Denver, a company that specializes in service dog training and disability advocacy. She is the co-author on a variety of articles and chapters related to transracial adoption and family communication. She has a Border Collie/Poodle mix service dog named Oso who assists with chronic pain and mobility.

x NOTES ON CONTRIBUTORS

Maude Bonenfant, PhD is a full professor, at the Department of Social and Public Communication, Université du Québec à Montréal. With a doctorate in semiotics, she specializes in social dimensions of communication technologies, social networks, big data, artificial intelligence, gamification, and video games. She holds a Canada Research Chair on Big Data and Gamer Communities, and she is also Co-director of the Research Laboratory for Social Media and Gamification and Director of the *Homo Ludens* research group on games and communication.

Emmeline Burdett, PhD is a co-editor of the blog journal Public Disability History. She is an independent scholar who has just finished working on a book about the use of the Nazi analogy in Anglo-US debates about euthanasia. She has also translated Pieter Verstraete and Christine van Everbroeck's book *Reintegrating Bodies and Minds*, from Dutch into English. The book was about the experiences of Belgian soldiers left disabled due to their service in World War I (1914–1918), and it was published in 2018 to coincide with the centenary of the end of the conflict.

Jennifer Chatsick, RSW, MSW is a professor in the Faculty of Health Sciences and Wellness at Humber College in Toronto, Canada. She has over 20 years of experience working with learners in community-based literacy programs and in a college setting. Her work focuses on providing accessible and inclusive education.

James L. Cherney, PhD is Associate Professor and the Director of the Communication Core in the Department of Communication Studies, and Faculty Associate in the Department of Gender, Race, and Identity, at the University of Nevada, Reno. He primarily researches the rhetoric of ableism by examining how it operates in public debates and influences popular media. His work includes his book *Ableist Rhetoric: How We Know, Value, and See Disability* (2019) and articles on disability sport and the visual rhetoric of disability in film.

Lauren E. Chu, BA is a PhD student in Biobehavioral Health and The Penn State University researching the biological embedding of stress and mitochondrial functioning. She has published in *Mitochondrian* and the *Psy Chi Journal of Psychological Research*. Her Goldendoodle service dog, Decker, had just retired but assisted with chronic pain, mobility, and stress intervention.

Kimberlee Collins, MA is a PhD student at the Dalla Lana School of Public Health, University of Toronto. Her research explores emotional responses to climate change and is supported by a Joseph-Armand Bombardier Canada Graduate Scholarship. She is an award-winning writer whose recent work has been published in *Journal of Literary & Cultural Disability Studies, Global Public Health,* and *Journal of Research in Arts Education*.

Joy M. Cypher, PhD is Professor of Communication Studies at Rowan University. She has grounded her scholarship at the intersection of communication, the body, and normalcy—bringing Disability Studies into conversation with the ethical enactments of our communicative worlds. She has developed courses in communication ethics, health, the construction of health, and a co-created course in the rhetoric of normalcy. She is the Founding Coordinator of the Health and Science Communication interdisciplinary program at Rowan University. She has won numerous teaching awards, including Rowan University's Lindback Award for Distinguished Teaching, and she was named Eastern Communication Association Teaching Fellow.

Whittney H. Darnell, PhD is an assistant professor at Northern Kentucky University and a member of the National Communication Association Interpersonal Communication Division's Diversity, Equity, and Inclusion Task Force. Her research focuses on understanding and improving the conversations people have about their health and wellness in everyday health contexts. Her work has appeared in academic journals, such as *Health Communication*, *Qualitative Health Research*, and the *Journal of International Research in Higher Education*.

Lisa J. DeWeert, MA is an adjunct communication professor at various Midwest universities. Her research focuses on the crossover between disability and interpersonal relationships, and she has presented her work at regional and national conferences. She focuses on the usefulness of translational work and the application of academic research in everyday life. She is a co-founder of Moxie Adaptive, for folks with limb differences, and she is a staff member of Young Life in Chicagoland.

Alexandra Dumont is a PhD candidate in Communication at the Université du Québec à Montréal. She is a research assistant for the *Canada Research Chair on Big Data and Gamer Communities*. Her research interest focuses on video games' social dimensions, such as representation, disability, and gaming communities. Other fields of interest include mobile games, monetization, and gambling mechanics.

Tracey Edelist, PhD researches societal norms and assumptions about speech, language, and hearing, and the lived consequences of those assumptions. She teaches disability studies courses at various Canadian universities and is completing a postdoctoral program at Université du Québec à Trois-Rivières, bringing critical disability studies perspectives to research within speech-language pathology. She served for five years on the Editorial Review Board of *Disability Studies Quarterly* and is a past board executive of the Canadian Disability Studies Association.

Jim Ferris, PhD holds the Ability Center Endowed Chair in Disability Studies at The University of Toledo. He is a poet and performance artist. He is the award-winning author of *Slouching Towards Guantanamo, Facts of Life*, and

The Hospital Poems. He has performed his poetry at the Kennedy Center and across the United States, Canada, and Great Britain. He is past president of the Society for Disability Studies and has published in dozens of publications, ranging from *POETRY* to *Text & Performance Quarterly,* from the *Georgia Review* to weekly newspapers.

Jordan Foster is a PhD candidate in the Department of Sociology at the University of Toronto. Jordan's research combines insights from across cultural sociology with work on consumption, new media studies, and inequality. This includes work on the representation of disability in mainstream and social media. Jordan's research has been published in such venues as the *Journal of Consumer Culture, European Journal of Cultural Studies,* and *Communications, Culture and Critique.*

Emily R. Gerlikovski, MA is a doctoral student, distinguished graduate fellow in the Humanities and Arts, and graduate teaching assistant at the University of Illinois at Urbana-Champaign. Her research interests center on interpersonal and family communication, often with a focus on LGBTQ+ individuals. She is also interested in sex education and sex communication, with her MA thesis highlighting the experiences of LGBTQ+ parents and how they talk about sex topics with their children.

Peter J. Gloviczki, PhD is a professor and chairperson of the Department of Broadcasting and Journalism at Western Illinois University. He is the author of *Mediated Narration in the Digital Age: Storying the Media World* (2021) and *Journalism and Memorialization in the Age of Social Media* (Palgrave Macmillan, 2015).

Gerard Goggin, PhD is Wee Kim Wee Professor of Communication Studies at Nanyang Technological University, Singapore. He is also Professor of Media and Communications at the University of Sydney. Gerard has published widely on disability and technology, with key books including with Christopher Newell, *Digital Disability* (2003) and *Disability in Australia* (2005); *Disability and the Media* (2015; with Katie Ellis); and the *Routledge Companion to Disability and Media* (2020).

Brian Grewe, PhD is the Director of Disability Access Services at Arapahoe Community College in Littleton, Colorado. His professional work centers on disability justice, access, and equity and student success through the lens of communication ethics. His research interests focus on the intersections of disability, education, and ethics within discourses of disability. He has served in different capacities as an adjunct instructor and visiting teaching assistant professor, teaching courses on disability, relational communication, and research methods.

Deion S. Hawkins, PhD is Assistant Professor of Argumentation and Advocacy and the Director of Debate at Emerson College in Boston, Massachusetts. As a first-generation college graduate, Deion has always been passionate about the power of education to promote advocacy, empathy, and dialogue. As a critical health communication scholar, he remains committed to advancing equity and fighting racism and other systems of oppression. His most recent research can be found in *American Behavioral Scientist, Frontiers in Health Communication,* and *Health Communication.*

Leah Heilig, PhD is Assistant Professor of Writing and Rhetoric at the University of Rhode Island. Her research interests include technical communication, disability studies and accessibility, user-centered design, and rhetorics of mental illness. Her work can be found in *Technical Communication Quarterly, Business and Professional Communication Quarterly,* and *Communication Design Quarterly,* among others.

Michael S. Jeffress, PhD is a full professor and school counselor at Medical University of the Americas in Saint Kitts and Nevis. He has been involved in disability advocacy work since the mid-1990s, after his son was diagnosed with Duchenne muscular dystrophy. He is an active member of the Disability Issues Caucus of the National Communication Association and is an author and editor of numerous books, chapters, and articles within the field of interdisciplinary disability studies. His latest edited volume is *Disability Representation in Film, TV, and Print Media* (2022).

Chelsea T. Jones, PhD is an award-winning writer and editor of numerous articles, books, and special issues. Her most recent work on disability, technology, and pedagogy has been published in *Technology in Society, International Journal of Education Through Art,* and *Journalism and Mass Communication Educator.* She is an assistant professor in the Department of Child and Youth Studies at Brock University in Toronto, Canada.

Amin Makkawy, PhD is an associate professor in the Department of Communication at California State University, Fresno. He builds connections between the field of communication studies and disability studies by researching how interactions between the disabled and the nondisabled within organizational contexts shape and are shaped by communicative acts. He leverages the resulting scholarly inertia to further develop as well as imagine theoretical and practical possibilities for both communication studies and disability studies. His most recent publications have appeared in the *Journal of Visual Impairment & Blindness* and *Communication Education.*

Aimee E. Miller-Ott, PhD is a full professor in the School of Communication at Illinois State University, where she has received the Outstanding University Teaching Award, the Outstanding College Teacher Award, and the Outstanding College Researcher Award. She has authored over 30 published research articles and book chapters. She explores ways through which people manage identity and information through their communication in the contexts of family health and non-traditional family types.

Shane T. Moreman, PhD is a full professor in the Department of Communication at California State University, Fresno. An intercultural communication scholar with a focus on anti-racism, he researches cultural identity expression using critical, humanities-based methods. His research, teaching, and leadership projects are never far removed from his Latinx, queer world making sensibilities. Growing up within a bilingual and bicultural South Texas context, he is eternally optimistic that collaborating across our differences provides us new ways toward unrealized social justice capacities.

Erin Sahlstein Parcell, PhD is Professor of Communication at the University of Wisconsin-Milwaukee where she is also Chair of the Department of Communication and Co-chair of the Institutional Review Board for Human Subjects. She co-edited *A Communication Perspective on the Military: Interactions, Messages, and Discourses* (2015). Her research has earned grants and awards including the 2019 Waterhouse Family Institute Research Grant and the 2017 National Communication Association Distinguished Article Award from the Family Communication Division.

David Pettinicchio, PhD is Associate Professor of Sociology and affiliated faculty at the University of Toronto's Munk School of Global Affairs and Public Policy. His research lies at the intersection of politics and inequality, with a focus on disability as global axis of exclusion and marginalization. He published the book *Politics of Empowerment* and is co-editing the *Oxford Handbook on the Sociology of Disability*.

Andrew Prahl, PhD is an assistant professor at the Wee Kim Wee School of Communication and Information at Nanyang Technological University, Singapore. His research addresses the consequences of replacing humans with machines. More broadly, Andrew's research investigates the effects of disruptive technologies on human communication and society.

Jeff Preston, PhD is Associate Professor of Disability Studies at King's University College at Western University where he teaches classes on disability, popular culture, and policy. A long-time advocate and public speaker, Jeff's work focuses on the intersection of disability, subjectivity, biopower, and culture. Jeff's first book, *The Fantasy of Disability*, was published in 2016.

Julie-Ann Scott-Pollock, PhD is Professor of Communication Studies at the University of North Carolina Wilmington (UNCW). Her areas of interest include performance ethnography and disabled embodiment and identity as performance. Her work can be found in journals such as *Text and Performance Quarterly, Qualitative Inquiry, Disability Studies Quarterly*, and *Departures in Critical Qualitative Research*. She has received numerous Top Paper awards from the National Communication Association and was the 2015 recipient of the UNCW Distinguished Scholarly Engagement and Public Service Award.

Tom Shakespeare, PhD is Professor of Disability Research in the Faculty of Epidemiology and Public Health at the London School of Hygiene and Tropical Medicine. He has been involved in the UK disability rights movement for more than 30 years. He spent five years at the World Health Organization and helped produce the *World Report on Disability* (2011). He has published more than 100 papers and chapters in the last 30 years, and his books include *Disability Rights and Wrongs* (2006) and *Disability—the Basics* (2018).

Liz Shek-Noble, PhD is a project assistant professor at the University of Tokyo in Japan. Her research areas include literary disability studies, adaptation studies, and media studies. Her work has appeared in publications including *Disability & Society*, *Genre*, and *Journal of Literary & Cultural Disability Studies*. She is working on a project funded by the Japan Society for the Promotion of Science on cultural representations of disability in contemporary Australian literature and society.

Dathan N. Simpson, MA is a doctoral student and graduate teaching assistant at the University of Wisconsin-Milwaukee. His research interests lie within interpersonal and health communication. He is researching how military families communicate about disability. His research also explores the experiences of LGBT service members.

Sarah Smith-Frigerio, PhD is Assistant Professor of Public Relations at the University of Tampa. Her research interests include crisis and health communication. Specifically, her work focuses on how we communicate about mental health concerns, as well as health advocacy and health activism. Her research has been published in *Health Communication*, *Qualitative Health Research*, and *Communication, Culture & Critique*.

Danielle Sparrow, MA is a global project manager with Clinical Edge, Inc. in Milwaukee, Wisconsin, where she works with sponsors and contract research organizations on clinical trials. She is a former Clinical Research Coordinator II in emergency medicine and surgery. Her research about microaggressions earned the inaugural 2018 Dawn O. Braithwaite award for qualitative research from the Interpersonal and Small Group Communication Interest Group of the Central States Communication Association.

Antonio L. Spikes, PhD is Assistant Professor of Communication Studies at Coe College in Cedar Rapids, IA, and Chair of the Diversity, Equity, and Inclusion Committee of Southern States Communication Association. His research focuses on the intersections of race, gender, disability, and sexuality. His most recent publication is a co-authored chapter on rachet feminism in *Badass Feminist Politics: Exploring Radical Edges of Feminist Theory, Communication, and Activism.*

xvi NOTES ON CONTRIBUTORS

Emily Stones, PhD is an associate professor at Regis University and resides in Arvada, Colorado, with her neurodiverse family. Her research interests include pedagogy, disability advocacy, nonprofit rhetoric, and the intersection of these areas. Her publications have appeared in journals such as *Humanities, Communication Teacher*, and *Teaching Media Quarterly* and in two edited volumes, *Pedagogy, Disability, and Communication: Applying Disability Studies in the Classroom* and *Disability Representations in Film, TV, and Print*. She received a Fulbright Award in 2022 and is slated to teach a disability history and culture class in 2023 at Nihon University in Japan.

Joshua St. Pierre, PhD is Canada Research Chair (Tier 2) in Critical Disability Studies and Assistant Professor of Political Science at the University of Alberta. Working at the intersection of critical disability studies, contemporary political theory, and feminist theory, his research focuses on the interplay of communication and disability within information societies. His first monograph is titled *Cheap Talk: Disability and the Politics of Communication*.

Shelby Swafford, MA is a PhD candidate in the School of Communication Studies at Southern Illinois University Carbondale. Her research engages feminist, queer, and crip theories through performance praxis and personal narrative methodologies. Her written work has appeared in *Text and Performance Quarterly, Cultural Studies ←→ Critical Methodologies*, and *Intercultural Health Communication*.

Craig R. Weathers, MA is a doctoral candidate in Communication Studies at the University of Denver. His research combines cultural studies and critical rhetorical approaches to study social movements, most often in educational contexts. Craig is an active member of the National Communication Association and the Association on Higher Education and Disability. His latest work (co-authored with Christina Foust) appeared in *The Rhetoric of Social Movements: Networks, Power, and New Media* (2020).

Anne Zbitnew, MA is the project lead on *Making Accessible Media*, an open access online course on access and inclusion in media production. She leads several disability arts and culture projects and is a professor in the Faculty of Media & Creative Arts at Humber College in Toronto, Canada.

Kuansong Victor Zhuang, PhD is a research fellow at the Wee Kim Wee School of Communication and Information at Nanyang Technological University where he is researching and co-writing a book exploring the intersections of disability and emerging technologies with Gerard Goggin. He is also working on a book project, based on his PhD research, tentatively titled *The Biopolitics of Inclusion: Disability and Capacity in the Singapore Nation*. He hopes to use his research to contribute to current debates about how inclusion happens both in Singapore and around the world.

LIST OF FIGURES

Fig. 21.1 A collection of ten different self-portraits, hand-drawn by members of "The CICE Team" in pen, pencil, marker, and pencil crayon. Some portraits are black and white, while others are very colorful. Each portrait is in a square box. Some show smiling figures with background objects such as a heart, a basketball, and an alligator. Other illustrations have text, including "I like Jonas Brothers." In each drawing, a figure of a podcaster is looking at the viewer   359

Fig. 21.2 A black and white hand-drawn self-portrait. In the portrait, the artist is facing the viewer and smiling, and appears to be standing beside a series of squares. The artist's image description is written on the right side: "I am wearing a black hoodie. I am wearing grey track pants. I wearing running shoes. I am wearing glasses"   360

Fig. 21.3 A black and white hand-drawn portrait. In the portrait, a figure is seated in a wheelchair and facing forward. The person is smiling and has their arms outstretched   361

Fig. 25.1 Conceptually illustrates the current findings. (Modified for the current study based on *Metamorphosis, 2020* by Annenberg School for Communication, USC)   428

LIST OF TABLES

Table 23.1	Use of force continuum table	389
Table 25.1	Parental caregiver demographic information	424

CHAPTER 1

Introduction

Michael S. Jeffress, Joy M. Cypher, Jim Ferris,
and Julie-Ann Scott-Pollock

DISABILITY STUDIES AND COMMUNICATION STUDIES: A COMPLICATED PURSUIT

By: The Editors

The Palgrave Handbook of Disability and Communication maps the course of two highly interdisciplinary academic disciplines. At the core of this *Handbook* is how we human beings make sense of disability as an identity and human phenomenon as we understand ourselves and others through personal introspection, daily interaction, our cultural artifacts, and our collective policies. Both disability and communication are expansive, everchanging, highly contextual, and well, complicated to study. We will briefly lay out these two highly interdisciplinary areas of intellectual inquiry before introducing the four editors of this *Handbook* and the outline of the sections and chapters.

M. S. Jeffress (✉)
Medical University of the Americas, Nevis, Saint Kitts and Nevis
e-mail: m.jeffress@mua.edu

J. M. Cypher
Department of Communication Studies, Rowan University, Glassboro, NJ, USA

J. Ferris
Department of Disability Studies, The University of Toledo, Toledo, OH, USA

J.-A. Scott-Pollock
Department of Communication Studies, University of North Carolina Wilmington, Wilmington, NC, USA

© The Author(s), under exclusive license to Springer Nature
Switzerland AG 2023
M. S. Jeffress et al. (eds.), *The Palgrave Handbook of Disability and Communication*, https://doi.org/10.1007/978-3-031-14447-9_1

Disability Is Complicated

Disability is complicated. The range of human circumstances that in this time we call *disability* presents in a wide variety of ways, with an exponentially broad array of impacts on the lives of people labeled *disabled* as well as the lives of everyone else.

Unlike other identity markers, disability is defined medically and socially by deviation from what normal embodiment, emotional response, and cognitive processing are considered to be (Garland Thomson, 1997). When one begins to research what it means to be disabled, several questions arise that are central to the design of any project: who is drawing the lines between disabled and nondisabled people, and for what purpose? How can the researcher offer a degree of objectivity when we all are implicated—whether we are aware of it—in what we might call the ability/disability continuum?

Disability is complicated. Who is considered disabled? What conditions count as disabilities? The perceptions of the degree of impairment as well as how affected people respond affect how we interact to negotiate with disability as an identity marker. People are considered disabled by others when their presences become disruptive to social spaces. People become "disabled" when they are perceived to be unable to do what is expected of a "normal" cultural participant.

For example, requiring glasses to see is not often perceived as a disability until corrective lenses are no longer available that enable a person to read the print required of them to be independent or able to travel independently by vehicle. Before literacy became an expectation and the majority of cultural members had access to printed material, whether one could read "normative sized print" did not determine whether one had a disability. Before vehicles, being unable to pass an eye exam attesting to a preferred level of visual acuity did not constitute a disruptive disability. Furthermore, in a world in which no human had eyes, no one would be blind. Not having eyesight would simply be a part of what it meant to be human. It is only with the application of normative expectations that people are labeled disabled or nondisabled.

If an individual has a job that requires employees to arrive at an office and sit at a desk from 8:00 a.m. to 5:00 p.m., and they are unable to fulfill this expectation due to chronic pain, mobility, or cognitive processing, then they become characterized as disabled. Their need for an alternative schedule makes them non-standard. Within that space, their bodyminds are characterized as disabled, unable to fulfill normative expectations and in need of accommodations (Price, 2011). In a job that did not require this constant presence, however, one would potentially not be deemed disruptive and potentially not be interpreted as disabled within the workplace by their supervisor and coworkers. As many workplaces shifted to remote settings during the Covid-19 lockdown, employees who needed place and time accommodations were no longer outliers and subject to stigma, because everyone needed accommodations.

Thus, the normative "center" against which disability is constrasted is always in flux.

Disability is complicated—and inherently, intrinsically, inescapably bound up in communication. The circumstances that we describe as disability do not exist outside of the communication around normative embodiment, processing normal human interaction across contexts. Because disability is always and unavoidably a product of comparison and contrast—what is normal in this space? with these people? doing this activity?—disability as a human identity is slippery and evolves with human experience. Disability is how we define when one does not meet the expectation of what "normal" should be. Of course, none of us truly meets this ideal for normal throughout our lifetimes. Injury, illness, and aging change our bodies, our minds, our emotional responses. We are at moments fulfilling this expectation of normal, or almost fulfilling it, or becoming complete disappointments. No one fulfills all the hopes and ideals that society lays upon us—and no one fulfills them for all that long. Disability is the human consequence of that truth articulated by Heraclitus more than two millennia ago: the only constant is change. Humans are mortal, and we will all become disabled—if we live long enough.

COMMUNICATION IS COMPLICATED

Communication is complicated too. For millennia practitioners and scholars have given careful thought to communication, with the greatest attention to the crafting and delivery of messages. In the last century this began to change, with scholars recognizing a much wider variety of ways we humans communicate as well as the importance of a host of factors that affect the communication that happens.

Communication plays a central role in the creation and dissemination of the norms that are crucial to the creation of the social experience of disability. For it is only in community that norms emerge, and it is only through community—which is impossible without communication—that norms are broadcasted and enforced. This central role of communication is less than fully explicated, although this *Handbook* takes us further along that path.

In the current era, communication as an academic discipline is part of the humanities, social sciences, fine arts, and professional programs across institutions. It is inherently interdisciplinary, drawing upon English, philosophy, anthropology, sociology, psychology, theater, creative writing, marketing, public relations, and more to grapple with what it means for human beings to make meaning with one another through interactions from intrapersonal processing to mass communication.

In the early 1990s there was precious little communication studies scholarship around disability. What scholarship there was seemed largely to content itself with received notions of disability, considering disabled people as deviants from norms which were clear, proper, and desirable. This deficit orientation was entirely in keeping with what we were just learning to think of as the medical model of disability. By this time, scholars in disability studies were articulating a competing social model of disability that explained how disability is not an objective diagnosis but a social construct in which cultural landscape and economy are created to exclude some bodies and minds; this model contends that a redesign of cultural architecture, expectations, and policy would eliminate the disparities of access, opportunity, and power that constitute disability. Over the course of the recent decades, disability studies has become interwoven into critical communication inquiry that understands the construct of disability as laden with cultural power. This cultural model of disability recognizes that disability is not inherent or natural to diagnose, treat, or manage; rather, it is created through our interactions, and subject to new understandings, meanings, and responses. The cultural perspective is a foundational understanding of communication scholars in this *Handbook*; it is situated at the intersections of gender, race, sexuality, and social class. The chapters of this volume draw upon the social and cultural models of disability and recognize how other identity markers interact in our understandings of disability and communication.

We can identify several distinct models or paradigms from which disability has been conceived, explained, and responded to. The earliest paradigm is often referred to as the moral model, which holds that the conditions considered as disabilities are indicators of moral flaws or caused by supernatural forces, for example, divine punishment or possession by demons. From this perspective, disability appears as punishment (or karma) for corruption, a test of faith, a metaphor for the debased human condition. From this perspective disability may also be considered the sign of a spiritual "gift," for example, the blind seer or the shaman whose seizures are understood as communication with the supernatural.

The second paradigm is often referred to as the medical or individual model, which attributes disability to biophysical causes and looks at people labeled disabled as patients needing treatment so that they can be restored to normal function and a normative role in society. This paradigm focuses on limitations in functioning and appearance; disability is considered a disease that should be cured. From this perspective the problems around disability are considered to arise only from impairments in function, never recognizing pervasive social and environmental barriers that disabled people face. In this paradigm, disability is seen as an individual problem, so solutions must be sought through individual rather than collective efforts. In this paradigm, disability is not a sign of a flawed identity but rather a form of deviance that must be remediated.

In response to the stigmatizing orientation of these paradigms, activists and scholars developed what might be grouped as a sociocultural paradigm. This paradigm recognizes disability as a social and cultural construct and regards disability as a social rather than an individual issue. To consider disability a construct is to fundamentally root it in the discursive world, where it is the product of relationships, cultural values, and ongoing negotiations of what constitutes normal, and thus, by default, disability. As a result, the sociocultural paradigm grounds disability as no longer inherent in individual bodies, but rather lived through social and enacted agreements and identities. Many variations of theorizing exist within this paradigm, including sociopolitical models that see disability as a unique minority group bound in its experience of oppression. Others focus on institutional constructs hegemonically normalized and inscribed as a means of social control and definition. Others still look at the interplay between embodied experience, performance, and discourse. What they all share in common, however, is the critical assumption that disability is negotiated and made meaningful in the world of social relation.

The sociocultural paradigm recognizes that communication is always implicated with disability. It is important to keep in mind, however, that the newer paradigms have not supplanted the earlier ones; the moral paradigm and the medical/individual paradigm are still commonly deployed, often in an unthinking reflexive way. In fact, the two earliest paradigms are still dominant in discourse—and in policy—around disability.

We come to think about disability from a variety of presuppositions and experiences; if as Shakespeare suggested, "what's past is prologue," it will be useful to consider what each of us has learned to think about bodies, minds, and this range of human circumstances that we call *disability*, as well as how we came to think critically about it. The four editors of this *Handbook* entered the fields of disability and communication at different times, with different backgrounds, trainings, and research questions that brought us to the intersections of these disciplines. In the following four sections each editor will disclose their locations and disciplines that merged to create this *Handbook* and explain where we see (and hope) scholarship moves from here.

JIM: CREATING THE VENUE FOR CRITICAL COMMUNICATION AND DISABILITY STUDIES

A moment in 1990 changed my life. I was following an intriguing citation I had found in a bibliography and stumbled across the only-just emergent field of disability studies. The *Journal of Social Issues* published a special issue in 1988 entitled "Moving Disability Beyond 'Stigma'," and I saw my experience reflected more clearly than I had ever seen before. I have been disabled since birth by what is often called a "lower limb deficiency" (note the presence of an unspoken norm here?), but it was only in that moment that I realized two crucial things: that the interpersonal weirdnesses that I had experienced most of my life really were happening (despite the best intentions of my nondisabled family to minimize or smooth things over: "No, she wasn't staring at you."); and that those weird encounters, which today we might call "microaggressions," were worthy of study.

In the early 1990s, a small group of young scholars came together through our interest in communication scholarship around disability. Beth Haller, Susan Fox, and I hunted out the conference panels at conferences and shared dismay not only at the paucity of attention that our field was giving to this powerful component of the social world but also at the narrow-minded, mechanistic, and outdated thinking that informed the scholarship. Of course, people with disabilities want to be able-bodied, the thinking seemed to be. Let's find ways to help them deal with the stigma that naturally attaches to their deviance.

It was in this environment that I tried to create a venue for cutting-edge scholarship in communication studies. In 1996 I began the petition drive that resulted in the creation of the Disability Issues Caucus (DIC) of the National Communication Association (NCA). I wanted to create a place for communication scholars in disability to come together and share their work. I wanted to encourage participation by disabled scholars in a largely inaccessible and unconsciously ableist field. And I wanted to push my communication studies colleagues to move away from the medical model and incorporate sociocultural perspectives in their work. I wanted to bring disability studies to communication studies.

Among the first people I reached out to were the most established scholars in the field who had shown an interest in disability: Teri Thompson and Dawn Braithwaite. Dawn particularly was concerned that a disability-related interest group would lead to a form of ghettoization of the work, which would make it easier for everybody else in communication studies to ignore disability-related scholarship. But I believed that creation of the group would lead not only to more scholarship but also to work that went beyond the dominant medicalized perspective that had been driving research and what little teaching there had been up to that point.

And the caucus had the effect I had sought. It led to research that moved beyond health and compliance-gaining to examine disability as a fact of humanity with profound implications for every area of concentration within the discipline. Today it is possible to find scholarship—possible if not common—that probes disability and identity, disability as rhetorical construction, the performance of disability and disability as performance, interpersonal and media questions around disability, and many of the other subdisciplines of communication studies. It has become much more common to find scholarship that recognizes disability as a useful and indeed important category of analysis like we have come to think about race, class, gender, and sexuality.

Joy: Finding a Community of Consequence

Like many others, writing and teaching have proven the means through which I navigate the thoughts and experiences of my world, and where I rediscover so many of my roots. As a child raised by a disabled mother, I learned early on the social frames through which she was viewed and upon which her value was determined. I learned my critical questioning from her and my father, and it fed my passion for justice and ethics, along with a recognition of the power and responsibility that comes from speech. But I didn't know that this passion would fuel my professional life—in part because I hadn't yet learned that the personal and the professional are not distinct, separate modes of being. It wasn't until my first disability studies reading in a graduate seminar that I finally heard my passion and my concerns echoed in the stories and theorizing on the page. A few years later, when I walked into the 1997 business meeting of the DIC, I found my community. Academe gave me words for what I saw and felt both growing up and as a scholar, for the hegemonic frames that loomed large, yet invisible, across my experiences. From that graduate seminar, through the 25 years in the DIC, to my classrooms today where interactions with students still forge a meaningful connection over bodies, normalcy, and discourse, I have found a home in the rich world of disability studies. Thus is the warp and woof of my scholarly and personal life—the intersections of embodiment, discourse, and ethics. I teach and write about a variety of topics that inhabit these spaces, and I am inspired by the thinking of Rosemarie Garland-Thomson, Michel Foucault, John Paul Sartre, and Lennard Davis when I do so. In my work, and in my person, I reside humbly where word, heart, and deed meet; and as such, I am honored to be a part of this project.

Julie-Ann: A Focus on Lived Embodiment

I did not consider myself a disability scholar when I began my PhD in 2004 at the University of Maine. It was not until 2006, when I attended my first National Communication Association Convention in San Antonio and met Jim, Joy, Bruce Henderson, and so many other communication and disability scholars that I realized that I was, in fact, a disability scholar. Of course, I had always known I was disabled, as you will read in my chapter included in this *Handbook*. I have a diagnosis of moderate, spastic cerebral palsy (CP). My body is noticeably atypical. And while, I have an obvious "CP gait" to anyone who knows anything about cerebral palsy, after six operations I am often interpreted as temporarily injured or sore and stiff from physical activity rather than having a chronic neuromuscular condition resulting from traumatic brain injury from birth. In addition to being disabled, I am also a writer, performer, and narrative researcher. I was nervous to disclose my disability as an early academic. I wanted to be known for my creative work and research, not my disabled body. Yet, my research questions continued to draw me toward embodiment, body image, and disability. As the stories I desired to hear from my research participants continued to focus on eating disorders, physical disability, memory loss, and seizures, I increasingly became aware that I am a communication studies and disability scholar, and while I stayed very close to performance studies and ethnography for my early conference presentations, I felt a pull toward the DIC at NCA. As an identity caucus we have become immersed in intersectionality and how disability is entangled in race, gender, sexuality, and class. I am grateful we are able to bring this volume together and look forward to how future additions can build on and expand the research into these complex questions.

MICHAEL: FINDING MY SCHOLARLY HOME WITHIN COMMUNICATION AND DISABILITY

I think most of us who pitch our tent in the area where the camps of disability studies and communication studies overlap do so because of our personal experience of disability and those with disabilities who have left indelible marks on our lives. Here, I will highlight five major influences for me. First, my son, Ryan, was diagnosed with Duchenne muscular dystrophy at age six in 1999; nothing has impacted my desire to change the narrative of disability in society and to champion disability justice more than the 20 years I spent as Ryan's dad. Second, my youngest daughter, Meleah, was diagnosed with osteosarcoma at age 11 in 2007 and became physically disabled from related treatments and surgeries. Watching her navigate adolescence into young adulthood with visible scarring, an atypical gait, and chronic pain from the prostheses in her leg and arm, has motivated me in profound ways to conduct research and engage in advocacy. Third, my adult diagnosis of "severe ADHD" came in 2008 at age—well, that is not important—and helped put my past experiences into perspective, not the least of which were the countless microaggressions I encountered toward my neurodivergence from the time I was in primary school and well into adulthood. The fourth and fifth events are connected and need their own paragraph...or two...or, well, please just keep reading.

In 2006 I enrolled in a doctoral program in communication studies having never taken a communication studies course, per se, beyond a few public speaking classes. I took to communication studies like a fish to water. My horizons expanded as I contemplated how basically everything communicates and anything can be studied through the lens of communication. The possibilities were endless, and the implications were awe-inspiring as I considered the role of communication—in its varied forms—in shaping and perpetuating cultures. In short, I realized everything is communication, and communication is everything.

The following year, my academic pursuits took a sudden turn. In the summer of 2007 Ryan discovered the adapted sport of power soccer. He soon became part of the first team started in Virginia, and the impact on Ryan's life and mine was immediate. Call it fate or serendipitous, but that same summer, I was enrolled in an ethnography course and needed a topic for my research project. I chose power soccer.

Prior to that first research project on a sport for disabled athletes, I did not know an academic discipline of disability studies existed. My literature review quickly expanded beyond adapted sport studies. I became interested in related broader issues of embodiment, identity, intersectionality, advocacy, and social justice, and I soon checked out of the library a copy of Rosemarie Garland Thomson's (1997) classic text on *Extraordinary Bodies*, and the rest is, as they say, history.

Then in 2008, I attended my first NCA conference to present my power soccer paper and discovered the DIC, where I saw a place to belong and develop my identity as a scholar. That first power soccer research effort grew into my dissertation, a top paper award at NCA in 2013, and my first academic book (Jeffress, 2015). I continue to be nurtured by the community of scholars within the DIC and make it my goal to offer scholarly contributions that showcase the rich interdisciplinary area for research and activism that emerges at the intersection of communication studies and disability studies. It is my hope that my role in this volume achieves that.

Notes on the Content and Structure

First, a note on language in this volume. How we talk about disability is as complicated as disability itself. Across chapters, you will encounter scholars who choose people-first language (people with disabilities) with a commitment to seeing the person before the inescapable stigma of disability. You will see other scholars who use identity-first language (disabled people) with a commitment to embracing disability as an identity marker that should be used like any other identifier (i.e., Black man, queer person, disabled woman, etc.). Both of these choices are valid, and we do not wish to force our authors to be uniform. We allowed each author to choose their language and how to talk about disability.

Now a word on the content of this volume. Beyond the introduction you are currently reading, this *Handbook* consists of an additional 26 chapters organized into five sections: "Language and Disability," "Identity and Intersectionalities," "Cultural Artifacts and Disability," "Institutional Constructs and Constraints," and "Advocacy, Policy, and Action." We will now briefly introduce each section and the chapters within them.

The five chapters of Section I explore important matters concerning the relationship between language and disability. In Chap. 2, Arciuli and Shakespeare discuss descriptive terms related to disability that may or may not have been considered acceptable at one time before becoming taboo. Yet, some of these "taboo words" have now been reclaimed by disability advocates as evidenced by the recent hashtag #CripTheVote. In Chap. 3, St. Pierre critiques simplistic models and systems of communication that focus on the quick and efficient flow of information. St. Pierre notes how communication systems are prone to communication accidents, which can be even more risky for dysfluent communicators, who often unintentionally communicate by accident. Next, Stones offers a timely theoretical discussion of the communication breakdowns between people of different neurotypes, the need to prioritize neurodivergent perspective, and lays out a path toward cross-neurotype communication competence. In Chap. 5, Sparrow et al give voice to the disabled participants they interviewed who provided their stories of microaggressions. The authors identify two sources for seven forms of disability microaggressions. In the final chapter of Section I, Ali offers a significant examination of the problem of compulsory able-bodiedness as it relates to communication and sexuality and the stigma and "desexualization" that accompany the fusion of the terms disability and sexuality.

The editors of this volume affirm that disability is a core identity marker. It is as much a part of one's identity as, for example, race, gender, sexual orientation, ethnicity, and class. Furthermore, disability is a marginalized identity, and people with disabilities collectively form a major minority group. As such, Section II spans Chaps. 7–12 and contains important discussions related to disability identity and intersectionality. We begin with a theoretical essay by Cherney, who demonstrates rhetorical parallels between ableism and other forms of discrimination against marginalized identities. He notes that as identities intersect, so do the forms of discrimination, but he suggests ways we can communicate to empower and support those who live with these intersectional identities. Scott-Pollock then provides an autoethnographic account of her embodied narrative as one who identifies as both a disabled woman and athletic (or a female "fitcrip"), thereby challenging the false dichotomy between fit and disabled. Chapters 9 and 10 continue in the autoethnographic vein. Swafford provides a balance of prose and poetry as she uses a medical pain scale as a framework to construct her personal narrative of chronic pain and illness in a nonlinear fashion that in her own words, "illustrates her disjointed, nonlinear experience of disability" (a.k.a., "criptime"). Next, Spikes explores the relationship between disability, gender, race, and class through narrative vignettes of his experience of being both Black and diabetic within the cultural context of the southern United States. Chapter 11 has DeWeert and Miller-Ott reporting on their interviews with heterosexual, cisgendered, disabled women, and the first time their disability became a topic of discussion with their romantic partners. Section II ends as it began, with a theoretical essay. Grewe and Weathers use a critical rhetorical approach to problematize ways disabled identity is co-opted and weaponized by others as a means to achieve selfish ends, such as preferred parking or seating, skipping waiting in lines, traveling with pets, and avoiding pandemic mask mandates.

Section III includes Chaps. 13–17 and covers selected topics within aspects of popular culture. Goggin et al get things started by contemplating the place of disability within the development and implementation of artificial intelligence (AI), which, they argue, is undergoing a crisis of legitimacy. In similar fashion, Dumont and Bonenfant focus attention on issues of inclusion related to three popular video games. In Chap. 15, Gloviczki uses posthuman critical theory to bring together autoethnography and media analysis of *Sports Night*, a late-1990s television comedy drama about a nightly cable-tv sports program. Specifically, Gloviczki focuses on the program's coverage of the body in two episodes that feature disability and racial violence. Chapter 16 has Preston applying his keen analysis to what has become a pervasive cultural artifact: the meme. To the point, Preston critiques the ableism and sexism in a viral meme known as, "I Can Count to Potato," which is based on a photo of a young woman with Down syndrome. Section III ends with a presentation by Foster and Pettinicchio of their research on viral videos created by users with disabilities on the social media platform TikTok. They suggest that platform norms make it less than democratic and inclusive—especially for disabled users; however, a select few register views in the hundreds of thousands, and even tens of millions. Sampling the top-100 most-viewed TikTok disability videos, Foster and Pettinicchio note the key themes and demonstrate ways in which the videos both challenge and reinforce stereotypes.

Chapters 18–22 comprise Section IV, which looks at broader systemic issues of discriminatory constructs and constraints entrenched in society communicatively through hegemonic notions of normalcy. Shek-Noble launches this section by presenting results from her comparative content analysis of how English-language news sources in the US and Japan covered post-disaster inaccessibilities and communication breakdowns experienced by people with disabilities in the wake of Hurricane Katrina and the 2011 Tōhoku Earthquake and Tsunami in Japan. In any society, government is a primary source for enshrining and exemplifying constructs and constraints. Burdett reminds us of this point in Chap. 19 as she applies a disability studies lens to critique the ableist rhetoric of "disability humor" in the political debates surrounding Brexit and discusses the implications for those who fight for disability justice. One legal policy has recently come under debate in the US centers around questions of who should have a service animal, and when and where a service animal should be permitted. In Chap. 20, Ballard et al distinguish between the legal and social access of service animals. Each of the authors is a service dog handler and draws upon lived experiences to recount vignettes of negative social interactions that unfold three insightful themes toward making society more just for service animal users. Next, Jones et al turn our attention to a place with tremendous potential to influence society, the educational system. The authors present their chapter alternating between dominant language and plain language to present an informative case study of a public pedagogy project involving intellectually disabled students producing eight podcasts at a Canadian college. Chapter 22 features Makkawy and Moreman interrogating a context known for its cultural constructs and constraints: the organization. As scholars who specialize in organizational communication, Makkawy and Moreman make a strong case for the field to adopt a "cripistemology" that would allow the full implications of disability to be realized and introduce innovation within organizational sensemaking and the construct of organizational capacity.

Section V is home to the final five chapters of this *Handbook*, and they call readers to a space that is the goal of good scholarship that encompasses communication studies and disability studies: the need for social change to achieve accessibility, inclusion, and equity for individuals with disability, in short, disability justice. Hawkins starts the conversation in Chap. 23 with his timely essay on the problem of police brutality toward people with disabilities. He shows that it is fundamentally a (mis)communication problem that calls for better police training. Chapter 24 is Heilig's astute review of the history of disability within the subdiscipline of technical communication. Beyond giving a helpful overview of the field, Heilig calls for reform in pedagogy and to move beyond an accommodations' paradigm to one of disability justice that focuses on inclusivity, human dignity, and sociospatial factors in designing technical communication. In Chap. 25, Darnell draws attention to a government assistance program offered by many states within the US for children with disabilities. She notes the struggles and information gaps that caregivers face in navigating these medical insurance programs and the types of communication within the community that would better serve these families. Next, Edelist offers a similar critique of a program in Canada for infants diagnosed at birth with hearing impairment. Edelist calls for reform that would result in language that does not problematize deafness and provide caregivers greater agency in the process. Chapter 27 takes aim at the epidemic of gun violence in America and the problematic rhetoric of mental illness associated with it. Smith-Frigerio examines the advocacy themes in social media posts trending with the hashtag #ImMentallyIllAndIDontKill in the wake of two 2019 mass shootings.

A FINAL WORD AND ACKNOWLEDGMENTS FROM LEAD EDITOR MICHAEL S. JEFFRESS

Although this volume ends after Chap. 27, we acknowledge that much is left to do. Putting this volume together was challenging to say the least. It grew out of a "Call for Chapters" (CFP) that I advertized in the summer of 2019. At the time, I was planning to edit one or two volumes on the theme of "discussing disability." Upon submitting the book proposal to Camille Davies at Palgrave Macmillan, I was given the option to proceed or to expand my proposal into a handbook project. Well, you know which option I chose.

At first, I thought I might solo edit the volume (You can't hear me, but I am laughing out loud right now as I reflect on the naivety of that fleeting idea). I had over 50 proposals for chapters, many of which you will find herein, and all systems seemed to be go. Then the pandemic happened, and productivity halted. My daughter, who had been cancer-free for ten years, was hit with a terminal diagnosis. Any project that went beyond my job description at the university was suspended as spending time with my daughter and trying to help her make the most of her final months became my main priority.

After about a year, my daughter seemed somewhat stabilized in her treatment and we were learning how to live, as they say, under "the valley of the shadow," and I was able once again to feel the internal self-goading to finish this important work and lift the ethical burden I felt to get feedback to those who submitted chapter proposals. I knew I needed help, and I could not have found any better than the three colleagues and mentors I have in Jim, Joy, and Julie-Ann. Thank you for partnering with me on this. Thank you for taking up the slack on the many occasions when I simply did not have the mental and emotional capacity to be productive. This project would have never made it to completion without the significant contributions of each of you. I offer the same gratitude to the contributors of this volume, many of whom have been waiting to see their work published for over three years now. Your patience and perseverance shall not be forgotten. Thank you! I also express deep gratitude to Camille Davies and her staff and colleagues at Palgrave. You provided nothing but empathy and support when I provided updates and more than once requested an extension.

Finally, I know I write for all the editors here, when I say that we hope this edition will motivate a new crop of scholars to discover their passion, conduct meaningful research, and expand the horizons within our interdisciplinary field of communication and disability. We acknowledge that our *Handbook* has gaps. Some of those gaps we earnestly tried to fill. We sought contributions, for example, from the Global South, but we simply did not receive any that matched the focus and scope of our project. We sought contributions from more scholars to represent even more intersectionalities among the editors and authors, but our attempts were unfruitful. We had some proposals that never translated into chapters or never made it beyond the first draft. I think this is largely in part because of how difficult times have been since the pandemic—especially for the marginalized voices we seek to empower here!

We hope that in future editions of this volume, we may succeed in areas where we fell short this time. However, we are proud to offer this volume to you. We believe it contains some important work, and we trust it will be viewed as a step in the right direction and that the next time we meet here on the written page, we will be wiser and our field will be stronger because of the work we have done together—the type of work exemplified in, carried out through, and we hope, inspired by this *Handbook*.

References

Garland Thomson, R. (1997). *Extraordinary bodies: Figuring physical disability in American culture and literature*. Columbia University Press.

Jeffress, M. S. (2015). *Communication, sport and disability: The case of power soccer*. Routledge.

Price, M. (2011). *Mad at school: Rhetorics of mental disability and academic life*. University of Michigan Press.

PART I

Language and Disability

CHAPTER 2

Language Matters: Disability and the Power of Taboo Words

Joanne Arciuli and Tom Shakespeare

Disability-related terms are powerful—so powerful that some have reached the status of taboo words. What do disabled people think of these words? As expected, there are differing views. Some choose to reclaim these words while others want them to disappear from everyday language. For example, the Twitter hashtag #CripTheVote was created by disability advocates to highlight issues which affect disabled people and their communities during election campaigns globally. Despite, or perhaps because of, the perceived offensiveness of the word *cripple*, these advocates have reclaimed a variant of it to suit their purposes. By contrast, campaigns against use of the "r-word"—in any form— have been instigated by individuals with disabilities, and their families and friends, all around the world. In this chapter, we discuss the nature of taboo words and provide some background on disability-related taboo words. We discuss the power of these taboo words and how they can be used not only negatively but also in positive ways.

J. Arciuli (✉)
Flinders University, Adelaide, SA, Australia
e-mail: joanne.arciuli@flinders.edu.au

T. Shakespeare
London School of Hygiene and Tropical Medicine, London, UK

© The Author(s), under exclusive license to Springer Nature
Switzerland AG 2023
M. S. Jeffress et al. (eds.), *The Palgrave Handbook of Disability and Communication*, https://doi.org/10.1007/978-3-031-14447-9_2

17

What Are Taboo Words?

As it happens, taboo words come in many forms. Here are just some of the descriptors associated with taboo words and phrases: bad words, foul words, curse words, obscenities, profanity, hate speech, slurs, insults, degrading language, abusive language, offensive language, irreverence, blasphemy, incivility, filth, slang, expletives, swearing, emphatic intensifiers, robust language.

According to an American study of 126 college students aged 18–38 years by Jay and Jay (2015), the top ten taboo words are: *fuck, shit, bitch, cunt, asshole, ass, damn, motherfucker, slut,* and *whore*. Interestingly, the top eight taboo words were the same for both male and female respondents in the study. In the UK, a 2016 Ofcom (media regulator) study asked 248 adults about taboo words to determine which are the most offensive culprits (Cameron & Stevenson, 2016). The aim was to establish a "barometer of offensive language." The most offensive words were *cunt, fuck,* and *motherfucker*; slightly more tolerable were *bastard, beaver, bellend, clunge, cock, dick, dickhead, fanny, flaps, gash, knob, minge, prick, punani, pussy, snatch,* and *twat*. Of particular interest in the disability space, the Ofcom study suggested that mental health and disability-related taboo words could be categorized as follows. "Mild" words included *loony, mental, nutter,* and *psycho*. Words with "medium" levels of offensiveness included *midget, schizo, special,* and *vegetable*. The word *"cripple"* was considered strong and generally unacceptable. The strongest words in this category—highly unacceptable at all times—included *mong, retard, spastic/spakka/spaz,* and *window licker*.

Contrary to widely held beliefs, the use of taboo words is not an indicator of limited language ability (Jay & Jay, 2015). These words have been a source of fascination for a very long time. For example, an English dictionary of slang titled "Classical Dictionary of the Vulgar Tongue" was published by Grose in 1785. A recent special issue of the journal, *Language Sciences*, showcasing 21 articles demonstrates that this topic is of interest in many disciplines such as linguistics, anthropology, philosophy, psychology, and sociology (Croom, 2015). Moreover, the special issue showed that the topic is a cross-linguistic concern with studies of multiple languages including English, Croatian, Hebrew, and Portuguese. A search of the articles in this special issue using the terms "disability" and "disabled" revealed that only one article contained the word "disabled"—the term appearing in a footnote (see Lycan, 2015). Another article listed some disability-related taboo words such as the r-word (Jay & Jay, 2015). We, like others in the disability field, consider that there is a lot to say on this topic in relation to disability-related taboo words.

Why Are Taboo Words So Powerful?

Taboo words seem to be highly salient stimuli for our brains. A study that asked people to read aloud swear words (e.g., "fuck"), euphemisms linked to swear words (e.g., "f-word"), and neutral words (e.g., "glue") found greater autonomic responses via electrodermal activity to swear words (Bowers & Pleydell-Pearce, 2011). People who can speak more than one language may express a preference for swearing, and react more strongly to taboo words, in their first language (see Dewaele, 2010; Harris et al., 2003; but see also Eilola & Havelka, 2007). In addition, soon after first learning these kinds of words they become highly salient for young children (Jay, 2018). Anyone who's been to a young child's birthday party has probably come across poo-bum-fart-wee references and jokes, often delivered at top speed while running away from the reaction. This is age-appropriate, at least in many groups within Western cultures.

Beyond developmentally predictable experimentation with taboo words, involuntary swearing or difficulty controlling swearing has been associated with certain forms of brain damage or deterioration and conditions such as Tourette's, among others. All of this evidence suggests that the brain may deal with taboo words differently from other words (Mackay et al., 2004; Meffert et al., 2011; Van Lancker & Cummings, 1999). So, yes, they're powerful. Why are mental health and disability-related taboo words offensive? One could argue that they are offensive because they are stigmatizing. Smith (2007) suggested that stigma can be defined as "a simplified, standardized image of the disgrace of certain people that is held in common by a community at large" (p. 464). Further, Smith argued that stigma communication fulfills several key aims: it distinguishes people, it categorizes these distinguished people as a separate social entity, it implies well-deserved placement in distinguished categories and that responsibility for placement lies with the distinguished people in question, and it links these distinguished people to peril.

In the disability sector, there are grassroots campaigns trying to raise awareness and discourage people from using certain taboo words. For example, campaigns against the "r-word" have been instigated by individuals with disabilities, and their families and friends, all around the world. According to an Australian website, therword.com.au, the r-word appears on social media approximately once every five seconds and is "incredibly offensive, hurtful and demeaning."

Shakespeare, who co-authored this chapter, has restricted growth (short stature) and has experienced many of the insulting words about dwarfism. He's overheard them in the bar, on the train, on the street. Words like: midget, a half-pint, Mekon, Munchkin, Oompa-Loompa, Mini Me, Wee Man, goblin, blob, short-arse, freak, and many more besides. Muttered, spoken, shouted. You could say that what's hurtful is the attitude that underlies them, rather than the words themselves. However, it's through words that you become aware of others' attitudes. For example, comedians who have banished racial slur words or sexist or homophobic slur words from their performances still too often resort to outdated and hurtful disability terminology, partly because they are so shocking, so outrageous. People with disabilities remain outsiders in many communities. The key point here is to educate people away from negative attitudes toward all differences, including disability, and to promote inclusion, so that there are no outsiders.

Which Words Are Acceptable to Disabled People?

As Shakespeare (2017) has discussed, anxieties about disabled people include anxieties about terminology: "But what should we call you?" Perhaps there is sometimes an implied fear that disabled people are very sensitive. Perhaps there is the implication that any worries about the status and treatment of disabled people are just another aspect of "political correctness." However, it is true that many simply do not wish to give offense. Disability rights is a relatively new domain—it has been called "the last liberation campaign." So well-minded people may struggle to keep up.

For some, the disability terminology debate is all about seeing people as persons first, rather than focusing on their medical condition(s). And this is very important. So, for example, rather than "epileptics" one might say "people with epilepsy" and rather than "schizophrenics" one might say "people with schizophrenia." The illness or impairment is just one aspect of their personality: they are "people first," like everyone else.

However, identity-first or disability-first language, rather than person-first language, is preferred by some disabled people. An example is "Deaf people," the capital D signifying that we are talking about a minority group with their own culture based around sign language, not just a group of people who can't hear. Similarly, there is often talk of "Mad Pride"—people with mental health conditions reclaiming a stigmatized label. Globally, the term "users and survivors of psychiatry" signifies that it is not the mental distress that defines people, but their negative experiences in the mental health system. People might reject the notion of mental illness completely, and consider themselves "different" but not ill or disabled.

Further complexity ensues when these terms differ across various contexts. We can agree that "mental retardation" and "mental handicap" are now outdated. Instead of "learning disabled people" one might say "people with learning disabilities," which is the term used in the National Health Service in the UK. But this comes up against another important principle: call people what they want to be called. So "people with intellectual difficulties" (US) and "people with learning difficulties" (UK) may be preferred by the people directly affected.

Words for short stature also differ across different countries. In the UK, the dominant term for many years was "restricted growth," as in "person of restricted growth." In Australia, "short stature" tended to be used. Whereas in the US, the dominant term has been "Little People." These labels are reflected in the dominant organizations representing these conditions—there are more than 200 causes of dwarfism, but regardless of specific diagnosis, Little People of America, Restricted Growth Association (UK), and Short Statured People of Australia will represent you. Then in the UK, a split within the community led to the formation of Little People UK—so different terms are not just about different nations, they might also be about different approaches within each setting. In this community, "dwarf" was for many years eschewed, but has now been reclaimed, particularly by younger generations unashamed of their different bodies.

In the world of autism, the rejection of pathologization was signaled by the creation of the term "Neurodiversity" by Judy Singer, whose family is affected by the condition. This phrasing celebrates the diversity of human beings, and rather stigmatizes "Neurotypicals," as the majority world are labeled. A study of 3470 UK residents explored preferences for terms used to describe autism (Kenny et al., 2016). Results revealed contention around person-first versus disability-first terminology. Professionals tended to prefer person-first language while adults with autism and parents of individuals with autism tended to prefer disability-first terminology such as "autistic" or "autistic person." Professionals are trying to indicate that autism is only one feature of a person; people with the condition are trying to say how important it is to them, and how it is fundamental to their identity. Many respondents felt that terms such as "low-functioning autism" and "high-functioning autism" were unhelpful and misleading. Possibly this is because people with milder impacts were more likely to respond, and do not want to be seen as "less real" than those with profound autism. The authors stated that (some of) the respondents viewed terms such as "disability," "deficit," or "disorder" as "value-laden terms" (p. 459) and that the term "diversity" may indicate efforts "towards actively de-stigmatising autism" (p. 459). Bailey and Arciuli (2020) noted that some Aboriginal and Torres Strait Islander people may have preferences for certain terms, or for avoiding certain terms, that refer to autism or disability. This is because conceptualizations of autism and/or disability may differ in some Indigenous communities by comparison with non-Indigenous communities.

We might also reflect on the ways that terminology can shift the emphasis to the ways how society treats disabled people, the so-called social model of disability: it is for this reason that "disabled people" is the preferred term in the UK, because many people want to emphasize how they are "disabled by society." Conversely, "impairment" refers to the underlying health condition(s): impairments may refer to things like being blind or deaf or having a mobility limitation or a cognitive difference. So, the query about terminology is a useful one, for a variety of reasons, and often reveals underlying political conceptualizations. Generally, it is a good idea to call people by the names they themselves prefer. And we may be able to use multiple terms, interchangeably, as a nod to individual preferences. For example, we could refer to "disabled people" as well as "people with disabilities" during discussions.

Words for Disabled People

But should there be a collective noun at all? Disability is very diverse. The idea that everyone with some sort of physical or mental impairment can be categorized together at all is rather new in human history. Prior to the early 1900s, it would have been unusual to have thought of all these people with so many different experiences as having anything in common. A variety of words were used—"feeble-minded," "cripple," "blind," "deaf and dumb," "lunatic," "insane." Back in 1915, the word "handicap" started to be used, mainly with reference to children, and in Britain and America it was more and more commonly employed to connote people with a range of impairments. Around the same time, "disability," which had previously signified legal restrictions such as affected women after divorce, was transferred for use as a collective noun. As the disability rights movement became stronger, so the term "handicap" became associated with out-dated approaches. A false etymology associated the word with begging, and by extension charity, to which the new disability activists were vigorously opposed. Whether or not there should be one collective noun is debatable partly because disability is very diverse. The body or mind can be damaged or limited or changed in many different ways. Some conditions are usually obvious at birth—for example cerebral palsy or Down syndrome. Some issues become evident when a child does not develop like other children—for example, autism.

Then there are traumatic injuries such as head injury or spinal cord injury that strike out of the blue, often affecting active young men who take risks or work in dangerous occupations. Some adult illnesses are episodic or degenerative—like depression or multiple sclerosis. Finally, there are conditions mainly associated with aging, such as stroke or dementia. As well as these differences of onset, it's also obvious that some impairments are visible—for example, restricted growth or phocomelia (a congenital condition causing limb defects, often associated with use of the drug thalidomide in pregnancy). Other conditions such as epilepsy, depression, and heart disease are not always visible.

This diversity of disability explains why it took centuries for "disabled people" to be considered as having something in common, regardless of differences. It's probably true to say that it took even longer for disabled folks themselves to think of themselves as one community. Why would someone with paraplegia think they had anything in common with someone who experiences mental illness? She might say to herself "I may not be able to walk, but at least my mind is working normally."

In general, not everyone who could be objectively thought of to be members of the disability community would consent to being classed with others facing functional restrictions. Research with people with restricted growth in the UK found that many of them insisted: "I am different, not disabled" (Shakespeare et al., 2009). A study for the UK Department of Work and Pensions (2003) found that more than half of those who could be defined as disabled did not think of themselves as disabled. Apart from the diversity of experiences, a key reason why people may not want to be labeled as disabled is because disability remains a stigmatized identity, a taboo word. Nobody wants to be categorized in a way which seems limiting or negative. They want to stress their similarity to others, not their differences; what they can do, not what they cannot do; their individuality, not their membership of a devalued community.

Indeed, some terminology attempts to avoid taboo words via euphemisms. However, this is not seen as a successful strategy by all. Well-intentioned efforts to be inclusive often fall flat. When people talk about "differently abled," it can feel like a slightly misguided attempt to say that everyone has things they are more or less good at, as if we could be relativist about functioning rather than rank better and worse forms of embodiment. "Diff-abled" fails because it is not just relativistic, it is also a clumsy neologism. "Physically challenged" also sounds like an awkward euphemism, implying that impairment is merely a difference, rather than often a real problem. Both these terms gloss over the reality that social barriers constitute some of the biggest problems for disabled people. The term "access inclusion seeker" as an alternative to the term "disabled" drew attention in Sydney, Australia, in 2019, and seems to highlight barriers. Apparently, the term was raised at a meeting of the Sydney City local council. Commentators, including some disabled people, dismissed the term as inappropriate. Here the problem seems to be that it is rather cumbersome— and euphemistic.

Gernsbacher et al. (2016) sampled 530 adults from the general population in the US to examine how positively people are viewed when described as having "special needs," having a "disability," having a certain disability, or with no label attached. Their results indicate that the term "special needs" is associated with more negativity than "disability" and that it connotes segregation. The authors stated: "Our data suggest that *special needs* has already become a dysphemism (a euphemism more negative than the word it replaces). *Special needs* will likely become a slur, if it is not already, and it might eventually become a dysphemistic metaphor, akin to *dumb, lame, crippled, deaf,* and *blind.* There is a cycle, where new words are devised, but in turn become deployed as insults. This suggests that the problem lies with social attitude towards the underlying condition, rather than the particular word used to label that condition. These linguistic transitions, along with the data here, recommend against using the euphemism *special needs* and instead using the non-euphemized term *disability*" (p. 10).

The Use of Taboo Words and Disability Terminology to Criticize High-Profile Figures

If disability terms become dysphemistic, then perhaps inevitably, they will be used as insults against significant public figures. But something more general is going on to do with the inherent negativity of disability terminology and the use of disability metaphors (Shakespeare, 1994). Disability is deployed as a metaphor for things not being good, for things going wrong, for people being incompetent. This happens particularly when it comes to mental health.

For example, there has been much speculation about the mental state of the 45th President of the United States. Does Donald Trump have narcissistic personality disorder, or dementia, or both? Is he in his "right mind"? Or, as

CNN (2018) framed it, "Even by President Donald Trump's frenetic standards, the events of the last 48 hours have been insane." Journalists and activists and even health professionals cannot resist making long-range diagnoses of Donald Trump's mental health.

Similarly, if someone perpetrates a terrible crime, like a high school killing, it seems a reflex action of some commentators to accuse them of being schizophrenic or on the autistic spectrum. While occasionally mental illness is associated with violence, this is the rare exception. Over a lifetime, 3 out of every 1000 people with schizophrenia commit murder (Fazel et al., 2010). A lifetime homicide risk of 3 per 1000 for people with schizophrenia is higher than the general population, although given that less than 1% of the general population has schizophrenia, this reinforces the point that the risk of a murderer being a person with schizophrenia is very low, and therefore the stereotype is misleading and harmful.

We resort to similar labels for political events. We describe a particular government decision as "crazy." Many talk of Brexit as "bonkers" or plain "mad." In all of these cases, we quite happily deploy the language of mental illness to connote the things we believe are wrong with the world and the way it is being managed. Particularly if a policy appears extremely dangerous, we reach for the mental illness metaphor to communicate our dissatisfaction. In fact, use of the mental illness metaphor is not new. Bernard Williams described Utilitarianism thus:

> There are certain situations so monstrous that the idea that the processes of moral rationality could yield an answer to them is insane: they are situations which so transcend in enormity the human business of moral deliberation that from a moral point of view it cannot matter anymore what happens. (1973, p. 92)

But the problem is that as soon as we start criticizing the use of words like "insane," we find ourselves doing it too. Still, whether it is backchat on Twitter, top flight philosophy, or idle conversation, we should surely feel uneasy about the use of the mental illness metaphor. It is ham-fisted and hurtful. The most obvious reason that it's wrong is that it trivializes the experience of mental illness.

We should not use words for diagnoses as everyday tactics of ridicule. If someone is very precise or cleans their house thoroughly, we call them OCD. If they appear fixated or regimented in their behavior or they do not follow conventions, we call them autistic, on the spectrum, or perhaps even "spectrumy." If they have too much energy and little concentration, we call them ADHD. When we use specific diagnostic labels to refer to everyday behaviors, we reduce damaging psychological conditions to silly personality traits. As a result, we may be less likely to take seriously the people who have significant problems of functioning. Because many of these conditions occur on a continuum, we think we know what they are like. But worry is a very different thing from generalized anxiety disorder. Mood swings are not bipolar disorder.

Sadness is not the same as depression. Again, we trivialize real illness, and stigmatize others.

Stigma and a profound lack of understanding toward people with mental health conditions is a large part of what makes it so difficult to have a psychotic illness, or a mental illness like anxiety or depression. We may think that mental illness pervades every aspect of a person's life, so they become untrustworthy, unreliable, or even dangerous. We may think that they make bad neighbors, partners, and employees. The print and broadcast media, social media, and the film and television industry are still full of this toxic stigma. One study of 20 years of movies with characters with schizophrenia found that most of them were depicted as violent, one-third of these violent characters engaged in homicidal behavior, and a quarter died by suicide (Owen, 2012).

In fact, mental illness is a common experience. One in three of us will experience some form of mental illness in our lifetime, even if only about 1% of the population has a serious illness like schizophrenia. Depression has one of the highest disease burdens of all medical conditions, affecting more than 300 million people worldwide (IHME, 2018). Twenty years ago, Kjell Magne Bondevik, then Prime Minister of Norway, experienced a profound bout of depression. He stepped down for three weeks until he recovered. Then he went back to his job. At no time did he do anything irrational. It's just another illness.

Harnessing the Power of Taboo Words in Positive Ways

So, as we have demonstrated, taboo words are powerful and can be used in negative ways. Then again, there are some arguments to be made that taboo words need not affect us in a negative way. One could argue that the opposite is true—that we can in fact harness the power of these taboo words in interesting and helpful forms to suit our purposes. Consider the following examples. Swearing seems to increase tolerance to pain. Scientists have set up experiments where people have to tolerate pain, for example, by putting their hand in ice-cold water (Stephens et al., 2009). During these kinds of experiments some people are told to swear while their hand is in the water while others are told to say neutral words. The swearing does seem to increase pain tolerance. And here's another example—taboo words can bring us together. A study conducted in a New Zealand soap factory examined the use of the word "fuck" in workers' interactions (Daly et al., 2004). The authors concluded that this taboo word was used to express positive politeness and in-group membership.

Of particular relevance here, another example of positive impact relates to the reclaiming of certain taboo words by minority groups (Croom, 2013; Galinsky et al., 2013). Think of a word like "queer." This used to be an insult, and associated even with "queer bashing," homophobic violence. Now, it reaches out to people who challenge "heteronormativity"—lesbian, gay, bisexual, trans, pansexual, and the whole alphabet soup of diversity. This word is now used with much pride by many, far from its past use as a term of derision.

Some ethnic and racial minorities have done the same with words such as "wog." So, these words are used to build a sense of identity: "we" can reclaim these words that "you" do not dare to use. We are cool, you are outsiders. Yet, to some gay or lesbian people, words like "queer" are still hurtful. For some ethnic and racial minorities "wog" is deeply offensive. These words can bring people together but can also divide communities.

"Cripple" or "Crip" has undergone a similar trajectory, used by the disability rights movement for decades to build a common identity. Most recently, the Twitter hashtag #CripTheVote was co-created in the US in 2016 by three disabled advocates—Alice Wong, Gregg Beratan, and Andrew Pulrang—to highlight issues which affect people with disabilities and their communities during election campaigns, a nonpartisan project to engage voters as well as politicians (Wong, 2016). Despite "cripple" being considered strongly offensive and generally unacceptable by many in the mainstream, these advocates have reclaimed a variant of this word to suit their purposes. It was used 1455 times on Twitter in the week prior to the US presidential election (Mann, 2018). More recently, as part of her 2020 presidential campaign, US Senator Elizabeth Warren interacted with disability advocates using this hashtag via a "Twitter town hall" with the hashtag trending during Warren's question and answer session. It is now used before, during, and after election campaigns around the world. Mann (2018) describes the #CripTheVote campaign as a new form of social movement (see Shakespeare, 1993, for evidence of the 40+ year history of disability rights). Incidentally, hashtags with the initial letter of each word capitalized, sometimes referred to as camel case, are preferred by people with disabilities because they can be read by automated screen readers.

However, as with "queer" and "wog," there is a risk that "Crip" does not reach everyone equally. Identity politics can be inward-looking and separatist (Shakespeare, 2006). Disability may not be someone's primary identification—they may prefer to be known as a woman, member of minority ethnic community, or simply as an individual. Approximately half the people affected by disability are older people, and they are less likely to identify as disabled, let alone to deploy the term "crip"; for them, illness and impairment are naturalized as part of getting older.

Conclusion

Language changes, and taboos change too. People with disabilities have been the butt of humor; they have been marginalized; they have been ignored; they have even been abused or murdered. In the twenty-first century, there is at last, for many, the prospect of inclusion, represented for many by the Convention on the Rights of Persons with Disabilities. Terminology is often the frontline of efforts to promote acceptance, and the boundaries of what is acceptable, what is hurtful, what is radical, and what is shameful change fast. It might be hoped that in future, disability is an unremarkable and unremarked-on part of someone's multifaceted identity. Stories of ethnicity, gender, and sexuality suggest that full acceptance is a long time coming, but that great changes can happen. Having disabled people as professionals; as academics; as journalists; as broadcasters; as comedians can only help, normalizing disability and difference as another dimension to the complexities and fascinations of life.

REFERENCES

Bailey, B., & Arciuli, J. (2020). Indigenous Australians with autism: A scoping review. *Autism, 24*(5), 1031–1046. https://doi.org/10.1177/1362361319894829

Bowers, J. S., & Pleydell-Pearce, C. W. (2011). Swearing, euphemisms, and linguistic relativity. *PLOS ONE, 6*(7), e22341. https://doi.org/10.1371/journal.pone.0022341

Cameron, D., & Stevenson, N. (2016). *Attitudes to potentially offensive language and gestures on TV and radio.* Research report. Retrieved January 16, 2020, from https://www.ofcom.org.uk/__data/assets/pdf_file/0022/91624/OfcomOffensiveLanguage.pdf

CNN (2018). 16 insane things that happened in Trumpworld in just the last 48 hours, *The Point.* Retrieved January 16, 2020, from https://edition.cnn.com/2018/02/28/politics/48-hours-trump-analysis/index.html

Croom, A. M. (2013). How to do things with slurs: Studies in the way of derogatory words. *Language & Communication, 33*(3), 177–204. https://doi.org/10.1016/j.langcom.2013.03.008

Croom, A. M. (2015). An introduction to the special issue on Slurs. *Language Sciences, 52*, 1–2. https://doi.org/10.1016/j.langsci.2015.08.001

Daly, N., Holmes, J., Newton, J., & Stubbe, M. (2004). Expletives as signals in FTAs on the factory floor. *Journal of Pragmatics, 36*(5), 945–964. https://doi.org/10.1016/j.pragma.2003.12.004

Department of Work and Pensions. (2003). *Disabled for life*, DWP, London.

Dewaele, J.-M. (2010). The emotional force of swearwords and taboo words in the speech of multilinguals. *Journal of Multilingual and Multicultural Development, 25*(2-3), 204–222. https://doi.org/10.1080/01434630408666529

Eilola, T. M., & Havelka, J. (2007). Emotional activation in the first and second language. *Cognition and Emotion, 21*(5), 1064–1076. https://doi.org/10.1080/02699930601054109

Fazel, S., Buxrud, P., Ruchkin, V., & Grann, M. (2010). Homicide in discharged patients with schizophrenia and other psychoses: A national case-control study. *Schizophrenia Research, 123*(2–3), 263–269. https://doi.org/10.1016/j.schres.2010.08.019

Galinsky, A. D., Wang, C. S., Whitson, J. A., Anicich, E. M., Hugenberg, K., & Bodenhausen, G. V. (2013). The reappropriation of stigmatizing labels: The reciprocal relationship between power and self-labeling. *Psychological Science, 24*(10), 2020–2029. https://doi.org/10.1177/0956797613482943

Gernsbacher, M. A., Raimond, A. R., Balinghasay, M. T., & Boston, J. S. (2016). "Special needs" is an ineffective euphemism. *Cognitive Research: Principles and Implications, 1*, 29. https://doi.org/10.1186/s41235-016-0025-4

Harris, C., Ayçiçeği, A., & Gleason, J. (2003). Taboo words and reprimands elicit greater autonomic reactivity in a first language than in a second language. *Applied Psycholinguistics, 24*(4), 561–579. https://doi.org/10.1017/S0142716403000286

Institute for Health Metrics and Evaluation (2018). Findings from the Global Burden of Disease Study 2017. IHME.

Jay, K. L., & Jay, T. B. (2015). Taboo word fluency and knowledge of slurs and general pejoratives: Deconstructing the poverty-of-vocabulary myth. *Language Sciences, 52*, 251–259. https://doi.org/10.1016/j.langsci.2014.12.003

Jay, T. B. (2018). Taboo language awareness in early childhood. In K. Allan (Ed.), *The Oxford handbook of taboo words and language* (pp. 96–107). https://doi.org/10.1093/oxfordhb/9780198808190.013.6

Kenny, L., Hattersley, C., Molins, B., Buckley, C., Povey, C., & Pellicano, E. (2016). Which terms should be used to describe autism? Perspectives from the UK autism community. *Autism, 20*(4), 442–462. https://doi.org/10.1177/1362361315588200

Lycan, W. G. (2015). Slurs and lexical presumption. *Language Sciences, 52*, 3–11. https://doi.org/10.1016/j.langsci.2015.05.001

Mackay, D. G., Shafto, M., Taylor, J. K., Marian, D. E., Abrams, L., & Dyer, J. R. (2004). Relations between emotion, memory, and attention: Evidence from taboo Stroop, lexical decision, and immediate memory tasks. *Memory & Cognition, 32 (3)*, 474–488. https://doi.org/10.3758/BF03195840

Mann, B. W. (2018). Rhetoric of online disability activism: #CripTheVote and civic participation. *Communication, Culture and Critique, 11*(4), 604–621. https://doi.org/10.1093/ccc/tcy030

Meffert, E., Tillmanns, E., Heim, S., Jung, S., Huber, W., & Grande, M. (2011). Taboo: A novel paradigm to elicit aphasia-like trouble-indicating behavior in normally speaking individuals. *Journal of Psycholinguistic Research, 40 (5–6)*, 307–326. https://doi.org/10.1007/s10936-011-9170-6

Owen, P. R. (2012). Portrayals of schizophrenia by entertainment media: A content analysis of contemporary movies. *Psychiatric Services, 63*(7), 655–659. https://doi.org/10.1176/appi.ps.201100371

Shakespeare, T. (1993). Disabled people's self-organisation: A new social movement? *Disability, Handicap and Society, 8*(3), 249–264. https://doi.org/10.1080/02674649366780261

Shakespeare, T. (1994). Cultural representation of disabled people: Dustbins for disavowal? *Disability and Society, 9*(3), 283–299. https://doi.org/10.1080/09687599466780341

Shakespeare, T. (2006). The social model of disability. In L. J. Davis (Ed.), *The disability studies reader* (2nd ed., pp. 197–204). Routledge.

Shakespeare, T. (2017). *Disability: The basics*. Routledge.

Shakespeare, T., Thompson, S., & Wright, M. J. (2009). No laughing matter: Medical and social factors in restricted growth. *Scandinavian Journal of Disability Research, 12*(1), 19–31. https://doi.org/10.1080/15017410902909118

Smith, R. A. (2007). Language of the lost: An explication of stigma communication. *Communication Theory, 17*(4), 462–485. https://doi.org/10.1111/j.1468-2885.2007.00307.x

Stephens, R., Atkins, J., & Kingston, A. (2009). Swearing as a response to pain. *Neuroreport, 20*(12), 1056–1060. https://doi.org/10.1097/WNR.0b013e32832e64b1

Van Lancker, D., & Cummings, J. L. (1999). Expletives: Neurolinguistic and neurobehavioral perspectives on swearing. *Brain Research Reviews, 31*(1), 83–104. https://doi.org/10.1016/S0165-0173(99)00060-0

Williams, B. (1973). A critique of utilitarianism. In J. J. C. Smart & B. Williams (Eds.), *Utilitarianism: For and against*. Cambridge University Press.

Wong, A. (2016). #CripTheVote: Our voices, our vote. Retrieved January 16, 2020, from https://disabilityvisibilityproject.com/2016/01/27/cripthevote-our-voices-our-vote/

CHAPTER 3

Communicating by Accident: Dysfluency, the Non-Essential, and the Catastrophe

Joshua St. Pierre

"To invent the sailing ship or steamer is *to invent the shipwreck*. To invent the train is *to invent the rail accident* of derailment. To invent the family automobile is to produce the *pile-up* on the highway" (Virilio, 2007, p. 10). Virilio's argument is now classic with the study of social acceleration. To invent a new technology of speed is also to invent its corresponding accident, which is to say, "the possibility of unintended and unfortunate outcomes" (Matthewman, 2013, p. 282). Yet time has its way of wearing accidents down to mundane statistics. Although getting in a car remains one of the riskiest activities available to humans, we fold this cost neatly into the benefits of modern life and get on with our busy day. As it is with transportation, so it is with communication.

Social acceleration is not a process reducible to new and faster technology, but technological advances certainly play a role. Hartmut Rosa (2003), one of the foremost theorists of social acceleration, ties the acceleration of transport and communication together, explaining that the "most obvious, and most measurable form of acceleration is the speeding up of *intentional* [emphasis added], goal-directed processes of transport, communication, and production" (p. 6). During the nineteenth century, accelerating both transport and communication to the speed of machines were considered linked projects. As James Carey (2009) explains, the term "communication" described at this time both the movement of material things (commodities or people) as well as the movement of immaterial ideas (information). While the twinned meaning of

J. St. Pierre (✉)
University of Alberta, Edmonton, AB, Canada
e-mail: jstpierr@ualberta.ca

© The Author(s), under exclusive license to Springer Nature Switzerland AG 2023
M. S. Jeffress et al. (eds.), *The Palgrave Handbook of Disability and Communication*, https://doi.org/10.1007/978-3-031-14447-9_3

"communication" has been lost to time, the coupling of thought remains such that the "transmission model of communication" today overshadows other models of communication (p. 15). Yet the imperial dreams of this model are old. "The center of this idea of communication is the transmission of signals or messages for the purpose of control. It is a view of communication from one of the most ancient of human dreams: the desire to increase the speed and effect of messages as they travel in space" (p. 12). In this model, "successful" communication is marked by a correspondence between the *intentional* idea of the sender encoded in the message and the idea reproduced in the mind of the receiver. This makes the process of communication brittle and prone to error, for the dream of imperial control it offers rests ultimately upon speeding the message, while protecting it from damage along the voyage.

This is background for what most people know, but dysfluent speakers know intimately: communication accidents—let's call them "miscommunications" (Mortensen 1997) or "misunderstandings" for now—course through our everyday lives. Words that accidently slip out, words misheard, or intentions misread are common to our experience. But I suggest these experiences are qualitatively different for the fluent speaker than the disabled one. At the level of lived experience, stutterers and communication accidents are intimate in ways revered for old dancing partners. One common experience of stuttering is feeling "out of control." The stutterer *feels* an accident oncoming, her body anticipates the next phoneme about to derail the speech act, but there is nothing much to do. When the moment of stammering happens, it often arrives with panic. Involuntary sounds and involuntary trembles of the body intended to shove the stutter into the common world draw stares from onlookers aware that the automaticity of social interaction has been broken. Feeling the weight of panic, the stutterer might push through the original intention, try to switch out the troublesome word, or even flee the accident in shame. These are well-worn experiences for people forced to navigate the rhythms of a fluent world.

We can thus understand the stutterer to be one who "communicates by accident" in two distinct ways. First, the stutterer communicates *by way of* the accident. In philosophy, "accidentals" refer to the metaphysical distinction of properties that *need not* exist in a specific object set in contrast to essential or substantive properties that *must*. Moreover, in literary studies, accidentals are those features of the text like typeface or marginalia that are not part of the text's substance. The syntax of a speech act is essential to its intended meaning, while accidentals like "um" or "er," stutters and blocks are ostensibly inessential. The stutter expresses an involuntary force of life—it often says things "by accident" the individual did not fully intend. Because accidentals distract rational communication from its intentional and goal-directed processes, this first sense of "communicating by accident" also means the stutterer is intimate with the pile-up. As an uncontrolled force, dysfluency is a virtual accident: an accident waiting to happen. But second, when the stutterer communicates, she can find it has happened "by accident." Communication happened (note the passive) in ways she did not quite understand or control.

These characterizations of stutterers as accidents-in-waiting are probably familiar for many who are used to being living scapegoats for the ills of information societies. Too often, anxieties about so-called communication accidents that ought to be cast toward structural conditions are instead centered upon individual selves made to carry the sins of miscommunication away from the polis and into the desert, the margin, of pathology. The first objective of this chapter is thus to retrace the accident within networks of force and power. While dysfluent subjects are indeed shuttles for cultural anxiety about information crashes, I argue this says more about our models of communication that expect *intentional* and *accurate* transmission of information and thereby prefigure the dysfluent accident into communication. The second objective is to rethink the scene of the dysfluent accident from what James Carey (2009) calls the model of communication as ritual, instead of the transmission model. I suggest that dysfluent accidents, and accidents of communication more generally, lose focus if we attend to communication too closely as transmission rather than a shared act of world-building. Approached from this register, dysfluent accidents might not be a matter of technical difficulty defined by narrow problems like entropy, but socio-cultural *dramas* that reveal contending forces and desires.

Accidents in Transmission

Dysfluent Breakdowns

Allow me to start by cataloguing a few kinds of dysfluent accidents (some of which overlap slightly). These are useful examples to have on the table, but also ideas that we will problematize as we go along:

- **The blurt.** Stutterers pepper their language with so-called fillers that ostensibly sit outside of, and even detract from, the message. We sometimes grimace and groan in the act of speech. In addition, we sometimes *find ourselves* in the midst of speaking sounds, words, or phrases we did not fully intend.
- **The misfire.** The phenomenon of stuttering includes both prolongation and repetition. Stuttering can extend the opening sounds of a message (e.g., aaaaaaaagree or bo-bo-bo-book), which an ableist grammar recodes as misfires that communicative parties can tacitly agree to ignore.
- **The stall.** A repetition can be a redundant redundancy (one that serves no discernable purpose), like repeating most of a sentence multiple times to get a "running start" on the difficult finish that was long ago anticipated by our impatient interlocutor. Or, in a hard block, the voice *suddenly and unexpectedly* runs dry. A word stops in your throat, and you must wait for infra-bodily traffic to clear while the absence of meaning gapes wide and dangerous in the social world.

- **Crossed wires.** A regular experience for stutterers, crossed wires describes the state of "talking past each other" that might begin when one party "mishears" the other and then feedbacks error into the conversation.
- **The swerve.** Clinicians prefer the term "avoidance" to describe the strategy stutterers employ when we sense an oncoming phoneme over which we expect to trip. I might, for example, begin to say "I agree" but change course, swerving around a potential misfire to substitute on the fly: "I do not know."
- **The cut-off.** This accident is one of attempted repair, caused when interlocutors or bystanders rush to the scene of an accident, interrupt, and reimpose order by attempting to predict and finish the stalled (or otherwise damaged) message according to a dominant grammar.
- **The gridlock.** Stuttering ferociously at the front of a queue, for example, halts the flow of information, people, and capital; it stalls a lane of traffic and tempts impatient honks in the form of tapped toes and glances, as everyone waits for an *undetermined time* until information and thus bodies will once again flow free.

When communication gets theorized, we usually start with its essential aspects—the intentional and constant—and, at best, work our way back to such accidents—the unexpected variations. In addition to the West's long-standing fixation with substance, the elision of the accident has to do with the transmission model of communication itself, in which, Lisbeth Lipari (2014) explains, "communication becomes a merely mechanical routine wherein things like the accuracy of the message, the efficiency of delivery, and the precision of reception are in the foreground …" (p. 10). Greater control over these variables is meant to quicken the *incident-free* relay of messages in the pursuit of greater instrumental power. To demonstrate this model, we can turn to systems theory and a purely functional definition of the accident.

System Failures

The sociologist of organization Charles Perrow (1999) defines an accident as "a failure in a subsystem, or the system as a whole, that damages more than one unit and in doing so disrupts the ongoing or future output of the system" (p. 66). Perrow's definition turns upon the meaning of antecedent terms—part, unit, subsystem, system—so let us work through an exemplary and truly spectacular accident of transmission described by James Gleik (2012):

> [O]n June 16, 1887, a Philadelphia wool dealer named Frank Primrose telegraphed his agent in Kansas to say that he had bought—abbreviated in their agreed code as BAY—500,000 pounds of wool. When the message arrived, the key word had become BUY. The agent began buying wool, and before long the error cost Primrose $20,000, according to the lawsuit he filed against the Western Union Telegraph Company. (p. 166)

In the instance above, the "system" to analyze is Primrose's mechanism of capital accumulation. The "subsystem" is his wool dealing, which, in turn, is comprised by an array of "units"—here, the relay of market information between Primrose and his agent. Finally, the unit consists of "parts" organized into the functional relation. The most relevant part to examine here would be the telegraphed message, the ostensible source of the accident. For Perrow (1999), an accident will always be triggered by component failure, often a part like a damaged value, inattentive operator (p. 71), or, in this case, damaged message. Yet to be an accident, and not merely what he calls an "incident," damage must extend to at least the register of subsystems. If, for example, Primrose received the damaged message too late to purchase 500,000 pounds of wool (and thus *not* damaged his future capacity to buy or sell wool), it would have been—at least for Primrose—an unremarkable incident; if anything, a "near miss."

Who or what was responsible for this accident? A modified or "damaged" message, sure, but this explanation is too general. If we analyze the functional system of the telegraph itself, the alteration of the message is already an accident regardless of downstream effects. Here, we could trace component failure to relevant subsystems of the telegraph: transmitter, channel, relay, and receiver. The common-sense answer might locate component failure in the channel (faulty copper wires) or maybe the relay station (human error in forwarding the message) and leave the question settled with repairs on the way. Indeed, conventional explanations for system failure include "operator error; faulty design or equipment; lack of attention to safety features; [or] lack of operating experience" (Perrow, 1999, p. 63). Yet many actants jostle in play. Three of the subsystems (transmitter, relay, and receiver) were telegraph offices, units themselves made of human bodies and minds, electromagnetism, copper, culture, sounding devices, speed, acoustics, protocols, codes, and ciphers.

Call it an irreducible feature of "vibrant matter" (Bennett, 2010), but components and processes do not always interact predictably. Bruno Latour (2007) would say that at moments of system failure, "completely silent intermediaries become full-blown mediators" (p. 81). The accident reveals components we thought compliant transmitters of force to be instead moonlighting schemers. "[E]ven objects, which a minute before appeared fully automatic, autonomous, and devoid of human agents, are now made of crowds of frantically moving humans with heavy equipment" (p. 81). That components can toggle between modes of mediator/intermediator, agent/automatic thing is important when it is time to assign responsibility for an accident. Maurizio Lazzarato (2014) is here instructive:

> Take the example of a corporation: salaried employees are [machinically] enslaved to the automatization of procedures, machines, and the division of labor, functioning as the "inputs" and "outputs" of the process. But when a breakdown, an accident, or a malfunction occurs, the subject function, consciousness, and representations must be mobilized in order to "recover" from the incident, explain it,

and mitigate its effects with a view to returning the automatic functions and enslavement procedures to their normal state. (p. 38)

Within the mode of "machinic enslavement" (a term borrowed from cybernetics) the speaking human becomes a mere input and output in the automated functioning of complex systems. Humans are governed as system components *up until* the moment of the accident, which throws automatic functions out of order. Now the subject—with all its robust volition and agency—is suddenly recalled, for only *persons* can be dragged before courts or boards and be held sufficiently responsible for breakdown.

This is precisely the conventional route taken by Frank Primrose when he damned all agency into the human subject and sued the Western Union Telegraph Company "for a *negligent mistake of the defendant's agents* [emphasis added] in transmitting a telegraphic message" (Primrose v. The Western Union Telegraph Co., 1894, p. 1). The defendants also deflected responsibility, pleading not guilty with two angles to their defense. First, they argued the message under question was both "a cipher and obscure" (p. 3). Gleik (2012) notes that ciphers had become popular at this time due to issues of secrecy and brevity (p. 160). Since telegraph companies charged by the letter, users quickly (to the ire of telegraph companies) formed shorthand to save money. The medium thus altered culture as people removed descriptive prose, context, and other redundancies from a message in order to transmit its presumptive essence with streamlined efficiency. Moreover, encoding the phrase "I have bought" as "BAY" serves to protect the message from unwanted eyes—say, rival wool buyers—as it travels through the common world. But the cost of controlling communication, of "increas[ing] the speed and effect of messages as they travel in space" (Carey, 2009, p. 12) is a system highly sensitive to error. Sandwiched between "B," and "Y," the encoded difference between "A" and "U" was only a single dot, a single pulse of sound. At speed and without context, the message is highly sensitive to change at multiple parts of its journey. Perrow (1999) would describe a telegraph system, much like a railway, as one "tightly coupled" (p. 92)—it lacks "slack" between its various parts and its rapid and linked processes. Such systems do not flex with shock and are especially prone to derailment.

Tacit recognition of this system vulnerability was active in the second part of the Western Union Telegraph Company's defense. Namely, the plaintiff was responsible for information damage if he ignored the terms of service written on the telegraph blank: "Errors can be guarded against only by repeating a message back to the sending station for comparison" (Primrose v. The Western Union Telegraph Co., 1894, p. 3). The repetition of a message (at another half the cost) would confirm its accuracy against the original. Put otherwise, this is a protocol to add redundancy to a tightly coupled system, *at the same time* as it transfers responsibility for its structural risks to the individual user.

While speed and accuracy are taken to be equal partners in the project of modern communication, the demands of speed often override those of accuracy in the decisive moment. We might think of Primrose, who not only did not consider the extra time and money to repeat the message worth the cost, but, according to the majority opinion, testified he had no memory of reading the small print. Or, to take an example closer to home, people with various communication disabilities are often accustomed, in varying degrees of intensity, to being misunderstood or having interlocutors approximate their message—a heavy-handed act of repair—because the time and labor needed to dig into the moment and wait for an indeterminate message to come into focus is deemed too costly.

After six years in lower courts, the US Supreme Court decided for the Western Union Telegraph Company. The user, Primrose, was found to knowingly incur the risks of sending a cipher without confirming its accuracy. There was a breach of implicit contract, for although Primrose did not recall the terms of service, Justice Grey argued in the majority opinion that "the terms on the back of the message, so far as they were not inconsistent with law, formed part of the contract between him and the company under which the message was transmitted" (Primrose v. The Western Union Telegraph Co., 1894, p. 25). Yet despite the verdict and the communicative contract it appears to uphold, this whole premise is nightmare material for stutterers. An accidental swerve, block, or misfire that occurs somewhere in bodily traffic to alter a $20,000 pulse of sound and cost my employer an additional six years of legal fees is a fear overstated, but a fear nonetheless. My hunch is that the threat of damaging flows of information invested with capital has worried many dysfluent speakers (and other non-normative communicators) who subsist within an informational economy. I think, for example, of a dysfluent friend, "E," who found employment at the Circulations Desk at the Columbia Law Library, where transferring incoming calls was a regular duty. E would sometimes receive a call, dial the extension, and then block *completely* when the second party answered. At this point, either the second caller would assume a bad connection and hang up, or E himself would disconnect the call in embarrassed frustration. Much like the "negligent" telegraph operator, E's non-intentional act breaks the automatic pulsations of the system. One significant difference between these examples is the degree of "interactive complexity" (Matthewman, 2013, p. 284) afforded by speed. Information systems that approach the speed of immediacy are made to interface with more systems, which makes the potential for breakdown more widespread. But in either case, components prone to flicker between thing and agent, intermediator and mediator, may be unreliable at the level of simple output, but redeem their value at the moment of breakdown as shock absorbers for unruly agency; as parts designed to break instead of the system.

Littered Speech

By calling attention to distributed agency, systems theory might alleviate some anxiety dysfluent folk experience for being risky objects. However, any aid is limited: perhaps the best systems theory can do for disability communities is call attention to risky components *and* risky systems. I agree with Perrow (1999) that individual failings cannot sufficiently explain "damage" to "symbols, communication patterns, legitimacy, or a number of factors that are not, strictly speaking, people or objects" (p. 64). As with the Primrose accident, the many fragments of agency that must join forces to transmit a message with both speed and efficiency can also "damage" a message with unthought speed. But insisting on the language of damage to describe a wandering or otherwise noncompliant message is where the usefulness of systems theory runs dry for disability studies.

A thought to move us in a different direction. Perhaps accidents are inelimible in a fundamentally untidy world. The late nineteenth-century pragmatist William James (1996) writes that "philosophers have always aimed at cleaning up the litter with which the world apparently is filled" (p. 45), which, for William Connolly (2005), means that James takes seriously "a place for something like an element of chanciness or volatility within [the world's] loose regularities and historical flows" (p. 73). Systems are accidents-in-waiting, but here, the problem for the communication engineer would run deep: systems can only be built with material hewn from an untidy universe. No matter the redundancies, no matter the guardrails we stake around "clear communication," intentions and meanings will go amiss. But misunderstandings in this world do not occur, as systems theorists and neo-Kantians might hope, due to insufficient parameters around either instrumental reason or rational deliberation, but because the world itself cannot be cinched up to such standards and, on the other side, because slippage of meaning is the common ground of understanding. In a move that tilts us from the transmission model toward the lived experience of stuttering, Rosi Braidotti (1994) suggests that "language is not only and not even the instrument of communication but a site of symbolic exchange that links us together in a tenuous yet workable web of mediated misunderstandings" (p. 14).

For those attached to order, the possibility of a world strewn with litter might quicken resentment against the world, bodies in which its unmasterability accrues, and even action itself. After all, in an untidy world, the actant is "a being or entity that makes a difference in the world *without quite knowing what it is doing* [emphasis added]" (Connolly, 2005, p. 72). This implies both that agency extends far beyond the human, and that when humans *do* act in concert with other entities, so many actants crowd the stage that "it's never clear who and what is acting" (Latour, 2007, p. 46). For instance, I might say a good class is one in which I communicate a concept well. Yet the passive voice is far more honest. A good class is when a concept gets communicated—I am never privy to why nor where nor when nor how an idea might ricochet and stick, nor, ultimately, to the affect-soaked meaning my words paint. That the meaning of our words never fully lies within our grasp is what Hannah Arendt (1958) calls the "suffering" of the word (p. 190). Speech *must* suffer to participate in a common world; it *must* be exposed to an unpredictable world to ignite chains of action.

Unfortunately, while dwelling with the ineliminability of suffering might help fold generosity and responsiveness into one's relations with dysfluent folk and thus change the conditions of the communication accident, the easier, and thus more likely response is to double down on the regulatory ideal of the self-mastered and intentional speech act, which presents ample opportunities to resent an untidy world that makes us suffer in order to act. An ableist "choreography" that reinstates dominant rhythms and modes of communication can serve such goals. Kevin Paterson (2012) writes that

> "[a] person with speech impairment 'dys-appears' because there is 'no slack' when negotiating the choreography of everyday life. One must keep 'in time' and 'in step' with the tempo of communication because slowness is the embodiment of failure and 'deficiency'. Disruptions (and distortions) arise in communicative encounters between people with and with-out speech impairment *because* the choreography of everyday life demands an exclusionary form of bodily performance and 'style' which does not reflect the carnal information of the former." (p. 169)

Perhaps the most striking aspect of this passage is the active role played by dominant choreographies to cast stutterers out of the communicative sphere. A slackless system, slowness coded as deficiency, and the demand that speakers embody fluent "styles" to be recognized as speakers is not just a functional but also a *moral* order that absolves the ostensibly fluent of their responsibility for disruptions in the communicative event.

Let us pause to note that the ground has already shifted under our feet. James (1996), Connolly (2005), Braidotti (1994), Arendt (1958), and Paterson (2012) have taken us from system protocols and system output to a distinctly different set of concerns around worlds, world-building, and the negotiation of differential rhythms.

Accidents of Ritual

The Ritual Model of Communication

The transmission model describes one mode of communication. Yet as Lipari (2014) explains, getting too invested in this model can cause us to miss other, and more interesting, aspects of communication (p. 10). As such, I wish to re-approach the dysfluent accident from another angle. For Carey (2009), the oldest and most enduring model of communication is that of *ritual*, a model that plucks the etymological resonance between the terms "communication," "commonness," and "communion" (p. 15). In this way, the model directs our attention "not toward the extension of messages in space but toward the maintenance of society in time; not the act of imparting information but the representation of shared beliefs" (p. 15). Communication in this mode emphasizes the shared act of *constructing, celebrating,* and *repairing* common worlds (Lipari, p. 12), and Carey famously suggests that communication is here akin to attending religious mass, where the point is not to transmit information but to draw people together in communion—to produce and maintain a shared view of the world through repeated practices. Pulling away from Protestant values, this view "downplays the role of the sermon, the instruction and admonition, in order to highlight the role of the prayer, the chant, and the ceremony" (Carey, p. 15). What makes the prayer, chant, and ceremony significant is their function as both social practices and techniques of the self. Through their repetition, we develop collective sensibilities and patterns of perception by which we can build common worlds.

Carol Padden (2015) takes up Carey's (2009) model to account for the rich complexity by which disabled people communicate. Ritual, she argues, emphasizes "performance, activity, and the materiality of communication itself. In this framework, meaning is not so much the definition of a word or sentence but instead is constructed *in situ,* in social and cultural activity" (p. 44). Unlike sending a message, meaning gets enacted in the very midst of unruly bodies that excrete "all levels of expression, from the minute details of discourse— from pitch, emphasis, gesture, head tilts, and eye gaze" (p. 44). Twitching bodies, stuttering tongues, signing fingers, and slurred lips (and all the affect they carry along) are no longer distracting "accidentals," but the very materiality of communion. Moreover, since communication happens "on site," time cannot be transcended or otherwise avoided with speed but must be lived through. The relative slowness of disabled communicators is a boon: meaning *composts* and develops over time. Communicating in crip time (Kafer, 2013; St. Pierre, 2015) generates eutropic conditions that are weird, messy, and bursting with possibility.

For Carey (2009), "[n]ews reading, and writing, is a ritual act and moreover a dramatic one. What is arrayed before the reader is not pure information but a *portrayal of the contending forces in the world* [emphasis added]" (p. 16). Like chanting in a mass, writers do not describe the world, but invite participants to share their view of its drama and thereby construct/maintain a commonality. This idea helps reform the communication accident.

Accident Redux

Consider the "crossed wire." So-called misunderstandings are often better understood as dramas of contending forces. It is perhaps not that my grumpy co-worker "misheard" my stuttered speech, but that he did not *want* to listen and did not *want* to belong in time to a common world with this disabled person. Similarly, in the mode of ritual, the "cut-off" is often a technique of boundary maintenance: either to protect a common world from outside influence or to reinstate hierarchies within. Ableism and disableism are forces of a titan scale that, of course, cut across other social dramas. Or take "the stall":

composer and writer Jerome Ellis explains that his general response to a blocked word is to look upward and freeze. "Part of it feels like my body goes into a kind of supplication or prayer almost. I have a friend who once referred to it as 'watching me ask for the word'" (Cole, 2020, n.p.). In the mode of transmission, meaning would flee this scene, yet in the mode of ritual, the frozen supplication is a link to the body's ancient relation to meaning and language, one in which we do not command but must together wait in the unexpected. Humans communicate by accident.

Finally, consider that the "misfire" can interrupt the *automaticity* of ritual. Chris Constantino (2016), a Speech-Language Pathologist and stutterer, writes:

> What strikes me about our stuttering is its ability to disrupt the expected flow of a conversation. Much of human communication is routine and automatic. People speak without actually saying anything, they engage in a ritualized exchange of mundane phrases in a rehearsed rhythm that requires little thought. Speaking is used to keep others at a distance rather than to bring us closer together. Heuristic phrases and trite clichés turn potentially new and exciting situations into familiar and rehearsed routines. We would rather act out a routine, "Hi, how are you," than actually speak to someone. (para. 3)

When I discussed this idea with Constantino, he offered the example of someone holding a door open while a stutterer tries to express their gratitude. What is supposed to be a routine interaction, an instrumental relation, unexpectedly becomes something unrehearsed and even intimate as two people are now locked in a moment of undecidability. Something new emerges on the scene that exceeds individual intentions. It is in such moments that thicker and more responsive social relations might grow:

> The unexpectedness of stuttering forces both listener and speaker into a space of trust and vulnerability. They must both give up control of the situation. The person speaking does not know when and for how long they will stutter. Likewise, the person listening does not know when to expect a stutter. In order for both people to communicate, they must trust one another. (para. 5)

Stuttering invites a renewed respect for the dialogical relationship opened between speaker and listener (St. Pierre, 2012; Cole, 2020). Arendt might say that the relationship of speaker and listener is, in general, characterized by weakness and suffering, since neither speaker nor listener controls the situation. Stutterers can experience this suffering in visceral ways. Constantino draws our attention to the way in which the shared moment of stuttering is defined and held together not by a pre-given contract, but by trust. Of course, Constantino is aware that some people will break trust which makes this kind of stuttering that *looks forward to* the unexpected an often-risky affair.

Conclusion

Within any community, some variation from norms of fluent speech is anticipated—adopting the language of Robert McRuer (2006), these are the "virtual failures" of compulsory fluency, those everyday stutters and tics that fumble the coherent performance of compulsory fluency, but that systems can nevertheless absorb. Everyone is virtually dysfluent. Put otherwise, everyone fails to perform fluency in a coherent and uninterrupted manner for even a short period of time (p. 384). These variations are blemishes that get smoothed over, despite being the frictious surface that makes language so creative and adaptive. "Critical" or "severe" failures of compulsory fluency are, on the other hand, uncontainable failures that dysfluent people take up to resist irresistible norms: a protracted block on a pivotal word becomes a void; a stumble becomes an unexpected event that onlookers can no longer ignore. But in turn, the block might become a ritual of waiting and listening; the stumble might shatter expectations and the automaticity of social rituals and thereby invite a new becoming. Nothing here is guaranteed. It is only by coming to terms with this fact that we might collectively build "tenuous yet workable web[s] of mediated misunderstandings" (Braidotti, 1994, p. 14). My hunch is that we all communicate by accident far more than our volitional selves would like to admit.

References

Arendt, H. (1958). *The human condition*. University of Chicago Press.

Bennett, J. (2010). *Vibrant matter: A political ecology of things*. Duke University Press.

Braidotti, R. (1994). *Nomadic subjects: Embodiment and sexual difference in contemporary feminist theory*. Columbia University Press.

Carey, J. (2009). *Communication as culture: Essays on media and society*. Routledge.

Cole, S. (2020, August 7). Made to be broken [Audio podcast episode]. In *This American life*. WBEZ Chicago. Retrieved March 11, 2021, from https://www.thisamericanlife.org/713/made-to-be-broken/act-one-10

Connolly, W. (2005). *Pluralism*. Duke University Press.

Constantino, C. (2016). *Stuttering gain* [Paper presentation]. International Stuttering Awareness Day Conference. Retrieved March 10, 2021, from http://isad.isastutter.org/isad-2016/papers-presented-by-2016/stories-and-experiences-with-stuttering-by-pws/stuttering-gain-christopher-constantino/

Gleik, J. (2012). *The information: A history, a theory, a flood*. Pantheon Books.

James, W. (1996). *A pluralistic universe*. University of Nebraska Press.

Kafer, A. (2013). *Feminist, crip, queer*. Indiana University Press.

Latour, B. (2007). *Reassembling the social: An introduction to actor-network-theory*. Oxford University Press.

Lazzarato, M. (2014). *Signs and machines: Capitalism and the production of subjectivity*. Semiotext(e).

Lipari, L. (2014). *Listening, thinking, being: Toward an ethics of attunement*. Penn State University Press.

Matthewman, S. (2013). Accidentology: A critical assessment of Paul Virilio's "Political economy of speed." *Cultural Politics, 9*(3), 280–295. https://doi.org/10.121 5/17432197-2346982

McRuer, R. (2006). *Crip theory: Cultural signs of queerness and disability.* New York University Press.

Mortensen, C. D. (1997). *Miscommunication.* Sage.

Padden, C. (2015). Communication. In R. Adams, B. Reiss, & D. Serlin (Eds.), *Keywords for disability studies* (pp. 43–45). New York University Press.

Paterson, K. (2012). It's about time! Understanding the experience of speech impairment. In A. Roulstone, C. Thomas, & N. Watson (Eds.), *Routledge handbook of disability studies* (pp. 165–177). Routledge.

Perrow, C. (1999). *Normal accidents: Living with high-risk technologies.* Princeton University Press.

Primrose v. The Western Union Telegraph Co., 154 U.S. 1 (1894). Retrieved March 11, 2021, from https://supreme.justia.com/cases/federal/us/154/1/

Rosa, H. (2003). Social acceleration: Ethical and political consequences of a desynchronized high-speed society. *Constellations, 10*(1), 3–33. https://doi.org/10.1111/1467-8675.00309

St. Pierre, J. (2012). The construction of the disabled speaker: Locating stuttering in disability studies. *The Canadian Journal of Disability Studies, 1*(3), 1–21.

St. Pierre, J. (2015). Distending straight-masculine time: A phenomenology of the disabled speaking body. *Hypatia, 30*(1), 49–65. https://doi.org/10.1111/hypa.12128

Virilio, P. (2007). *The original accident* (J. Rose, Trans.). Polity.

CHAPTER 4

Cross-Neurotype Communication Competence

Emily Stones

Communication competence is generally understood as how people successfully manage personal and professional relationships by adapting one's communication and behavior to a variety of situations based on one's understanding of oneself, one's interpersonal goals, the other person, the environment, and the relationship (Wilson & Sabee, 2003). The qualities associated with communication competence include, but are not limited to, supportive and empathetic communication (Wiemann, 1977), communication that promotes equality and dialogue (Baxter & Montgomery, 1996), motivation to understand the perspectives of others (Spitzberg & Cupach, 1984), and the awareness of identity and cultural values on communication preferences (Ting-Toomey, 1993).

Cross-neurotype communication competence applies these same principles and goals in cross-neurotype contexts, or situations in which persons with neurological differences communicate to make meaning and promote mutual understanding. The development of cross-neurotype communication competence remains an essential component of the neurodiversity movement (Hillary, 2020; Walker, 2012), a social and cultural movement primarily aimed at providing people with neurological differences a voice to describe their own experiences and direct their own lives, and to challenge socially constructed notions of normalcy that have severely harmed and stigmatized neurological minorities throughout time (Bertilsdotter Rosqvist et al., 2020).

The initial thrust of the neurodiversity movement came from autistic persons who claimed that the neurological differences and traits associated with autism were central to their identity. These early activists promoted the

E. Stones (✉)
Regis University, Denver, CO, USA
e-mail: estones@regis.edu

© The Author(s), under exclusive license to Springer Nature Switzerland AG 2023
M. S. Jeffress et al. (eds.), *The Palgrave Handbook of Disability and Communication*, https://doi.org/10.1007/978-3-031-14447-9_4

45

"neurodiversity paradigm" as a replacement for the "pathology paradigm," the prevailing framework through which society viewed autism as a disorder requiring treatment and curing (Walker, 2012, p. 155). As the movement grew, additional voices joined the conversation including people with conditions "currently known as ADHD, Tourette's, dyslexia, hearing voices, bipolar disorder, Down syndrome, and dementia," although these categories and terminology remain in flux, in part due to the self-distancing of some groups from problematic and discriminatory diagnostic terms used to explain their personhood (Bertilsdotter Rosqvist et al., 2020, p. 2). Bertilsdotter Rosqvist et al. articulated the shared characteristics within this diverse group as differences in "sensory, affectual and cognitive processing" and the commitment of movement members to decentering the norms that paint these differences as deficits (2020, p. 2).

This chapter's approach to cross-neurotype communication competence supports the goals expressed by Bertilsdotter Rosqvist et al. (2020) and others (Kapp, 2013; Russell, 2020; Yergeau, 2010) to expand the way we discuss sensory, affective, and cognitive differences in non-pathological contexts and to promote mutual understanding, tolerance for difference, and equity across neurotypes. The use of the terms "neurotype" and "neurotypes" (as people can claim multiple neurotypes, like ADHD and autism) throughout this chapter denotes difference without hierarchy, with emphasis on one's performed and self-perceived neurological differences in the context of one's social and institutional experiences. This chapter builds on the work of scholars who draw connections between disability, culture, and communication (Braithwaite & Braithwaite, 2011; Emry & Wiseman, 1987; Hillary, 2020), to identify culturally significant patterns of thinking and acting within the neurodiversity movement. Recognizing that individuals are greater than their culture and that cultural patterns are integrated, dynamic, and contradictory, this analysis isolates cultural categories that emerge from neurodivergent narratives as significant areas of miscommunication between people of different neurotypes. In illuminating these cultural categories and the possible range of orientations to them, this chapter aims to break down binary thinking about preferences and create space for cross-neurotype "metacommunication," or communication about communication (Craig, 2016, p. 1; see also Bertilsdotter Rosqvist et al., 2020, p. 166).

Prioritizing Neurodivergent Perspectives

The following review of 68 essays that privilege neurodivergent perspectives reveals four categories of cultural significance including interest systems, sensory sensitivity, affect display, and social interaction. The essays included in this review all addressed perceived communication barriers and additionally met at least one of the following three criteria: (1) the author(s) identified as neurodivergent, (2) the essay explicitly stated support for the neurodiversity movement, (3) the essay prioritized the self-reported experiences and perspectives of interviewed neurodivergent individuals. These essays reveal cultural categories that highlight neurodivergent experiences and behavioral preferences in social contexts. Indeed, this chapter attends to social interaction and avoids problematic diagnoses about what is "happening in the heads of individuals" (Hipólito et al., 2020, p. 206). Cross-neurotype miscommunication often occurs when there exists a paucity of intercultural competence, or competency comprising of "knowledge" that increases understanding, "motivation" to communicate effectively, and "skills" needed to appropriately enact one's knowledge and motivation in specific contexts (Ting-Toomey, 1998, p. 410). For example, the choice to privilege cultural categories that emerge from neurodivergent standpoints reflects an intentional effort to build knowledge apart from the neurotypical perspectives that dominate communication theory and practice (Hillary, 2020; Stenning, 2020; Yergeau, 2010).

This chapter offers these cultural categories as an initial groundwork for disciplinary research and teaching of cross-neurotype communication competence. The move to expand the available vocabulary around cross-neurotype communication is further motivated by studies showing that neurotypical communicators using inclusive language reduce uncertainty for people identifying as neurodivergent (Mann, 2020). To contextualize the forthcoming discussion of categories, this chapter elaborates on the importance of developing a theory and practice of cross-neurotype communication competence. First, it explores the usefulness of these communication practices to navigate intersectional experiences within the movement itself. Second, it outlines the centrality of social stigma to the experience of neurodivergence and argues that "successful social engagement is a joint responsibility" (Hipólito et al., 2020, p. 206). This section includes a discussion of neuro-shared and neuro-separate spaces to demonstrate how cross-neurotype communication can function within neuro-shared spaces, but without replacing other safe and supportive communicative spaces. After discussing the cultural categories, the chapter concludes with additional thoughts for advancing a research agenda on cross-neurotype communication competence.

Cross-Neurotype Communication within the Neurodiversity Movement

Neurodiversity rose as a concept in the late 1990s through a combination of autobiographical academic writing (Singer, 1999), burgeoning online autistic communities through sites like Autism Network International (Sinclair, 2010) and Austics.org (Tisoncik, 2020), and coverage in *The Atlantic* magazine (Blume, 1998). A new reality emerged as participants "began to realize how much autistic people have to offer" themselves and their peers (Sinclair, 2010, para 12). The neurodiversity movement paralleled the early thoughts of the broader disability rights movement (Baggs, 2020). The interconnected factions drew from the social model of disability to define disability as a natural human variance—a part of our biodiversity—and identified society's limited thinking about disability as the primary source of problems for people with disabilities (Shakespeare, 2010). Members of the neurodiversity movement supported this view of difference by evoking rhetoric to distinguish "neurotypical" persons (i.e., the normative, dominant group) from "neurodivergent" persons (i.e., the divergent, minority group) and they produced a cultural framework that gave meaning to individual preferences and experiences apart from medical models that pathologized and problematized neurological differences (Walker, 2012, p. 159).

Present-day, the neurodiversity movement mobilizes around the cultural values of neuro-variation and self-representation, but also recognizes that this understanding of neurodiversity primary reflects the thoughts of white autistic males with average-to-high intelligence and low support needs (Bentley, 2017; Hughes, 2021; Matthews, 2019). The perceived homogeneity of the movement prompts additional questioning about "normalcy both within the [neurodiversity movement] and outside" (Bertilsdotter Rosqvist et al., 2020, p. 7) and beckons the need for cross-neurotype communication competence within the movement itself. For example, the prevailing understanding of neurodiversity often leaves out the intersectional experiences of oppression specifically faced by neurodivergent queer and BIPOC individuals and groups (Brown et al., 2017). Continuing efforts in the movement to include intersectional standpoints and narratives have deepened the movement's understanding of how cultural ableism intertwines with sexism, homophobia, racism, and xenophobia (Brown et al., 2017; Heilker, 2012; Matthews, 2019; Woods et al., 2018).

Individuals and families of neurodivergent people with higher care needs and with health co-conditions that negatively impact their quality of life also critique the neurodiversity movement for undermining the experiences of people with a more fraught relationship with neurodivergence (Hughes, 2021). These critics worry that claims of neuro-variation make it more difficult to secure resources and health care for those who need them (Jaarsma & Welin, 2012). In response, members of the movement have emphasized the value of self-representation and dignified treatment, and they have encouraged the intentional collaboration between health providers, researchers, and neurodivergent people. As a result, these fields are seeing a positive correlation between quality health care and culturally "sensitive" approaches that value traits associated with neurodivergence, incorporate patient perspectives, and utilize strength-based (rather than deficit-focused) therapeutic approaches (Bradshaw et al., 2021; Kapp, 2013, p. 1; Mottron, 2017; Nicolaidis et al., 2015). Additionally, members with lower care needs often avoid rigid non-interventionist perspectives of neurodiversity and increasingly express support for educational services that build language and social skills, remaining opposed primarily to providers that frame such services "in unnecessarily medical or clinical ways" that devalue personal needs and preferences (Bertilsdotter Rosqvist et al., 2020, p. 7).

Social Stigma

The neurodiversity movement calls into question the cultural norms and assumptions that have long contributed to neurodivergent people's experiences of social stigma. At its worst, the stigmatization process involves the removal of neurodivergent people from mainstream society and placement in psychiatric institutions, nursing homes, special education facilities, and prisons where people can be monitored, controlled, and treated (Evans, 2014). Outside of these institutions, which disproportionately affect individuals with higher care needs and fewer spoken communication skills, neurodivergent people can struggle into adulthood to sustain friendships, participate in social events, and maintain healthy romantic relationships (Ellis, 2017; Gelbar et al., 2014; Sarrett, 2018; Sinclair, 2010). Neurodivergent people often find themselves "out of place" (Kitchin, 1998, p. 345) in a world dominated by neurotypical biases that paint neurodivergent people as "terrible at communicating" (Harrington, 2017, p. 33). Furthermore, many individuals are treated as "undesirably different" in social contexts—feared, stereotyped, and excluded (Coleman Brown, 2017, p. 157). Early scientific research blamed cognitive, affective, and sensory differences as the barriers in social relationships in two primary ways: first, by condemning neurodivergent people for not communicating "normally" and, second, by claiming that neurodivergent people do not *want* social relationships. Yet, subsequent research and first-person testimonies reveal the fallacy of these two arguments.

Neurotypical culture often pathologizes the communication preferences of neurodivergent people, claiming that their cognitive deficits cause behavioral problems that require professional intervention to correct (Kapp, 2013). The stigma attached to social perception of neurodivergent behaviors negatively affects neurodivergent people's opportunities for, and gratification from, social encounters (Butler & Gillis, 2011). Confusion in cross-neurotype interpersonal encounters traditionally blames the neurodivergent person for this occurrence, even when evidence demonstrates the limits of both participants. For example, the mutual struggle to empathize between people with different experiences remains a "double empathy problem" that shows the limits of social interactions bound by narrow social norms, rather than located in any one individual (Milton, 2012, p. 884).

A pronounced example of the double-empathy problem occurs when non-speaking individuals are unable to participate in a primarily spoken "communication system" (Rubin et al., 2001, p. 410) and thus the dominant group deems them unintelligent, non-communicative, or even "non-persons" (Baggs, 2007). In this scenario, the dominant group laments someone else's failure to learn a speaking language, but sees their own "failure to learn a [non-speaking] language" as acceptable and "natural" (Baggs, 2007). In a lower stakes' situation, the idea that communication difficulties span both ways applies to the "awkwardness" of some cross-neurotype interactions, which represent a bi-directional limit of both communicators "to adapt to the others timing" in a given social interaction (de Jaegher, 2013, p. 12). Likewise, the "mutual difficulties" in neurotypical and neurodivergent people understanding each other in mixed neurotype communication situations proves the importance of increasing awareness and understanding of these differences and the contexts in which they occur (Kapp, 2013, para 1).

A second assumption is that some neurodivergent people do not want to socialize, a sentiment historically reinforced by scientific studies of autism. Kanner (1943) provided the first scientific definition of autism as a social disorder, claiming that the behaviors he observed among autistic children demonstrated a "powerful desire for aloneness and sameness" (p. 249). His influential essay established a framework for interpreting nonverbal and verbal autistic communication as a sign of social disinterest or a lack of social motivation. This dominant presumption blames an already socially stigmatized population for their minority status, despite first-person testimonies that claim it an inaccurate diagnostic conclusion. While some autistic people do claim to enjoy solitude (Brown, T., 2017), others explain how they adapted to it to escape painful relationships and interactions. Raymaker's (2020) testimony below explains how they adjusted to solitude to cope with the toll of painful interactions that framed their differences as inadequacies.

> Growing up, I had been the stupid one, the confused one, the damaged, scary, aloof, broken, worthless, lazy, crazy, alone, alone, alone, one-of-a-kind, never-trying-hard-enough, busted, always alone one—and I had made peace with that. I had learned to love it, and worn it for a skin. Then, in 1999, with the tsunami-like smack of a co-worker's incorrect assumption that I already knew what I was, I learned I was none of those things. I was Autistic. (2020, p. 133)

Raymaker's personal experiences reflect a broader trend, especially in autistic communities, of members expressing an interest in creating and sustaining relationships (Cresswell et al., 2019; Jaswal & Akhtar, 2018; Jones & Meldal, 2001) and discovering that they enjoy social interaction in welcoming and "safe" places that support their personhood (Bertilsdotter Rosqvist et al., 2015, para 12; see also Bertilsdotter Rosqvist et al., 2020). This narrative also reveals a type of "acculturation" (Braithwaite & Braithwaite, 2011, p. 477) into the autistic community and autistic culture that reframes the characteristics once viewed deficits, now seen as accepted and valued strengths.

Underlying these two arguments—that neurodivergent people do not communicate correctly and/or do not want social interaction—is a third misconception, that neurotypical communication practices are helpful and productive for everyone who uses them. This faulty logic suggests that once someone learns to communicate in the dominant way, they are "cured" of their deficits and will begin reaping the benefits of neurotypical communication.

First-person accounts refute this perspective, claiming that suppressing preferred behaviors, mimicking neurotypical communication, and thus, "passing" in certain social situations, causes a number of negative effects on neurodivergent people including increased anxiety, physical and mental exhaustion, and lowered self-esteem (Ellis, 2017; Fistell, 2016; Valencia, 2017; Milton & Sims, 2016; Strauss, 2017; Yergeau, 2013). The disconnect between how one wants to act versus how one is expected to act can also make one "more acutely aware of their own minority status within a majority neurotypical society" which leads to "feelings of inadequacy and shame" (Crompton et al., 2020, p. 1445; see also, Fistell, 2016). Furthermore, these mimicking behaviors, also referred to as "masking" (Milton & Sims, 2016, p. 528), "camouflaging" (Belmonte, 2020, p. 174), or "acting abled" (Filteau, 2017) prolongs the idea that behaviors deemed problematic can be "fixed" and that the burden of change falls solely on the shoulders of the neurodivergent. In other words, the pressure on one-directional change toward a neurotypical communicative ideal remains harmful even for those capable of making such changes.

Neuro-Separate and Neuro-Shared Spaces

Cross-neurotype communication competence coincides with communicators creating and sustaining *neuro-shared* spaces, meaning "spaces made socially and physically accessible for both NTs [neurotypicals] and [neurodivergent] people" (Bertilsdotter Rosqvist et al., 2013, p. 369). A neuro-shared communicative space enables neurotypical and neurodivergent communicators to interact without privileging the communication preferences of either participant over the other.

Neuro-shared spaces stand in contrast to *neuro-separate* spaces, or spaces dominated by people of a similar neurotype (Bertilsdotter Rosqvist et al., 2013). Neuro-separate spaces dominated by neurotypical communicators are evidenced by the privileging of verbal and nonverbal communication norms associated with traditional public speaking and argumentation, the physical appearance of self-control, and the exchange of culturally bound pleasantries in casual conversation. While some of these norms are explicitly stated and even taught across schools (such as public speaking), others are implicit and more difficult to discern, with neurodivergent people learning them instead through observation, trial and error, and "I guess, osmosis or something," as one autistic person sarcastically put it (Gross, 2020). Neurodivergent people often experience neurotypical spaces as hostile and confusing and feel pressured to conform to neurotypical preferences (Ellis, 2017; Bertilsdotter Rosqvist et al., 2015; Sinclair, 2010). These neuro-separate spaces exacerbate the marginalization and Othering of neurominority groups.

Research documents the importance of accessible neuro-shared spaces for neurodivergent people (Bertilsdotter Rosqvist et al., 2013; Jones & Meldal, 2001; Ryan & Räisänena, 2008). Yet, the neuro-shared spaces that this chapter envisions as constitutive of cross-neurotype communication competence should not devalue the equal importance of available neuro-separate spaces controlled by neurodivergent people. The autistic community, specifically, benefits from the maintenance of autistic spaces that allow members to interact in more comfortable and preferable ways. Autistic people view these neuro-separate spaces as a welcome departure from a society governed by neurotypical communication preferences. Annual overnight retreats for and by autistic people like Autreat and Autscape provide excellent examples of face-to-face spaces in which "autistic people are ordinary, not special" (Leneh Buckle, 2020, p. 109). In these spaces, autistic persons can share experiences, explore an autistic identity, build friendships and community, develop an advocacy narrative, question medical frames and prescribed treatments, and criticize neurotypical norms. Autistic people often feel better understood, accepted, and "at ease" with other autistic peers in these spaces (Crompton et al., 2020, p. 1444).

The notion of physically and socially accessible neuro-shared spaces supports cross-neurotype communication competence, but should not be considered a replacement for all neuro-separate spaces. Reflection on how these spaces function and who benefits from them is key to discerning the value, utility, and ethics of such spaces. For example, some spaces created "for" autistic people in which autistic people make up the majority of its participants, such as special education classrooms and group therapy programs, in reality reflect the neurotypical biases of the neurotypical people who created them (Sinclair, 2010, para 22). In addition to this caveat, one must avoid adhering to formulaic and idealistic notions of neuro-shared communicative space. In practice, neuro-shared spaces are full of contradictions and tensions that participants must manage. People of all neurotypes have different capabilities in different situations and at different times in their lives. Additionally, such spaces should not rely on a self-diagnosed or medically diagnosed neuro-identity that causes one to side with one group over another. While self-identification may happen, cross-neurotype communication competence focuses on the mutual consideration of values and preferences.

Cross-Neurotype Cultural Categories

An approach to cross-neurotype communication competence pulls from principles of intercultural communication to focus on communicative behavior, implicitly understanding that all behavior consists of "goals, motivations, or reasons" (Hillary, 2020, p. 103). The idea that behavior is communication, and shifting attention to what is being communicated, echoes a neurodivergent rallying call to cease diagnostic explanation and instead react competently to the neurodivergent person and the context in which the communicative behavior occurs.

The traits and preferences of neurodivergent people fluctuate greatly and contradict each other regularly, but cultural discourse from the studied texts reveals patterns of thinking about certain communicative behaviors that are useful to this chapter including interest systems, sensory sensitivity, affect display, and social interaction. Under each category, I offer two opposing orientations to show the breadth and depth of behaviors discussed by the essays and emphasize that people's life experiences often fall on various points across each continuum and with different intensities. Importantly, one's behavior and values are not static—they remain fluid and are impacted by multiple factors such as environment, context, relationship, and mood. Dialogue is the best defense against the binarization possible with this type of representation, and I present these categories as a way to jumpstart reflection, conversation, and additional disciplinary development of cross-neurotype communication competence. The categories provide reference points for navigating cross-neurotype interactions and help communicators to make sense of experiences and preferences.

This next section of the chapter provides an expanded discussion of the four cultural categories and the value orientations that give meaning to situational behaviors. In addition to generating further knowledge about cross-neurotype communication, this section points to skills needed to appropriately enact one's knowledge and motivation in specific neuro-shared contexts.

Interest Systems

Neurodiversity literature reveals that the identification of shared interests is gratifying and leads to relational bonding, but also recognizes that people engage in their interests differently (Belmonte, 2020; Bertilsdotter Rosqvist et al., 2015; Cresswell et al., 2019; Murray, 2019). From the studied texts, *interest systems* emerge as the first cultural category of importance in cross-neurotype communication. Interest is not only what draws our attention, but also how one engages with their interests, that is, one's "interest system" for learning, remembering, and making sense of one's interests (Murray, 2019, p. 45). Although originally discussed through a brain-based framework of cognition (Murray et al., 2005), increasingly neurodiversity essays allude to interest systems to describe lived experiences and explain behavioral patterns in social interaction (Jurgens, 2020; Murray, 2019; Stenning, 2020). The theoretical concepts of polytropism and monotropism describe the scope of individual orientations within the broader cultural category of interest systems.

Polytropism "involves having many, but less focused attention patterns" and is often associated with neurotypicality (Jurgens, 2020, p. 75). Individuals engaged in polytropic behavior prefer to spread processing resources across multiple items of interest, expending energy in drawing connections between interests and/or generating new interests rather than putting all of one's energy into one particular interest. An individual who embraces a polytropic approach may show a preference for multitasking and organization, even when surrounded by distractions and interruptions. They can excel at initiating and facilitating interaction, and even find pleasure in shifting seamlessly between topics. Polytropic behavior is best demonstrated in informal social situations characterized by unstructured "small talk" and mingling and in formal situations that emphasize efficiency and productivity. A person who prefers a polytropic approach may find it tedious to focus too long on any one activity/subject and may hold the expectation for themselves and others to generate (or feign) interest in a variety of topics presented.

Monotropism refers to "the tendency for our interests to pull us in more strongly" (Murray, 2019, p. 44). A person engaged in monotropic behavior may find themselves in a hyper-focused "attention tunnel" (p. 45) that feels fluid, comfortable, and stable. Some describe this feeling as a "flow state" (McDonnell & Milton, 2014, p. 38), explaining that "[b]eing in the flow means the body and mind follow their own pace and an emotional drive without being hindered by anything internal or external" (Bertilsdotter Rosqvist et al., 2020, p. 161). This focus and deep engagement produce a more complex understanding of the item or subject at hand and a recognition of patterns that a less focused observer may miss (Kapp, 2013). Monotropic behavior is typically associated with autistic persons (Murray et al., 2005), although components of monotropism like "hyperfocusing" is also associated with schizophrenia and ADHD (Ashinoff & Abu-Akel, 2021, p. 1), and the idea of high-performance flow appears in literature on the ideal neurotypical workplace (Csikszentmihalyi, 2008). A surplus of free time, physical isolation, and the threat of a deadline may spur monotropic behavior, even in those who consider themselves oriented toward polytropism.

Focused attention provides pleasure and stability, but competing demands on one's attention can increase anxiety and frustration. The pulling in of interests creates an accompanying inertia, or "resistance to a change in state: difficulty starting, stopping or changing direction" (Murray, 2019, p. 45). Thus, someone engaged in a monotropic approach to their interests may perceive interruptions negatively or find interruptions "jarring" (Pate, 2017, p. 233) and, consequently, respond with behaviors that help ease anxiety adjust to the environment, or shift focus (Murray, 2019). Stigmatizing attitudes toward some adaptive behaviors associated with neurodivergent people, such as repetitive movement like stimming and flapping, overlooks their benefits to the person using them and their communicative function in social situations (Bascom, 2011; Yergeau, 2018). A person who prefers a monotropic approach may find polytropic small talk and pleasantries "superficial" (Dekker, 2020, p. 45) and may find it difficult to pay attention to, or generate interest in, things outside of their current focus.

Sensory Sensitivity

Needs and preferences around *sensory sensitivity* consistently emerge as a dominant theme in the studied texts and often accompany discussions about environmental accessibility (Bertilsdotter Rosqvist et al., 2020; Leneh Buckle, 2020; Sinclair, 2010). The cultural category of sensory sensitivity draws attention to the ways people experience a range of visual/ tactile/olfactory/auditory stimuli in a given environment. Importantly, degrees of sensitivity vary between people and also within individuals across a variety of sensory modalities, as some people experience a heightened awareness of a single sense (as is the case with people who experience misophonia or synesthesia) rather than across all senses. Conversely, people may feel less sensitive to certain senses across a range of modalities, enhanced by bodily variation, illness, or mood, or outside forces such as drugs and other stimuli.

The sensory sensitivities of neurodivergent people have been heavily politicized and pathologized, despite the universality of sensory experiences. An explanation for this disconnect between theory and experience is a reliance on a dominant, neurotypical language to define the range and experience of "normal" sensory experiences (Jackson-Perry et al., 2020, p. 125). To escape the language of deficit, this chapter highlights two orientations to sensory sensitivity—"sensory-seeking" behaviors and "sensory-defensive" behaviors (Sinclair, 2010, para 15). In identifying the breadth of behavior in relation to sensory sensitivity, we also open up a space to discuss "sensory management strategies" that allow the consideration of personal needs and preferences as well as environmental factors that contribute to sensory experiences (Jackson-Perry et al., 2020, p. 134).

People enact sensory-seeking behavior when looking for additional sensory stimulation to generate pleasure, connect with others, or tap into other sensory experiences (Jackson-Perry et al., 2020). Individuals who engage in sensory-seeking behavior may stand close when talking to others or touch their surroundings, as this engagement allows one to react and interact more fully with ones' surroundings (Baggs, 2007) and may be perceived as enjoyable (Wick, 2017). People can intentionally use sensory-seeking strategies to alter a mood, spark a memory, or increase comfort in an uncomfortable environment.

Sensory-defensive behavior occurs when people experience sensory stimuli intensely and find this experience overwhelming. Individuals who engage in sensory-defensive behavior may avoid touching people and prefer to be in quieter, non-crowded environments. These preferences might occur regularly or intermittently, depending on one's mood, situation, or environment. Someone feeling sensory-defensive may be reluctant to try new foods, expose themselves to strong scents, or wear uncomfortable clothes. Murray (2019) argued that sensory-defensive behavior can be connected to a monotropic hyperfocus, in that one's focused attention may amplify a particular sensory experience to a heightened degree, to a point of feeling overwhelmed by it. An attunement to sensory-defensive behaviors naturally leads to an increased awareness of the environment in which social interactions take place. The facilitation of equitable and enjoyable social interreactions depends on understanding how the environment impacts the sensory experiences of participants (Leneh Buckle, 2020; Sinclair, 2010).

Affect Display

Affect display emerges as a third cultural category of interest to neurodivergent people, in part because of the awareness that affect display matters greatly in a neurotypical world (Fistell, 2016; Hillary, 2020; Seidel, 2020; Yergeau, 2013). Affect display refers to verbal and nonverbal displays of emotion, ranging from facial expressions and eye contact to paralinguistic cues such as vocal tone.

Functionally, it is useful to separate affect display from feelings on the premise that culture primarily governs the performance and interpretation of affect display, although in actuality, feelings remain culturally bound too, even if thought to be experienced "internally."

Gender and racial biases in the dominant culture are well-documented, such as the expectation that women express positive, reassuring emotional cues (Brody & Hall, 2000; Villepoux et al., 2015) and the "forecasting" that the affect displays of people of color communicate anger (Moons, et al., 2017, p. 140). Among neurodivergent people of color, there are dire consequences to the dominant culture's (mis)identification of behavior as aggressive including being labeled "emotionally disturbed" (Asasumasu, 2017, p. 82) or called a "psychopath" for not complying with normative, neurotypical behavior (Brown, L.X.Z., 2017a, p. 141). These assumptions may be accompanied by institutionalization, institutional punishment (Juarez, 2017), and police brutality (Brown, L.X.Z., 2017b; Onaiwu, 2017a). Another example of how the dominant culture categorizes "correct" and "incorrect" forms of affect display is in the claim (and criticism) toward neurodivergent persons of color that, "You don't act [your race]" (Stephan, 2017, p. 156; see also COBRA, 2017; Christian, 2017; Onaiwu, 2017b; Xurd, 2017). The discussion of affect display as a cultural category offers an opportunity to explore complex intersectional experiences around affective preferences, behaviors, and expectations.

Based on the studied texts, this chapter identifies an orientation toward high affect display and an opposing orientation toward low affect display, again caveating that one's orientation to affect display may change and intensify depending on the context of an interaction. High affect display refers to a higher value placed on the production and reception of affective cues. People with this orientation to affect display depend more explicitly on nonverbal cues to communicate with others, assign meaning and motivation to nonverbal cues, and feel uncertain when they don't understand someone else's nonverbal behavior. They may also place more trust in nonverbal communication than in verbal communication, generating meaning from nonverbal cues when incongruencies (i.e., contradictions between verbal and nonverbal messages) occur.

Low affect display refers to a lower value placed on the production and reception of affective cues. People preferring low affect display may see nonverbal communication as not necessarily purposeful or meaningful, such the case with tics (Fistell, 2016; Nasim, 2010). A person who values low affect display may "find tiring the amount of energy needed" to read nonverbal cues (Crompton et al., 2020, p. 1442), find the cues confusing and "idiosyncratic" (Hillary, 2020, p. 97), or refer to the interpretation of affect display as "mindreading" (Hipólito et al., 2020, p. 205). People preferring low affect display may emphasize literal communication—to communicate plainly, concretely and clearly—and struggle to understand figurative, abstract, or sarcastic communication. Correspondingly, a person may prefer to communicate via written communication, which includes less nonverbal communication cues. People who prefer low affect display may use information inductively, generating meaning from social interactions from the "bottom-up," rather than drawing conclusions from a previously established set of ambiguous social rules (Bertilsdotter Rosqvist et al., 2020, p. 157).

Social Interaction

The final cultural category this chapter will discuss as emerging from the studied texts is *social interaction*—or one's preferences for interacting with others. This chapter's earlier discussion of social stigma identified that interest in social interaction varies across neurotypes and that research often misunderstands the social preferences of neurodivergent people. For example, a "shutdown" to sensory overload and/or feeling overwhelmed can be interpreted as social disinterest (Sinclair, 2010, para 15), as can failed attempts to engage a person while they are monotropically focused on an interest (Murray, 2019). Even in these instances, a "stuck" person may want another person to initiate or facilitate social interaction (Sinclair, 2010, para 55) or they may welcome someone interacting around a common point of interest (Murray, 2019; Sinclair, 2010). There is a lot of complexity within this category, but two orientations to social interaction that arise from the studied texts include structured sociality and unstructured sociality.

Unstructured sociality privileges spontaneity and responsiveness, and may coincide with other polytropic behaviors and value placed on high affect display. People who prefer polytropic approaches often have "multiple interests aroused at any time, pulling in multiple strands of information, both external and internal" and can discern a path forward through this highly interactive process with other people and the environment (Murray, 2019, p. 46). People who prefer monotropic approaches may also enjoy unstructured sociality, especially if the interaction occurs around an interest of theirs (Sinclair, 2010). A person demonstrating a preference for unstructured sociality may find the lack of constraint freeing and exciting.

Structured sociality privileges predictability and stability. People who prefer structured sociality may struggle to understand social cues and find it tiring to interpret the "unpredictable behaviors" that unstructured sociality elicits (Crompton et al., 2020, p. 1443). They may dislike abrupt transitions (HarkenSlasher, 2017), prefer advance warning of activities, or want more explicit rules around interaction. A person who values structured interaction may also want additional time to observe activities to better understand what is involved in the activities before joining them. A person may use echolalia, the repetition of words or phrases, or "scripting," to rehearse for a potential interaction, to express themselves, to process thoughts, or to self-regulate in an uncomfortable social situation (Phair, 2017, p. 339; see also Pate, 2017; Sturgeon, 2017). This person may also value low affect display, wishing people "to say what you mean" and not leave one to guess what one wants or needs (Sinclair, 2010, para 62). The literalness of structured social interaction may be disorienting to someone who prefers unstructured interaction and cause confusion about other people's intentions and feelings toward them (Sinclair, 2010). A person's preference for structure may also change with the predictability of the environment and/or the familiarity of people present.

A structured orientation to social interaction is well-represented by the "interaction badge system" started at Autreat and now frequently used in disability inclusive and autistic-friendly spaces (Leneh Buckle, 2020, p. 112). With the interaction badge system, participants wear colored badges (or nametags) to explain and facilitate social interaction. The instructions on the individual badges read,

Red: Please do not approach me. I do not wish to socialize with anyone.
Yellow: Please do not approach unless I have already told you that you may approach me while I am wearing a yellow badge.
Green: I would like to socialize, but I have difficulty initiating. Please feel free to approach me. (p. 112)

The repetition of this badge system across events and the explicit instructions written on the badges assists those who prefer structured sociality to be more comfortable in new and stimulatory environments.

CONCLUSION

An analysis of 68 essays that privilege neurodivergent perspectives shows that people who identify as neurodivergent recognize the significance of four cultural categories in their social lives including interest systems, sensory sensitivity, affect display, and social interactions. This chapter frames these categories in non-medical ways in order to facilitate more narratives, more nuances, and generally more productive and dialogic communication about neurological differences. Additionally, the orientations discussed in conjunction with these cultural categories are not finite or static—they inform, but do not determine, how one views and interacts in the world.

Communication scholarship can offer much to the study of cross-neurotype communication competence. This chapter took a step in that direction, but additional work is needed. There are three primary limitations to this study that future research can address. First, this study focused on written and published narratives and future work could consider how neurodivergent people are sharing their stories/experiences/perspectives via podcasts, social media platforms, and other virtual spaces. Given that the roots of the neurodiversity movement grew from online forums and virtual interactions, subsequent research should consider the richness and relevance of these mediums. Second, this study reflects the autistic bias of the neurodiversity movement, as autistic narratives make up a disproportionate percentage of the studied texts. It is entirely possible that the proposed categories will evolve or new categories will emerge with the robust inclusion of more neurological differences and social experiences. Indeed, I encourage future research to push the number and the complexity of these categories forward, based on additional neurodivergent perspectives. Finally, the intersectional components of cross-neurotype communication competence, including the ways that neurodivergence interconnects and impacts the experiences of queer, BIPOC, disabled, immigrant, and other socio-political categories to which people belong. An ethical and reflective theory of cross-neurotype communication depends on the inclusion of a myriad of experiences.

Cross-neurotype communication competence is required within the movement itself, in order to assist members in navigating people's a range of care needs and intersectional experiences. It is also a necessary ingredient for cross-neurotype collaboration in non-profit organizations, health-care initiatives, and research endeavors that seek to incorporate neurodivergent perspectives into these institutions and spaces. There exists a plethora of long-term benefits of robust and widespread cross-neurotype communication competence, including improved familial and non-familial interpersonal relationships, accessible and environmentally conscious social events, equitable workplaces, and inclusive communities. To reap these benefits, scholars must conduct additional studies of texts that discuss cultural differences, analyze human communication practices that demonstrate cross-neurotype communication competencies, and create opportunities for dialogue in our classrooms in order to prepare subsequent generations for a more equitable society.

REFERENCES

Asasumasu, K. A. (2017). Things about working with "emotionally disturbed" children that will break your heart. In L. X. Z. Brown, E. Ashkenazy, & M. Giwa Onaiwu (Eds.), *All the weight of our dreams: On living racialized autism* (pp. 76–84). DragonBee Press.

Ashinoff, B. K., & Abu-Akel, A. (2021). Hyperfocus: The forgotten frontier of attention. *Psychological Research, 85*(1), 1–19. https://doi.org/10.1007/s00426-019-01245-8

Baggs, A. (2007, January 14). *In my language* [Video]. YouTube. https://www.youtube.com/watch?v=JnylM1hI2jc&list=PL70BB95AC2A07D6B2&index=3&t=0s

Baggs, M. (2020). Losing. In S. K. Kapp (Ed.), *Autistic community and the neurodiversity movement: Stories from the frontline* (pp. 77–86). Palgrave Macmillan. https://doi.org/10.1007/978-981-13-8437-0

Bascom, J. (2011, November 23). On "quiet hands." *Just Stimming.* http://www.thinkingautismguide.com/2011/11/on-quiet-hands.html

Baxter, L. A., & Montgomery, B. M. (1996). *Relating: Dialogues and dialectics.*

Belmonte, M. K. (2020). How individuals and institutions can learn to make room for human cognitive diversity. In H. Bertilsdotter Rosqvist, N. Chown, & A. Stenning (Eds.), *Neurodiversity studies: A new critical paradigm* (pp. 172–190). Routledge.

Bentley, S. (2017). The silencing invisibility cloak. In L. X. Z. Brown, E. Ashkenazy, & M. Giwa Onaiwu (Eds.), *All the weight of our dreams: On living racialized autism* (pp. 299–305). DragonBee Press.

60   E. STONES

Bertilsdotter Rosqvist, H., Brownlow, C., & O'Dell, L. (2013). Mapping the social geographies of autism—Online and off-line narratives of neuro-shared and separate spaces. *Disability & Society, 28*(3), 367–379. https://doi.org/10.1080/0968759 9.2012.714257

Bertilsdotter Rosqvist, H., Brownlow, C., & O'Dell, L. (2015). "What's the point of having friends?": Reformulating notions of the meaning of friends and friendship among autistic people. *Disability Studies Quarterly, 35*(4). https://doi.org/10.18061/dsq.v35i4.3254

Bertilsdotter Rosqvist, H., Chown, N., & Stenning, A. (Eds.). (2020). *Neurodiversity studies: A new critical paradigm.* Routledge.

Bertilsdotter Rosqvist, H., Örulv, L., Hasselblad, S., Hansson, D., Nilsson, K., & Seng, H. (2020). Designing an autistic space for research: Exploring the impact of context, space, and sociality in autistic writing processes. In H. Bertilsdotter Rosqvist, N. Chown, & A. Stenning (Eds.), *Neurodiversity studies: A new critical paradigm* (pp. 156–171). Routledge. https://doi.org/10.4324/9780429322297-15

Blume, H. (1998). Neurodiversity. *The Atlantic.* http://www.theatlantic.com/magazine/archive/1998/09/neuro diversity/305909/

Bradshaw, P., Pickett, C., van Driel, M. L., Brooker, K., & Urbanowicz, A. (2021). 'Autistic' or 'with autism'? Why the way general practitioners view autism matters. *Australian Journal of General Practice, 50*(3), 104–109. https://doi.org/10.31128/ajgp-11-20-5721

Braithwaite, D. O., & Braithwaite, C. A. (2011). "Which is my good leg?": Cultural communication of people with disabilities. In J. Stewart (Ed.), *Bridges not walls* (11th ed., pp. 470–483). McGraw Hill.

Brody, L. R., & Hall, J. A. (2000). Gender, emotion, and expression. In M. Lewis & J. Haviland (Eds.), *Handbook of emotions* (2nd ed., pp. 447–460). Guilford Press.

Brown, L. X. Z. (2017a). Why the term "psychopath" is racist and ableist. In L. X. Z. Brown, E. Ashkenazy, & M. Giwa Onaiwu (Eds.), *All the weight of our dreams: On living racialized autism* (pp. 137–144). DragonBee Press.

Brown, L. X. Z. (2017b). Too dry to cry. In L. X. Z. Brown, E. Ashkenazy, & M. Giwa Onaiwu (Eds.), *All the weight of our dreams: On living racialized autism* (pp. 112–123). DragonBee Press.

Brown, L. X. Z., Ashkenazy, E., & Giwa Onaiwu, M. (Eds.). (2017). *All the weight of our dreams: On living racialized autism.* DragonBee Press.

Brown, T. (2017). The moon poem. In L. X. Z. Brown, E. Ashkenazy, & M. Giwa Onaiwu (Eds.), *All the weight of our dreams: On living racialized autism* (pp. 41–43). DragonBee Press.

Butler, R. C., & Gillis, J. M. (2011). The impact of labels and behaviors on the stigmatization of adults with Asperger's disorder. *Journal of Autism Development Disorder, 41*(6), 741–749. https://doi.org/10.1007/s10803-010-1093-9

Christian, Y. (2017). They said I didn't act like a black. In L. X. Z. Brown, E. Ashkenazy, & M. Giwa Onaiwu (Eds.), *All the weight of our dreams: On living racialized autism* (pp. 195–198). DragonBee Press.

COBRA—Confessions of a black rhapsodic aspie. (2017). You think I don't notice? In L. X. Z. Brown, E. Ashkenazy, & M. Giwa Onaiwu (Eds.), *All the weight of our dreams: On living racialized autism* (pp. 215–216). DragonBee Press.

Coleman Brown, L. M. (2017). Stigma: An enigma demystified. In L. Davis (Ed.), *The disability studies reader* (5th ed., pp. 145–159). Routledge. https://doi.org/10.432 4/9781315680668-18

Craig, R. T. (2016). Metacommunication. In K. B. Jensen, R. T. Craig, J. D. Pooley, & E. W. Rothenbuhler (Eds.), *The international encyclopedia of communication theory and philosophy* (pp. 1–8). John Wiley & Sons. https://doi.org/10.1002/9781118766804.wbiect232

Cresswell, L., Hinch, R., & Cage, E. (2019). The experiences of peer relationships amongst autistic adolescents: A systematic review of the qualitative evidence. *Research in Autism Spectrum Disorders, 61,* 45–60. https://doi.org/10.1016/j.rasd.2019.01.003

Crompton, C. J., Hallett, S., Ropar, D., Flynn, E., & Fletcher-Watson, S. (2020). "I never realized everybody felt as happy as I do when I am around autistic people": A thematic analysis of autistic adults' relationships with autistic and neurotypical friends and family. *Autism: The International Journal of Research & Practice, 24*(6), 1438–1448. https://doi.org/10.1177/1362361320908976

Csikszentmihalyi, M. (2008). *Flow: The psychology of optimal experience.* HarperCollins.

De Jaegher, H. (2013). Embodiment and sense-making in autism. *Frontiers in Integrative Neuroscience, 7,* 1–19. https://doi.org/10.3389/fnint.2013.00015

Dekker, M. (2020). From exclusion to acceptance: Independent living on the autistic spectrum. In S. K. Kapp (Ed.), *Autistic community and the neurodiversity movement: Stories from the frontline* (pp. 41–49). Palgrave Macmillan. https://doi.org/10.1007/978-981-13-8437-0

Ellis, P. E. (2017). Blood, sweat & tears: On assimilation. In L. X. Z. Brown, E. Ashkenazy, & M. Giwa Onaiwu (Eds.), *All the weight of our dreams: On living racialized autism* (pp. 23–29). DragonBee Press.

Emry, R., & Wiseman, R. (1987). An intercultural understanding of nondisabled and disabled persons' communication. *International Journal of Intercultural Relations, 11*(1), 7–27. https://doi.org/10.1016/0147-1767(87)90029-0

Evans, B. (2014). The foundations of autism: The law concerning psychotic, schizophrenic, and autistic children in 1950s and 1960s Britain. *Bulletin of the History of Medicine, 88*(2), 253–285. https://doi.org/10.1353/bhm.2014.0033

Filteau, A. (2017). Acting abled, acting white. In L. X. Z. Brown, E. Ashkenazy, & M. Giwa Onaiwu (Eds.), *All the weight of our dreams: On living racialized autism* (pp. 217–220). DragonBee Press.

Fistell, S. (2016, November 23). My life with Tourette's Syndrome. *New York Times.* https://www.nytimes.com/2016/11/23/opinion/my-life-with-tourettes-syndrome.html

Gelbar, N. W., Smith, I., & Reichow, B. (2014). Systematic review of articles describing experience and supports of individuals with autism enrolled in college and university programs. *Journal of Autism and Developmental Disorders, 44*(10), 2593–2601. https://doi.org/10.1007/s10803-014-2135-5

Gross, Z. (2020, April 23). *Autism acceptance month and promoting neurodiversity in the workplace with ASAN.* [Webinar]. Partners for youth with disabilities. https://learn.pyd.org/webinars/#webinar-recordings-general

HarkenSlasher. (2017). 'Autistic' name calling: How and why it hurts an Autistic. In L. X. Z. Brown, E. Ashkenazy, & M. Giwa Onaiwu (Eds.), *All the weight of our dreams: On living racialized autism* (pp. 45—50). DragonBee Press.

Harrington, E. (2017). Portable shame. In L. X. Z. Brown, E. Ashkenazy, & M. Giwa Onaiwu (Eds.), *All the weight of our dreams: On living racialized autism* (pp. 33–36). DragonBee Press.

Heilker, P. (2012). Autism, rhetoric, and whiteness. *Disability Studies Quarterly, 32*(4). https://doi.org/10.18061/dsq.v32i4.1756

Hillary, A. (2020). Neurodiversity and cross-cultural communication. In H. Bertilsdotter Rosqvist, N. Chown, & A. Stenning (Eds.), *Neurodiversity studies: A new critical paradigm* (pp. 91–107). Routledge. https://doi.org/10.4324/9780429322297-10

Hipólito, I., Hutto, D. D., & Chown, N. (2020). Understanding autistic individuals: Cognitive diversity not theoretical deficit. In H. Bertilsdotter Rosqvist, N. Chown, & A. Stenning (Eds.), *Neurodiversity studies: A new critical paradigm* (pp. 193–209). Routledge. https://doi.org/10.4324/9780429322297-18

Hughes, J. A. (2021). Does the heterogeneity of autism undermine the neurodiversity paradigm? *Bioethics, 35*(1), 47–60. https://doi.org/10.1111/bioe.12780

Jaarsma, P., & Welin, S. (2012). Autism as a natural human variation: Reflections on the claims of the neurodiversity movement. *Health Care Analysis, 20*(1), 20–30. https://doi.org/10.1007/s10728-011-0169-9

Jackson-Perry, D., Bertilsdotter Rosqvist, H., Layton Annable, J., & Kourti, M. (2020). Sensory strangers: Travels in normate sensory worlds. In H. Bertilsdotter Rosqvist, N. Chown, & A. Stenning (Eds.), *Neurodiversity studies: A new critical paradigm* (pp. 125–140). Routledge. https://doi.org/10.4324/9780429322297-12

Jaswal, V. K., & Akhtar, N. (2018). Being vs. appearing socially uninterested: Challenging assumptions about social motivation in autism. *Behavioral and Brain Sciences, 42*, 1–84. https://doi.org/10.1017/S0140525X18001826

Jones, R. S. P., & Meldal, T. O. (2001). Social relationships and Asperger's syndrome. A qualitative analysis of first-hand accounts. *Journal of Intellectual Disabilities, 5*(1), 35–41. https://doi.org/10.1177/146900470100500104

Juarez, J. (2017). Understanding the challenges facing autistic children in higher education. In L. X. Z. Brown, E. Ashkenazy, & M. Giwa Onaiwu (Eds.), *All the weight of our dreams: On living racialized autism* (pp. 54–60). DragonBee Press.

Jurgens, A. (2020). Neurodiversity in a neurotypical world: An enactive framework for investigating autism and social institutions. In H. Bertilsdotter Rosqvist, N. Chown, & A. Stenning (Eds.), *Neurodiversity studies: A new critical paradigm* (pp. 73–88). Routledge. https://doi.org/10.4324/9780429322297-8

Kanner, L. (1943). Autistic disturbances of affective contact. *Nervous Child, 2*(3), 217–250. http://simonsfoundation.s3.amazonaws.com/share/071207-leo-kanner-autistic-affective-contact.pdf

Kapp, S. K. (2013). Empathizing with sensory and movement differences: Moving toward sensitive understanding of autism. *Frontiers in Integrative Neuroscience, 7*(38), 1–6. https://doi.org/10.3389/fnint.2013.00038

Kitchin, R. (1998). 'Out of place,' 'knowing one's place': Space, power and the exclusion of disabled people. *Disability & Society, 13*(3), 343–356. https://doi.org/10.1080/09687599826678

Leneh Buckle, K. (2020). Autscape. In S. K. Kapp (Ed.), *Autistic community and the neurodiversity movement: Stories from the frontline* (pp. 109–122). Palgrave Macmillan. https://doi.org/10.1007/978-981-13-8437-0

Mann, B. W. (2020, November 11). *Theorizing intersectional stigma management communication at the crossroads: LGBTQIA+ and Autistic subjectivities* [Conference presentation]. National Communication Association.

Matthews, M. (2019). Why Sheldon Cooper can't be black: The visual rhetoric of autism and ethnicity. *Journal of Literary & Cultural Disability Studies, 13*(1), 57–74. https://doi.org/10.3828/jlcds.2019.4

McDonnell, A., & Milton, D. (2014). Going with the flow: Reconsidering "repetitive behaviour" through the concept of "flow states". In G. Jones & E. Hurley (Eds.), *Good autism practice: Autism, happiness and wellbeing* (pp. 38–47). BILD. https://doi.org/10.1080/00909882.2010.490841

Milton, D. E. M. (2012). On the ontological status of autism: The 'double empathy problem'. *Disability & Society, 27*(6), 883–887. https://doi.org/10.1080/09687599.2012.710008

Milton, D., & Sims, T. (2016). How is a sense of well-being and belonging constructed in the accounts of autistic adults? *Disability and Society, 31*(4), 520–534. https://doi.org/10.1080/09687599.2016.1186529

Moons, W. G., Chen, J. M., & Mackie, D. M. (2017). Stereotypes: A source of bias in affective and empathic forecasting. *Group Processes & Intergroup Relations, 20*(2), 139–152. https://doi.org/10.1177/1368430215603460

Mottron, L. (2017). Should we change targets and methods of early intervention in autism, in favor of a strengths-based education? *European Child & Adolescent Psychiatry, 26*(7), 815–825. https://doi.org/10.1007/s00787-017-0955-5

Murray, D., Lesser, M., & Lawson, W. (2005). Attention, monotropism and the diagnostic criteria for autism. *Autism, 9*(2), 139–156. https://doi.org/10.1177/1362361305051398

Murray, F. (2019, August). Me and monotropism. *Psychologist,* 44–48. https://thepsychologist.bps.org.uk/volume-32/august-2019/me-and-monotropism-unified-theory-autism

Nasim, R. (2010). Yahav's story: My way of living with Tourette's. *International Journal of Narrative Therapy & Community Work, 4*, 23–42.

Nicolaidis, C., Raymaker, D. M., McDonald, K. E., Baggs, W. A. E. V., Dern, S., Kapp, S. K., Weiner, M., Boisclair, C., & Ashkenazy, E. (2015). "Respect the way I need to communicate with you": Healthcare experiences of adults on the autism spectrum. *Autism, 19,* (7), 824–831. https://doi.org/10.1177/1362361315576221

Onaiwu, M. G. (2017a). Don't let them be Autistic. In L. X. Z. Brown, E. Ashkenazy, & M. Giwa Onaiwu (Eds.), *All the weight of our dreams: On living racialized autism* (pp. 85–87). DragonBee Press.

Onaiwu, M. G. (2017b). Preface: Autistics of color: We exist....we matter. In L. X. Z. Brown, E. Ashkenazy, & M. Giwa Onaiwu (Eds.). *All the weight of our dreams: On living racialized autism* (pp. x–xxii). DragonBee Press.

Pate, E. (2017). The middle, or—The Mestiza and the coffee shop. In L. X. Z. Brown, E. Ashkenazy, & M. Giwa Onaiwu (Eds.), *All the weight of our dreams: On living racialized autism* (pp. 221–240). DragonBee Press.

Phair, D. (2017). Unpacking the diagnostic TARDIS. In L. X. Z. Brown, E. Ashkenazy, & M. Giwa Onaiwu (Eds.), *All the weight of our dreams: On living racialized autism* (pp. 336–344). DragonBee Press.

Raymaker, D. M. (2020). Shifting the system: AASPIRE and the loom of science and activism. In S. K. Kapp (Ed.), *Autistic community and the neurodiversity movement: Stories from the frontline* (pp. 133–144). Palgrave Macmillan. https://doi.org/10.1007/978-981-13-8437-0

Rubin, S., Biklen, D., Kasa-Hendrickson, C., Kluth, P., Cardinal, D. N., & Broderick, A. (2001). Independence, participation, and the meaning of intellectual ability. *Disability & Society, 16*(3), 415–429. https://doi.org/10.1080/09687590120045969

Russell, G. (2020). Critiques of the neurodiversity movement. In S. K. Kapp (Ed.), *Autistic community and the neurodiversity movement: Stories from the frontline* (pp. 287–303). Palgrave Macmillan. https://doi.org/10.1007/978-981-13-8437-0

Ryan, S., & Räisänena, U. (2008). "It's like you are just a spectator in this thing": Experiencing social life the "aspie" way. *Emotion, Space and Society, 1*(2), 135–143. https://doi.org/10.1016/j.emospa.2009.02.001

Sarrett, J. C. (2018). Autism and accommodations in higher education: Insights from the autism community. *Journal of Autism & Developmental Disorders, 48*(3), 679–693. https://doi.org/10.1007/s10803-017-3353-4

Seidel, K. (2020). Neurodiversity.com: A decade of advocacy. In S. K. Kapp (Ed.), *Autistic community and the neurodiversity movement: Stories from the frontline* (pp. 89–107). Palgrave Macmillan. https://doi.org/10.1007/978-981-13-8437-0

Shakespeare, T. (2010). The social model of disability. In L. Davis (Ed.), *The disability studies reader* (3rd ed., pp. 266–273). Routledge. https://doi.org/10.432 4/9780203077887-25

Sinclair, J. (2010). Cultural commentary: Being autistic together. *Disability Studies Quarterly, 30*(1). https://doi.org/10.18061/dsq.v30i1.1075

Singer, J. (1999). "Why can't you be normal for once in your life?" From a "problem with no name" to the emergence of a new category of difference. In M. Corker & S. French (Eds.), *Disability discourse* (pp. 59–67). Open University Press.

Spitzberg, B. H., & Cupach, W. R. (1984). *Interpersonal communication competence.* Sage.

Stenning, A. (2020). Understanding empathy through a study of autistic life writing. In H. Bertilsdotter Rosqvist, N. Chown, & A. Stenning (Eds.), *Neurodiversity studies: A new critical paradigm* (pp. 108–124). Routledge. https://doi.org/10.432 4/9780429322297-11

Stephan, B. (2017). My experience. In L. X. Z. Brown, E. Ashkenazy, & M. Giwa Onaiwu (Eds.), *All the weight of our dreams: On living racialized autism* (pp. 155–159). DragonBee Press.

Strauss, J. (2017). Passing – and passing. In L. X. Z. Brown, E. Ashkenazy, & M. Giwa Onaiwu (Eds.), *All the weight of our dreams: On living racialized autism* (pp. 187–191). DragonBee Press.

Sturgeon, J. (2017). Sometimes I wonder if I'm being masochistic. In L. X. Z. Brown, E. Ashkenazy, & M. Giwa Onaiwu (Eds.), *All the weight of our dreams: On living racialized autism* (pp. 72–75). DragonBee Press.

Ting-Toomey, S. (1993). Communicative resourcefulness: An identity negotiation theory. In R. L. Wiseman & J. Koester (Eds.), *Intercultural communication competence* (pp. 72–111). Sage.

Ting-Toomey, S. (1998). Intercultural conflict competence. In J. N. Martin, T. K. Nakayama, & L. A. Flores (Eds.), *Readings in cultural contexts* (pp. 401–413). Mayfield Publishing.

Tisoncik, L. A. (2020). Austistics.org and finding our voices as an activist movement. In S. K. Kapp (Ed.), *Autistic community and the neurodiversity movement: Stories from the frontline* (pp. 65–76). Palgrave Macmillan. https://doi.org/10.1007/ 978-981-13-8437-0

Valencia, D. (2017). Passing without trying. In L. X. Z. Brown, E. Ashkenazy, & M. Giwa Onaiwu (Eds.), *All the weight of our dreams: On living racialized autism* (pp. 246–253). DragonBee Press.

Villepoux, A., Vermeulen, N., Niedenthal, P., & Mermillod, M. (2015). Evidence of fast and automatic gender bias in affective priming. *Journal of Cognitive Psychology, 27*(3), 301–309. https://doi.org/10.1080/20445911.2014.1000919

Walker, N. (2012). Throw away the master's tools: Liberating ourselves from the pathology paradigm. In J. Bascom (Ed.), *Loud hands: Autistic people, speaking* (pp. 154–162). The Autistic Press.

Wick, K. G. (2017). Love letter to my autism. In L. X. Z. Brown, E. Ashkenazy, & M. Giwa Onaiwu (Eds.), *All the weight of our dreams: On living racialized autism* (pp. 124–127). DragonBee Press.

Wiemann, J. M. (1977). Explication and test of a model of communicative competence. *Human Communication Research, 3*(3), 195–213. https://doi.org/10.1111/j.1468-2958.1977.tb00518.x

Wilson, S. R., & Sabee, C. M. (2003). Explicating communicative competence as a theoretical term. In J. O. Greene & B. R. Burleson (Eds.), Handbook of communication and social interaction skills (pp. 3–50). Lawrence Erlbaum Associates. https://doi.org/10.4324/9781410607133-7

Woods, R., Milton, D., Arnold, L., & Graby, S. (2018). Redefining critical autism studies: A more inclusive interpretation. *Disability & Society, 33*(6), 974–979. https://doi.org/10.1080/09687599.2018.1454380

Xurd, N. S. (2017). Raceabelism. In L. X. Z. Brown, E. Ashkenazy, & M. Giwa Onaiwu (Eds.), All the weight of our dreams: *On living racialized autism* (pp. 148–149). DragonBee Press.

Yergeau, M. (2010). Circle wars: Reshaping the typical Autism essay. *Disability Studies Quarterly, 30*(1). https://doi.org/10.18061/dsq.v30i1.1063

Yergeau, M. (2013, January 7). But I never think of you as disabled! Accessing paternalism, erasure, and other happy feel-good theories. *Autistext.* http://autistext.com/2012/01/07/but-i-never-think-of-you-as-disabled-accessing-paternalism-erasure-and-other-happy-feel-good-theories/

Yergeau, M. R. (2018). *Authoring autism: On rhetoric and neurological queerness.* Duke University Press.

CHAPTER 5

Microaggressions Toward People with Disabilities

Danielle Sparrow, Erin Sahlstein Parcell, Emily R. Gerlikovski, and Dathan N. Simpson

In 1970, Psychiatrist and Harvard Professor Chester Pierce introduced the concept of microaggressions, which he defined as subtle forms of racism that occur daily. He wrote, "Most offensive actions are not gross and crippling. They are subtle and stunning...the cumulative effect to the victim and to the victimizer is of an unimaginable magnitude" (pp. 265–266). Sue (2010) has since broadened the definition of microaggressions to "brief, everyday exchanges that send denigrating messages to certain individuals because of their group membership" (p. xvi). With a dominating focus historically on race, microaggressions research has expanded to include other socially marginalized groups, such as gender and sexuality minorities (Roffee & Waling, 2016; Sue, 2010). People with disabilities (PWD) also experience microaggressions (Keller & Galgay, 2010). As one of our participants shared, "Everyday. Everyday something. There's a look. There's a comment" (Trisha, a woman with Progeria).

Microaggressions come in a variety of forms, ranging from overt assaults to "subtle snubs or dismissive looks, gestures, and tones" (Sue et al., 2007,

D. Sparrow
Clinical Edge, Inc., Milwaukee, WI, USA

E. S. Parcell (✉) • D. N. Simpson
University of Wisconsin-Milwaukee, Milwaukee, WI, USA
e-mail: eparcell@uwm.edu

E. R. Gerlikovski
University of Illinois at Urbana-Champaign, Champaign, IL, USA

© The Author(s), under exclusive license to Springer Nature
Switzerland AG 2023
M. S. Jeffress et al. (eds.), *The Palgrave Handbook of Disability and Communication*, https://doi.org/10.1007/978-3-031-14447-9_5

p. 273). These acts can be intentional; however, they are frequently unintentional and unrecognized (Suárez-Orozco et al., 2015; Sue, 2010; Sue et al., 2007), and for PWD they can have significant negative effects over time (Keller & Galgay, 2010; Lett et al., 2020). Keller and Galgay (2010) identified ten forms of microaggressions against PWD (denial of identity/experience, denial of privacy, helplessness, second-class citizenship, secondary gain, spread effect, patronization/infantilization, de-sexualization, exoticization, and spiritual intervention). Olkin et al. (2019) confirmed their typology and identified two others (disbelief of symptoms by medical professionals and discounting of disability by others). While past research has furthered an understanding of microaggressions against PWD, "there remains a need for more nuanced research" of these experiences (Kattari, 2019, p. 401). In this chapter we share our findings from a qualitative interview study where we sought to expand the research on the experiences of microaggressions for PWD.

METHOD

After receiving our university's Institutional Review Board approval, our first author posted a recruitment message to Facebook groups dedicated to those with disabilities. Participation in this study was open to anyone 18 years of age or older with a congenital or acquired disability, and who was cognitively able to understand the study and their participation in it.

Potential participants contacted our first author to set up their interviews, and she conducted ten semi-structured interviews [nine through Skype or Facetime, and one through Facebook Messenger with a participant who is Deaf (Sam)]. During the interview, she asked questions based on a set of planned topics. Participants answered questions about their experiences with microaggressions (e.g., "Can you recall types of everyday moments where you feel marginalized or othered?", "Is there a specific time you can tell me about?") as well as background information about their disabilities (e.g., type and whether it is congenital or acquired) and demographic information (e.g., age, gender, race). Interviews lasted between 15 to 35 minutes and were transcribed resulting in 112 double-spaced pages for analysis. Participants chose a unique pseudonym that was used throughout memos, transcriptions, and the final report. There was no follow-up communication with the participants after data collection.

To begin the analysis, our first and second authors immersed themselves in the data by reading the transcripts from the first five interviews several times. Next, they initiated an inductive open-coding process that included descriptive and NVivo coding (Saldaña, 2016). They then began a second phase of coding through which they identified themes (i.e., sources, and types of microaggressions). At this point, the first author conducted an additional five interviews to confirm the initial findings and provide additional examples. The entire team then familiarized themselves with these transcripts and engaged in a process of comparing the initial findings with the new data. We decided at this point in the analysis to use Keller and Galgay's (2010) typology as a reference point for the forms of microaggressions identified in our participants' experiences. Once we finalized our findings, we identified exemplars from the data choosing the most evocative examples when more than one existed. Throughout the process we engaged in a set of practices that underwrite the trustworthiness of our findings (e.g., audit trail, multiple researchers, referential adequacy; Lincoln & Guba, 1985).

FINDINGS

Several themes emerged in our analyses. We focused our findings on the sources (kids vs. adults, and inside/outside the Disability community) and forms of microaggressions, which confirmed previous research as well as made unique contributions.

Sources of Microaggression

Kids vs. Adults
One issue discussed by participants was who commits microaggressions. They shared stories of being targets of microaggressions coming from strangers, acquaintances, co-workers, friends, romantic partners, and family; however, one key distinction they made was between the actions of children versus adults. They excused and/or treated as acceptable children's behaviors. Sarae has osteogenesis imperfecta (OI), which is a genetic disorder that affects her bones, making her short in stature and a wheelchair user. Sarae described how she perceives the behaviors of children versus adults:

> You know a lot of people think…that kids are the issue, but in reality I've had some of the best experiences with kids and the worst experiences with adults…adults tend to feel sorry for me a lot more than kids do. Kids I'll often hear [them] ask their parents like, "Why can't she walk?"…But [the kids] don't think of it as like something sad. I think they just have questions because they don't know…and so, I think kids are a lot more curious and they ask "Why?" a lot. "Why can't she do this?" and "Why is she in a wheelchair?"

Sarae also contrasted her experiences with adults who stare versus children who do the same. "Where [kids often ask questions], adults, they don't often say much. They just kind of look. And I've had people look for a very long time, let's just say that." Another participant, Trisha, shared similar experiences. "People stare at me constantly. Kids do it [but] I don't mind…because [their stares] are innocent curiosity." Trisha was born with progeria, also known as Hutchinson-Gilford Syndrome, which is an extremely rare rapid-aging disease that also causes major growth delays. Trisha, who is just over three feet tall, described how kids talk to her versus adults:

Kids ask me, "Can you come out and play" and I am like, "Yeah! One minute!" But yeah to the lady at the grocery store, same checkout lady who has seen me there, God knows how many times, and she cannot help herself but say, "Oh I thought you were a little kid." Every single time I am there.

For our participants, interactions with adults and children differed significantly, and they interpreted children's behaviors as less negative than adults "who should know better."

Microaggressions from Within Disability Communities

While our participants' experiences with microaggressions often involved participants without (at least visible or known) disabilities as the aggressors, participants also shared stories of microaggressions committed by other PWD. For example, Sam, who is deaf, works as a teacher for the hearing impaired. "The crap doesn't just come from the able-bodied," he said. "Deaf people born to Deaf families who grew up using [American Sign Language] and went to deaf schools…and have…generations of Deaf people in their families…look down on the rest of us (hearing families, mainstreamed, etc.) as 'too Hearing.'" Sam lost his hearing slowly over time, so he was not raised using ASL (American Sign Language) but rather had to learn it later in life. He recalled a situation where he signed in front of a large group at work and used English instead of ASL. Another person who was deaf called him out for not using "'pure' ASL…and scathingly asked [him], her every pore oozing contempt, what [he] had just said, and when [he] told her, she corrected [him], in front of over 100 [people]…That kind of shit…This community eats its own alive." Her behaviors displayed for him that microaggressions can come from anyone and are more egregious when they come from within his community. Rose, who is blind, also described instances of within-community microaggressions as a form of projection:

> [Microaggressors] usually have some type of person with disability [in their lives], or a *disability that they are dealing with*…Something that they are not okay with. And that they are working through. It's like an ignorance, either willful or otherwise.

Experiences such as this, where the aggressor is someone from within the disability community, are frustrating for PWD like Sam and Rose because the aggressors' actions reflect an internalized ableism that invalidates their identities and creates tension within their interpersonal interactions.

Types of Microaggressions for PWD

Consistent with previous literature, participant experiences fell into types of microaggressions (i.e., denial of identity, denial of privacy, helpless treatment, spread effect, patronization, exoticization, and social distancing/isolation).

Denial of Identity

This form can be teased out into two subcategories: denial of personal identity and denial (or minimization) of experience. We identified in our data *denials of personal identity* occurs when a PWD is not treated with a person-first approach, and their identity is primarily, if not entirely, based on their disability. These types of microaggressions focus on the disabled part of a person's identity and disregards other aspects and/or their accomplishments, expertise, and knowledge. For example, when Sam told his ASL interpreter, who is not deaf, that he had secured a teaching position at a top school, she replied with, "Oh yeah, I hear [they are] hiring a lot of deaf people these days." Sam felt she minimized his value and abilities with a comment that insinuated he was hired only because of his disability. Likewise, Agatha, who has cerebral palsy, shared that people say to her, "I would have never guessed [you were disabled]!" She said, "...there's like those people who like you can tell who are genuinely surprised but then there are those other people who are just saying it because they want to be nice. [They say things like], 'Oh, I didn't realize!'" Susan, another participant who is blind aptly captured her frustration with these types of microaggressions when she said, "Who am I? I am a mother, a Mexican-American, an artist, and I am blind." Her identity is not located only in her blindness, but she is often treated as such in her daily life.

The second type of denial of identity, *denials of experience,* was also evident in our participants' recollections. Rose, who is legally blind and has ADHD (attention deficit hyperactivity disorder), expressed frustration with her husband, who repeatedly asks her to explain her behavior. She explained:

> He would just say, "Why?" Kind of like in a very assertive, pushy manner...To me the answer is very clear. The reason why was because I forgot or I got distracted by something else or my anxiety about my ADHD-related anxiety was through the roof, so I could finish that other thing today, or that one thing got left off my to-do list or you know?...The answer is that I have ADHD, but that answer isn't good enough for [him or other] people, because they don't understand ADHD.

Situations like Rose's reflect challenges that PWD experience with feeling misunderstood and the ableist assumptions circulating in the culture and in their personal relationships. Charmaz and Rosenfield (2006) noted that when invisible disabilities are made known to others, this disclosure does not always result in understanding the disability. Those not experiencing the invisible disability might make false assumptions about the disability and the experiences that come with it (Charmaz & Rosenfield, 2006). Rose felt her husband did not fully understand ADHD and how it impacted her life. Charmaz and Rosenfield explain that invisible disabilities often elicit disbelief by others.

Another way our participants experienced denial of experience microaggressions, which is not reflected in Keller and Galgay's (2010) typology, is *toxic positivity* (i.e., communicating that PWD should maintain a positive mindset). For example, Olivia shared how a previous mentor, who was also physically disabled, would encourage her to minimize her struggles and not focus on them. When Olivia would share her frustrations with not being able to access different activities due to her inability to walk, her mentor would tell her to, "Look on the bright side." Olivia explained that this kind of talk "very much minimalized the pain and the suffering that are a normal part of the process for coping with a disability." Olivia also described microaggressive comments from others, such as, "God doesn't give you more than you can handle." She shared that people "think of [these comments] as a compliment," but she does not see them as such as they invalidate her feelings about her situation. She also experiences the same microaggressions from nondisabled people who might say things like, "'Everything happens for a reason' [and the like]...as coping mechanisms for their own lives." Olivia says that it is these "coded comments that are meant to be well-meaning[ed] that are actually the most offensive" because they dismiss her perspective and material reality in their attempts to "stay positive."

Denial of Privacy

Denial of privacy microaggressions are experiences where PWD are expected or asked to share "private information about their bodies, their health, their treatment...to gain access or just because they are in public" (Weeks Schroer & Bain, p. 232). In these instances, PWD are treated as if they do not have a right to privacy because they are disabled and so they should disclose information freely. Agatha shared a story of how a high school gym teacher violated her privacy boundaries:

> My teacher, she's like, "Why? Are you okay? Why are you limping?" and I'm like, "I'm fine, I always limp." I was literally just trying to get out the room...and this lady just kind of kept drilling me..."Well I looked in your file and I didn't see anything about a limp or anything" and I am like, "Wait, what? Like, you looked at my file? Like, that doesn't sound like something you can just do," and I just kind of left it at that because I had to leave...I was embarrassed but like I was more like, "Really? So, is that your place to say anything?"

Agatha recognized that, depending on the situation, she will choose to share a level of information about her cerebral palsy (CP) with someone:

> ...People will ask why I limp all the time, and...I'll either say I have CP or depending on the situation I'll just be like, "I've always had it, I am fine, everything is good." And most of the time people just leave it at that. They realize, "Maybe she doesn't really want to talk about it."

But sometimes people become intrusive and expect her to share information with them. She had a different teacher demand in front of other students that Agatha explain why she was walking a certain way:

...the exam was still going on, and she asked fairly loudly..."Why are you limping?" And I was like, "It's fine. I always limp. It's okay," and I just walked out of the room. And the next day she was like "No really, why do you limp?" and I [thought], "Really lady? Are we doing this right now [with other people around]?"

Agatha said that she often tried to manage her privacy boundaries by, "...com[ing] up with excuses" for why she was limping. "I remember using the excuse, 'Oh my foot just fell asleep,' or something like that. And I mean, the teachers weren't dumb, but most of them caught on that it wasn't just that."

Rose reported being asked to disclose her disability on almost a daily basis. She shared one story that involved a fellow bus rider who, without a valid reason, asked her why she was reading her phone so close to her face:

> ...I didn't want to get my glasses out because I was about to get on the bus, and I had my phone about three inches away from my face because I was checking the bus schedule. [They asked], "You smelling your phone?"...People say that stuff to me all the time. Usually what I do, and in this circumstance what I did, instead of getting mad because what's the point, I actually looked at him and took a deep breath, because this isn't my first rodeo and I said, "Well, no, actually. I can't see very well, so I need to put my phone close to my face to see it." ...this person just felt really bad, so they just started asking me questions about my vision and stuff, which I happily answered.

Rose recognized how some PWD manage these denials of privacy by heading them off at the pass:

> I have heard the phrase, "Excuse me but I can't see very well." All the time. If you just ask the flat question, "What does that say?" or "What is that over there?", or even when I am at a restaurant or ordering food from McDonalds or wherever I'll ask, "What does that say?" but I have to qualify it by saying, "I am blind," which is ridiculous. I shouldn't have to qualify it by saying I am blind. Why can't someone just help me if I am asking?

Denial of privacy in these cases reflects ableist assumptions that create the context where PWD are forced to explicitly explain, for example, why they walk a certain way or why they need help, when answers to such questions are unnecessary. Such experiences reflect how PWD are forcibly discourse dependent (Galvin, 2014) in an ableist society (see Calder-Dawe et al., 2020 for a recent study where PWD talked about ableist interactions in their daily lives).

Helpless Treatment

These microaggressions [previously labeled helplessness by Keller and Galgay (2010)] are actions that offer PWD unsolicited help or advice, which treat PWD as if they cannot take care of themselves. Ruth is a 52-year-old woman who acquired fibromyalgia, an invisible disability, approximately ten years ago. Ruth experiences varying degrees of chronic pain that limits the activities she can participate in. In the interview, she described how her loved ones speak to her regarding her fibromyalgia, "I often get attacked from loved ones that I don't know what I'm talking about and that if I would just do these X, Y, and Z things, [the pain] would go away." Ruth shared that she doesn't want to take opiates for her pain because while medication might make activities more bearable, she describes herself as having "a completely different personality" on opiates and how "that confuses [my loved ones] even more."

Rose shared stories of when people ask her questions about her behavior (e.g., why she cannot read something) when it is none of their business and they do not need to know the information. After she tells them she is blind,

> They will [sometimes] say, "Well, wear your glasses." And like [I think], "This has nothing to do with you, and literally is none of your business. Why do you think [you can say that to me]?…You've heard the term mansplaining. Essentially, it's able-explain[ing]. It's ableism."

Trisha also shared that, "People ask me all the time, 'How come you don't have a disability sticker on your car? You could park closer.' [I don't] because, I am not disabled [in a way that I need one]!" Others assume that she has not thought to use a disabled placard (to her advantage). They might offer such unsolicited advice because they think she isn't intellectually capable of thinking of it because she looks like a child to them (i.e., spread effect discussed later).

One type of helpless treatment that previous research has not recognized is *pitying*. Rose said when others try to help her, she cannot help but feel "it's because [she is] being pitied [for being blind], not just because they want to help." Sarae has also reported feeling pitied:

> They see my size and so they have that kind of wakeup call of like, "There's this girl and she deals with a lot probably [because of her osteogenesis imperfecta]." And then it goes back to feeling sorry for me and just being like, "Oh like look at her," and I think that's a huge problem.

They say things to her like, "I want you so bad to be able to walk," which she sees as them taking pity on her. She continued:

> And it's weird because I think people think we go around having our disability as like, in our minds all the time like, "Oh I have OI. I have osteogenesis imperfecta." And I am like, "I just live my life. Yeah, I happen to have OI, but I live my life just like you do. I live it differently, but don't we all live it differently?" So, I think it's just like, it's not on the forefront of my mind all the time. Not that I am trying to forget. Right? I can never forget it, but it just is what it is. I don't think about it as a burden and as something that holds me back. It's just, these are my circumstances, and this is how I go through daily life…and that's how I manage.

Pitying appears a particularly cutting form of helpless treatment given its underlying assumptions that PWD do not like certain aspects of themselves or even their entire existence. These assumptions are borne out of ableist notions of ideal bodies, relationships, and lives.

Spread Effect

Spread effect occurs when individuals relate to PWD as if their disability (e.g., blindness) is connected to other disabilities (e.g., hearing difficulties). These microaggressions are born from incorrect understandings of PWD. Olivia, a 21-year-old female who was born with a visible disability called spastic quadriplegia (a type of CP), described how others treat her as if her disability means she is cognitively disabled:

> I've had a lot of people, sometimes they're not even verbal comments, but sometimes... the old ladies at my church will go up to me and start stroking me on the arm or on the head, like patting me and I find it very condescending, even though I know they mean it to be like an act of endearment, but you wouldn't go up to a person that you only see from church and just start patting them if they were able-bodied.

Rose lamented, "...people assume that if you have ADHD you are dumb, which is the opposite usually." Trisha described how people take advantage of her based on her size, "I think people like that, target people like me. A lot of people do think, 'Oh she is little, so she must not be very smart'... sometimes people treat you like you're just dumb as rocks. I don't know what else to say." Like Trisha, Sarae shared how others think her disability means she is "dumb as rocks," and they treat her as such (e.g., talking to her in a condescending way like she is a child). She is, "always surprised with the amount of people that think that a physical disability and like a cognitive like mental condition goes (sic.) hand in hand." Sarae stated:

> Like obviously they don't expect a 22-year-old to be my size and so they think that my brain must function differently, or I must have a different level of comprehension or awareness. I get all the time...I mean, God bless them, but older people, they will talk to me like, "How old are you"? It's just like nails on a chalkboard and I am like get me out of this social interaction, I don't like this... just because you have a OI like does not mean that my mind is not affected...I'm always surprised with the amount of people that think that a physical disability and like a cognitive, like mental condition goes hand in hand...I think more often than not they don't, and I think people need to be more aware of that for sure...The biggest assumption that people make about me is not even really based on my disability but just the fact that I am cognitively not there.

Charmaz and Rosenfield (2006) explained those without a disability "treat the body as a comparative and normative looking glass, separated from self and situation. Their taken-for-granted comparative images and normative standards result in unitary judgments imposed upon ill and disabled individuals" (p. 39). Sarae explains that people look at her, and seeing a physical disability, make a judgment about her whole existence.

Patronization

According to Keller and Galgay (2010), patronization has two subcategories: false admiration and infantilization. Our participants voiced experiences with the latter. For example, Trisha recalled a time when she went to get her car's oil changed, "This girl talked to me like I was seven years old." She also shared how she, "was at a bar once, and [a man] just picked me up...Picked me up like I was a little kid...People have no awareness. Or like [they say], 'You're so cute!' I am like, 'Ugh.'" Sam also experienced infantilization when his college ASL interpreter treated him like her misbehaving child. He shared, "Okay she one day was saying stuff like I had to pay attention...get my feet down...etc and this was crossing a line, this felt like mothering." Trisha's and Sam's experiences with infantilization reflect ableist assumptions that disabilities equate with lower maturity levels.

Exoticization

For this microaggression type, individuals hypersexualize PWD and/or treat them as objects of their sexual fantasies. Trisha shared these things have happened before and that some people have "no filter" for their thoughts. She relayed a disturbing story of how a man targeted her in a bar and her disbelief over his actions:

> He walked up to me and...I just knew he was going to say something, I just didn't know what it was, but I could just feel it. He was looking at me up and down, and I am like, "Oh god here it comes." He goes, "You know what I want to-do to you?"

Exoticization microaggression like this can be considered the interpersonal parallel of what Garland Thompson (2002) called exotic visual rhetoric that "presents disabled figures as alien, distant, often sensationalized, eroticized, or entertaining in their difference" (p. 65) and circulates in the public sphere. Whether at the proximal (interpersonal) or distal/cultural (rhetoric), PWD experience being objectified.

Social Distancing/Isolation

Like Lee et al. (2019), participants in our study reported experiencing social distancing/isolation as a form of microaggression. They shared stories of these moments of indirect microaggression when peers at school did not involve them in social activities like birthday parties and/or sharing the same lunch table. As adults they also experienced these microaggressions when friends, family, or co-workers did not invite them to do things with them outside their home. Sam shared:

Esp[ecially] if you are disabled, people stigmatize you when you are disabled. Not **because** you are disabled, it's not the fault of the disability, or you, but WHEN you are disabled. they pair up. Automatically. Disablity/weakness. [People] feel contempt for weakness and as a result you are often isolated. you dont usually have a normal social life, esp if you are mainstreamed and the only disabled person in the school.

Other participants shared similar experiences of social distancing/isolation. Susan talked about a time when she was excluded from a group outing to the movies. The interviewer asked her if she thought that they intentionally did not invite her. She replied, "Yeah, I do, or at least they didn't think to invite the blind lady because well, 'She can't see [the movie].'" Susan described how it felt to be left out of the group due to the assumptions others make of her, "It sucks because I want to live a normal life, but I guess you could say that I am often excluded. Sometimes [other moms] invite me but it really depends on what they are doing that day."

Like Susan, Sarae also talked about how microaggressions could be the unintentional *absence* of action and yet still have the same isolating effects as direct verbal assaults. She recalled:

[Kids in school] weren't mean. They never said anything mean…It was like the whole high school went along and then there was me…People are like, "You must have been bullied," and like I'm like, "Not really." No, like they didn't, they didn't say anything or do anything. They weren't being bad people…That's what made it really awkward. It was that nothing nothingness.

Participants also shared how their own (in)actions had isolating effects. Ruth, for example, reported feeling isolated because of her disability and how it affects her motivation and ability to socialize with others. "[My fibromyalgia] definitely affects [my social life]. I cancel things a lot [because I am not up to doing them on the day]." She talked about how her loved ones (i.e., husband, daughter, brother) become angry with her when she cancels plans due to her disability. Charmaz and Rosenfeld (2006) noted that physical disability can lead to PWD feeling invisible and being relegated to a liminal space where their sense of self is diminished.

DISCUSSION

PWD are socially devalued and subtly discriminated against through daily microaggressions (Keller & Galgay, 2010; Sue, 2010), and they live in a world where society often defines them by a medical model of disability viewed through the lens of ability (Siebers, 2008), which leads to acts of microaggressions. In this study, we sought to make contributions to the existing research about the microaggressions by exploring those committed against PWD.

The findings of our qualitative interview study identified sources of microaggressions (kids vs. adults, and those outside and within PWD communities) and reinforced existing typologies for microaggressions (Keller & Galgay, 2010; Lett et al., 2020). Two new forms of microaggressions emerged in our analysis: toxic positivity and pitying. *Toxic positivity* covers microaggressions that focus on reiterating and encouraging adapting a positive attitude towards one's situation ("At least you're alive") and reflects surface-level advice that ignores the unique situations individuals with disabilities experience by assuming "problems" can be minimized by being positive. *Pitying* occurs when microaggressors express patronizing concern for PWD ("Bless your heart. I'm sorry you have to live this way"), which reflects ableist assumptions that PWD are in constant state of wishing they were "normal."

Limitations

We must note study limitations. First, while our participants' stories are rich and reveal several different sources and forms of microaggressions for PWD, these data likely do not exhaust the possibilities. We identified new subcategories of microaggressions (i.e., toxic positivity and pitying) in these data, but scholars should continue adding to the existing typologies (Keller & Galgay, 2010; Olkin et al., 2019). Relatedly, the participants, while representing a relatively diverse set of disabilities, are not particularly diverse in other ways (e.g., race). To address this limitation, researchers should actively recruit PWD with varied demographics.

Implications for Future Studies

Our study indicates that microaggressions for PWD have not been exhausted and research should continue in this area. We have several ideas for future inquiry. First, our participants discussed their theories for why others commit microaggressions, and we urge other researchers to take up this line of inquiry in the future. Our participants cited such reasons as microaggressors' naivety and distorted assumptions/beliefs about disabilities and PWD. If a model of microaggressions for PWD is to be developed, the source(s), and influences on them, are important factors in the process. We also recommend that researchers consider going into depth on different contexts for ableist microaggressions (e.g., the classroom: Tigert & Miller, 2021; cases with service dogs present: Ballard et al., 2023).

Also, although communication researchers have previously studied privacy challenges for PWD (e.g., Braithwaite, 1991), our findings bring into bold relief the varied experiences around denials of privacy as forms of microaggressions. We urge scholars to revisit privacy and disclosure issues potentially bringing theoretical perspectives, such as communication privacy management (Petronio, 2002), to bear on their work. Another theoretical approach that would help expand microaggressions research, and specifically about those committed against PWD, is relational dialectics theory (RDT) (Baxter, 2011). A critical theory, RDT is well positioned to help identify, expose, and potentially change the cultural and personal discourses circulating related to PWD. Framed from RDT, microaggressions against PWD are reflections, in part, of dominant discourses about ability, gender, and race. Given the emerging area of intersectionality within microaggressions (Yep & Lescure, 2019) and disability studies research (Olkin et al., 2019), we encourage researchers to explore this issue. Our participants' experiences reflected the intersection of disability with other aspects of their identities (e.g., gender), and we see much promise for this line of inquiry. We take a disability justice approach, which recognizes how systems of oppression such as ableism, racism, sexism, and homophobia, are intertwined and uphold each other (Piepzna-Samarashina, 2018). By addressing ableism through the study of microaggressions against PWD, we can also make contributions toward the work seeking to dismantle systems of oppression.

Conclusion

Our study's findings add to the existing literature of disabilities studies and microaggressions. The ten PWD we interviewed shared their experiences interacting with individuals who communicated in ways that denied their identities and privacy, treated them as helpless, incorrectly connected their disabilities with other forms, patronized and exoticized them, and socially distanced or isolated them. We encourage researchers to continue studying ableist microaggressions to expand our understanding and increase awareness around how PWD are marginalized in everyday talk and from what sources (e.g., children as well as adults; people within and outside disability communities). We hope future research incorporates theoretical perspectives such as communication privacy management, relational dialectics theory, and/or intersectionality theory to help make sense of the microaggressive experiences of PWD in ways that might offer transformative possibilities.

References

Ballard, R. L., Ballard, S. J., & Chue, L. E. (2023). Invisible marginalizations of service-dog handlers: The tensions of legal inclusion and social exclusion. In M. S. Jeffress, J. M. Cypher, J. Ferris, & J.-A. Scott (Eds.), *The Palgrave handbook of disability and communication*. Palgrave.

Baxter, L. A. (2011). *Voicing relationships: A dialogic approach*. Sage.

Braithwaite, D. O. (1991). "Just how much did that wheelchair cost?" Management of privacy boundaries by persons with disabilities. *Western Journal of. Speech Communication, 55*(3), 245–274. https://doi.org/10.1080/10570319109374384

Calder-Dawe, O., Witten, K., & Carroll, P. (2020). Being the body in question: Young people's accounts of everyday ableism, visibility, and disability. *Disability & Society, 35*(1), 132–155. https://doi.org/10.1080/09687599.2019.1621742

Charmaz, K., & Rosenfeld, D. (2006). Reflections of the body, images of the self: Visibility and invisibility in chronic illness and disability. In P. Vannini & D. Waskul (Eds.), *Body/embodiment: Symbolic interaction and the sociology of the body* (pp. 35–49). Taylor & Francis.

Galvin, K. M. (2014). Blood, law, and discourse: Constructing and managing family identity. In L. A. Baxter (Ed.), *Remaking 'family' communicatively* (pp. 17–32). Peter Lang.

Garland-Thomson, R. (2002). The politics of staring: Visual representations of disabled people in popular culture. In S. L. Snyder, B. J. Brueggemann, & R. Garland-Thomson (Eds.), *Disability studies: Enabling the humanities* (pp. 56–75). Modern Language Association.

Kattari, S. K. (2019). The development and validation of the Ableist Microaggression Scale. *Journal of Social Service Research, 45*(3), 400–417. https://doi.org/10.108 0/01488376.2018.1480565

Keller, R. M., & Galgay, C. E. (2010). Microaggressive experiences of people with disabilities. In D. W. Sue (Ed.), *Microaggressions and marginality: Manifestation, dynamics, and impact* (pp. 241–267). Wiley.

Lee, E.-J., Ditchman, N., Thomas, J., & Tsen, J. (2019). Microaggressions experienced by people with multiple sclerosis in the workplace: An exploratory study using Sue's taxonomy. *Rehabilitation Psychology, 64*(2), 179–193. https://doi.org/10.1037/ rep0000269

Lett, K., Tamaian, A., & Klest, B. (2020). Impact of ableist microaggressions on university students with self-identified disabilities. *Disability & Society, 35*(9), 1441–1456. https://doi.org/10.1080/09687599.2019.1680344

Lincoln, Y. S., & Guba, E. G. (1985). *Naturalistic inquiry.* Sage.

Olkin, R., H'Sien, H., Schaff Abbene, M., & VanHeel, G. (2019). The experiences of microaggressions against women with visible and invisible disabilities. *Journal of Social Issues, 75*(3), 757–785. https://doi.org/10.1111/josi.12342

Petronio, S. S. (2002). *Boundaries of privacy: Dialectics of disclosure.* State University of New York Press.

Piepzna-Samarasinha, L. L. (2018). *Care work: Dreaming disability justice.* Arsenal Pulp Press.

Roffee, J., & Wailing, A. (2016). Rethinking microaggressions and anti-social behavior against LGBTIQ+ youth. *Safer Communities, 15*(4), 190–201. https://doi. org/10.1108/SC-02-2016-0004

Saldaña, J. (2016). *The coding manual for qualitative research* (3rd ed.). Sage.

Siebers, T. (2008). *Disability theory.* University of Michigan Press.

Suárez-Orozco, C., Casanova, S., Martin, M., Katsiaficas, D., Cuellar, V., Smith, N. A., & Dias, S. I. (2015). Toxic rain in class: Classroom interpersonal microaggressions. *Educational Researcher, 44*(3), 151–160. https://doi.org/10.310 2/0013189X15580314

Sue, D. W. (2010). *Microaggressions and marginality: Manifestation, dynamics, and impact.* Wiley and Sons.

Sue, D. W., Capodilupo, C. M., Torino, G. C., Bucceri, J. M., Holder, A. M. B., Nadal, K. L., & Esquilin, M. (2007). Racial microaggressions in everyday life: Implications for clinical practice. *American Psychologist, 62*(4), 271–286. https://doi.org/1 0.1037/0003-066X.62.4.271

Tigert, M. K., & Miller, J. H. (2021). Ableism in the classroom: Teaching accessibility and ethos by analyzing rubrics. *Communication Teacher.* https://doi.org/10.108 0/17404622.2021.2006254

Yep, G. A., & Lescure, R. (2019). A thick intersectional approach to microaggressions. *Southern Communication Journal, 84*(2), 113–126. https://doi.org/10.108 0/1041794X.2018.1511749

CHAPTER 6

"When We Say That It's Private, a Lot of People Assume It Just Doesn't Exist": Communication, Disability, and Sexuality

Ameera Ali

DISABILITY AND SEXUALITY

When considering the terms disability and sexuality, what comes to mind? You may think of these as distinct terms, or perhaps you may think of them as overlapping. Whichever way you initially perceive these terms will largely be influenced on how you conceive of each of them more intricately. The ways in which we communicate and understand these terms are located in complex interpretive relations as language and discourse are value-laden and reflect the broader socio-cultural world. Indeed, language and discourse may appear to be value-neutral; however, they fundamentally reflect beliefs embedded within various socio-cultural contexts. In Western contexts, the fusion of the terms disability and sexuality is often met with much resistance and stigma within broader social, popular, and cultural communication. This chapter considers the particular meanings evoked when these terms are communicated together.

Defining Disability

To begin, let us briefly define and operationalize these terms to gain an understanding of the intricacies and undertones encapsulated within them. The term disability has never been defined in one, single, universal manner as it is a complex term which carries multiple meanings (Gill, 2015). How one defines and

A. Ali (✉)
York University, Toronto, ON, Canada

© The Author(s), under exclusive license to Springer Nature
Switzerland AG 2023
M. S. Jeffress et al. (eds.), *The Palgrave Handbook of Disability and Communication*, https://doi.org/10.1007/978-3-031-14447-9_6

conceives of disability will vary based on their understanding of the term, their personal relationship to it, and disability discourses or schools of thought with which they align themselves. As such, due to the varying ways it is understood, there is no clear consensus as to how disability can or should be defined. Traditionally and contemporarily, "dominant definitions of disability have served to exclude and 'other' persons who are characterized as deviating from socially constructed norms" (Davidson & La Monica, 2011, p. 403). Indeed, disability is often constructed as a "difference" namely to be understood as juxtaposed against a contrasting state of normalcy (Davidson & La Monica, 2011; DeWelles, 2019; Grue, 2015; Titchkosky & Michalko, 2009).

These understandings are often in-line with the individual [or medical] model of disability which medicalizes and conceives of disability as a problem which resides within an individual and is in need of being fixed or cured (Oliver, 1983, 1996). This chapter transcends such conceptions of disability and, rather, defines it in accordance with the field of critical disability studies wherein disability is neither isolated from an individual nor from the broader socio-cultural world, and does not exist in relation to a standard form of "normality" (Titchkosky & Michalko, 2009). This understanding of disability is also in alignment with the social model of disability which emphasizes the social, systemic, and attitudinal barriers that disable individuals (Oliver, 1983, 1996). Indeed, this chapter acknowledges disability as relational and constituted within social communication, social institutions, and social relations.

Defining Sexuality

Similar to disability, the term sexuality evokes many different understandings based on academic conceptions, personal experiences, and social discourse. There are varied disciplinary conceptualizations of sexuality, some of which include: medicalized conceptions in science and psychiatry, developmental understandings pertaining to psychology and human development studies, and socio-historical understandings in the humanities and social sciences (see Parker, 2009). Social and cultural understandings of sexuality also vary with some contexts positioning sexuality as varied, fluid, and non-binary, with others understanding sexuality as embedded within specific rules, limits, and contingencies. This chapter defines sexuality as one's experience of sexual identity, desire, and expression "within the context of the personal identity of the individual," and that which is "heavily influenced by past cultural learning, one's self-image, and the expectations that others have of the person" (Trieschmann, 1988, p. 159). Sexuality is often conceived of as solely intrinsic and isolated from external factors; this definition, however, eloquently underscores how various idiosyncratic facets such as identity, self-image, and the conceptions of others are involved in constituting one's sexual subjectivity. Importantly, these elements may further influence one's sense of sexual expression, agency, and "worth."

The Salience of Communication

Returning to the points made at the outset of this writing, what can be observed through these operationalized definitions of disability and sexuality, is that each of these terms is not only contingent upon individual factors but also embedded within social and cultural dynamics. Thus, rather than conceiving of disability and sexuality as individualized experiences, these definitions also position them as socio-culturally constituted. It is through these definitions that we can gain an understanding of the ways that meanings associated with both disability and sexuality influence the ways they are communicated not only individually, but, more importantly, when they are fused together. Surely, then, communication surrounding disability and sexuality influences the ways they materialize in the lived subjectivities of disabled people. When considering this from a subjective perspective, it is critical to have a direct account of this experience.

This chapter will entail a case study of Shane Burcaw—a disabled author and YouTube personality who is well-known for actively speaking of the infantilization, dysfunction, and "difference" that are incessantly attributed toward him regarding his sexuality as a disabled person, conceptions that he himself also occasionally internalizes. I will discursively analyze how disability is communicated in the context of sexuality both through Burcaw's lived experiences and through his socio-cultural context. The discourse analysis I embark on troubles notions of "normalcy" and "difference" and aims to explore the ways in which dominant discourses of sexuality and disability can fundamentally shape understandings of these terms. In particular, a Foucauldian lens will be utilized wherein an emphasis on the power of discourse in constructing notions of sexual propriety (Foucault, 1978) will be underscored. As Hall (2004) asserts in reference to Foucault, we come to understand ourselves and others through historically contextual categorizations of "truth," propriety, and normality. As such, this chapter observes discourse analysis' fundamental objective to deconstruct notions of power and ideology while exposing how discourses serve to naturalize and pathologize particular conventions, wherein they fortify normality and difference, and privilege and oppression (Wodak, 2001). In other words, I uncover the ways in which discourses can reinforce dominant understandings of normalcy, which subsequently also reinforces notions of difference. Through this, the chapter will fundamentally draw forth the desexualization of disabled individuals and the ways this is profoundly grounded in both compulsory sexuality and compulsory nondisabledness. I then discuss how desexualization attempts to forcibly naturalize asexuality for disabled people and I elucidate the ways discursive communications of disability and sexuality fundamentally serve to reify the stigmatization of disabled individuals as sexual beings.

Disability and Sexuality: The Experiences of Shane Burcaw

Introducing Burcaw

Author and YouTube personality Shane Burcaw is well-known for publicly speaking about disability and sexuality through his own subjective experiences as well as in relation to broader understandings of this topic. Burcaw's experience with Spinal Muscular Atrophy (SMA) throughout his life has caused a substantial weakening of his muscles over time, meaning that he requires assistance with many daily tasks. His nondisabled long-term partner—Hannah Aylward—happily supports him with his day-to-day activities. Burcaw and Aylward's relationship has incited much curiosity from viewers of their YouTube channel, readers of Burcaw's books, and unsurprisingly, strangers in public.

On the couple's YouTube Channel, *Squirmy and Grubs*, as well as in two of his published books: *Laughing at My Nightmare* (Burcaw, 2014) and *Strangers Assume My Girlfriend is My Nurse* (Burcaw, 2019), Burcaw discusses his experience with SMA along with the stigma and discrimination he faces from others due to being in an intimate relationship with Aylward. For example, the very caption of the banner for their YouTube channel reads: "once upon a time, a boy with no muscles fell madly in love with a beautiful girl who had plenty of muscle to spare. The townsfolk gasped with horror at the sight of their disgusting interabled[1] relationship, but they didn't care." The "gasping" referenced here reflects the confounded, astonished, and even horrified responses others have expressed regarding their relationship. On their channel, Burcaw and Aylward regularly share anecdotes regarding these types of responses to their relationship, which often entail disability appearing as tragedy, misfortune, loss, and, contrastingly, inspiration.

Disability and Sexuality: The Public Gaze

Given that YouTube is fundamentally a space of participatory culture (Burgess & Green, 2009), Burcaw and Aylward not only share their experiences, but also engage with commentary and inquiries from their viewers. The couple mentions that upon others learning of their relationship, the most common inquiries they receive overwhelmingly pertain to Burcaw's sexuality. Burcaw states that "many of the questions show that there is a lot of misinformation [and] a lot of stigma about disability and intimacy" (Squirmy and Grubs, 2020b). When discussing this more explicitly in his book, Burcaw states that society "has a disturbing infatuation" with his sexual life and goes on to mention the questions most frequently asked involve "the functions of [his] reproductive system" (Burcaw, 2019, p. 141). Burcaw emphasizes that the confusion over whether his genitals "work" is something that has perplexed him for some time. This fixation on the functionality of his body is unsurprising; however, as when disability and sexuality are discussed together, disability often appears in terms of incapacity, inefficiency, and dysfunction (Orange, 2009). Burcaw and Aylward regularly take to their YouTube channel to respond to such inquiries from viewers. Their disability-and-sexuality-themed videos tend to be the most popular on their channel, and, as Aylward notes, "these videos [...] have a ton of views and that's amazing because there's not a lot of resources to find information about disability and sexual health" (Squirmy and Grubs, 2020d). In discussing their choice to discuss the intimate details of their relationship, Aylward states: "unfortunately when we say that it's private, a lot of people assume it just doesn't exist. And that's a really damaging stereotype for all disabled people when you assume that disabled people aren't sexually active" (Squirmy and Grubs, 2020b). As such, Burcaw and Aylward utilize their platform to counter disability myths and stigmas, and to raise awareness surrounding disability and sexuality—both from their personal experiences as well as more broadly.

Disability and Sexuality: Discursive Paradoxes

In one of their videos discussing the topic, Burcaw mentions the way how disability appears as lack, loss, and dysfunction wherein he notes that "people assume that people with disabilities don't have a libido. I do" (Squirmy and Grubs, 2020a). This misconception is one that is unfortunately profoundly common as sexuality is very seldom assumed to be a "natural" occurrence for disabled individuals (Richards et al., 2006). Disabled people regularly disappear from normative conceptualizations of sexuality and are frequently positioned as infantilized, asexual, sexually undesirable, and incapable of possessing sexual agency (Payne et al., 2016; Philaretou & Allen, 2001; Shah et al., 2015). Indeed, notions of sexuality in the context of disability are fundamentally stigmatized and conceived of as taboo (Benedet & Grant, 2007; Whittington-Walks, 2018; Yoshizaki-Gibbons & O'Leary, 2018). In the rare instances where disabled people are recognized to be sexual beings, this is too often met with a paradoxical discourse of them as *hyper*sexual, which also stems from the infantilization of disabled people and is equally as harmful. Indeed, although beyond the scope of this chapter, it is important to note that despite discourses of disabled people "lacking" sexuality, there is curiously a concurrent antithetical postulation of disabled individuals as hypersexual (see Brodwin & Frederick, 2010; Perlin & Lynch, 2016; Yoshizaki-Gibbons & O'Leary, 2018). Still, the prevailing discourse within the fusion of disability and sexuality, is that of the disabled person as an asexual being.

In response to Burcaw's comment above, Aylward attests: "there's a spectrum, and people with disabilities fall—separately from their disability—on wherever they are on the spectrum" (Squirmy and Grubs, 2020a). Here, Aylward generates what Foucault (1978) refers to as "reverse" discourse. Reverse discourse seeks to deconstruct and counter dominant discourses and "enable the production of new, resistant discourses" (Weedon, 1987, p. 110). Indeed, Aylward transcends dominant discourses of libido as contingent upon one's identity as disabled or nondisabled, and rather, positions virility as part of a broad spectrum of sexuality. Aylward's emphasis on the spectrum of sexuality de-centers disability as the focus, and instead allows disability to appear as peripheral to Burcaw's sexuality. Moreover, Aylward eschews "normalizing" discourses which position disability as "akin to" nondisability in the context of sexuality (i.e., "we're the same"). Rather, she suggests that both sexuality and disability are diverse and that one cannot be reduced to the other.

Aylward's usage of reverse discourse is salient to consider as she uses the couple's platform to dispel harmful dominant misconceptions of disability and sexuality in an attempt to overthrow them. As Weedon (1987) notes, "resistance to the dominant at the level of the individual subject is the first stage in the production of alternative forms of knowledge or where such alternatives already exist" (p. 111). Thus, Burcaw and Aylward's critical accounts are especially salient in countering taken-for-granted discourses and communication surrounding disability and sexuality given their subjective nature. Indeed, YouTube provides Burcaw with a platform to disrupt misconceptions of disability and sexuality that are pervasive in the general public, culture, and media through critically sharing his positionality. YouTube, being a user-generated space for both popular culture and self-representation, allows creators to engage in self-expression and communication without the mediation and gate-keeping that is part-and-parcel of more traditional forms of media (Saul, 2010). As such, Burcaw and Aylward have much more choice and fluidity which allow for increased agentic and authentic communication. Through their channel, viewers are able to gain exposure to representations otherwise omitted from Western popular culture, while taken-for-granted discourses are reconstituted in meaningful ways (Saul, 2010). Importantly, YouTube provides an avenue through which others can gain awareness of disparaging socio-cultural constructs [of disability and sexuality] and how these can be both resisted and reified by those whom these constructs target (Saul, 2010).

Disability and Sexuality: Navigating and Internalizing Discourse

Although the couple attempts to disrupt dominant discourses and de-center disability from Burcaw's sexual subjectivity, the primacy that others place on his disabled identity in relation to his sexuality has nonetheless influenced the ways he publicly navigates his intimate relationship with Aylward, and perhaps accounts for some of the popularity of the couple's YouTube channel. The unsolicited attention the couple receive can often resemble that of constant surveillance which can precipitate apprehension when in public. In speaking of his initial discomfort of even holding hands with Aylward in public, Burcaw attests "I was like self-conscious about any kind of attention-drawing behaviour […] not that holding hands is that, but I took it too far" (Squirmy and Grubs, 2020a). Thus, the responses of others have a direct influence on his approach to public intimate behavior. Vaz and Bruno (2003) discuss experiences of surveillance in stating that instances of perceived surveillance are correlated with experience of *self-surveillance*, which refers to the attention to and alteration of one's behavior in the actual or perceived observation of them by others. Further, self-surveillance involves identifying "threats" and establishing practices for restraining them (Vaz & Bruno, 2003); which has been demonstrated through Burcaw's resistance to public displays of affection due to the threat of unwarranted attention and discomfort.

In the following passage, Burcaw expresses how strangers' responses to his sexual agency have also influenced the ways in which he perceives his own sexual subjectivity:

> Everyone seemed so impressed that "someone like me" could and did engage in sexual activity. I felt special, like a rare breed of the disabled population who had overcome the social stigmas surrounding disability to such an exceptional degree that I was worthy of sex. (Burcaw, 2019, p. 141)

Here, Burcaw explicitly mentions social stigmas of disability as constituting his sense of sexual worth as a disabled person. The term stigma is described as an attribute or state of being that is conceived of as "different," inferior, or abnormal (Goffman, 1963). Stigmas are communicated and dictated by constructed socio-cultural norms which influence understandings of one's merit and worth. To "successfully" embody and exemplify these socio-cultural norms signifies worth and value, whereas to "fail" at assuming them signifies deviance and futility (Goffman, 1963). In Burcaw's passage above, it is evident that "successfully" fulfilling the Western cultural norm of having an active sexual life is noted as successfully overcoming the [sexual] stigmas and "difference" of being a disabled person.

This sentiment of being "worthy" of sex that Burcaw mentions is reflective of compulsory sexuality—the notion that social life functions around the presumption that sexuality is desirable, "natural," and "healthy" (Emens, 2014; Przybylo, 2016). By proclaiming his sexual subjectivity, Burcaw is able to evade the assumptions of him as asexual and position himself as a sexual subject, allowing disability to appear as aptitude rather than lack. Yet, although Burcaw has acquired a sense of sexual "normalcy," it is important to acknowledge that conditions for normative social life also demand particular normative expectations that all participants must efficiently uphold (Goffman, 1963). In other words, to be sexually active is one aspect of acquiring a sense of "normalcy" through evading sexual stigmas and stereotypes of asexuality, yet there are additional expectations within this sense of "normalcy".

Indeed, compulsory sexuality does not solely dictate that *anyone* may attain sexual agency as it works to legitimize *specific* bodies and relationships (Emens, 2014; Przybylo, 2016). More specifically, compulsory sexuality is deeply tied to the notion of what Robert McRuer terms "compulsory able-bodiedness"— the conception of "able-bodiedness" as being normative and desirable (McRuer, 2006). I adapt McRuer's term to that of compulsory *nondisabledness* to underscore the social model of disability, as the term "able-bodiedness" can imply a universal state of bodily "normalcy," creating an "us" versus "them" discourse inferring that disabled people are corporeally deficient and subsidiary to nondisabled individuals. Interestingly, in one of his books where he discusses his very first intimate relationship with a woman, Burcaw makes reference to the "able-body" in a passage where he states:

> After eighteen years of believing I would never find someone who didn't care about my disease, my tiny arms, my weak muscles, my wheelchair, my dependency on others, my inevitable decline, my death, and now here lay Jill, caressing me and kissing me and acting like I was the sexiest, most able-bodied boy she had ever met. (Burcaw, 2014, pp. 186-187)

Here, Burcaw uses the notion of the "able-bodied" (i.e., the nondisabled) as standard and desirable, wherein disability appears as subsidiary. Intriguingly, despite the fact that he mentions Jill's acceptance of his disabled body, he nonetheless juxtaposes himself against that of the "sexy able-body." In other words, rather than stating that Jill made him feel desirable in his own skin, his understanding of her affinity toward him is through a normative nondisabled prototype. Indeed, the term "able-body" is often used in a polarizing manner to create a rift between the disabled body and its mythical "able-bodied" Other (Inahara, 2009). Through this polarization, disability is defined in opposition to a privileged "able-bodied" norm wherein the [physically] disabled body is constructed as inferior, lack, and/or excess (Inahara, 2009).

Through this dichotomy, nondisabled people are universally defined by only one, single, fixed, "able" body whereby disability and disabled bodies are consequently conceptualized in opposition to this (Inahara, 2009). Moreover, the "able-body" is constituted by wholeness whereas disabled bodies are transient and fluid, thereby disrupting the construction of the able-bodied whole (Brodwin & Frederick, 2010; Inahara, 2009). Disability, then, is understood in relation to nondisabledness, and, as such, disability becomes denigrated through the accentuation of nondisability. Perceived deviations of disabled bodies from the "able-body" are often read as failing to meet the standard of a "normal" and desirable nondisabled body which can precipitate sentiments of being sexually inferior (Liddiard, 2014). Indeed, when disabled bodies are perceived as lacking and inferior, they are constructed as less "worthy" and less "capable" of sexual engagement. This sentiment is taken up further by Burcaw in an alternative passage where he discusses his sexual subjectivity:

> Early on it tortured me that I couldn't be a "better" sexual partner. My head was filled with damaging ideas about the importance of a man being able to perform in bed, and at times in my life, I was convinced that no woman [...] would ever want to be intimate with me. (Burcaw, 2019, p. 146)

Disability and Sexuality: Transgressing Discursive Confines

As is evident through Burcaw's quote, discourses of a nondisabled standard, not only influence nondisabled people's conceptions of him but also his own.

What is also interesting from Burcaw's quote is that his conception of "better" sexual efficiency is engrained in both compulsory nondisabledness as well as discourses of masculinity and virility. Burcaw mentions the "importance of a *man* being able to perform in bed" which reflects how his subjective experience with disability also influences his identity as a man. This is unsurprising as in Western contexts, sexuality has often been seen as a form of power, agency, and liberation, particularly for [nondisabled] males (Philaretou & Allen, 2001)—traits that are in direct contrast to the ways that disability is dominantly characterized. Indeed, disabled men are often regarded as "half men" with subordinate masculinity, virility, and sexual proficiency (Philaretou & Allen, 2001). Fortunately, Shane has since disassociated himself from such discourses as he states:

> Once I abandoned the idea that sex needs to conform to society's narrow and ignorant guidelines—man dazzles woman by how hard and strong and fast he can gyrate his hips into hers—my sex life became much healthier and enjoyable. (Burcaw, 2019, p. 146)

For Burcaw and Aylward, who have stated that their sexual encounters are less conventional than what society generally deems acceptable, gendered benchmarks are quite exclusionary and have little relevance to their sexual endeavors. To be clear, the couple has stated that Burcaw requires significant assistance with maneuvering his body which entails Aylward having to do much of the physical work during acts of intimacy. As such, Burcaw's involvement in intimacy may be perceived as more of a passive role, even though he is equally as active in the endeavor. Since facilitated sex is particularly taboo in Western societies, this invalidates the ways that Shane as well as many other disabled people achieve sexual agency (Perlin & Lynch, 2016). As such, the allegiance to rigid notions of womanhood and manhood becomes challenged by disability and may subsequently prompt constructions of disabled individuals as less than "whole" (Brodwin & Frederick, 2010), which is also connected to the notion of the "lacking" disabled body in contrast to the "whole" able-body as underscored earlier.

Burcaw and Aylward have avidly discussed this on their YouTube channel where Aylward has expressed to Burcaw: "I really don't feel like the dominant one in the relationship. I think you have a very outgoing personality, and you communicate a lot verbally [...] you'll be like [...] 'give me your forehead' and you'll give me a kiss" (Squirmy and Grubs, 2020b). Burcaw expands by stating to viewers: "since I am not physically able to initiate a kiss [...] I show her my lips [...] which means like 'hey, come down to my level'" (Squirmy and Grubs, 2020c). Through the ways they describe their intimate relations, Burcaw and Aylward acknowledge disability in their communication, yet it seldom appears as deficiency, limitation, or lack, but rather, it appears in terms of innovation and subversion. Together, they transgress rigid understandings of intimacy, as well as Western taboos associated with facilitated sex (Perlin & Lynch, 2016), and instead, create narratives of mutual exploration and learning.

In responding to Burcaw's mention of the ways he initiates intimacy by signaling to Aylward (either verbally or non-verbally), Aylward responds: "I do that to you though also, like before I come over, I'll do that to you from across the room" (Squirmy and Grubs, 2020b). Aylward attempts to soften the binary between disability and nondisability here, where she emphasizes that initiating intimacy is an activity that they both approach in ways that are specific to their relationship, rather than specific to disability. As Burcaw concurs, "we have found ways that we can both provide for the other" (Squirmy and Grubs, 2020b). The couple's attempt at subverting disparaging conceptions of disability is apparent. In the following quote Aylward speaks to how disability has also allowed them to transcend normative approaches to intimacy:

> We need to use more communication than able-bodied couples [pause] I don't even know if I agree with that statement, like we do use more communication […] but I don't think that able-bodied people shouldn't do that […] our intimate life does benefit from that and saying what both of us want and figuring out how to get it, because I think a lot of times if you're doing like cookie-cutter whatever, it might not be completely what both people are dreaming of having. (Squirmy and Grubs, 2020b)

Speaking to Burcaw, she expresses: "you've taught me to talk more about my feelings. I think because we have to talk about it, it's wonderful" (Squirmy and Grubs, 2020b). Here, the couple's reality of disability and sexuality fundamentally challenges allegiance to rigidly unidimensional ("cookie-cutter") approaches to intimacy upon which normative expectations of sexuality are often built. Aylward's discussion of communication and facilitation allows disability to appear as desirable and constructive to their intimate relationship.

As has been elucidated through this case study, through their narratives, the couple eschews notions of sexual ableism— "a system of imbuing sexuality with determinations of qualification to be sexual based on criteria of [dis]ability, intellect, morality, physicality, appearance, age, race, social acceptability, and gender conformity" (Gill, 2015, p. 3), wherein sexuality becomes valorized and ascribed with very particular characteristics and criteria, which often explicitly exclude disabled people. This is where the intersections between compulsory sexuality and compulsory nondisabledness become further apparent. Indeed, compulsory sexuality and compulsory nondisabledness correspondingly share a symbiotic relationship, wherein one is always contingent upon the other (Kim, 2011). In order for one to be perceived as sexually apt in a "healthy," "natural," or "desirable" manner, this must be in alignment with society's understanding of what constitutes a "normative" sexual subject.

The Significance of Discourse and Communication

Focusing on the lived experiences of a disabled individual underscores the ways that disability and sexuality materialize in the lives of disabled people, through the social relations, communications, and discursive processes which inform and constitute them. These dynamics play a key role in a disabled person's access to and experience with sexual agency; both in terms of their sexual subjectivity as well as other's conceptions of them as sexual agents. Through Burcaw's self-representation, disability eludes discourses of deficiency, calamity, and subordination, and instead, is reconstructed as autonomous, subversive, and innovative. This representation, however, also subsequently becomes juxtaposed against the perceptions of viewers, readers, and strangers who continually privilege nondisability and thus center disability in terms of lack, loss, and difference.

It is important to note that as activism and awareness surrounding disability have developed, representations of disabled people as having sexual agency have progressed. While there are indeed [marginal] representations of disabled individuals as sexual beings in popular discourse and the media, this is largely overshadowed by the gross overrepresentations of them as asexual (and at times, hypersexual). Thus, there exists little nuance between these two misrepresentations of disability and sexuality. As such, disability continues to appear in discourses of sexual lack, deficiency, and dysfunction, and disappear in discourses of sexual desire, competence, and agency. The inaccurate postulation that disabled individuals are inevitably incapable of precipitating, possessing, and expressing sexual desire, should not be conflicted with disabled people themselves positioning themselves as asexual, however. Desexualization as a process imposed by systems of power, and asexuality as a claimed and embodied identity, are fundamentally distinct; yet they share many power-laden similarities.

Disabled individuals who have been desexualized have had their "intrinsic" sexual subjectivities stripped from them in being categorized as asexual, while those who self-identify as asexual have been stigmatized and deemed as abnormal precisely due to *not* experiencing an "intrinsic" sense of sexual desire. The fact that disabled individuals have been desexualized in an attempt to *naturalize* asexuality for disabled people, works in opposition to those who identify as asexual but are seen as deviant and *unnatural*. Indeed, since asexuality has been historically pathologized and invalidated as a legitimate sexual orientation (Bogaert, 2006; Cerankowski & Milks, 2010; Przybylo, 2011, 2016), when individuals claim asexuality as an orientation and identity, they are deemed abnormal; yet when asexuality is imposed onto disabled individuals, it is conceptualized as a "normal" part of their identity. In other words, for disabled individuals the "abnormal" is seen as "natural," while with the asexual community the "natural" is seen as "abnormal."

What is critical to consider here is the salience of discourse and communication in constructing understandings of disability and sexuality. If disability is perpetually conceived of in terms of deficiency, and sexuality is perpetually conceived of as demanding a particular sexual subject, it is clear that disabled people will continue to be characterized (by others) in ways that desexualize and position them as unworthy of sexual agency. A further critical implication when considering the desexualization of disabled people is that it is built upon a discursive foundation of "normalcy" and "difference." Through stereotypes of them as asexual, disabled individuals are fundamentally constructed as inferior, deficient, and Other in relation to a socio-culturally constructed normative sexual subject. In this way, discourses of "normalcy" versus "difference" materialize (Inahara, 2009).

Another salient point to consider is that normalcy does not exist as a "natural" phenomenon, but is rather socio-historically constructed (Davis, 1997). As such, conceptions of abnormality and difference are solely possible due to constructions of "normalcy" (Warner, 1999). As Goffman (1963) articulately states: "the role of normal and the role of stigmatized are parts of the same complex, cuts from the same standard cloth" (p. 130). In other words, normalcy *depends* on difference as difference depends on normalcy in order to thrive. Indeed, as discourses both constitute and are constituted by other discourses (Foucault, 1980), discourses of normalcy fundamentally depend on discourses of difference in order to prevail as they cannot exist on their own. If there exists no standard discourse or prototype of "normal," "difference" cannot be defined. Accordingly, Inahara (2009) writes "I wonder whether, if physical ability for all individuals was not limited to a simple conception of able-bodiedness, we would no longer have a single definition of what constitutes physical difference" (pp. 55–56). Although speaking specifically to physical disability and "able-bodiedness," Inahara evokes the salience of shifting how we conceive of and communicate difference (and normalcy). Thus, if we are to deconstruct and reconceptualize taken-for-granted understandings of difference and normalcy, the ways in which we conceive of disability and sexuality would, too, become reconceptualized.

Concluding Thoughts

Returning to the opening remarks of this chapter, the ways in which we each conceive of disability and sexuality will largely be shaped by the broader meanings we associate with these terms. As has been evoked through this chapter, dominant discourses of disability and sexuality are communicated in very particular ways. Specifically, the appearance of disability in relation to sexuality is commonly embedded within notions of deficiency, infantilization, and inferiority, while its observed disappearance is crystallized through discourses of sexual autonomy, independence, and sovereignty. This relationship stems from the overwhelming and spontaneous assumption of disabled persons as asexual beings wherein notions of sexuality in the context of disability are stigmatized and constructed as taboo (Benedet & Grant, 2007; Whittington-Walks, 2018; Yoshizaki-Gibbons & O'Leary, 2018). Indeed, sexuality is very seldom assumed to be a natural occurrence for disabled individuals (Richards et al., 2006), and disabled people regularly disappear from normative conceptualizations of sexuality (Payne et al., 2016). This contributes to the incessant stigmatization of disability as disabled people are positioned as asexual, sexually undesirable, and incapable of engaging in sexual relations or possessing sexual agency (Payne et al., 2016; Philaretou & Allen, 2001; Shah et al., 2015).

Accordingly, the promise in critically reflecting on the ways we communicate about and conceive of disability and sexuality should never be overlooked. In doing so, we may choose to adopt Titchkosky's (2003) "politics of wonder." A politics of wonder encourages us to move from explanation to exploration. It encourages us to make the familiar strange and question our taken-for-granted assumptions as to the certitude of what we know about disability. It also "leads us to ask if we might come to know disability differently by wondering how people have already come to know disability with certainty" (p. 16). Reflecting in such ways allows us to avoid reifying and reproducing misrepresentations of disabled life. It emphasizes the salience of possibility, "new" ways of understanding disability and what this can mean for the lives of disabled and nondisabled people, and encourages us to deconstruct what we may think of as "truth." Disability has the potential to transform the ways we conceptualize sex, through "creating confusions about what and who is sexy and sexualizable, what counts as sex, and what desire 'is'" (Mollow & McRuer, 2012, p. 32). Indeed, sexuality can undeniably be a "source of oppression for disabled people" yet it can also be "a profoundly productive site for invention, experimentation, and transformation" (McRuer, 2018, p. 476). Let us consider this transformation together, through a politics of wonder.

NOTE

1. The term "interabled" here refers to their relationship as it is comprised of Burcaw, who identifies as a disabled person, and Aylward, who is understood by the couple to be "able-bodied." It is critical to note that the terms "interabled" and "able-bodied" are terms that are highly contested within the disability community. While some members identify with and utilize these terms, many others problematize them as they infer a universal state of "normalcy" among non-disabled people which positions disabled people as inferior and deficient in comparison.

REFERENCES

Benedet, J., & Grant, I. (2007). Hearing the sexual assault complaints of women with mental disabilities: Consent, capacity, and mistaken belief. *McGill Law Journal, 52*(2), 243–289. https://lawjournal.mcgill.ca/article/hearing-the-sexual-assault-complaints-of-women-with-mental-disabilities-consent-capacity-and-mistaken-belief/

Bogaert, A. F. (2006). Toward a conceptual understanding of asexuality. *Review of General Psychology, 10*(3), 241–250. https://doi.org/10.1037/1089-2680.10.3.214

Brodwin, M. G., & Frederick, P. C. (2010). Sexuality and societal beliefs regarding persons living with disabilities. *Journal of Rehabilitation, 76*(4), 37–41.

Burcaw, S. (2014). *Laughing at my nightmare.* Roaring Book Press.

Burcaw, S. (2019). *Strangers assume my girlfriend is my nurse.* Roaring Book Press.

Burgess, J., & Green, J. (2009). *YouTube: Online video and participatory culture.* Policy Press.

Cerankowski, K. J., & Milks, M. (2010). New orientations: Asexuality and its implications for theory and practice. *Feminist Studies, 36*(3), 650–664, 699–700. https://www.jstor.org/stable/27919126

Davidson, D., & La Monica, N. (2011). Disability definitions. In M. Z. Stange, C. K. Oyster, & J. E. Sloan (Eds.), *Encyclopedia of women in today's world* (Vol. 1, pp. 402–405). Sage.

Davis, L. J. (Ed.). (1997). *The disability studies reader.* Routledge.

DeWelles, M. (2019). Just like but unlike: Sameness, difference, and disability in children's storybooks. *Journal of Teaching Disability Studies*, Issue 1. Retrieved April 7, 2020, from https://jtds.commons.gc.cuny.edu/just-like-but-unlike-sameness-difference-and-disability-in-childrens-storybooks/

Emens, E. F. (2014). Compulsory sexuality. *Stanford Law Review, 66*(2), 303–386. https://doi.org/10.2139/ssrn.2218783

Foucault, M. (1978). *The history of sexuality. Volume 1, An introduction.* Penguin.

Foucault, M. (1980). Truth and power. In C. Gordon (Ed.), *Power/knowledge: Selected interviews & other writings by Michel Foucault, 1972–1977* (pp. 109–133). Vintage Books.

Gill, M. (2015). *Already doing it: Intellectual disability and sexual agency.* University of Minnesota Press.

Goffman, E. (1963). *Stigma: Notes on the management of spoiled identity.* Prentice-Hall.

Grue, J. (2015). *Disability and discourse analysis.* Routledge.

Hall, D. E. (2004). *Subjectivity.* Routledge.

Inahara, M. (2009). This body which is not one: The body, femininity, and disability. *Body and Society, 15*(1), 47–62. https://doi.org/10.1177/1357034X08100146

Kim, E. (2011). Asexuality in disability narratives. *Sexualities, 14*(4), 479–493. https://doi.org/10.1177/1363460711406463

Liddiard, K. (2014). The work of disabled identities in intimate relationships. *Disability and Society, 29*(1), 115–128. https://doi.org/10.1080/09687599.2013.776486

McRuer, R. (2006). *Crip theory: Cultural signs of queerness and disability.* New York University Press.

McRuer, R. (2018). *Crip times: Disability, globalization, and resistance.* New York University Press.

Mollow, A., & McRuer, R. (2012). Introduction. In R. McRuer & A. Mollow (Eds.), *Sex and disability* (pp. 1–36). Duke University Press.

Oliver, M. (1983). *Social work with disabled people.* Macmillan Education.

Oliver, M. (1996). *Understanding disability: From theory to practice.* Macmillan Education.

Orange, L. M. (2009). Sexuality and disability. In M.G. Brodwin, F.W. Siu, J. Howard, & E.R. Brodwin (Eds.). *Medical, psychosocial, and vocational aspects of disability* (3rd ed., pp. 263–272). Elliott & Fitzpatrick.

Parker, R. (2009). Sexuality, culture and society: Shifting paradigms in sexuality research. *Culture, Health & Sexuality, 11*(3), 251–266. https://doi.org/10.1080/13691050701606941

Payne, D. A., Hickey, H., Nelson, A., Rees, K., Bollinger, H., & Hartley, S. (2016). Physically disabled women and sexual identity: A photovoice study. *Disability & Society, 31*(8), 1030–1049. https://doi.org/10.1080/09687599.2016.1230044

Perlin, M. L., & Lynch, A. J. (2016). *Sexuality, disability, and the law: Beyond the last frontier?* Palgrave Macmillan.

Philaretou, A. G., & Allen, K. R. (2001). Reconstructing masculinity and sexuality. *The Journal of Men's Studies, 9*(3), 301–321. https://doi.org/10.3149/jms.0903.301

Przybylo, E. (2011). Crisis and safety: The asexual in sexusociety. *Sexualities, 14*(4), 444. https://doi.org/10.1177/1363460711406461

Przybylo, E. (2016). Asexuals against the Cis-tem! *Transgender Studies Quarterly, 3*(3-4), 653–660. https://doi.org/10.1215/23289252-3545347

Richards, D., Miodrag, N., & Watson, S. L. (2006). Sexuality and developmental disability: Obstacles to healthy sexuality throughout the lifespan. *Developmental Disabilities Bulletin, 34*(1-2), 137–155.

Saul, R. (2010). KevJumba and the adolescence of YouTube. *Educational Studies, 46*(5), 457–477. https://doi.org/10.1080/00131946.2010.510404

Shah, S., Wallis, M., Conor, F., & Kiszely, P. (2015). Bringing disability history alive in schools: Promoting a new understanding of disability through performance methods. *Research Papers in Education, 30*(3), 267–286. https://doi.org/10.1080/02671522.2014.891255

Squirmy and Grubs. (2020a, June 22). *Does Shane's disease affect his sex drive? Intimacy and disability Q&A part 3.* [Video]. YouTube. Retrieved April 7, 2020, from https://www.youtube.com/watch?v=3LJJnULUyFY

Squirmy and Grubs. (2020b, May 20). *Intimacy & disability—How we make it work—Q&A part 1.* [Video]. YouTube. Retrieved April 7, 2020, from https://www.youtube.com/watch?v=8iBROcohmxk

Squirmy and Grubs. (2020c, May 10). *Physical affection and intimacy in our relationship.* [Video]. YouTube. Retrieved April 7, 2020, from https://www.youtube.com/watch?v=5tq83yqreU0

Squirmy and Grubs. (2020d, June 9). *Sexual function and Shane's disease—intimacy and disability Q&A part 2.* [Video]. YouTube. Retrieved April 7, 2020, from https://www.youtube.com/watch?v=P_CbYrTTUdo

Titchkosky, T., & Michalko, R. (2009). Introduction. In T. Titchkosky & R. Michalko (Eds.), *Rethinking normalcy: A disability studies reader* (pp. 1–15). Canadian Scholars' Press.

Trieschmann, R. B. (1988). *Spinal cord injuries: Psychological, social, and vocational rehabilitation.* Demos Medical Publishing.

Vaz, P., & Bruno, F. (2003). Types of self-surveillance: from abnormality to individuals 'at risk'. *Surveillance & Society, 1*(3), 272–291. https://doi.org/10.24908/ss.v1i3.3341

Warner, M. (1999). Normal and normaller: Beyond gay marriage. *GLQ: A Journal of Lesbian & Gay Studies, 2,* 119–171. https://doi.org/10.1215/10642684-5-2-119

Weedon, C. (1987). *Feminist practice and poststructuralist theory.* Blackwell.

Whittington-Walks, F. (2018). "One of us" or two? Conjoined twins and the paradoxical relationships of identity in American Horror Story: Freak Show. In J.L. Schatz & A.E. George (Eds.), *The image of disability: Essays on media representations* (pp. 11-27). McFarland & Company, Inc.

Wodak, R. (2001). What CDA is about: A summary of its history, important concepts and its developments. In R. Wodak & M. Meyer (Eds.), *Methods of critical discourse analysis* (pp. 1–13). Sage Publications.

Yoshizaki-Gibbons, H. H., & O'Leary, M. E. (2018). Deviant sexuality: The hyper-sexualization of women with bipolar disorder in film and television. In J. L. Schatz & A. E. George (Eds.), *The image of disability: Essays on media representations* (pp. 93–106). McFarland & Company.

PART II

Identity and Intersectionalities

CHAPTER 7

Ableism and Intersectionality: A Rhetorical Analysis

James L. Cherney

Perhaps disability studies will lead to some grand unified theory of the body, pulling together the differences implied in gender, nationality, ethnicity, race, and sexual preferences. Then, rather than the marginalized being in the wheelchair or using sign language, the person with disabilities will become the ultimate example, the universal image, the modality through whose knowing the postmodern subject can theorize and act.
—Davis (1997, p. 5)

Disability functions as a multivalent trope, though it remains the mark of otherness.
—Garland-Thomson (1997, p. 9)

Intersectionality, established by Crenshaw's (1991) groundbreaking black feminist analysis of black women's lives, "enables a complex understanding of the ways in which race, gender, class, sexuality, and ability among other dimensions of social, cultural, political, and economic processes intersect to shape everyday experiences and social institutions" (Naples et al., 2019, p. 5). People at intersections of marginalized identities face layered or compounded discrimination because they are excluded on more than one criterion. Simply put, the racist and sexist discrimination experienced by a black woman is doubly problematic compared to the racist discrimination experienced by a black man or the sexist discrimination experienced by a white woman.

J. L. Cherney (✉)
University of Nevada, Reno, Reno, NV, USA
e-mail: jcherney@unr.edu

© The Author(s), under exclusive license to Springer Nature Switzerland AG 2023
M. S. Jeffress et al. (eds.), *The Palgrave Handbook of Disability and Communication*, https://doi.org/10.1007/978-3-031-14447-9_7

Most forms of bigotry find their targets in, on, or through bodies. Calling attention to specific physical or material characteristics, and making these into markers of difference, is the first stage in the development of systematic discrimination. Such marks become the basis for practicing oppression and subordination by identifying what those bodies lack—for example whiteness, maleness, ablebodiedness—as justification for subordination. When a body's lack of something makes it less and subjects it to institutionalized inequities, the form of bigotry at work is at least in part ableist. In a sense, ableism operates within every form of discrimination that targets bodies.

Extending my earlier work on ableist rhetoric, this chapter contends that rhetorical practices associated with various forms of discrimination share similar characteristics and premises. Revealed, those similarities can illuminate intersections between ableism, racism, sexism, heterosexism, cissexism, classism, and the like. In particular, I contend that the rhetorical warrants that underly an ableist orientation also sustain and perpetuate many other discriminatory perspectives. This thesis directs attention to the rhetoric found at the specific locations that facilitate layering subordinated subjectivities on different people, which I argue offers a unique perspective on how intersecting discrimination operates and empowers groups that meet in them.

Intersections with Disability

A growing amount of research explores the ways how disability intersects with race and gender (Bailey & Mobley, 2019; Bell, 2011; Brown & Moloney, 2019; Naples et al., 2019; Pickens, 2019). Unsurprisingly, this research shows significant connections and parallels between these marginalized groups, for example, inequities such as economic insecurity compound and extend marginalization of disabled, raced, and gendered populations (Maroto et al., 2019; Miles, 2019). The practice of identity politics as a way of confronting such inequities also unites disability with race and gender. The disability rights movement in the US, like the political projects centered on race and gender, has been explicitly tied to identity (Cherney, 1999, 2019; Davis, 2002; Dolmage, 2014; Linton, 1998, Samuels, 2014). By extension, these identities connect via attempts to enact "recognitive and distributive justice," which "interlock in ways that make them inseparable, especially given how ableism, ageism, racism, and other forms of oppression and marginalization are jointly constructed" (Guidry-Grimes et al., 2020, p. 28).

Intersections between disability and other marginalized identities have a long history in Western culture. For example, as Jay Timothy Dolmage (2018) has shown, immigration policies in the US and Canada beginning in the nineteenth century have entangled disability with race, ethnicity, and gender through practices of scrutiny and beliefs that treated these as inherently linked. Similarly, eugenics, and the eugenics laws enacted in the US in the early twentieth century, assumed that various inherited disabilities were biologically tied to race, poverty, and gender (Pernick, 1996; Stubblefield, 2007). Through practices like these, the contemporary categories of disability, race, ethnicity, and gender—and the discriminatory regimes that target them—were created and refined in relation to each other.

The Holocaust presents one of the most recognizable and repugnant cases where ableist thinking informed and supported discriminatory activity against people deemed "degenerate" but otherwise ablebodied. Henry Friedlander's (1995) extensive history of the Nazi "Final Solution" documents that the early phase of the Nazis' program of mass executions and eugenic genocide—before it focused on Jews and "gypsies"—killed at least 70,000 physically and mentally disabled adults prior to 1941 (p. 85). Cloaked in the rhetoric of "euthanasia" and "mercy death," this initial phase of executions—known as the T4 program—built upon the logic of the prewar mass eugenic sterilizations of a conservatively estimated 300,000 disabled adults (p. 30). The killing of institutionalized children began even before T4 and continued after Hitler suspended the murder of disabled adults in the killing centers, but records of this activity are less complete and the methods employed (such as overdoses of medication that might be interpreted as medical error and failed medical procedures that were presented as potentially therapeutic) make quantification more difficult. Nonetheless, Friedlander estimates that at least 5000 mentally and physically disabled children were killed by the Nazis during this period (pp. 39–61). His work establishes that these programs of executing the disabled "proved to be the opening act of Nazi genocide" (p. 22) as it laid the foundations for the murderous campaign carried out against 6 million Jews and other targeted populations. With the T4 program the Nazis created killing centers in which they invented techniques used in the gas chambers and crematoria, developed procedures for selecting and isolating victims, and perfected means of subterfuge to hide mass exterminations. T4 also provided the mental training for those who would run the death camps. As Friedlander notes, "The killers who learned their trade in the euthanasia killing centers of Brandenburg, Grafeneck, Jartheim, Sonnenstein, Bernburg, and Hadamar also staffed the killing centers at Belzec, Sobibor, and Treblinka" (p. 22). Normalizing the extermination of disabled people efficiently desensitized those who would later kill millions more deemed undesirable.

T4 reveals the key rhetorical basis used to justifying the Nazi genocide. This program and the execution of tens of thousands of disabled people institutionalized human inequality and created a policy of exclusion that easily expanded from isolating those viewed as incurably abnormal and defective to ostracizing anyone labeled "'unproductive' and 'unworthy'" (Friedlander, 1995, p. 17). This required and generated a concept of human "degeneration" that could be applied with equal maleficence to Jews and "gypsies" as well as the mentally and physically disabled. Encapsulated in the term *lebensunwerten Lebens* ("life unworthy of life") the Nazi practice of deeming some humans defective and degenerate—sanctioned and justified by the ableist rationale that a disabled life is less worth living—became the essential rhetorical move behind the Holocaust. Reclassified as unworthy lives, the various groups that the Nazis sought to

102   J. L. CHERNEY

eliminate became legitimate targets for mass murder. Their blood could be shed because it might otherwise pollute the German people; their lives could be taken because they might otherwise be a burden on others and the state.

Despite the nearly universal rejection of the Nazi ideology and agenda, and the public shame for the widely practiced eugenics policies of the twentieth century, the COVID pandemic that began in 2020 demonstrates that the logic behind the doctrine of *lebensunwerten Lebens* persists. As Lennard Davis put it, the pandemic "like a skilled taxidermist, lifts off the skin of the kind of discrimination to find the invidious structural armature that gives it shape and form" (p. S139), and what it reveals is that the "ideology of health is deeply imbued with ableist notions of the normal and abnormal" (p. S140). Faced with potentially limited resources, some medical professionals and policy makers developed guidelines for patient triage that used a patient's disability as a decisive factor. The state of Washington "recommended giving limited resources only to younger, healthier people, not to older patients," Alabama "specified that people with intellectual disabilities 'are unlikely candidates for ventilator support,'" and Tennessee excluded from critical care "people with spinal muscular atrophy who need assistance with activities of daily living" (Davis, 2021, p. S140). Seen as naturally less likely to enjoy a high quality of life even if they recovered, specifically targeting aged and disabled people was normalized as a rational decision. As Davis points out, when making life-or-death decisions, this exclusion and reduction of those whose lives are less worthy revives the "Lives Unworthy of Living" rhetoric of the Holocaust (p. S141).

Ableist Rhetoric and Other Bigotry

In earlier work (2011, 2019) I analyze ableist rhetoric as an orientation shaped by particular ways of understanding disability. Here I use "understanding" in a broad sense to include how disability is known, valued, and seen. Ableist culture transmits this perspective to those who grow up under its influence through different lessons, but a rhetorical approach reveals the commonplace assumptions that inform how most of these work. To comprehend various different events that demand interpretation and explanation, individuals rely on basic concepts to frame their meaning. They learn these concepts as necessary ways of making sense of complicated situations, which they encounter articulated as narratives, engaged as debates, recorded as data, displayed as performances, or otherwise presented as "texts." In my analysis, individuals encounter texts as things that can (and are expected to) be understood, so in working to understand them they adopt and learn fundamental guidelines, generalizable assumptions, and interpretive norms that inform ways of making something inexplicable or novel into something meaningful. When encountering a disability or engaging in a disability-related situation, the ableist perspective employs basic ideas like these to comprehend it.

In my research, I identify three of these ideas: that deviance from an expected norm signals the presence of something unquestionably wrong, that ability is a function of bodies instead of social structures that privilege particular skills, and that normalcy is a natural state as essential as natural law. As a rhetorician, I conceptualize these as "warrants," which are the assumed rules of interpretation that link any set of information to a conclusion. Warrants work like the major premise of a syllogism by validating the logic that allows one to deduce a conclusion from something accepted as accurate. In the classic categorical syllogism "Socrates is human, humans are mortal, therefore Socrates is mortal," the major premise—the generalizable rule—"humans are mortal" warrants the conclusion "Socrates is mortal" based on the accepted grounds that "Socrates is human." Adopting the same syntactic structure, I express the three ableist ideas noted above as simple equivalencies: *deviance is evil, body is able,* and *normal is natural.* Called and recalled into action by such texts as stories of demonic possession, rules governing organized sport, and public debates over appropriate medical procedures, these warrants become commonsense foundations that dictate an ableist perspective.

Rhetorically analyzing the operation of other discriminatory perspectives reveals that these same warrants appear at work in such orientations as sexism, racism, and cissexism. For example, discrimination against trans people employs *normal is natural* by claiming that a binary (two-sex) model of sexuality is the natural arrangement for most animals, and that it has evolved over the years as a normal extension of natural selection (Shaffer, 2007). When used as a warrant for understanding trans bodies, the idea that *normal is natural* presents trans people as abnormal and therefore unnatural. Similarly, assumptions about the threat posed by their "deviant" bodies ranges from unfounded assertions that trans people are likely to engage in sexual assault if allowed to share bathrooms (Borello, 2016) and that gender-affirming medical care is an unholy affront to a Christian God (Lindell, 2021). As with ableism, these primary warrants frequently entwine to give cissexists a sense of coherence. Some religious opponents to trans-supportive legislation who equate "God's law" with natural law conclude that attempting to "normalize" trans identities poses a harmful threat even to trans people, which demonstrates how *normal is natural* and *deviance is evil* can become mutually supportive bases for bigotry (e.g., Family Policy Alliance, 2021). The warrant *body is able* plays a similar role by firmly ascribing the development of gender to biological sex, so that one's physical genitalia—conveniently reduced by *natural is normal* from a demonstrably complex set of possibilities to a simple dichotomy of female vagina or male penis—dictates one's identity.

The widespread history of such ableist ideas in virtually all discriminatory perspectives suggests the central role that views of disability play in orienting most forms of bigotry. One prime example is the way gender has been constructed in relation to disability. As Rosemarie Garland-Thomson (1997) notes, throughout western history the "equation of femaleness with disability is common," and prominent examples range from "Freud's delineating femaleness in terms of castration to late-nineteenth-century physicians' defining menstruation a disabling and restricting 'eternal wound' to Thorstein Veblen's describing women in 1899 as literally disabled by feminine roles and costuming" (p. 19). Early iterations of this idea can be found in texts surviving from the ancient Greeks. In her analysis of Aristotle's work, Garland-Thomson points out that "the father of Western taxonomy" articulates a connection between disabled and female bodies by describing "'the female as it were a deformed male' or—as it appears in other translations"—"a mutilated male" (p. 20). In other words, in Aristotle's system the human male stood as the standard of physical perfection and any other body "is really in a way a monstrosity. .. The first beginning of this deviation is when a female is formed instead of a male" (p. 19). Garland-Thomson reads this seminal move as "initiat[ing] the discursive practice of marking what is deemed aberrant while concealing what is privileged behind an assertion of normalcy" (p. 20). In this step Aristotle lays the groundwork for the invisibility of prejudices rooted in such assertions, and provides possibly "the original operation of the logic that has become so familiar in discussions of gender, race, or disability: male, white, or able-bodied superiority appears natural, undisputed, and unremarked, seemingly eclipsed by female, black, or disabled difference" (p. 20).

In other words, Aristotle's (ca. fourth century B.C.E./1942) *Generation of Animals* provides one of the earliest known examples of the ableist logic that *normal is natural*, as it relies on the warrant that whenever abnormality appears, that "Nature has in a way strayed from the generic type" (p. 401). Aristotle makes the equivocation even more explicit when he argues that whenever "some violence is done contrary to what is normal. .. that *ipso facto* means something contrary to Nature, because in the case of things which admit and do not exclude the possibility of being other than they are, *'normal' and 'natural' are identical*" (emphasis added, p. 475). Aristotle's text does not merely craft the idea of the normal, but naturalizes it, thus establishing *normal is natural* as a rule of interpretation that carries the ethos of natural law. In his logic, the natural physiological "superiority" of the male body creates a norm that differentiates the female body as inferior, and any attempt to challenge this idea violates the natural order. Even if not directly connected to these Aristotelian roots—although many would agree the patriarchal society of the ancient Greeks has played some role in the development of contemporary sexism—the ableist rhetoric at the intersection of disability and the female body remains pervasive and potent.

In her study of what she aptly names "fantasies of identification," Ellen Samuels explores attempts to ameliorate cultural anxieties that undermined discriminatory practices by establishing firm ground for identifying a person's sex or race. Such fantasies include the logic of court cases that worked at "discovering, inventing, or simply recognizing the presence of bodily marks that could be read as the truth of racial and personal identity" (p. 84) to address concerns about racial ambiguity that threatened the slaveocracy of the antebellum Southern United States. In Samuels' analysis, these fantasies' invocation of physiological characteristics as definitive markers of identity reveals the action of the "overmastering fantasy" that "disability is a knowable, obvious, and unchanging category" (p. 121). Grounding identification in the physical body—the social practice Samuels names "biocertification" (p. 122)—allows the "fantasy that race is knowable" (p. 97). Exposing the entwined strands of race and disability in the history of identification by fingerprinting, Samuels shows how the latter *realizes* the former, as "race is crucially mediated through the evocation of physical disability, which stands for the *truly* absolute bodily difference" (p. 99). Via practices of biocertification, the intersection of race and disability becomes firmly tied to ableist thinking.

Similarly, in his analysis of the practice of "cure" as a mechanism for maintaining the medical model of disability, Eli Clare reveals another way how the ableist rhetoric that *normal is natural* pervades racist and sexist perspectives. When enacted, cure "pushes us toward normality" (p. 180) through the eradication of defect, which justifies the practice because in an ableist culture "many of us have been seduced into believing that the need to eliminate disability and 'defectiveness' is intuitively obvious" (p. 27). As Clare notes, "In a world without ableism, *defective*, meaning the 'imperfection of a bodily system,' would probably not even exist" (p. 23). As racist and sexist orientations make the straight able-bodied white male the center of a hierarchy of normalcy, any body-mind that deviates from these norms becomes defective and effectively in need of being cured. Clare explains that "Whether focused on repairing disabled body-minds or straightening kinky hair, lightening brown skin or making gay, lesbian, and bi people heterosexual, cure aims to make us as *normal* and *natural* as possible." The presumed "consequences and dangers" posed by "defects" creates intense pressure to cure "correct" physical "defects," and Clare concludes that "This nonsense wouldn't exist without the threat of *unnatural* and *abnormal*" (p. 173). The logic of cure and its application in the contexts of race and gender rely on the warrant that treats normalcy as a natural condition.

Undermining Discriminatory Rhetorics
at the Intersections

Exposing Flawed Arguments

The rhetorical approach I employ here complements existing analyses of intersectionality by articulating strategies that promote anti-discrimination and undermine bigotry. For example, the rhetoric of disability rights and work of disability studies have crafted two powerful arguments from which to challenge the ableist warrant *normal is natural*. First, disability studies research documents the historical rhetoric that empowers the artificial (and changing) fiction of the normal body that has come to be naturalized as the unquestionable (and stable) fact upon which ableist discrimination depends. Davis (1997) explains that using the word "normal" to mean "the common type" only appeared in European languages around the mid-1800s. As a guideline for evaluating bodies, the norm replaced the much older concept of the "ideal." The ideal, traditionally understood as an unattainable abstraction only truly reachable by gods, tends to equalize human differences because "in a culture with an ideal form of the body, all members of the population are below the ideal" (p. 10). With the invention of the norm, the aesthetic pinnacle of an ideal is replaced by the bell curve of statistics, and being average, paradoxically, becomes itself a kind of ideal state of being. Davis points out that the initial project of identifying and establishing the statistical averages of physical characteristics was inextricably tied to the project of eugenics, and that one thing that almost all early statisticians had in common was that they were eugenicists. He maintains that "Statistics is bound up with eugenics because the central insight of statistics is the idea that a population can be normed." Applying a norm to a population immediately identifies abnormal or nonstandard people, and—when being normal is the desirable state—the "next step in conceiving of the population as norm and non-norm is for the state to attempt to norm the nonstandard—the aim of eugenics" (p. 14).

This and similar work effectively reverse the ableist warrant that articulates normal as a naturally occurring category, and shows that a more coherent and legitimate way of thinking is that—as an artificial human creation—*normal is* un*natural*. Exposing the rhetorical move that invents the normal body while denying its manufacture reveals what Garland-Thomson (1997) named the "normate," which is "the veiled subject position of cultural self, the figure outlined by the array of deviant others whose marked bodies shore up the normate's boundaries. The term *normate* usefully designates the social figure through which people can represent themselves as definitive human beings" (emphasis in original, p. 8). The normate is inherently a "constructed identity" that provides a position of authority and power to those whose "bodily configurations and cultural capital" allow them to adopt it, but its power relies on the invisibility of its operation. The normate becomes visible "only when we scrutinize the social processes and discourses that constitute physical and cultural otherness" to see how mark*ings* reveal the presence of mark*ers*. Tracing the lines of power that identify and marginalize others shows how "their cultural visibility as deviant obscures and neutralizes the normative figure that they legitimate." By illuminating "the processes that sort and rank physical differences into normal and abnormal," and examining how disability is thus "inflected by race, ethnicity, and gender," we can explore how bigotry rests on establishing "corporeal difference as deviance." As a result, "theorizing disability and then examining several sites that construct it" allows us to "uncover the complex ways that disability intersects with other social identities to produce the extraordinary and the ordinary figures who haunt us all" (pp. 8–9). Exposing the unmarked and privileged center to scrutiny removes the invisibility that protects its power, allowing it to be interrogated, challenged, and redistributed.

Second, anti-ableist rhetoric makes the strong case that ab*normal is natural*, as deviation from an artificial norm is the natural state of any single body (Clare,

2017). No two bodies are completely alike, so there cannot be a single body that is in everything the arithmetic mean against which bodies could be defined as normal. If there were, that one body's uniqueness would make it different from all other bodies, and its normalcy would collapse as inherently paradoxical. Even if we relied upon statistical analysis to expand the "sameness" of bodies to include ranges instead of a specific point on a metric (as in "the normal height for an adult human male is between 68 and 70 inches") the infinite number of metrics upon which such ranges could be determined makes it all but impossible for someone to fit in all of them at one time. Additionally, these ranges would constantly fluctuate across time and place depending on things like economic status and nutrition that impact the population for which the statistics were derived, which makes any definition of normalcy based upon them inherently ephemeral. Even if these ranges were somehow stabilized, our bodies naturally change as they grow and age, and if any body ever were to fit into all the "normal" ranges for a moment in time, that moment would eventually pass. Fitting someone into the normal range of any metric upon which bodies can be assessed requires adjusting those ranges to bracket all the conditions that would otherwise make the person appear abnormal: the 68–70 inch range of "normal" height only applies to a body of a specific sex (male), of a specific state of development (adult), from a specific historical period (contemporary/modern), and a specific race (Caucasian), with a specific ability status (ablebodied), etc. Change any of these characteristics, and the "normal range" changes with it, so identifying a body as normal requires setting aside all those things that would otherwise make it unique. We produce normalcy by artificially excluding natural differences.

Treating the metrics themselves as "natural" categories obscures the ways that the choices involved in their production reflect the operation of power and privilege. The practice of measuring some things and ignoring others—and the scales used to measure them—enacts a selection of traits based upon a chosen value system. Stuart Hall (1996) described such systems as "ideology," which is "the mental frameworks—the languages, the concepts, categories, imagery of thought, and systems of representation—which different classes and social groups deploy in order to make sense of, define, figure out and render intelligible the way society works" (p. 26). Through ideology, a group of people maintain "its dominance and leadership over society as a whole" by stabilizing forms of power through which to "reconcile and accommodate the mass of the people to their subordinate place in the social formation" (p. 27). What is the normal color of human skin? What is the normal type of hair? What is the normal level of optimism? What is the normal amount of fear? The choice of things that we decide to evaluate (or not) as normal reflects our values and biases, but this is a choice we make and not the dictates of biological necessity or natural law. Simply put, no body is, or can ever be, completely normal. A discriminatory regime based on the natural existence of the normal body cannot be coherently sustained once people recognize the fallacies of the ableist warrant that makes it seem reasonable, commonsensical, and obvious.

Neuroqueering as Rhetorical Solution

Along with exposing the flaws in the rhetoric that presents ableism as logical, disability studies scholars also provide critical techniques that flip the discriminatory operation of intersections. Taking advantage of links between disability and other oppressed characteristics produces paths to activism by radically reconfiguring relationships between bodies and the power. While this practice is not new, "disability studies offers as much to its [interdisciplinary] predecessors as it borrows from them" (Sandahl, 2003, p. 25). For example, starting around the early 2000s, such scholars as Clare (1999), Carrie Sandahl (2003), Robert McRuer (2006), and Alison Kafer (2013) explored the intersection of "the productive reciprocity between queer theory and disability studies, queer identity and crip identity, queer activism and crip activism" (Sandahl, 2003, p. 25). One practice of identity politics that grows out of this is the neuroqueer.

The term *neuroqueer* and practice of *neuroqueering* was coined by Nick Walker in 2008 to describe a political project explicitly situated at the intersection of neurodivergent and queer identities. As Walker (2021) explains, neuroqueering involves "engaging in practices intended to undo and subvert one's own cultural conditioning and one's ingrained habits of neuronormative and heteronormative performance" (para. 162). Several scholars have adopted and popularized a neuroqeer approach as a means to reveal and challenge ableist and cis-heterosexist privilege, hierarchies, and discrimination (Enger, 2019; Yergeau, 2018). Like crip and queer theory, neuroqueering rhetorically recovers words meant to stigmatize to empower a two-pronged attack against straight neurotypical hegemony.

Neuroqueering thus enacts what Foucault (1973/1994) described as uncovering what "systematizes" the things people say "from the outset, thus making them thereafter endlessly accessible to new discourses and open to the task of transforming them" (p. xix). What systematizes slurs is the certainty that even the people they target agree with the negative connotations of being a crip or queer. What Simi Linton (1998) calls "claiming disability" directly rebuts the ableist assumption that even the disabled must want to escape life with a disability and long to be ablebodied. From an ableist perspective, the most incomprehensible claim of Joseph Shapiro's (1994) report on the 1988 Deaf President Now protests at Gallaudet University is John Limnidis' declaration that "I'm proud to be deaf. If there was a medication that could be given to deaf people to make them hear, I wouldn't take it. Never. Never till I die!" (p. 85). Similarly, Eli Clare (2017)—whom the "medical-industrial complex" labels with the diagnosis of "cerebral palsy"—proclaims "the simple truth that I'm not broken. Even if there were a cure for brain cells that died at birth, I'd refuse. I have no idea who I'd be without my tremoring and tense muscles, slurring tongue" (pp. 5–6). Proudly claiming an identity as neurodivergent as well as queer or trans rhetorically disproves the assumptions of the "cisgenderist-ableist paradigm" that marks these as undesirable "co-morbidities" (Shapira & Granek, 2019, p. 494), and simultaneously decouples the warrant *normal is natural* from two directions at once. Exploiting the intersection of queer and neurodivergent identities, the neuroqueer identity rejects the doubly-privileged position of the straight neurotypical subject and demonstrates "the potential of intersectional analysis to expose how the production of 'normal bodyminds' operates" (Shapira & Granek, 2019, p. 508). As Lydia X. Z. Brown (2017) points out, neuroqueering simultaneously rejects the desexualization of disabled bodies and the pathologizing of queer/trans bodies, thus exposing "interlocking systems of injustice" (Oswald et al., 2021, p. 7) at the core of the neuroqueer nexus.

Closing Thoughts

As my explanation of neuroqueering suggests, the shared rhetorical dimensions of many intersections reinforce modes of discrimination that might otherwise appear to be distinct. In my analysis, intersections appear in the common rhetoric found in the center where two or more oppressed identities cross. To paraphrase what the late Chris Bell (2011) explained in a conversation we shared in 2006, what matters most at an intersection is not the paths of the roads that cross or the people and vehicles that travel upon them, but what happens in the shared space the roads occupy but do not own. When roads intersect, they create a new location that generates new rhetorical possibilities.

Since rhetorical theory's ancient origins, shared ideas have been viewed as the *places* for constructing positions from which to advocate and persuade. We preserve that idea today in the words "location" and "topic" which are derived from the Latin word *loci* and its Greek counterpart *topoi*, which names the "commonplaces" that can be relied upon to make sense of and argue claims about a specific issue or area of concern. One important type of such commonplaces are warrants, as these reflect the shared rules underlying logical inferences. As a basis for understanding and reasoning about what meets at an intersection, the warrants employed there apply to all of the identities involved. In this analysis, the ableist ideas that *normal is natural, deviance is evil*, and *body is able* are the same warrants that inform such discriminatory regimes as sexism and racism. They provide the logic that marginalizes the intersection, locating places where the angry impulse to translate fear into the oppression of others congeals into a pseudo-coherency that some mistake for reasonable thinking. As such, they are at the same time places from which to attack bigotry and advance the project of emancipation.

References

Aristotle. (1942). *Generation of animals* (A. L. Peck, Trans.). Harvard University Press. (Original work published ca. 4th century B.C.E).

Bailey, M., & Mobley, I. A. (2019). Work in the intersections: A black feminist disability framework. *Gender & Society, 33*(1), 19–40. https://doi.org/10.1177/0891243218801523

110   J. L. CHERNEY

Bell, C. M. (Ed.). (2011). *Blackness and disability: Critical examinations and cultural interventions.* Michigan State University Press.

Borello, S. (2016, April 22). Sexual assault and domestic violence organizations debunk 'bathroom predator myth.' *ABC News.* Retrieved December 17, 2021, from https://abcnews.go.com/US/sexual-assault-domestic-violence-organizations-debunk-bathroom-predator/story?id=38604019

Brown, L. X. Z. (2017). Ableist shame and disruptive bodies: Survivorship at the intersection of queer, trans, and disabled existence. In A. Johnson, J. Nelson, & E. Lund (Eds.), *Religion, disability, and interpersonal violence* (pp. 163–178). Springer International Publishing. https://doi.org/10.1007/978-3-319-56901-7_10

Brown, R. L., & Moloney, M. E. (2019). Intersectionality, work, and well-being: The effects of gender and disability. *Gender & Society, 33*(1), 94–122. https://doi.org/10.1177/0891243218800636

Cherney, J. L. (1999). Deaf culture and the cochlear implant debate: Cyborg politics and the identity of people with disabilities. *Argumentation and Advocacy, 36*(1), 22–34. https://doi.org/10.1080/00028533.1999.11951635

Cherney, J. L. (2011). The rhetoric of Ableism. *Disability Studies Quarterly 31*, 1–16. http://www.dsqsds.org/article/view/1665.

Cherney, J. L. (2019). *Ableist rhetoric: How we know, value, and see disability.* Pennsylvania State University Press.

Clare, E. (1999). *Exile and pride: Disability, queerness, and liberation.* South End Press.

Clare, E. (2017). *Brilliant imperfection: Grappling with cure.* Duke University Press.

Crenshaw, K. (1991). Mapping the margins: Intersectionality, identity politics, and violence against women of color. *Stanford Law Review, 43*(6), 1241–1299. https://doi.org/10.2307/1229039

Davis, L. J. (2002). *Bending over backwards: Disability, dismodernism, and other difficult positions.* New York University Press.

Davis, L. J. (Ed.). (1997). *The disability studies reader.* Routledge.

Davis, L. J. (2021). In the time of pandemic, the deep structure of biopower is laid bare. *Critical Inquiry, 47*(S2), S138–S142. https://doi.org/10.1086/711458

Dolmage, J. T. (2014). *Disability rhetoric.* Syracuse University Press.

Dolmage, J. T. (2018). *Disabled upon arrival: Eugenics, immigration, and the construction of race and disability.* Ohio State University Press.

Enger, J. E. (2019). "The disability rights community was never mine": Neuroqueer disidentification. *Gender & Society, 33*(1), 123–147. https://doi.org/10.1177/0891243218803284

Family Policy Alliance (2021). *Transgenderism and gender dysphoria: God created mankind male and female, in his image and likeness, which cannot be changed.* Retrieved December 17, 2021, from https://familypolicyalliance.com/issues/sexuality/transgender/

Foucault, M. (1994). *Birth of the clinic: An archaeology of medical perception.* (A. M. S. Smith, Trans.). Vintage Books. (Original work published 1973).

Friedlander, H. (1995). *The origins of Nazi genocide: From euthanasia to the Final Solution.* University of North Carolina Press.

Garland-Thomson, R. (1997). *Extraordinary bodies: Figuring physical disability in American culture and literature.* Columbia University Press.

Guidry-Grimes, L., Savin, K., Stramondo, J. A., Reynolds, J. M., Tsaplina, M., Burke, T. B., Ballantyne, A., Kittay, E. F., Stahl, D., Scully, J. L., Garland Thomson, R., Tarzian, A., Doron, D., & Fins, J. J. (2020). Disability rights as a necessary framework for crisis standards of care and the future of health care. *Hastings Center Report, 50*(3), 28–32. https://doi.org/10.1002/hast.1128

Hall, S. (1996). The problem of ideology: Marxism without guarantees. In D. Morley & K. H. Chen (Eds.), *Stuart Hall: Critical dialogues in cultural studies* (pp. 24–45). Routledge.

Kafer, A. (2013). *Feminist, crip, queer.* Indiana University Press.

Lindell, C. (2021, May 18). "My God makes no mistakes": Texas Senate oks ban on gender-affirming care for young Texans. *Austin American-Statesman.* Retrieved December 17, 2021, from https://www.statesman.com/story/news/2021/05/18/after-debating-theology-senate-oks-gender-care-ban-young-texans/5150720001/

Linton, S. (1998). *Claiming disability: Knowledge and identity.* New York University Press.

Maroto, M., Pettinicchio, D., & Patterson, A. C. (2019). Hierarchies of categorical disadvantage: Economic insecurity at the intersection of disability, gender, and race. *Gender & Society, 33*(1), 64–93. https://doi.org/10.1177/0891243218794648

McRuer, R. (2006). *Crip theory: Cultural signs of queerness and disability.* New York University Press.

Miles, A. L. (2019). "Strong black women": African American women with disabilities, intersecting identities, and inequality. *Gender & Society, 33*(1), 41–63. https://doi.org/10.1177/0891243218814820

Naples, N. A., Mauldin, L., & Dillaway, H. (2019). From the guest editors: Gender, disability, and intersectionality. *Gender & Society, 33*(1), 5–18. https://doi.org/10.1177/0891243218813309

Oswald, A. G., Avory, S., & Fine, M. (2021, March 2). Intersectional expansiveness born at the neuroqueer nexus. *Psychology & Sexuality.* Advance online publication. https://doi.org/10.1080/19419899.2021.1900347

Pernick, M. S. (1996). *The black stork: Eugenics and the death of "defective" babies in American medicine and motion pictures since 1915.* Oxford University Press.

Pickens, T. A. (2019). *Black madness: Mad blackness.* Duke University Press.

Samuels, E. (2014). *Fantasies of identification: Disability, gender, race.* New York University Press.

Sandahl, C. (2003). Queering the crip or cripping the queer? Intersections of queer and crip identities in solo autobiographical performance. *GLQ: A Journal of Lesbian and Gay Studies, 9*(1-2), 25–56. https://muse.jhu.edu/article/40804

Shaffer, A. (2007, September 27). Pas de deux: Why are there only two sexes? *Slate.* https://slate.com/human-interest/2007/09/why-are-there-only-two-sexes.html

Shapira, S., & Granek, L. (2019). Negotiating psychiatric cisgenderism-ableism in the transgenderautism nexus. *Feminism & Psychology, 29*(4), 494–513. https://doi.org/10.1177/0959353519850843

Shapiro, J. P. (1994). *No pity: People with disabilities forging a new civil rights movement.* Three Rivers Press.

Stubblefield, A. (2007). "Beyond the pale": Tainted whiteness, cognitive disability, and eugenic sterilization. *Hypatia, 22*(2), 162–181. https://doi.org/10.1111/j.1527-2001.2007.tb00987.x

Walker, N. (2021). *Neuroqueer heresies: Notes on the neurodiversity paradigm, autistic empowerment, and postnormal possibilities.* Autonomous.

Yergeau, M. R. (2018). *Authoring autism: On rhetoric and neurological queerness.* Duke University Press.

CHAPTER 8

Performing FitCrip in Daily Life: A Critical Autoethnographic Reflection on Embodied Vulnerability

Julie-Ann Scott-Pollock

This critical autoethnography draws upon the performance of daily life and existential phenomenology to problematize the artificial, ableist binary between fit and disabled through embodied narrative. Through telling personal stories we live through our disabled bodies. Personal stories allow us to map how our communicating bodies create and re-create shared cultural understandings through our ongoing daily communicative encounters. Ableism and athleticism seem constant and natural but are co-created and struggled over through human interaction and vulnerable to challenge and dismantlement as they emerge and re-emerge across cultural spaces.

My Fit, Disabled Body: An Overview

1985: Snipped

I wake up in a hospital bed, groggy, nestled in my arm is a yellow and brown animal crocheted by a hospital volunteer. Maybe it's a giraffe. It is also wearing two leg casts with an IV. The doctor looks at my anxious mother. They just snipped my Achilles tendons, lengthening them, dropping my heels to the floor. The doctor looks at my mother, "Don't worry. She's so strong. She'll recover."

J.-A. Scott-Pollock (✉)
Department of Communication Studies, University of North Carolina Wilmington, Wilmington, NC, USA
e-mail: scottj@uncw.edu

© The Author(s), under exclusive license to Springer Nature Switzerland AG 2023
M. S. Jeffress et al. (eds.), *The Palgrave Handbook of Disability and Communication*, https://doi.org/10.1007/978-3-031-14447-9_8

113

I do. I always did, but it took time and left scars.

I have spastic cerebral palsy. I did not walk until I was two years old. Once I did, my back was hunched as I perched to balance on turned-in toes. At age four, after six months of recovery, my heels drop to the floor, but my back remained hunched in order for me to balance with my feet facing each other.

1993: Sawed

I wake up in a hospital bed screaming. There's blood on the sheets. The epidural fell out of my back post-surgery so they had to tie me to the bed to "ride out" the pain since going back up to the required medication could cause my body to go into shock. I can't stretch beyond the three-inch length of the nylon bands constraining me so I won't disrupt my broken legs in traction.

The doctor assures my mother. "Don't worry. She's strong and she's on too much medication and under too much stress for her brain to remember this."

I remember it. At age 12, they sawed my femur bones in half, rotated them thirty degrees, and nailed them back together. The pain and the desperate feeling of being tied down in agony awakened sudden moments of paralysis followed by panic. That was the beginning of my anxiety.

1994: Removed

I wake up in a hospital bed. My legs feel heavy. The bolts are gone.

The doctor says to my mother. "She's strong, her bones almost pulled those bolts out. She's probably a few inches shorter than she would've been if we hadn't had to bolt her legs during a growth spurt. Shame to lose those inches when she's already so small but if you look, she's still proportionate."

At age 13, they sliced back into the still purple scars on my thighs, prying my quad muscles to the side to remove the bolts that had held my bones together as they healed. I did not know how to hold my back or move my legs on my now straightened hips. Six months later, with hours of physical therapy, I left my crutches behind. I learned to walk again with a straight back and feet.

2005: Fused

I wake up in a hospital bed and wince. The hardware is on the outside this time. Bolts and screws stick three inches out of my big toe bones. The gauze is soaked with blood. I can't move my big toe. The doctor looks at my mother.

"She's strong. This is nothing compared to the other operations. She'll recover quickly."

At 24, they cut and re-lengthened my Achilles tendons to alleviate the pressure of my involuntary spasming muscles on my toes that were causing hairline fractures throughout my foot. That effort was unfortunately negated by the snipping, adding stiff scar tissue. In response, the doctors fused my big toe, making it immobile to help brace my foot for the constant spasms on my left side. This caused my other toes on that foot to curl under, spasming against the fused toe, but the pain is manageable if I wear shoes with large toe boxes.

Today, with my bones rotated, my tendons lengthened, and my toes fused in place, I stand straight with my feet facing forward. My knees and ankles are still stiff. My gait is atypical but my noticeable limp does not disrupt cultural spaces. My stamina is above average despite chronic pain. My muscles are defined from the constant involuntary signals my brain sends to my skeletal muscles throughout the day and night to tighten.

Anxiety and My FitCrip Embodiment

I am disabled and I need to move. I require physical therapy to maintain mobility. I also live with anxiety, and I dislike the side effects of medication. I use endorphins from cardiovascular exercise to manage my body's fight or flight urges. Exercise keeps me focused and centered. I seek out fitness opportunities. From a very young age, this has included public exercise classes and congregating with people for cardiovascular activities. In these spaces there are often instructors who provide guidance on how to move one's body efficiently. Instruction offers assurance that I am well and safe. I find the presence of an exercise authority comforting.

I am repeatedly noticeably and publicly *both* fit *and* disabled.[1] I am a FitCrip.[2] This seemingly contradictory identity is continually negotiated across my daily interactions as my body ages, moving in and out of different cultural spaces and social roles. How people communicate with me and to each other about my disabled body changes with time. Operations, age, relationships, and status entangle with discourses of ableism. A fit, disabled body that does not seek out athletic spaces reserved exclusively for disabled bodies becomes a fleshed contradiction of the terms, "fit" and "disabled."

Para-athletics designed for atypical bodies categorize and organize disabled bodies for formal competition. Collective fitness culture does not offer these formal adaptive spaces. Fitness activities for the disabled involve able-bodied volunteers helping disabled bodies experience surfing, skiing, and swimming as charity events. Fitness activities for disabled bodies tend to stay within the realm of medicalized cultural spaces and discourses, focusing on physical therapy for personal treatment and maintenance. Yet, as my stories will illuminate, the contradiction in these terms is fragile, constituted by an ableist society that desires to divide disabled bodies from "normal" bodies. This artificial divide is porous. It allows counter meanings to seep through. My disabled fitness remains forever open to re-negotiation, dependent on the social situation that interprets how others interpret my body. As a performance of identity scholar, I see each communicative encounter as a co-struggle over meaning as cultural members seek to understand what it means to perform who we are through our bodies with each other.

When a fitness space and community values strength and endurance, my body often is valued as well. When agility and flexibility are valued, my body is not. The acceptance and value of my body grows less binary as I enter an age demographic where bodies are noticeably wearing down. Bodies that are negotiating the build-up of injury and illness over the course of decades are less questioning of my restricted sharp movements. My stiff, disabled gait grows increasingly "normal" across my fitness encounters of white, middle class, heteronormative presenting women in their 30s–40s. Others in my demographic have acquired injuries from athletic activities and daily living. Pain and restricted movement are now part of their embodied stories and daily performances of self. As their shoulders, knees, wrists, and ankles wear out, I'm more familiar to them than I was as a child and young adult. At this moment in my story, aging and disability begin to merge with one another. My FitCrip identity is no longer so jarring. This evolution reveals how if our culture embraced the inevitability of mortality, we could communicate about and interact with disabled fitness and fit disabled bodies with ease. This ease can extend across identity categories as we acknowledge that all unease is culturally constituted, situational, and open to new encounters that offer opportunities for connection and inclusion.

THE CRITICAL AUTOETHNOGRAPHIC DISABLED GAZE IN DAILY PERFORMANCE AS METHOD

I use autoethnographic writing as a method of inquiry because it allows me as a researcher to situate my body in relation to others to comprehend cultural realities (Scott, 2018). Methodologically, the term combines autobiography and ethnography, calling for the "turning of the ethnographic gaze inward on the self (auto), while maintaining the outward gaze of ethnography, looking at the larger context wherein self-experiences occur" (Denzin, 1997, p. 227). This gaze allows me to navigate the gaze of culture. I gaze back at them as they gaze at me and also gaze *with* them *at* me. Autoethnography allows me to write my body's lived knowledge. Drawing from existential phenomenology, our bodies experience what it means to be ourselves living in the world (Merleau-Ponty, 1962). We gather knowledge of the experiential realities of our bodies interacting with others in time and space, negotiating what it means to be who we are through our ongoing human encounters with other bodies, through which we are continually categorized, interpreted, and re-understood (Langellier & Peterson, 2004). I interpret these ongoing encounters as *performances of daily life* through which we become who we are through interpreting others' responses and applying that understanding to future interactions (Langellier & Peterson, 2004).

Autoethnography allows me to reflect on my daily performance of self and to map how meanings and understandings surrounding identity surface and are struggled over through my lived, embodied experience. I am perpetually aware of performativity, the process through which cultural power, meaning, and understanding emerge and are struggled over across my daily encounters (see

Butler, 1993). Ableism, the pervasive cultural devaluing of my diagnosed disabled body, becomes tangible and open to resistance through my interactions. I engage this awareness through applying a critical lens to my stories (Boylorn & Orbe, 2014). "Critical autoethnographic stories not only uncover marginalization, stigma, and prejudice in our personal stories, but also look towards means to resist it" (Scott, 2018, p. 3). Through the stories of my lived experience of being a FitCrip—disabled, strong, with endurance—I am able to expose a manufactured, binary contradiction as fragile. Through our daily performances of self (from personal storytelling to daily encounters) we can dismantle ableism and co-create inclusive cultural understandings. Communicative responses to disabled fitness can shift us to a cultural space of ease as we witness *any*body embracing the pleasure that comes from physical movement in shared cardiovascular health spaces.

Disability as the Negation of "Normal," "Healthy," and "Fit"

Rosemarie Garland-Thomson (2009) asserts that the able-bodied cultural gaze demands the story of the disabled body. Medicalized discourse defines my body as the opposite of normal. Unlike race and gender that have observable predictable markers, my disabled body is simply embodied abnormality (Garland-Thomson, 1997). To be normal is to lack the diagnoses, appearance, and/or experience of the disabled body. McRuer (2006) builds upon Rich's (1980) term "compulsory heterosexuality" to coin the term "compulsory able-bodiedness." Rich (1980) argues that to grasp heterosexuality as the "natural order of things," there needs to be a tangible embodiment of deviance. Queer bodies' daily performances of self are highlighted and stigmatized. The queer body is positioned as deviant so that bodies that are not defined as queer are "normal." Normal bodies are only defined by the contrast of the abnormal body. Like queer bodies, disabled bodies provide the contrast for "normal" (e.g., healthy bodies). Society needs embodied representations of deviance from "normal." The disabled body's abnormality is a necessary antithesis to normality. Normality cannot exist without my body to serve as a representation of what normal is not. Compulsory able-bodiedness is arguably even more pervasive in contemporary society than compulsory heterosexuality because the medical community diagnoses disabled bodies as malfunctioning and in need of correction. Disability is the disruption of healthy, good embodiment. To be disabled is to fall short of preferred embodiment. Disabled people are unapologetically labeled as lesser, deficient in our ongoing performances of self.

Compulsory able-bodiedness is entangled in the definition of fitness. To be fit is to be in good health, especially because of regular exercise (Merriam Webster Dictionary). To be disabled "to have a physical or mental condition that limits movements, senses or activities" (Merriam Webster Dictionary). Strength, fitness, and limitations are all dependent on cultural members' expectations of the bodies interacting in the specific situation. Bodies that are deemed disruptive to the dominant aesthetic and experience of the fitness space are not "fit." Interpretations of my body have changed across time and contexts. This change illuminates the power of performativity and vulnerability of meaning. In each communicative encounter, new meanings can emerge that challenge pervasive marginalization. I offer snapshots of me within fitness spaces—as a young child, a teenager, a young adult, and finally as a middle-aged adult—to highlight how disability and aging change how we interpret personal embodied performance. This evolution highlights the fragility of pervasive marginalization of disabled bodies as deficient and opens a space for us to learn to embrace and value *all* bodies across cultural spaces as long as we are here.

1986: But I Want to Roller Skate

I am in kindergarten. We just finished reading time on the classroom carpet. I am excited because it is Tuesday. Tuesday is gym day. I take my place in our class's alphabetized line between Juliana and Kate. With a bit of concentration, I am able to keep up with my straight-footed classmates to the school gym. As I catch the swinging blue door before it falls on me, I feel familiar jitters of anticipation. I know that the 45 minutes of movement will help me feel centered and calm for the rest of the day. The gym teacher, Mr. Bishop, has red plastic milk crates holding dozens of pairs of red-wheels attached to metal clamps designed to clutch children's sneakers so we can spend the class cruising in circles around the orange safety cones set out to make a large oval on the gray and white flecked linoleum floor that doubled as our school cafeteria. I watch as other children quickly scoot from the floor to standing and join the skating ring. I can't stand up. Each time I try, I fall back down. My feet face each other, and when I try to move forward, my skates' stoppers catch, and I fall. I look around the room for help. The gym teacher, Mr. Bishop, stands on the other side of the room. He is tall, lanky, with curly brown graying hair and a closely trimmed beard. Every time I think I have his attention he looks away. I want to skate. I like to go fast, and long for any opportunities to move in a fluid, smooth motion. It took almost a month for me to learn, but once I could finally swing my tight, spasming leg over my little pink bike and balance my body, I took off. I love how wheels allow my body to move. They quiet the interruptions of my constantly spasming limbs. I ride my bike in circles for hours around the country mile block my house sits on. I think roller skates can offer me that same feeling of both exhilaration and centeredness. I hope there is a way to stop my turned-in feet from entangling my skates. Maybe there is a different way to do it. As an academically inclined five-year-old who enjoys learning, I have faith in any teacher's ability to help so I crawl over to the wall and paw my way up it to a standing position. I attempt to lean against it to reach Mr. Bishop since I can't seem to catch his eye. I fall half a dozen times before making it to his feet.

"Mr. Bishop, I can't do it. Can you show me how to roller skate?"

He tilts his head toward me, only briefly making eye contact. "Listen, this isn't something you're going to be able to do. That's okay. Just take your skates off. You can stay here if you want or we can have you do something else. Do you want to get a book from the library or just watch?"

My face grows hot with embarrassment and shame. I sit down against the wall, looking at the metal skates clutching my orthopedic Stride Rite sneakers. I don't want to take them off. Mr. Bishop walks away to tell a few boys in the class to stop touching each other. He is finished interacting with me. I sit with my skates on my feet, watching my classmates wiz by me in circles, deeply desiring the calmness I know that repetitive movement would bring. I don't want to go sit and read. We just finished sitting and reading before I came. I want to move with everyone else. I like organized fitness spaces, even if my body makes people uncomfortable in them.

My disabled body, 35 years later still remembers that feeling of embarrassment and longing on the gym floor. My chest grows tight. I try to breathe deeply to loosen the knots. I go on my elliptical in the basement before returning to this essay. I feel better. At the time, I thought Mr. Bishop walked away, refusing to make eye contact because he was disgusted by my inability to roller skate, but now, I think he was also uncomfortable and embarrassed. I think what it must have been like looking into the eyes of a hopeful little girl who wanted to participate in his planned activity. He had no solution of how to help my turned in feet glide on skates like the rest of my classmates. In that moment, in that fitness space, the answer was to remove my disabled body from that context. My disabled body made gym teachers uncomfortable. I grew used to watching other kids do activities like skating and gymnastics. I learned there were no adaptations for me. With time, I realized that the former child athletes had ignored and mocked bodies like mine as children grew up to be physical education teachers. They did not design the fitness spaces for me. I diligently worked to not be too disruptive in a group fitness so that I could move with and among without getting in the way of others. I hoped that if I avoided being disruptive, I could continue drawing on the energy of group cardiovascular activity and grow from the direction of experts, even if they would not adapt the activity to my disabled body's ability.

1996: But I Want to See How I Have Improved

Ten years later I am enrolled in the required high school physical education class. I am recovered from my bone rotation and the subsequent hardware removal. A combination of physical therapy and hours a day of jumping on a trampoline to increase balance and mobility in my ankles and knees means that my body is light and strong, with above average cardiovascular endurance. At the start of the semester, we are required to take a fitness test and then work to improve on our weakest area for half of class throughout the year.

The first evaluation focuses on strength. My peers stand in amazement around me in the crowded weight room. It lacks ventilation and smells like body odor, but I am at ease and happy. I have been strength training in physical therapy since I was two years old and the constant involuntary tremors of my disabled body makes my muscles strong and dense. I am able to lift over 100 pounds in the deadlift, which is more than my weight. My leg lifts and barbell curls are also in the 99th percentile. I am stronger than all of the other girls and two-thirds of the boys. Mr. Lewia is clearly startled. He raises his eyebrows and double checks the numbers of the weights. Mr. Lewia is compact, and trendy in his 1990s black wind pants and oversized maroon t-shirt that highlight our school colors. He does not smile much. He stares at his clipboard a lot. He is also the boys' football and basketball coach and tends to not speak to the girls in the class any more than necessary while continually conversing with boys in his teams throughout our 90-minute class.

We move on to the endurance test. I am excited to see how I do. I can jump for hours on my large trampoline. I can hike for miles. I am sure that I will do well. The test requires stepping up onto a bench fused to the wall and then stepping back down as many times as possible in five minutes. As I attempt to step up my leg locks in a spasm, cerebral palsy shortens and thickens my muscles, restricting movement. What makes me great at dead lifts makes me terrible at stepping up on a high bench. I manage to hold my leg in place until the spasm passes and then hoist my other leg up. I hold the wall at the top to steady myself before stepping down. I do this about 12 times in five minutes. My classmates are flushed and breathing heavily. I am not. I don't have the range of motion or balance to effectively use this activity to test my cardiovascular endurance. Mr. Lewia lets me know that I am below the fifth percentile, so I will be working on endurance. All of the other girls in the class scored higher in endurance than strength. I look around and realize that I will be doing a mixture of running and aerobics classes with a group of boys. I am the only girl who will not be working on strength. My brief moment of collective, fit identity and belonging in the weight room is over. I feel awkward and out of place.

Over the course of the next months, I take training seriously. I am much slower than everyone else, but I work hard, concentrate on bending my stiff knees and ankles enough to ensure that I do not fall and I go further and faster every week. While the boys make fun of the aerobics class with the cheerleading coach that we are required to take for the first 20 minutes of each class, I concentrate on mastering the movements and my coordination improves. I like controlled, ordered moving. It is calming and helpful to me. I look forward to repeating the sequence twice a week followed by jogging. I know that I'm getting faster and more coordinated.

I hesitantly approach Mr. Lewia at the end of class in May. I am worried and hoping he will ease my mind. "Um, Mr. Lewia, will the endurance test be stepping up on that bench again? Because I know that I'm improving my endurance. I'm so much less tired than I was when we started running, but um, with my cerebral palsy I'm worried that I can't get my foot up there and balance very well. So, because of that it's not really my endurance that makes my score so low."

"Your grade in the class is based on how much you are here and participating. Don't worry about how your endurance is. You aren't graded by how fit you are."

"Yeah, but I'd really like to see how much my endurance has improved. I just don't think the step-up test is the way to figure that out. You know?"

"That's the test. Don't worry about it. Like I said, it won't impact your grade given your um, your situation."

"Okay." I look away, my face hot with shame and embarrassment just as it was ten years earlier on roller skating day. I want to be able to see how much I have grown from all of my work. Two weeks later, my changes are marginal. I cannot lift my foot high enough to complete the assessment with enough speed to test my cardiovascular health. I still receive an A in Physical Education (given my situation). I decide I am not going to participate in organized exercise in public anymore. My body is disruptive, and ultimately, I am excluded.

For the next decade I avoid any sort of group fitness activity. I still find repeated cardiovascular movement soothing, but my larger body can no longer balance and swing my tight spasming leg over a bicycle seat and hold the bike steady at the same time, so I spend hours jumping on my trampoline at home, and once in college, on elliptical machines at the gym. I swim, hike, and canoe outdoors, but always by myself or with a trusted friend or two who are at ease with my body's movements. When I finally opt to try once again to allow group discussion and evaluation of my disabled, fit body, it does not go well.

2006: But I Want to Stretch

I am 25 years old, in graduate school, and I fell in love at the gym. My boyfriend, Evan, tore his hamstring playing in an intramural soccer league and spent months recuperating on the elliptical next to me. He convinces me that anyone who can go on an elliptical as long as I can, can do other fitness activities with other fit people (mainly him). I believe him. We start road biking. At first, he steadies the bike as I climb on. Then, we transition to a tandem bike that he can steady while I climb onto the back seat and then swing my leg over. I'm strong and fast. We bike for miles every day through the Summer and Fall. In Winter, I take up downhill skiing. Learning is painful. I cannot do "Pizza-French Fries." (Pizza-French Fries is a beginner's skiing method. Skiers keep their feet straight in "French Fries" and to turn them to a "Pizza slice" to slow down.) Because the doctors rotated my feet forward, I cannot turn my toes in to slow down. Evan's friend, Nick, tries to tell him it isn't safe for me to learn to ski if I cannot do Pizza-French Fries but Evan is undeterred. To stop, I just fall. Skipping Pizza-French Fries accelerates my learning and I can shift to the edges of my skis, balancing on the icy Maine mountains in a matter of weekends. I keep up with Evan and Nick on black diamond runs within a month while Nick's girlfriend Jessica is still doing Pizza-French Fries on the beginner green slopes.

I enjoy the graceful gliding that both skis and bicycles offer my tight cerebral palsied limbs. Moving through the Maine mountains is soothing for me. In both biking and skiing spaces my personal performance of athleticism momentarily passes for "normal." Those around me attribute my limp to soreness after miles on a bike and everyone sort of limps in ski boots. I grow at ease exercising in public and being interpreted as fit. I am stronger with more endurance than most people I encounter. My anxiety is lower because of my constant opportunities to move.

One night, while having a glass of wine with my best friend Kasey and complaining that I felt stiff after a long day of skiing, she convinces me to take a yoga class with her at the university gym. I tentatively agree. "You're so fit. You'll be great and it's centering. It will help you stretch more." Kasey has just started getting into fitness herself and has shared how uncomfortable she feels at her larger size in fitness spaces, but has found the benefits are worth the awkwardness. Knowing that she knows embodied marginalization, I trust her assessment. We decide to go to yoga after my graduate seminar.

I show up at the dimly lit yoga class in my bootcut deep purple pants and a cropped white tank top. My stomach is flat, my muscles are defined. My outfit mirrors the majority of the other undergraduate and graduate students in the room. My hair is up in a similar messy bun. The toes of my scarred bare feet are painted a glossy black and match the other young women in the room desiring a "winter polish." Aesthetically, standing still, I blend, except of course for the fact that my shuffling stiff gait means that my pants are soaked to halfway up my calves from walking through the snow outside. I unroll my blue yoga mat that I checked out at the front desk next to Kasey's. I am late and the only spots left are in the front of the room. I feel the familiar tightness of anxiety around my heart and lungs and stomach. I hold my bare midriff for a moment, then touch my collar bone. My arms attempt to shield the parts of my body where my anxiety coils. Kasey knows me well. She sees my anxiety and smiles encouragingly but I'm unsure of my decision. Yoga is about flexibility, balance, and grace. I'm strong with great cardiovascular health, but the constant firing of my brain to tighten my muscles means I'm awkward and stiff. My face grows hot as I see the women around me touch their foreheads to their toes with their legs splayed open in butterfly stretches. I take a deep breath and sit at the edge of my mat and smile nervously at Kasey, picking at the soggy hem of my pants rather than revealing my restricted motion by stretching.

The yoga instructor enters. She looks about 20 years old, with curly, dirty blond hair. Her crop top and low-slung yoga pants are similar to mine. She smiles, breathes deeply, and says "Namaste." She bows, and takes her spot at the front of the room. I also take a deep breath. The entangled nerves loosen. She begins. We start with three sun salutation sequences. I can touch my toes, jump my feet back, lower to a hovering push-up, arch my back, and stretch my heel cords. It feels good. I'm glad to be here. She follows this warm-up by telling us to stand in "mountain pose" with our palms facing forward to begin a "warrior sequence." The first warrior pose begins in a lunge position. Everyone else does it effortlessly. I fall to the side. I can't spread my legs far enough apart in either direction to balance. I am careful not to stumble into the woman next to me. Kasey smiles. We both laugh nervously as I try to get my balance. The woman on my other side glares. The instructor snaps, "If you are not taking this seriously, you can just leave."

"I'm taking it seriously. I'm sorry. I'm nervous. My balance isn't very good."

"Well, this is the easiest pose we are going to do today, so if you can't do it, you may just want to do something else with your time." She looks angry. Maybe she thinks I am being disruptive on purpose.

My face burns. Kasey snaps at the instructor. "She has cerebral palsy and she's never done this before. She's a student here and entitled to be in this class."

The woman next to me snaps back at Kasey, "Well, she looks like she's in better shape than most of this class. She should be able to hold a warrior pose for a few seconds without falling into someone. If she took it seriously, she could."

"I really can't do it. I'll leave." My face burns. My lungs are tight. My breaths are shallow. My brain spins with anxiety. This is no longer centering. I need to move. I look at Kasey and then toward the door.

"You're all a bunch of assholes," Kasey calls over her shoulder as we walk out, leaving our university borrowed yoga mats in the middle of the floor.

Kasey and I head to the locker room to grab our shoes before heading up to the ellipticals upstairs to peddle our frustrations away. The familiar repetitive cardio movement calms me. My chest unravels. I can breathe freely. Kasey and I decide to sign up for the spinning class the following night. I can independently climb on a bike that is securely balanced on a stand and with my feet clipped into the peddles I can peddle longer, faster, and at a higher level than many of the people around us. My body is welcomed and revered. A few months later, Evan and I take up a 5:00 AM spinning class together every morning to train first for long days of skiing and then our adventure honeymoon in Costa Rica.

In my 20s, my body performs a cultural conundrum in fitness spaces, challenging the normative cultural performance of group fitness. I am thin and toned from hours of cardiovascular and strength building activity, but still tight, sore, and awkward. How people communicate about my body changes across fitness spaces. People smile and offer compliments on ski slopes, biking trails, and spinning class. My embodied performance is accepted and revered as fit. However, as a FitCrip, I am not welcomed in able-bodied athletic spaces where competition is a primary goal rather than personal speed, agility, and fitness milestones.

2007: They'd Rather Forfeit

I meet Evan for a midday coffee in the University library cafe. He looks upset.

"What's going on?"

"I talked to Bjorn and Nick about why they forfeited yesterday instead of asking you to play. Guess what they said?"

"What?" I clutch my skim pumpkin latte a little too tight. The cover pops off and hot foam spills onto my thumb.

"They said they thought that it may be too dangerous for you to run around with other people. You might fall. You fell on a Black diamond with Nick and you were totally fine. He knows how strong you are. I don't get it. I mean we needed one more girl to play, and they forfeited instead of asking you."

"I know. I'm glad you didn't push it. I would've just been uncomfortable if they didn't want me there."

"I know, but it sucks. They suck. You're so athletic. Way more athletic than either of their girlfriends. Jess can run for like 2 minutes without stopping."

"I'm fit, Evan, but I'm not really an athlete. I don't compete in anything."

"Well, you could. You're so strong. They're stupid."

Evan sips his coffee with a frustrated crease in his forehead. I wonder if I should explain that my fit body with its atypical movement just isn't welcome in dominant competitive sports spaces. I'm not a para-athlete competing among other atypical bodies. I have no desire to perform a competitive athletic identity. I like to move to manage my body and emotions, not to win. I agree that it seems absurd that his coed intramural soccer team forfeited rather than ask me to play. I look down as my defined leg muscles tremor with a spasm and then look outside. I'd rather ski or bike than play soccer anyway. I'm relieved when Evan opts to not play soccer the following year so we can spend more time doing these activities together.

I have multiple stories from this time in my life. My peak physical fitness was also the time when I was constantly unsure and vulnerable whenever my stiffness and lack of balance were on display. I tended not to stretch at the gym. I waited until the evening when Evan could balance my legs on his shoulders, pushing gently to try to get the stiff muscles to first shake, and then release, allowing my leg to move to a 90-degree angle before going to sleep when the involuntary spasms will once again reduce my range to 60 degrees by morning, and then 45 degrees by the end of the day. I assume all of my fitness activities will remain outside of structured, collective spaces. I pursue the soothing emotional and physiological rewards of cardiovascular movements with Evan on our bike, swimming, hiking, and skiing for the next decade and a half, until I reached an age and cultural space that caused fitness spaces to open to the performance of my tight, spastic, strong body.

2019: And I Want to Heal

I'm 38. I feel panicked but hopeful. It's been years since I have been on a bicycle or skis. Being a professor and a mother leaves so little time to prep the necessary equipment and coordinate travel to suitable places to ski or bike. I tried running to keep in shape, but my atypical gait meant that my hips and knees were perpetually sore. Once my knee started to swell, I stopped running. A month later I was pregnant with my third son. A year and a half later, I was pregnant with my fourth son. My only sources of exercise are a home elliptical and walking and swimming with my four children ranging from an infant to eight years old. My body, while at a deemed "healthy" weight by my doctors is heavier than it was in my 20s, my torso is wider from my abs separating while I carried my third son, with increased damage from my fourth. I found out on a forum for women with cerebral palsy that barre classes can increase range of motion, balance, and flexibility while the signature "tucking" clenching of muscles can heal the deep abdominal muscle separation from pregnancy.

I go to the website for the chain Pure Barre and immediately feel anxiety coiling around my lungs and stomach. My toes curl under with spasms. The women in the ads are beautiful and thin with their hair in the familiar buns and ponytails of those who rejected my presence in that yoga class years ago. They stand next to what looks like a ballet bar, all holding the same pose. I'm nervous, years of being isolated and rejected in group fitness activities, particularly those that require grace and flexibility, flood back. Still, I am desperate for more mobility. My body is still muscular and strong. My cardiovascular health is good. I wonder if maybe it is worth a try. I sign up for a complimentary class.

I arrive in my purple lululemon leggings and pink tie dye tank top, my hair pulled up in the familiar messy bun. Tan socks with sparkles on the top and sticky soles hide the scars on my feet and my gnarled stiff toes. Like the majority of the room, I am in my 30s, white, thinnish, with an income that allows me to consider the $120 a month membership. There are women who are younger, older, BIPOC, and plus sized, but they are in the small minority. Almost everyone here looks like me, except I limp and they do not. I know that my balance and flexibility are nowhere near the average of the room, but they won't know that until the workout begins. I hold the small exercise ball, resistance bands, and set of two-pound weights required for the workout. A woman, also with a messy bun, who looks strikingly similar to the yoga instructor who kicked me out of class years ago, (except 15 years older, with blond highlights concealing new gray hair), smiles.

"Did you hurt your leg? I pulled a muscle in here a few days ago. It was killer, but great, like every barre class, right?"

"Um, actually I always limp. I have cerebral palsy. It makes my muscles tight and my gait kind of stiff and jerky. I don't have a lot of range of motion."

"I'm so sorry. Is it progressive? My sister has Multiple Sclerosis. I know how hard that can be."

"No. It's not progressive. It's a brain injury. It won't get worse but I'm getting older and had four babies in seven years. I'm hoping this will help increase my balance and flexibility."

"It definitely will. So many of us are hurt in here. You'll blend right in with all of our bad knees, and bad ankles, and arthritis, carpal tunnel, back problems, bunions. Gosh we're all breaking down, aren't we? Aging is awful."

I smile back at her. The knot in my chest begins to unravel. Maybe it will be fine.

And it is. Heather, with her bouncy blond ponytail and muscular legs, tests her head mic before taking us through cardio and strength series followed by stretching. Throughout the workout there are modifications for people who cannot round their backs for crunches, feel unstable on one foot, cannot support their weight on their wrists for triceps dips, or balance on their toes. My balance and range of motion are limited, but modifications are readily available and not disruptive among the aging bodies around me. The fact that my leg is not as high as others and that I must press the heel of foot into the carpet and flex rather than stand on one foot is not questioned. Many people use a variety of accommodations. In addition, my whiteness, my middle-class income, and my size allow my disabled body to blend in this fitness space. My embodied performance meets their aesthetic. Pure Barre features me on their social media, first for my local studio and then for the national chain, to showcase how bodies like mine are welcomed alongside the other featured members. As a mother of four in my late thirties, I am finally accepted in a group fitness space. I deeply value my time with the other women at the studio and the support and guidance of the instructors. The mixture of cardio, strength, flexibility, and endurance help my body heal. I grow stronger and leaner. My anxiety is manageable despite my hectic life as an academic mother. The first time I venture off of my property during Covid-19 lockdown is to go to an open-air socially distant barre class. Everyone is happy to see me. My cerebral palsied body's performance of fitness belongs among theirs. I share enough of their cultural markers to be among them. As their bodies age and change, mine is no longer jarring.

Hopes for Our Mortal Changing Bodies

My disabled body, at this moment in time, occupies places of privilege. I am categorized as noticeably disabled, but also middle aged, white, thin, professional, and middle class. My aging body's performance is accepted as familiar in fitness spaces with others that share these identity markers. Compulsory able-bodiedness and the cultural gaze are not disrupted in my personal performance of disability. I am noticeably disabled, but also familiar. The bodies around me are at ease due to the changes in their own ability over time. In turn, my anxiety lessens and my mobility improves. As my body continues to age and change with time, rejection may follow. Cultural meanings and relationships surrounding our ongoing performances of self are unstable, but in this cultural moment, I fit.

The evolution of how others perceive my personal performance over time reveals that fitness and disability are not inherently opposite but culturally negotiated, situational, open to merge, and diverge across interacting bodies with varying identity markers. The term FitCrip is uncomfortable. It makes people's brows furrow. Defined simply as the antithesis of normal, stories of disabled bodies illuminate that identity categories are culturally created, interpreted through communicating bodies situated in culture and open to change. As other bodies break down, fitness adaptations for my disabled body become comfortable and familiar.

People communicate about me and my body with ease within fitness space. Of course, this acceptance and familiarity largely stem from my body meeting other criteria that allows one's personal performance of self to be welcomed in the Pure Barre studio at this moment in time. My race, weight, perceived socioeconomic status, and normative performances of gender and sexuality, coupled with athletic, fit bodies navigating sports injuries in their twenties to fifties, allow my disabled body to be non-disruptive to the collective performance of "Pure Barre." I am accepted and valued in this particular context.

Disability, defined only as the diagnosed deviation from normal, highlights how what is normal is not inherent or natural but radically contextual and open to change based on the expectations of other bodies in those spaces. Our need for deviant, non-normative bodies to reject is culturally created through communicative repetition that allows performativity surrounding ableism to emerge and be reiterated. Each encounter also offers us an opportunity to resist and dismantle ableism, co-constituting inclusion through our interactions.

This understanding extends across stigmatized embodiments. Bodies marked and marginalized by size, race, ethnicity, socioeconomic status, age, sexuality, and gender are also included and excluded based on our understandings of how those bodies relate to ours, in the particular communicative spaces and moments that we move through. As cultural members we must work to realize that our biases toward marginalized bodies are culturally compelled, situational, and open to reinterpretation across our communicative interactions. Each encounter is a performance of self with others with an opportunity to co-constitute new understandings.

With this knowledge, we can collectively work to resist the desire to reject bodies that we categorize as not belonging in a particular cultural context through our daily communication practices. Rather than assuming this desire to reject is "natural" and that the body is disruptive to a cultural space, we can work to open contexts. This action acknowledges communication as the foundation of our shared meaning-making. Through this communicative shift, we have the potential to grow more at ease with the bodies we are in, the bodies we are becoming, and the bodies around us, without the need to restrict when and where we allow bodies to move among and with us.

All bodies change over time, and are vulnerable to be interpreted differently in different cultural spaces. Acknowledging the power of how we communicate about bodies offers the opportunity to transform our culture to flex around and adapt to all bodies. And this transformation offers the opportunity to embrace embodied experience across time, contexts, and situations, allowing us to be included in spaces that bring us happiness and joy for as long as our bodies are here.

NOTES

1. A note on my word choice. I reject person-first language. I am not a woman with whiteness. I am a white woman. I am not a woman with straightness. I am a straight woman. I refuse to defy the common grammatical rules of how we use adjectives in the English language to talk about my body. I am disabled. It is just another identity marker for me.

2. I use the term "crip" to denote that I claim and embrace disabled identity and that I am committed to infusing disabled consciousness and standpoint into dominant cultural understandings, values, rituals, and narratives. I use the term "Fit" strategically. I toyed with the terms Criplete (a play on athlete) or Crip Jock. Criplete implies that I formally compete in sports. I do not. Jock implies a performance of masculinity and/or anti-intellectualism which are not part of my experience. Fit, denoting a perception of cardiovascular and physical health and endurance, is the most accurate term to describe my identity. Parathlete and Super Crip literature do not speak to my lived experience because I am not a competitive athlete. I do not desire to join a space designed for disabled bodies to train and compete. Desiring the physical cardiovascular activity for embodied experience is different than the desire to compete in organized sports and requires a separate line of inquiry.

References

Boylorn, R. M., & Orbe, M. P. (2014). *Critical autoethnography: Intersecting cultural identities in everyday life*. Left Coast Press.

Butler, J. (1993). *Bodies that matter: On the discursive limits of sex*. Routledge.

Denzin, N. (1997). *Interpreting ethnography: Ethnographic practices for the 21st century*. Sage.

Garland-Thomson, R. (1997). *Extraordinary bodies: Figuring physical disability in American culture and literature*. Columbia University Press.

Garland-Thomson, R. (2009). *Staring: How we look*. Oxford University Press.

Langellier, K. M., & Peterson, E. E. (2004). *Storytelling in daily life: Performing narrative*. Temple University Press.

McRuer, R. (2006). *Crip theory: Cultural signs of queerness and disability*. New York University Press.

Merleau-Ponty, M. (1962). *Phenomenology of perception*. Routledge.

Rich, A. (1980). Compulsory heterosexuality and lesbian existence. *Signs, 5*(4), 631–660.

Scott, J.-A. (2018). *Embodied performance as applied research, art and pedagogy*. Palgrave Macmillan.

CHAPTER 9

On a Scale of One to Ten: A Lyric Autoethnography of Chronic Pain and Illness

Shelby Swafford

> This is a story about you, about your body in the world around you, about the edges to these sacks of flesh, these bags of blood and bone, of meat and gristle, of lymph and lyricism we all walk around in. Or don't walk around in. (Ferris, 2008, p. 242)

I am in pain. But if you asked me where I hurt, I couldn't tell you. I can't locate it in a precise part of my body, though my attention may be drawn to a particular part, a particular pain, in any particular moment in time—a shooting pain in my shoulders, a stabbing pain down my legs, an aching pain that gathers in my lower back with the weight of each day's end. Sometimes, late at night (or early in the morning), before I am finally able to will my body to sleep, I try to remember what a painless body felt like, and I become less and less convinced that such a thing ever really exists—in any stable sort of way, at least. Maybe it's because the longer you live in pain, the harder it is to imagine the possibility of living without it. Or maybe it's because, for me, imagining the possibility of living without it is sometimes too painful to bear.

I am in pain. I am *constantly* in pain. I repeat those words because sometimes they are all I have; all I can grasp on to. If you asked me where I hurt, or why I hurt, or how I hurt, I couldn't tell you. I can't locate it in language, though my attention may be drawn to a particular word, a particular phrase, in any particular moment in time—a long-awaited diagnostic label, a doctor's orders, a symptom descriptor that finally feels *right*. Sometimes, late at night

---

S. Swafford (✉)
Southern Illinois University Carbondale, Carbondale, IL, USA
e-mail: sswafford@siu.edu

© The Author(s), under exclusive license to Springer Nature Switzerland AG 2023
M. S. Jeffress et al. (eds.), *The Palgrave Handbook of Disability and Communication*, https://doi.org/10.1007/978-3-031-14447-9_9

130   S. SWAFFORD

(or early in the morning), before I am finally able to will my body to sleep, I try to put into words what my pained body feels like, and I become less and less convinced that the language to explain it ever really exists—in any stable sort of way, at least. Maybe it's because the longer you live in pain, the harder it is to imagine the words to describe living with it. Or maybe it's because, for me, imagining such descriptions seems like too much weight for any words to bear.

I've lived in this version of my body—my pained body, my sick body—for years now. It's hard to pinpoint a beginning, a precise point of time my body began to live this way, because there is no clean, clear divide between "before" and "after" in my body's memory. To story it that way would be a disservice to the reality of living in my body and dishonest to my body's orientation to time. It would be a narrative infused with "a *compulsory nostalgia* for the lost able mind/body, the nostalgic past mind/body that perhaps never was" (Kafer, 2013, p. 42, original emphasis). Compulsory nostalgia animates dominant "curative" frameworks of time, constructed futures in which "the only appropriate disabled mind/body is one cured or moving toward cure" (p. 28). The curative frameworks that fuel compulsory nostalgia assume a "before" self and "after" self for those with acquired disabilities, "with a cultural expectation that the relation between the two selves is always one of loss, and of loss that moves in only one direction. The 'after' self longs for the time 'before,' but not the other way around" (pp. 42–43). But my body is not bifurcated, and it does not only move in one direction; chronic conditions can trouble the very concept of a cure.

In this chapter, I attempt to explore the "crip time" of living with chronic pain and illness through lyric autoethnography, to tell a story of my body that resists compulsory nostalgia, curative frameworks, and ableist temporalities. To do so, I first review the theoretical foundations of crip time in recent disability studies literature. Next, I discuss autoethnographic methods within disability studies research, and particularly the use of lyric autoethnography to blend poetics and personal narrative, center the embodied experiences of disabled people, and textually construct crip time. I then include my own lyric autoethnography in the form of ten poetic and narrative vignettes, using the numerical rating pain scale as a heuristic for writing through my memories of chronic pain and illness. Through this method of critical/creative storytelling, I highlight the communicative construction of disability—how we come to understand disability from the stories we are told and the stories we tell about and by disabled bodies.

"Bending the Clock" with Crip Time

Disability is often framed in the language of time, and disability studies scholars have carefully attended to this temporal dimension of disability. As Kafer (2013) notes, "Familiar categories of illness and disability—congenital and acquired, diagnosis or prognosis, remission and relapse, temporarily able-bodied and 'illness, age, or accident'—are temporal; they are orientations in and to time...and could be collected under the rubric 'crip time'" (p. 26). A subversion of normative frameworks of time—"ableist time" or "straight time"—crip time taps into the disability community's reclamation of *crip* as a site of identification, politicization, and academic inquiry (McRuer, 2006). Related to queer theory and the concept of queer time (Halberstam, 2005; Muñoz, 2009), crip time troubles linear constructions of time with firm delineations between past/present/future. Kafer (2013) further explains:

> Crip time is flex time not just expanded but exploded; it requires reimagining our notions of what can and should happen in time, or recognizing how expectations of "how long things take" are based on very particular minds and bodies. We can then understand the flexibility of crip time as being not only an accommodation to those who need "more" time but also, and perhaps especially, a challenge to normative and normalizing expectations of pace and scheduling. Rather than bend disabled bodies and minds to meet the clock, crip time bends the clock to meet disabled bodies and minds. (p. 27)

This description of crip time "bending the clock" points to a temporal reorientation away from normative/ableist/straight time and toward disabled subjectivities. In this way, as Sheppard (2020) notes, crip time is "messy and untidy and moves in unexpected ways, just as crip bodyminds can be messy and untidy and move in unexpected ways" (p. 45).

Samuels (2017) reflects on her perspective of crip time in six ways. She first positions crip time as "time travel," as she argues that "disability and illness have the power to extract us from linear, progressive time with its normative life stages and cast us into a wormhole of backward and forward acceleration, jerky stops and starts, tedious interval and abrupt endings" (para. 5). Second, crip time is "grief time," or "a time of loss, and the crushing undertow that accompanies loss" (para. 10). Samuels is careful here to situate this loss not as a wish for a cure, or as a manifestation of curative frameworks, but as a "wish to be both myself and not-myself, a state of paradoxical longing that I think every person with chronic pain occupies at some point or another" (para. 11). Third, crip time is "broken time," as it "requires us to break in our bodies and minds to new rhythms, new patterns of thinking and feeling and moving through the world" (para. 13). Disrupting capitalist notions of productivity, crip time "insists that we listen to our bodyminds so closely, so attentively, in a culture that tells us to divide the two and push the body away from us while also pushing it beyond its limits" (para. 13). Fourth, Samuels says "crip time is sick time," particularly for the United States, in which "you have to work hard to earn the time to be sick" (para. 17). Fifth, "crip time is writing time" (para. 21); writing *about* crip time often means writing *in* crip time, when our bodyminds are well enough to wrangle the words. Finally, for Samuels, crip time is "vampire time," the "time of late nights and unconscious days, of life schedules lived out of sync with the waking, quotidian world" (para. 25).

Crip time challenges compulsory nostalgia in cultural narratives of disability, disrupting the kind of "cure-driven future [that] positions people with disabilities in a temporality that cannot exist fully in the present, where one's life is always on hold, in limbo, waiting for the cure to arrive" (Kafer, 2013, p. 44). Kafer further articulates a desire for crip futures, "futures that embrace disabled people, futures that imagine disability differently, futures that support multiple ways of being" (p. 45). This "critical crip futurity" is essential because of the cultural insistence on erasing disabled people from the future and positioning disabled bodies as "the future no one wants" (p. 46). As Kafer argues, our pasts and presents in which disabled people—especially disabled people of color, queer disabled people, disabled women, poor disabled people, and/or people with developmental and psychiatric disabilities—"have faced sterilization, segregation, and institutionalization; denial of equitable education; health care and social services; violence and abuse; and the withholding of the rights of citizenship" make exploring disability in time and imagining crip futures crucial (p. 46).

WRITING IN CRIP TIME WITH LYRIC AUTOETHNOGRAPHY

I approach writing my experience of chronic pain and illness in crip time through autoethnography. Autoethnography embraces the connection between personal narratives and the social, cultural, and political contexts which inform our understandings of them. As Ellis (2007) notes, "doing autoethnography involves a back-and-forth movement between experiencing and examining a vulnerable self and observing and revealing the broader context of that experience" (pp. 13–14). This pendulum process pivots on a hinge between the "auto" (self) and the "ethno" (culture), highlighting this ever-present relationship between personal narratives and larger cultural systems. As a research methodology, autoethnography recognizes the critical potential of evocative, self-reflexive storytelling for critiquing and challenging dominant cultural narratives of identity.

Holman Jones et al. (2013) identify four distinguishable characteristics of autoethnographic writing: "purposefully commenting on/critiquing of culture and cultural practices, making contributions to existing research, embracing vulnerability with purpose, and creating a reciprocal relationship with audiences in order to compel a response" (p. 22). In combining these four elements, autoethnography compels social change by illuminating the political and cultural dimensions of our personal experience, akin to the feminist consciousness-raising mantra "the personal is political." As Silverman and Rowe (2020) argue, it is "in the moments of vulnerability, of the body on the page, of exposing individual truths against the backdrop of universal claims, that we begin to change ideas about which research matters and whose voices are worth being heard" (p. 94). Gingrich-Philbrook (2007) further maintains that autoethnography exists in an epistemic/aesthetic double-bind, or between the demand to create knowledge on the one hand and the demand to create art on the other. The autoethnographer's task is to work within both ends of this double bind, or "perform between them" (p. 312), attending to both the epistemic value of storytelling and the aesthetic value of craft. In short, auto-ethnography is a way to textually perform the aesthetic/epistemic poetics of our personal/political stories.

Autoethnography and Disability Studies

Disability studies scholars have illustrated the potential of autoethnography as a research method for critically storying embodied experiences of disability (Birk, 2013; Esposito, 2014; Huell & Erdely, 2020; Kasnitz, 2020; Morella-Pozzi, 2014; Richards, 2008; Scott, 2013, 2020). In her autoethnographic account of kidney failure, transplantation, and recovery, Richards (2008) offers a helpful typology of three kinds of illness autoethnographies: testimony, eman-cipatory discourse, and destabilized narrative. The destabilized narrative in par-ticular, those which "show how messy and contingent reality can be [and] invite the reader to cocreate meaning" (pp. 1723–1724), Richards argues, "might empower [health care providers and lay people] to question their beliefs and attitudes to illness and disease and thereby come to new negotiated mean-ings of their positions" (p. 1726). Because of this destabilizing potential, auto-ethnography offers a way into describing the "messy" and "contingent" realities of disabled bodies living in crip time.

Some scholars have turned to autoethnographic methods to explore their experiences of chronic pain, making visible the invisibility of living with chronic pain while responding to the contestation of chronic pain conditions within dominant medical discourses. As Birk (2013) argues, "What I hope to demon-strate is that chronic physical pain—despite its traditionally being seen as the most private and personal of experiences—is also a public, even political issue" (p. 391). By telling her story of chronic pain, Birk exemplifies the complexities of diagnosis, performing pain, and the inability of the medical establishment to recognize her pain as real. In the hinge between "auto" and "ethno," Birk troubles the line between public and private in chronic pain discourse. Similarly, Huell and Erdely (2020) co-created their autoethnographic performance about back pain, self-care, empathy, and the U.S. medical system, *I Got Your Back (IGYB)*, to "challenge the conceptualization of pain as interior, demon-strating the relations between empathy and performance" (p. 385). They argue:

> Experiences of chronic pain are subjugated knowledges meant to be hidden and locked away, disguised and dismissed by the wearer. *IGYB* attempts to meet the call to co-performative witnessing by crafting an empathy that oscillates between what is told and what is not, what our bodies can and cannot do, will or will not say or do. (p. 393)

Autoethnography offers a methodological orientation to this oscillation, cen-tering embodied epistemologies and emphasizing aesthetic possibilities for writing experiences of pain, illness, and disability.

Crip Poetics and Lyric Autoethnography

Poetry is one such aesthetic possibility for autoethnographic inquiry. Autoethnographers, and qualitative researchers broadly, have recognized the potentials of poetic inquiry as a creative, critical, and embodied methodology (Faulkner, 2016, 2017, 2020; Pelias, 2021; Prendergast et al., 2009; Speedy, 2015). Building on extensive literature on poetic inquiry, Faulkner (2017) defines poetic inquiry as "the use of poetry crafted from research endeavors, either before a project analysis, as a project analysis, and/or poetry that is part of or that constitutes an entire research project," and argues that "the key feature of poetic inquiry is the use of poetry as/in/for inquiry" (p. 210). Disability studies scholars have recognized the possibilities of poetic inquiry for writing their bodies in crip language, for capturing the particularities of living in a disabled body through poetics. In his ars poetica, *The Enjambed Body*, Ferris (2004) explores his body's relationship to poetry to articulate a crip poetics, one that recognizes "the body is not just an important image *in* poetry, it is also an important image *of* poetry" (p. 219, original emphasis).

Poetic inquiry offers a method of "language in play" for scholars to study experiences of chronic pain (Kuppers, 2007, p. 95). For example, Esposito (2014) uses poetic autoethnography to explore her understanding of embodiment after acquiring chronic pain. Rather than rely on traditional narrative structure to tell her story, she translates her autoethnographic journals into poems, with the hope that the poetic voice "enables multiple readers to identify and, perhaps, to trouble their own notions about the body and mind" (p. 1180). Similarly, Ferris (2008) uses the poetic voice to explore the idiosyncrasies, intimacies, and relationality of pain, written as a lyric address that constructs "the iterative and iterable performance of an event in the lyric present, in the special 'now' of lyric articulation" (Culler, 2015, p. 226).

As a particular thread of poetic inquiry, lyric inquiry "is based on a conviction that using expressive and poetic functions of language creates the possibility of a resonant, ethical, and engaged relationship between the knower and the known" (Neilsen, 2008, p. 94). Neilsen (2008) argues that the term *lyric* has "the roomy capacity to include the expressive, the poetic, and the phenomenological in our scholarship" while disrupting false dichotomies between "literary or academic, subjective or objective, science or art, humanities or social sciences" (p. 94). In this chapter, I use the term *lyric autoethnography* to describe this kind of roominess, this blend of the expressive, poetic, and phenomenological. In choosing this term, I follow Neilsen's assertion that "Lyric…is embodied language: the self (and selves) of our personal landscapes embodied in aesthetic forms of writing" (p. 95). Faulkner (2020) further notes that the lines between lyric poetry and narrative poetry are blurry, and that "we can talk about lyric elements in narrative poetry and vice versa" (p. 79). I approach my autoethnography in this chapter leaning into this bleeding boundary between narrative and lyric.

In what follows, I include poetic and narrative fragments of my embodied experience of chronic pain and illness. In an effort to textually represent the crip time of living with chronic pain and illness, I employ a layered account approach, a technique that Ronai (1995) argues offers "an impressionistic sketch, handing readers layers of experience so they may fill in the spaces and construct an interpretation of the writer's narrative" (p. 396). I use the numeric pain scale as a heuristic for writing through these experiences, layering poetic and narrative fragments marked with non-linear numerical headings to signify the messy and arbitrary linguistic process of communicating pain and illness.

On a Scale of One to Ten

Seven

On a scale of one to ten, with one being no pain and ten being the worst pain imaginable, how much pain are you feeling right now? I can imagine a lot of pain. (Ferris, 2008, p. 243)

I waited almost two months to see the first rheumatologist after insisting for almost two months that the doctor at my University's health center who diagnosed me with mono was wrong. I told her I had mono before, and this was different. I told her I was in pain. Constantly. I told her all of my lymph nodes were swollen most of the time. I told her I was exhausted. I told her it felt like I was going to burst out of my body.

She didn't believe me.

I was persistent.

I think she gave in and wrote me the referral just to get me off her back, to pass me along as someone else's problem. And honestly? That's fine with me. After weeks of dragging myself into the health center to see her—to insist to her that I knew my body better than she did at this moment—I was too sick and too tired to keep fighting her much longer.

I didn't really know what rheumatologists were or what they did, but when I finally received the referral, I felt like I had won.

That feeling didn't last long.

After a physical examination and about 15 minutes of questions and answers—most of which he spent cutting me off, deciding for me when I had said enough, too much, and it was *his* turn now—he diagnosed me with fibromyalgia and prescribed me a regimen of medications that was so expansive I can't recall them all now. I do recall, though, that they added up to 63 pills per week.

I saw him only twice more after my initial diagnostic visit. When I tried to schedule my third follow-up appointment, his office never returned my call.

One

It started with small red spots. They began to appear, like magic, all over my body. I noticed them on my forearms first—clusters of deep maroon dots, collecting in constellations on my otherwise pale skin.

It's January, late afternoon, and I've been wearing my coat all day so I don't know how long they've been there. But once I see them, I can't look away. Sitting at my dining room table, arms turned out in front of me as if to receive a gift or a hug or a child, I stare at them, tracing their patterns around the curve of my hands, my wrists, my elbows, trying to make sense of where they came from and what they mean.

"I think I'm having an allergic reaction," I tell my husband, inviting him to join me in my inspection. It seems as if he can hear the twinge of concern in my voice; he moves quickly to take my arm in his hand. He turns it, gently, running the tip of his finger down my skin as if he's trying to trace the clusters, too.

"Call the doctor."

He says this with a sense of urgency I haven't yet thought to feel. It's been a few months since my first diagnosis and we're both still learning how to live with my body's unfolding uncertainties. It's past 4 p.m.; the University health center where my primary care physician is located will be closing soon. My fingers shake and stumble as I dial the number in my phone.

Eight

> This is where
> I'd write a poem –
> about the ocean
> or the stars
> or my grandmother's kitchen –
> if only my hands
> didn't hurt.

Two

"Student Health Services. How can I help you?" I recognize the voice on the other end of the line as one of the regular receptionists; she is warm and helpful and kind. I feel myself exhale into the receiver.

"Hi, yes. I know the health center is closing soon, but I just noticed red spots appearing all over my body, and I'm not sure what they are, but I might be having an allergic reaction." My confusion shifts to panic as I realize it's Friday. They aren't open on weekends, and the only after-hours care in the area is the local hospital emergency room. I glance at the clock. 4:15. "I can't afford another fucking ER visit," I think to myself. "Is there any way I could come in and get checked out?"

"Sure, honey. I'll let the doctor know you're coming. Can I put you on hold just a moment?" Her voice is calming, grounding, reassuring. Exhale.

"Of course," I say, hoping she can hear my smile. "Take your time."

4:16.

4:17.

4:18.

4:19.

"Okay, honey. The doctor knows you're coming. She won't leave before you get here." She says this with a giggle, as if she can feel the tension through the phone, as if she could relieve the pressure with her laughter. Exhale. "Can you tell me, so I can tell the doctor—these dots, are they on the palms of your hands or the soles of your feet?"

I turn my arms out again, ready to receive, and see the spots are still spreading.

"Yes. My palms." I reach down and rip my boots off, then socks, until my feet are bare and I can search the soles of them for the stars my body is creating.

4:21.

"Soles, too."

Exhale.

"Alright. Okay. That's okay, honey." (For whatever reason, I don't believe her when she says these words, but I receive them, as one would a gift or a hug or a child.) "You live far from campus? How soon can you get here?"

4:22.

Time seems to stop and start speeding up, all at once.

"I'll be there in ten."

Six

Right now, in this moment, I'd give it a five. Maybe. I guess it really depends on what you mean by "one" and "ten"—what you think of when you think of "unimaginable pain," what you imagine when you imagine a body existing with no pain at all.

Right now, in this moment, I can bear it, and that has to count for something. Some days, it reverberates through my body with such intensity I can hear it in my head, completely consuming my every thought, as if my nerve endings are raging against my skin, ravaging through bone and blood to burst out of me, as if my body cannot contain it.

Some days—most days—pain is the first sensation I feel when I wake in the morning, made better or worse by the shallowness or depth of sleep, by how far my body is willing to let me wade into the waters of my subconscious. All the experts have told me not sleeping worsens the pain. None of them have told me how to sleep through the pain.

So, some days, when I wake from struggled sleep, when pain is the first sensation, I feel waking from struggled sleep, when the pain I first feel waking from struggled sleep is overwhelming, I lay in bed a little longer.

Some days, I lay in bed all day.

Three

On a scale of one to ten, with zero being nonexistent and ten being, well, use your imagination, how would you rate your karma? (Ferris, 2008, p. 246)

After the first test,
the doctor thinks there has been a mistake.
"We have your results, but they can't be correct.
Your numbers just aren't adding up.
Something must be wrong with the machine."
A poppy blooms in my arm's crease, deep
red, swollen, petals wilted at the edge.
It took three nurses five tries to get the needle in.
To find a vein that would hold its weight,
that could hold its weight without collapsing
in on itself. "You bruise like a peach," the third says
and I can almost taste summer in my grandmother's kitchen.

After the second test,
I lose count of the number of vials they need
because my numbers just aren't adding up,
because there has been no mistake,
because they have my results, and they are correct,
and there is nothing wrong with the machine.
The doctor says my blood vessels are bursting, beneath
the blooming poppy, beneath the crimson stars, beneath
the scars and freckles and birthmarks.
"Petechial hemorrhages," she calls them,
before sending me for test three.

Four

In normal blood—healthy blood—platelet counts range from 150,000 to 450,000 per microliter. Platelets allow our blood to clot, stopping the bleed. Our bodies send platelets signals when our vessels are damaged, and with a kind of evolutionary magic, these tiny plate-shaped cells extend themselves outward, growing tentacles to latch onto broken vessels, like an octopus swimming through the depths of our inner oceans in search of shipwrecked remains. Our bodies, too, are a carefully balanced ecosystem. Too many platelets and your blood spontaneously clots, usually in the arms or legs, which can cause heart attacks or strokes. Too few and you will bleed out.

My first test read 2000.

My second, zero.

Ten

On a scale of one to ten, with one being completely alone, truly unique, new, fresh, solo, out there, and ten being peas in a pod, kernels in a sea of corn, drops in an undifferentiated ocean, photons in a galaxy of suns, moments in a universe of eternity—how do you live with yourself? (Ferris, 2008, pp. 250–251)

There are a lot of things I don't know, but one thing I think I do know now is the thin membrane between life and death, between breath and not; how death can be so close you can feel it brush against your skin. It's the sensation of saline pumped into your bloodstream through a catheter in your right arm's artery; the faint taste of chemicals on your tongue from the casings of the poisons that save you; that glimmer of pity people get in their eye when they think you're dying. Or when they know you're dying. It's your veins collapsing under the weight of your skin; the hollow ringing in your left ear right before you hit the floor; the poppy blooming in the crease of your arm. It's falling asleep to an image of the person you love waking up in a pool of your blood. It's waking up in a pool of your sweat instead. It's the tower in your dreams, built tall, of plastic orange prescription bottles. It's you locked away—safe, still breathing—up top. It's your body, committing suicide on a cellular level.

And then it's you deciding if you even want to stop it.

Nine

The doctor at my health center tells me I need to go to the ER and that she is calling an ambulance. "I can't fucking afford an ambulance," I think to myself but actually say aloud. "I'm sorry. I'm flustered. The numbers just aren't adding up. But I'm a graduate student, and you've seen our insurance, and I really *can't* afford an ambulance. It's only a few blocks. I'll be okay to drive myself."

I think I say this aloud, or something like this aloud, but if I'm being honest, all I really remember is that somehow I convinced her to let me drive myself to the hospital, because the next thing I know, I am laying in the ER while no less than three nurses try no less than five times to get an IV needle to prick into the poppy in the crease of my arm.

And I know I didn't get there in an ambulance. I would remember the bill.

I remember wearing a powder blue gown, but don't remember how I got it on. I remember shivering from the cold, though I had no less than three blankets, because I remember a nurse, a woman who was warm and helpful and kind, checking on me to ask if I was comfortable. I remember someone—I don't remember who—asking me about do-not-resuscitate orders and next of kin. I remember my husband was there then, because I remember this person that I do not remember asking us how long we had been married. I remember when we said "almost six months," she chuckled and joked that we "were just jumping right in with that 'in sickness or in health' vow, huh?" I remember that every prick of that needle into my poppy hurt more than I would've ever thought possible.

I remember seeing no less than two doctors—the ER physician and the on-call hematologist. I remember MRI scans and CT scans and EKGs. I remember one blood transfusion, then two. I remember the hematologist telling me about the IVIG treatments I would receive, but all I really remember from that conversation is that he said something about them being derived from the stem cells of bunnies. I remember him telling me that, considering all of the tests they had done so far, there were two causes that seemed most likely in my case: a rare blood disease called ITP, or leukemia.

I remember the moment he told me I don't have cancer.

I remember each minute waiting to hear those words felt eternal.

I remember the relief.

I remember being admitted for more transfusions, more bunny stem cells, to replenish the octopuses in my blood. I remember finishing my last treatment a little before 4 a.m., and I remember thinking this was the longest 12 hours of my life. I remember remembering how surprised I was when I learned that the lifespan of an octopus is so short.

I remember that a little after 4 a.m., after all the tests and transfusions and IVIGs, when the numbers started to add up again and the commotion settled, I insisted on being discharged.

I remember saying, "I've been here too long. I need to go home." I remember saying, "I can't sleep here." I remember thinking, "This will cost too much. I need to go home." I remember thinking, "I will burst out of my body if I stay here."

I remember the hematologist, sleepy-eyed from the excitement, coming into my room to ask me why I needed to leave, if I was sure I needed to leave. I remember telling him I had PTSD, and was panicking, and wouldn't be able to rest. I remember him asking me how far I lived from the hospital. I remember how quickly I said "two blocks."

I remember his reluctance when he agreed, and how he gave me his personal cell phone number to call in case my skin started showing signs of bursting blood again. I remember the sternness in his voice as he instructed me to report back on Sunday for another blood test.

I remember wincing at the wilted petals of my poppy.

I remember the sweetness of a peach.

I remember being wheeled out of the hospital, per protocol, just before the break of dawn. I remember ranting to the aide about Michel Foucault and panopticons and the medical gaze.

I wish I remembered exactly what I said.

I remember collapsing into bed that morning and imagining thousands of tiny vessels collapsing along with me. I remember sleeping for what felt like the shortest 12 hours of my life. I remember I dreamt I was an octopus, swimming alongside a rabbit in an ocean of blood.

Five

On a scale of one to ten, with zero being the concrete beneath your feet and ten being your own crown chakra, how much does your mind weigh? (Ferris, 2008, p. 253)

"On a scale of one to ten, dear, how bad is the pain today?" She smiles at me when she asks this, and I think it's because by now she knows what I'm going to say. The perks of having a favorite nurse at your favorite doctor's office. She's the kind that doesn't chastise me when I admit I haven't taken my meds every morning or haven't kept up with the stretches during stretches of bad pain days; she listens and takes notes when I tell her why.

She believes me.

She is rare.

"Well, I know you know that I struggle with this question every time I see you," I say to her, turning my arms out, as if to receive something, anything, in the bulky sleeve of the blood pressure monitor she slips around my upper arm. "I can walk and talk and I got out of bed this morning, and that has to count for something."

She laughs, as if to relieve the pressure. I wince at the tug of the sleeve on my skin, at the shooting pain in my shoulders, the stabbing pain down my legs, the aching pain that gathers in my lower back with the weight of each day's end. And then I remember bursting blood vessels, and cells growing tentacles, and a three-foot catheter pulled from a pic line in my right arm.

"Let's just call today a four."

CONCLUSION

We need stories about disability. We need stories about disability from disabled storytellers. We need crip stories. We need to witness, document, and tell crip stories because to do so is to invest in crip futures, futures that include disabled people—and I mean that literally. Even in the midst of the COVID-19 pandemic, a mass disabling event in which disabled and chronically ill folks have been particularly vulnerable to disease and death, the tired logics of capitalist ableism continue to prevail. As I struggle to find a way to conclude this experiment of writing in crip time, I realize that part of this struggle stems from the stories currently being told about disabled bodies like mine. Just yesterday, for example, the director of the Centers for Disease Control and Prevention, Rochelle Walensky, proudly told reporters at a COVID-19 press conference that "the overwhelming number of deaths, over 75 percent, occurred in people with at least four comorbidities. So these are people who were really unwell to begin with, and yes, really encouraging news in the context of Omicron" (cited in Spocchia, 2022, para. 3–4). I think about what it means to be "encouraged" by the deaths of so many disabled and chronically ill people. Who does such news encourage? How is that statement meant to inspire hope? And why am I supposed to have confidence in what can and should only be described as eugenics?

When I heard Walensky's comment, my first thought was about all the disabled people who were not only just told that their lives were expendable, but that their deaths would be encouraging. My second thought was about all the people who listened to that statement without so much as a flinch; those who see themselves, at best, as unaffected, and at worst, those who were, in fact, encouraged. So, we need crip stories. I repeat those words because sometimes they are all I have; all I can grasp on to. As Kafer argues, "It is my loss, our loss, to not take care of, embrace, and desire all of us. We must begin to anticipate presents and to imagine futures that include all of us" (p. 46). Storying my experience of chronic pain and illness is my way of contributing, in small part, to this anticipation and imagination.

Like Samuels (2017), I have been writing my experience of chronic pain and illness in crip time, over many years, collecting fragments of stories and poems in journals and notebooks and on scraps of loose-leaf paper, "wonder[ing] if I will ever get it done" (para. 21). As I write *in* crip time, I hope to capture crip time in my writing. Through lyric autoethnography, I was able to collect these various fragments into a narrative frame, layering them in and out of time, releasing my body's story from the limitations of linear, chronological structure to resist the compulsory nostalgia of curative temporal frameworks. Following the crip poetics of disabled poets, I lean into the lyric voice, relying on expressive, evocative, and phenomenological language. By doing so, I hope to illuminate the embodied and cultural complexities of living with chronic pain and illness so readers might develop a deeper understanding of such experiences (if they do not also already live with chronic pain and illness themselves). This is not to suggest that my experiences stand in for all experiences of disability, or all experiences of chronic pain and illness—such embodiments are intimately individual and shaped by a variety of cultural factors like race, class, gender, sexuality, nationality, diagnostic status, visibility of disability, and more. But it is to say that telling disabled stories in this hinge between "auto" and "ethno" offers a way to explore and challenge the intricacies of ableism as it manifests in our daily lives.

References

Birk, L. B. (2013). Erasure of the credible subject: An autoethnographic account of chronic pain. *Cultural Studies↔Critical Methodologies, 13*(5), 390–399. https://doi.org/10.1177/1532708613495799

Culler, J. (2015). *Theory of the lyric.* Harvard University Press.

Ellis, C. (2007). Telling secrets, revealing lives: Relational ethics in research with intimate others. *Qualitative Inquiry, 13*(1), 3–29. https://doi.org/10.1170/780040947

Esposito, J. (2014). Pain is a social construction until it hurts: Living theory on my body. *Qualitative Inquiry, 20*(10), 1179–1190. https://doi.org/10.1177/1077800414545234

Faulkner, S. (2016). *Poetry as method: Reporting research through verse.* Routledge.

Faulkner, S. (2017). Poetry is politics: An autoethnographic poetry manifesto. *International Review of Qualitative Research, 10*(1), 89–96. https://doi.org/10.1525/irqr.2017.10.1.89

Faulkner, S. (2020). *Poetic inquiry: Craft, method and practice* (2nd ed.). Routledge.

Ferris, J. (2004). The enjambed body: A step toward crippled poetics. *The Georgia Review, 58*(2), 219–233. https://www.jstor.org/stable/41402415

Ferris, J. (2008). Just try having none. *Text and Performance Quarterly, 28*(1–2), 242–255. https://doi.org/10.1080/10462930701754499

Gingrich-Philbrook, C. (2007). Autoethnography's family values: Easy access to compulsory experiences. *Text and Performance Quarterly, 25*(4), 291–314. https://doi.org/10.1080/10462930500362445

Halberstam, J. (2005). *In a queer time and place.* New York University Press.

Holman Jones, S., Adams, T. E., & Ellis, C. (2013). Introduction: Coming to know autoethnography as more than a method. In S. Holman Jones, T. E. Adams, & C. Ellis (Eds.), *Handbook of autoethnography* (pp. 17–48). Left Coast Press.

Huell, J. C., & Erdely, J. L. (2020). Crafting empathy in *I got your back: A one(ish) person show exploring pain, empathy, and performance. Text and Performance Quarterly, 40*(4), 384–396. https://doi.org/10.1080/10462937.2020.1853213

Kafer, A. (2013). *Feminist, crip, queer.* Indiana University Press.

Kasnitz, D. (2020). The politics of disability performativity: An autoethnography. *Current Anthropology, 61*(21), S18–S25. https://doi.org/10.1086/705782

Kuppers, P. (2007). Performing determinism: Disability culture poetry. *Text and Performance Quarterly, 27*(2), 89–106. https://doi.org/10.1080/10462930701251066

McRuer, R. (2006). *Crip theory: Cultural signs of queerness and disability.* New York University Press.

Morella-Pozzi, D. (2014). The (dis)ability double life: Exploring legitimacy, illegitimacy, and the terrible dichotomy of (dis)ability in higher education. In R. M. Boylorn & M. P. Orbe (Eds.), *Critical autoethnography: Intersecting cultural identities in everyday life* (pp. 176–194). Left Coast Press.

Muñoz, J. E. (2009). *Cruising utopia: The then and there of queer futurity.* New York University Press.

Neilsen, L. (2008). Lyric inquiry. In J. G. Knowles & A. L. Cole (Eds.), *Handbook of the arts in qualitative research* (pp. 93–102). Sage Publications.

Pelias, R. J. (2021). *Lessons on aging and dying: A poetic autoethnography.* Routledge.

Prendergast, M., Leggo, C., & Sameshima, P. (2009). *Poetic inquiry: Vibrant voices in the social sciences.* Sense.

Richards, R. (2008). Writing the othered self: Autoethnography and the problem of objectification in writing about illness and disability. *Qualitative Health Research, 18*(12), 1717–1728. https://doi.org/10.1177/1049732308325866

Ronai, C. R. (1995). Multiple reflections of child sex abuse: An argument for a layered account. *Journal of Contemporary Ethnography, 23*(4), 395–426. https://doi.org/10.1177/089124195023004001

Samuels, E. (2017). Six ways of looking at crip time. *Disability Studies Quarterly, 37*(3) https://dsq-sds.org/article/view/5824/4684

Scott, J.-A. (2013). Problematizing a researcher's performance of "insider status": An autoethnography of "designer disabled" identity. *Qualitative Inquiry, 19*(2), 101–115. https://doi.org/10.1177/1077800412462990

Scott, J.-A. (2020). Disrupting compulsory performances: Snapshots and stories of masculinity, disability, and parenthood in cultural currents of daily life. In A. L. Johnson & B. LeMaster (Eds.), *Gender futurity, intersectional autoethnography: Embodied theorizing from the margins* (pp. 24–36). Routledge.

Sheppard, E. (2020). Performing normal but becoming crip: Living with chronic pain. *Scandinavian Journal of Disability Research, 22*(1), 39–47. https://doi.org/10.16993/sjdr.619

Silverman, R., & Rowe, D. (2020). Introduction. Blurring the body and the page: The theory, style, and practice of autoethnography. *Cultural Studies↔Critical Methodologies, 20*(2), 91–94. https://doi.org/10.1177/1532708619878762

Speedy, J. (2015). *Staring at the park: A poetic autoethnographic inquiry.* Routledge.

Spocchia, G. (2022, January 9). *"My disabled life is worthy": CDC prompts backlash for comments on Omicron deaths."* The Independent.. Retrieved January 10, 2022, from: https://www.independent.co.uk/news/world/americas/cdc-omicron-covid-disabilities-deaths-b1989524.html

CHAPTER 10

On Being a Diabetic Black Male: An Autoethnography of Race, Gender, and Invisible Disability

Antonio L. Spikes

One…
Two…
Three…
Four…
One hour…
Forty-five minutes…
Thirty minutes this time…
One hour again. Maybe I am getting better…

These were the thoughts that were coursing through my mind days before the most monumental event in my life. During this period, I was a part-time hourly wage worker at the now-defunct grocery store in Georgia called BI-LO. I noticed my body was going through changes such as frequent urination. The symptom was so gradual that I had not noticed it until I realized that I had not drunk any water for two hours and was still going to the bathroom. Not to mention that I found myself drinking more water, which only aggravated the increased urination symptom. It felt like I was turning myself into an irrigation system.

A. L. Spikes (✉)
Coe College, Cedar Rapids, IA, USA
e-mail: aspikes@coe.edu

© The Author(s), under exclusive license to Springer Nature Switzerland AG 2023

M. S. Jeffress et al. (eds.), *The Palgrave Handbook of Disability and Communication*, https://doi.org/10.1007/978-3-031-14447-9_10

145

This particular symptom scared me, but not because of the novelty. I was afraid due to the familiar terror of these symptoms, which are related to diabetes. This disorder runs in my family. I am very knowledgeable about increased urination and increased thirst symptoms. My mother experienced these symptoms in her diabetes management when she had consistently high blood sugar levels. The signs were so bad that she had to wear adult diapers towards the end of her life. The thought that I could potentially receive the same disease that killed my mother and many other Black people before or just after their fiftieth birthday made me cringe.

As a result, I thought ignoring the symptoms was preferable to confronting the reality that I had type one diabetes. Whenever I had the urge to urinate, I would tell my bookkeeping manager that I have to resume another task, though I was going straight to the restroom. Unfortunately, some coworkers have noticed my bathroom habits and reasonably inquired if I was okay. My symptoms were even noticeable to some of our regular customers.

One night as I was working at the cash register, a tall Black woman wearing a black formal dress outfit topped with a black netted hat and glasses came to my lane register. I smiled at her because she was one of our regulars. Because of that, she began to inquire about my health. I remember the conversation going as such:

"Son, you lost a lot of weight!" she said with surprise in her voice.

"Why, thank you!" During this time, I was working on weight loss, and I loved my progress.

"No, no. I'm concerned. You lost a lot of weight in a short time."

"Well, I've been working hard at it, ma'am."

"No...I don't think that's what it is." She said this hesitantly. In the South, we have an implicit custom that we only step into someone's business (or involve ourselves in someone else's affairs) if it is urgent. Otherwise, we stay out of people's business. For those who do not understand the term "business," it typically means personal matters. She was struggling with this cultural norm until she ultimately broke it.

"I don't mean to get too personal, but do you have diabetes in your family?"

I remember thinking, "Damn!" because at this point, I was fully aware that I most likely had the disease. Again, I was hoping that by ignoring it, the symptoms would go away. But this nice woman had other plans.

I answered the question. "Yeah, my great-grandmother had it. My mother died from it in 2004."

"Oh, I'm so sorry," she said sweetly and mournfully. "I asked because diabetes runs in my family too, and seeing you like this reminds me of what my family members looked like before their doctors diagnosed them." She grabbed her bags from the end of the register counter and placed them in her buggy (or "cart," if you prefer). She looked at me all of a sudden with a visual sternness. "All I'm saying is you may want to get yourself checked. Diabetes is not something to ignore or play with. Have a good evening."

That short conversation stuck with me throughout the entirety of my pre-"diabetic diagnosis" journey. Over time, my symptoms worsened. I could drink almost a gallon jug of water and would still be thirsty. Excessively drinking water only exasperated my symptoms. I would urinate every two hours, to every hour, to every 45 minutes. The constant urination would not stop when I slept at night. I had very little sleep to the point that I was sleepwalking throughout my home, knocking on the door of my stepbrother and asking him what he was doing in his room. Esteemed readers, waking up from your sleep-walking episode is not pleasant at all! It was also embarrassing, considering I rarely talked to my stepbrother.

I told my father what I had feared, and his answer was my own: ignore it. Since we were a Black lower-income family that lacked health insurance, we had to pay the total cost of healthcare. Money was a constant concern in our household. When I pressed him about my fears, he asked, "Do you have doctor money? No? Then don't worry about it. You'll be fine." I tried to do what he said since this was my initial response to my symptoms.

The following day, I could barely move. I felt like death. The fatigue was so much that even sleep could not alleviate it. A couple of minutes after eating breakfast, I could not keep it down. I vomited in the toilet in a manner you would see in a movie: on my knees, head very much in the toilet bowl, empty-ing the contents of my stomach. I sluggishly grabbed our home cordless phone and told my dad what happened. To my surprise, back then, he came back home from work and took me to the doctor. It was at this point that I received the most unfortunate news that I had type one diabetes.

This essay is an autoethnography about my life as a person with type one diabetes. However, this will be an autoethnography that highlights how racial, gender, and class identity issues affected the processing of my diagnosis, my lifelong treatment, and how my family adjusted to it. I support these stories with research into race and disability. I hope that you, esteemed reader, will become more knowledgeable about living as a Black male diabetic. Perhaps, depending on who you are, you may feel a particular connection.

RACE AND DISABILITY AND DIABETES

Researching about race and type one diabetes is simultaneously an illuminating and frustrating experience. While researching this topic, I often feel like I am made invisible twice: by the automatic assumption that diabetes is type two diabetes and the reflexive belief that only white people have type one diabetes. It is true that type one diabetes primarily affects white people (Mayer-Davis et al., 2009). Still, I hardly find this fact justifiable to exclude people of color's perspectives about this disease from research.

Scholars have shown that Black people are more likely to develop type two diabetes than type one (Goad, 2018). Because of this reality, some people assume Black people were more likely to develop this disease due to our genes. However, Spanakis and Golden (2013) have shown no genetic differences between Black and white people's risk of contracting type two diabetes. This discovery has led some people to suggest that the difference is due to the racism that Black people experience, which in my experience leads to added stress, which also leads to high blood sugar levels.

Looking at the research, I again do not see myself. I feel that I need to incorporate myself into a category of a disability that does not fit my reality. It is this reality of invisibility that made me realize how people racialize diabetes. As Bennett (2018) noted in his study about how politicians socially constructed Justice Sonia Sotomayer at the nexus of disability and race, diabetes is as much a disability concept as it is a racialized concept. What he noted has stuck with me about the relationship between people of color and notions of diabetes. He briefly stated that people often assume that Gloria Anzaldua had type two diabetes when she had type one diabetes. Before Sotomayer clarified the distinction, people had thought she had type two diabetes as well.

It is essential to understand the difference between type two and type one and the common racialized and ableist assumptions people attach to the causes. Type two diabetes is what people are most familiar with as caused by insulin resistance. Essentially, this disorder is characterized by the body becoming resistant to accepting insulin for glucose conversion (diabetes.org). The body does not use insulin to convert carbohydrates into energy, allowing blood glucose to stay in the blood. People usually correlate insulin resistance with an increase in body weight because research states that body weight can increase insulin resistance, though this is not always the case (Hardy et al., 2012). In other words, what became cultural gospel is that being overweight makes you more susceptible to type two diabetes.

Type one diabetes, however, is characterized as an autoimmune disorder that involves the body's immune system attacking the beta cells on the pancreas responsible for the production and deployment of insulin. Eventually, the immune system kills these cells and renders the body incapable of producing insulin. Even though these differences are very known, it is still astonishing to think about these differences. Type one and type two diabetes are essentially two completely different diseases that share a typical result. Type two is characterized by the failure to process insulin, while doctors describe type one as the inability to produce insulin.

Type two is often assumed to be caused by irresponsible actions and laziness, meaning that one has not exercised and dieted enough to avoid the disorder (Yan, 2021). Type one, when recognized as such, is considered not the fault of the individual due to its autoimmune nature (Mulvey, 2020). Considering this, one can see a pathway in which diabetes becomes racialized. Because the research often positions people of color as more likely to develop type two diabetes than white people, we are often assumed to have type two diabetes (diabetes.org). Also, people think Black type two diabetics are responsible for developing the disease due to our presumed nutritional and recreational ineptitude. It is pretty interesting to see how out of touch people are with the research on type two diabetes which has seen people of all sizes developing the disease (George et al., 2015). Moreover, because people of color are often stereotyped as lazy and irresponsible, research states that people of color are more often developing type two; people of color are often assumed and stigmatized as type two.

As a type one Black diabetic, people often think I have type two diabetes due to irresponsible dieting and exercise. The latter isn't usually evident in interpersonal communication. However, people often assume that my body has become resistant to insulin absorption because of race and diabetes. In this manner, society at large doubly invisibilized me by an otherwise invisible disability.

It is this automatic assumption of race and disability that reminds me of the DisCRT framework. DisCRT is an acronym of a subdiscipline within the critical race theory framework that brings disability studies and critical race theory into a conversation (Annamma, Connor, & Ferri, 2013). To remedy this, they created DisCRT to talk about how ability and race mutually construct each other. A typical example that reveals the relationship between race and disability is how schools often place children of color in special education units at disproportionate rates (Annamma, Connor, & Ferri, 2013).

Looking at this example, I can see how some people within the education system unconsciously link race and disability. For instance, my third-grade language arts teacher recommended to my mother that I should be in special education, even though I had stellar grades in my other classes. I remember having a difficult time in her classroom, particularly due to her calling me out and holding me as an example of what not to do. I remember struggling over concepts I learned in a previous grade. Sometimes, I doubted if I ever learned concepts such as generalization and context clues.

One night, after the parent-teacher conference, my mother and I had a conversation about my language arts teacher.

I remember asking, "What did Mrs. Lane say?"

My mother sighed exasperatedly. "She thought you would do better in a special education class"

I remember being shocked by her suggestion. Then my mother added, "I asked her why she thought you should be in a special education class when you had good grades in your other classes She couldn't answer. Then I told her about how she mistreats you in class and the effect that may have on your school performance."

My mother smirked. I asked her, "What did she say?"

"She didn't say anything. She couldn't say anything. But, I did ask her why your unpreparedness equated to you having a mental disorder. I simply told her that she should not mistake your unpreparedness for lack of intelligence. And she should be nicer to you."

I didn't think this was a pleasant conversation because Mrs. Lane equated mental disorders to lack of intelligence. This was a sore spot for us since we have someone in our family with a mental disorder. Luckily, my mother understood what was happening and essentially told her that my being unprepared does not equate to a disability. Also, having my unpreparedness raised as a bad example to other students to gain compliance from them did not help either. Once my mother brought this up to her, things became better.

Moreover, the connection with race and disability is what I could connect with as a type one diabetic. From the puzzling lack of prescription medication, the automatic assumptions of what type I have, the cause of my health status, and the early resistance I have had with family members, race has been critical to constructing my disability status. Race has also been integral to how I understood my disability status, to the point that I did not think I had a disability despite clearly having one. In the following sections, I will discuss how my race and disability mutually constructed each other through my vignettes. Additionally, society's construction of race is integrally involved with the intersections of class and gender. The point in these vignettes is to understand how race, class, gender, and disability mutually constructed each other in creating specific situations I faced regarding my type one diabetic status.

Story One: "Let's Hope You Have Type Two"

My father and I have butted heads on many issues, including those that involve gender, class, culture, and race, though more rarely than other issues. We even clashed with the topic of diabetes. How does this happen? Well, reader, it happens like this.

My father drove me to a clinic that I never knew existed in our small town. It is funny the things you overlook when you don't rely on them to survive. I mentioned my unfamiliarity with this clinic to my father, and he stated this is the place he goes to for medical care. As a 19-year-old college student, I thought I didn't have to think about medical care until this incident. Being extremely tired, urinating frequently, suffering severe dehydration, and vomiting qualifies as a medical care emergency.

My father paid the uninsured fee, and the medical attendant immediately took me to the back. Even though I rarely go to the doctor, I knew this was weird considering that there was a waiting room for people there before me, also waiting for medical care. We walked to the back and entered the room. The room had the typical setup with a cushioned table/bed with a sheet of paper traveling in the middle and chairs, sinks, and biohazard containers where they dispose of used needles. The nurse that came in was a tall dark-skin Black woman whom I recognized immediately.

"I think I saw you before," I said, unsure if I had seen her before.

"Yeah, you have. I used to see your mother when she was in the hospital. Nice to see you again." She said this with an ironic smile. It was nice to see a familiar face. Since my hometown is small, it is pretty easy to see people in various business and institutional settings that you have noticed before. However, watching the person who took care of my mother now about to confirm my worst nightmare did not create the comfort that familiarity usually breeds.

"So, what brings you here?"

"Go on and tell her what you told me. Maybe she can make sense of it." My dad said this in a tone that indicated his frustration and puzzlement. At the time, my dad believed that much of my sudden symptoms were a figment of my imagination. It also didn't help that I had a habit of overthinking and worrying about things.

"Yeah, I've been drinking a lot of water because I've been thirsty. And, I've also been tired a lot despite not doing much. Also, I've been going to the bathroom more often than normal every hour. Sometimes even less than that. The constant thirst and urination had been going on for almost two weeks, then I finally vomited just a couple of minutes ago because I was extremely nauseous. Do you know what this is about?" I asked earnestly, though I knew what the answer was.

"Yes, sounds like you have diabetes." She said this in a prompt manner that still stunned me though I knew what her answer would be. This announcement surprised my father as well. I was correct for a change. I brought up the possibility that I could have diabetes after researching my symptoms. However, he quickly dismissed it as me imagining things. Despite this being extremely frustrating on my part, it kind of felt good and scary to know what was finally going on from a professional.

"However, to make sure, let me check your blood sugar."

I hated this. Seeing my mother have her fingers constantly pricked when she was alive made me wish I never had to do this for myself. I remembered the first time my mother checked my blood sugar, and the pain was so intense I was close to tears. The same pain came back again as the nurse checked my blood sugar.

Let's talk about blood sugar levels for a sentence. Healthy blood sugar levels vary from professional/organization to professional/organization. Some say that the range for blood sugar levels should be between 80 mg–120 mg. Some also say it should be between 70 mg–130 mg. The blood sugar monitor registered my level at 440.

"Yeah, you have diabetes." the nurse answered affirmatively. "The question now is determining what type of diabetes you have. You are familiar with type one and type two, correct?"

"Yeah, somewhat similar. Type one is where you need insulin, and type two is where you need pills, correct?"

"Yes and no, it's more complicated than that. Type one means your pancreas no longer produces insulin, and type one means that your pancreas still produces insulin, but your body no longer responds to it because it has become insulin resistant. I will do a C-Peptide test, which will determine whether or not there is insulin present. If there is none, you have type one, and you will have to take insulin for the rest of your life. If you have type one, then we can start you on pills to reduce your insulin resistance. Either way, we are going to give you insulin now because your body urgently needs it."

I was certainly not excited about having a shot since I was scared of needles. But interrupting this thought process was my dad.

"Which one is more expensive to treat?" my father stated concernedly.

"Well, by the numbers, type one is due to the cost of insulin. Pills are often cheaper than insulin, though, on the whole, diabetes is still pretty expensive. One vial of insulin often costs hundreds of dollars."

I remember thinking: just fucking great. My part-time cashier job does not pay me enough to take care of a chronic illness. At this point, I remember reading information about diabetes and how Black people are more likely to get it and die from it. It also uncomfortably made me remember my time with my mother. Before I lived with my father, my life was the typical one you would see in over-dramatized movies on the Black Entertainment Television network and Lifetime: the child of a poor single Black mother on EBT/SNAP benefits, Medicaid, and later on disability benefits. Despite these federal programs, we were far from living the life; and there were times when she struggled to pay for anything. I remember thinking that her health probably worsened due to inadequate care or simply the stress of poverty. As a child, I used to see insulin vials in her refrigerator. As a preteen, I stopped seeing them. Hearing the cost of insulin, I was starting to wonder if I stopped seeing them because she could not afford them.

"I'm going to draw your blood, and then the doctor will come in and tell you what your next steps are going to be, depending on what the results are."

The nurse's words brought me out of my reverie. I was back in the present. After the nurse left, I told my dad that I don't think I can finance my existence now.

"It will be okay. Let's hope you have type two then. I don't know if I can afford your insulin since you can't." My father's comment represents one of the things I simultaneously found inspiring and annoying at times. Even after I say something about not financing my existence, he still tells me not to worry. Though I would like to find comfort in his easygoingness, I still struggled with figuring out my financial life and imminent physical survival.

At this point in my life, I was making minimum wage at a part-time cashier job in a grocery store. The minimum wage was $5.85 at the time of my diagnosis: July 2, 2008. Days afterward, the federal minimum wage would slightly jump to $6.55. Despite the raise, it still was not enough for me to independently afford my insulin. I began to look at myself as an odd medical commodity that I had to pay for and could not dispose of readily. For disposing of myself would end my life, painfully I imagined back then. It became pretty daunting to me that the job that I worked hard to secure in my teenage years would not pay me enough to live. No amount of Christmas gift cards and employee appreciation days were going to help me financially. Despite how astonishing this was, I decided to push that aside and focus on getting better. It was the only thing I could think of without making myself lose my mind.

A tall white woman entered the room with a smile on her face. "Hello, Mr. Spikes."

"Hello," I said.

"I've gone over the notes your nurse gave to me, and we are going to give you insulin now."

As she gave me an insulin shot and gave me instructions on how to do this myself, I asked her, "when will you know whether or not I am type one or type two?"

"In a couple of days. I will call you and let you know."

"The thing is, I can't afford the insulin. I don't have insurance because my job doesn't offer it, and private insurance usually excludes pre-existing conditions, which I now have. Is there a way for you to provide me with affordable insulin?" At this point, I was uncomfortably fumbling with words because I was ashamed that I could not finance my existence.

"Don't worry. You're not the only one I see that struggles with affording insulin." She said with a smile. "I'm going to send you home with a vial of Lantus so that you can continue medicating yourself."

"What is Lantus?"

"It's the insulin I just gave you. You only need one shot per day. I'm also going to give you a blood sugar monitor and a prescription for test scripts. I'll warn you, though. Blood sugar test scripts can be expensive. The monitor I will give you has ten scripts already in it, but you will need more since you have to test at least four times a day."

After a while, she told me how to afford insulin on my low income, more information about how to use insulin, test scripts, when to test, the normal range, and what the follow-up visit will look like. Though she hit me with an avalanche of information, I was slightly relieved that I finally knew what was happening to me. However, I was still terrified of feeling sick like this again due to mismanagement or, quite simply, lack of funds.

"You Used to Be a Fat Boy? Oh, I Know." Automatic Assumptions of Disability Categories

Before I attended a four-year university, I enrolled in a community college. It was after one year of college that I received my diabetes diagnosis. It was so immediate that I wondered if I somehow contracted the disease on my own. I mean, geez. I heard of the freshman 15, but I lost 15 pounds and still gained diabetes. It was almost like a cruel joke.

For most of my life until this point, I was an overweight person. People in my life often shamed me into losing weight. As a kid, I wanted to have a joyous life, not frequent reminders of my impending diabetic death. Unfortunately, I had such a childhood where people thought making me aware of risk factors for early death could get me to acclimate to the dominant image of Black boyhood masculinity and play on the court. I began losing weight in other ways. When I finally lost weight, I was happy. However, then I realized that the weight loss was due to me getting diabetes. And type one diabetes is not caused by being overweight, nor is type two. In other words, it was diabetes all along.

In my second year of college, I was excited to room with my cousin. He had a habit of bringing people from our hometown and the campus we were on into his room. He would often introduce them to me, stating that I need to meet more people. This was one of these occasions where I just waltzed into his room and met a familiar crowd of people.

There were three men and one woman in his dorm room, all Black and all familiar. His male friends were people I have seen on and off in his room. However, the woman was a past classmate I had in a unique classroom where only four students enrolled, including myself. During those times, I would regularly visit my cousin's dorm room. Like many dorm rooms, our rooms were connected by a shared bathroom, which allowed us to have our own space without sharing a room. At that point, and even today, privacy and distance were significant to me.

"Hello, everyone," I greeted routinely. My cousin and his friends welcomed me routinely as well. From my memory of that day, it was a typical afternoon. My cousin would talk about the people he respected and disliked. His male friends would agree with him, and the female friend would sometimes chime in if she knew who they were. I would often use this time to examine the communication habits of my cousin and his friends. It may sound awful to say this, but seeing how he emulates dominant masculinity within his communication habits, how his friends do it, and how the female friends and girlfriends often contribute to this dynamic was fascinating. I have always been drawn to communication analysis.

Suddenly the conversation went to talking about torture in the U.S. Yes, the sudden topic switching was standard, especially if my cousin or I thought the previous conversation wore itself out or it wasn't exciting. I remember making the quip: "All you have to do to threaten my life is strap me to a chair and feed me a chocolate cake."

He and his usual male friends laughed. They knew of my diabetic diagnosis. However, my former classmate was confused. I saw her confused look and said, "I'm a diabetic. That's why I said that."

"Oh! That makes sense. I was thinking, how on earth chocolate cake would be torture?" she said, laughing.

We laughed for a minute until she asked a question I remember to this day.

"Did you used to be fat?" She asked this with a mix of curiosity and certainty.

I didn't know how to answer that at first until my cousin interjected with the answer. Never to mince words, he said, "Oooh, yes, he used to be."

All laughed. Then another friend chimed in. "Tim, I remember you talking about how much weight he lost."

"Yeah, being overweight causes diabetes. That's why I asked." the woman said. "I know because I got family who has it, and they got it due to not eating right and not exercising."

I deadpanned. "Yeah, I used to be overweight, and I used to think I got diabetes due to me being overweight, but that's not what happened."

"Wait, so how else can a person have diabetes?" she said, puzzled.

I described that I had type one diabetes and that my body's immune system attacked my pancreas. She had a different facial expression of puzzlement.

"I've never heard of that!"

"That's what the doctor told me. And I got the proof in my refrigerator where I store my insulin. I can't go a day without it."

I remember her apologizing for making that assumption. Though I accepted her apology and didn't hold that against her, I still think about it sometimes. I partly don't fault her for her statement because most people's understanding of diabetes is based on information about type two diabetes. I remember seeing brochures about the benefits of losing weight to avoid diabetes and very little about the threat of an autoimmune attack. So, when I break the news to people about a disease that could impact you no matter the body type, they are often surprised. I also remember my cousin's friend saying that her family members have diabetes. I would not be surprised if people informed her that, as a Black woman, she is most likely to contract and die from diabetes. Such information does not include the effects of medical racism and discrimination on people's mortality.

So Now You Are a Vegetarian?: Racialized Conflict in Managing Diabetes with Diet

"Tony, you know we are not going to change our eating habits for you, right?"

My eating habit was one of the many arguments I would have with my father and my stepmother about my diet. Due to my trauma over my sickness, I metaphorically dove headfirst into the information about healthy eating and exercise. Essentially, a healthy diabetic diet was considered a healthy diet overall, except with fewer carbs. A low-carb diet is what I found to help me manage my diabetes. Many foods I usually ate, such as white flour products, were considered an absolute no-no. My conscious exclusion of these products was also a no-no for my family.

After my diagnosis, I had received so much advice from my family members and friends. I have heard advice such as avoiding pork products, eating fried chicken but without salt, eating fried chicken by taking the skin off, and eating lots of green leafy vegetables (the only correct advice I heard). As you can see, much of my family's recommendations were either based on ignorance about the disease or impractical. Instead of taking their advice to heart, I appreciated that the suggestions came from a place of concern and good intentions.

My father and my stepmother struggled to accommodate my new diet demands. Part of that accommodation process, I believe, was fear about changing their habits or perhaps being forced to do so. It was honestly weird. I could not understand whether their resistance to my new eating style was out of concern or through perceived coercion. For instance, my stepmother would say that I had to buy food that acclimated to my own dietary needs. So, I did.

Unfortunately, this had led to more questions about the necessity of the changes:

"I'm not asking you all to change your eating habits drastically. You have noticed I eat most of your food, just less of it."

"Yes, I noticed that," my stepmother said. "Sometimes, I wondered if you have eaten."

"No, he didn't." My dad interjected from the living room.

"Yes, I did!" I said frustratingly. "Why do you always question whether or not I eat?"

"I'm questioning whether or not you eat enough!" my dad said.

"The amount I'm eating is normal for me and is a normal amount of food recommended by a whole bunch of organizations, dad."

"What I'm saying is that you need to survive off of more than just rabbit food," he said with a chuckle that just utterly annoyed me.

The conversation turned away from the original topic. I remember feeling that my father was now alluding to something that bothered him. The term that stuck out to me was rabbit food. I remember knowing full well what he meant by the word, but I wanted him to say what he meant.

"What do you mean by rabbit food?"

"I only ever see you eating vegetables. Rarely anything else."

I remember sighing heavily. "Dad, I eat meat too. I'm still the carnivore you remember. But, I eat more vegetables in comparison to meat because of my high cholesterol." I said this with a smirk.

"You be eating like those white girls on the reality shows. You know, those anorexic girls."

I sighed heavily with this. This isn't the first time my father brought up the subject of anorexia. My stepmother also brought up the issue as well as other family members. For much of my life, I had a bigger body than they were accustomed to. It must have been a shock to see me at 160 pounds instead of being above 200 pounds. I try to convey that this is an average weight for me, but they did not listen to me.

But I realized that it wasn't just about me. It was about our whole family and our community's understanding of what health looks like. For as long as I have been a member of the Black community, we have had a different version of health that was separate from mainstream society's imagination of the thin body. Black and queer people have created inclusive body spaces so that our bodies will be accepted and celebrated instead of derided (Cameron et al., 2018). These political movements have infiltrated the everyday lives of Black people by affecting the way we see the health of a body. For my Black family, our vision of a healthy body was a big body. Skinny bodies were not derided in our families, for we accepted them as well. However, I believed that my family's resistance to my body was due to their unfamiliarity with me having a smaller body and their own racialized understanding of what a healthy body can be.

"Dad, perhaps you are so used to seeing bigger bodies that you don't see a body like mine as, well, normal."

He sighs. "I don't know."

I remember being so furious about my father's statement that I could not continue the conversation. I went back to my room to contemplate what just happened. Food and body size have been an issue between my folks and me for a while. They believed I was intentionally starving myself while I knew that wasn't the case and eating the appropriate amounts of food. I was also aware that I was eating quite differently for them, such as fresher vegetables and whole grains. Interestingly, they used this moment to racialize it.

Eerie Similarities to Medical Racism Stories

"You know, doctors typically give two types of insulin to people with your disease: long-acting and rapid-acting. You know this, right?"

I could feel the confusion on my doctor's face. I was a graduate student at this time at a midwestern university. I was going to the university doctor because I was having a potentially dangerous issue with my diabetes management: wildly swinging blood sugar levels. My blood sugar levels were rarely within range (70–130) most of the time. They were either high (250–300) or low (55–69). As a person with diabetes, this is very bad. However, I began to realize how under-medicated I was as a T1 diabetic.

"Yes, I know. This discovery is why I came to you. I need rapid-acting insulin to stabilize my blood sugar levels."

"But," my doctor said with still a confused look. "I'm looking at your charts, and your doctor diagnosed you when you were 19 in 2008. It is 2014, and you were never given rapid-acting insulin? Was it even a conversation with your previous doctor?"

"It was a conversation, but they never gave it to me. I honestly don't know why."

"Hmm," he ruminated. "Though they never gave you rapid-acting insulin, as you should, it seems you still have relatively good A1C levels. Perhaps they thought that adding rapid-acting insulin would expose you to dangerously low blood sugar levels...."

"But I'm having them now. Since I will use rapid-acting insulin for food, then I don't see how that would be an issue."

"I agree with you," the doctor said with renewed perkiness. "I'm going to prescribe you Apidra. This insulin is coming from the same company that produces your long-acting insulin, so filling out the patience-assistant forms won't be a problem."

"Thank you!" I said as I left the examination room and made my way toward the waiting room.

If you are the average reader who does not understand the medical terminology employed, allow me to give you a brief definition of each of them. First, long-acting insulin (or Lantus) is insulin that T1 and T2 diabetics administer to themselves to cover our background insulin needs. The primary purpose of insulin (both natural and artificial) is to convert glucose (produced by carbohydrates) into energy to be placed into your cells. Our liver continuously delivers glucose into our bloodstream so we can have a source of energy. Long-acting insulin converts this background glucose stream into energy so that our blood sugar levels will remain stable (Healthwise Staff, 2021).

Since 2008, this was the only insulin that I have had. Long-acting insulin only needs to be administered once a day because it lasts 24 hours. However, long-acting insulin cannot convert the glucose provided by meals into insulin because it is not fast enough. This is where rapid-acting insulin (Humalog, Apidra, and Novolog) is designed to do so that diabetics can have a stable rise in blood sugar levels during their meals. I did not have rapid-acting insulin. Because of this, I had blood sugar levels that swung so wildly that they often placed my life in danger.

This severe lack of medical care made me question the prior relationship I had with my doctors, and the perspectives they may have had of me, and the experiences that my mother had with diabetes. One of the reasons I was so scared of having diabetes was my mother's ordeal with it. By the time my mother died, she had congestive heart failure, liver failure, kidney failure, vision loss, and had both of her legs amputated. Seeing my mother go through this and discovering I had the same disease in 2008 made me terrified of my future. The swinging blood sugar levels did not help matters either.

In grad school, I focused increasingly on intercultural communication. Moreover, diversity, equity, inclusion, and justice became more paramount as a sub-focus within intercultural communication. As time went on, I have become more interested in the stories of medical racism. I have primarily heard of stories from Black women about how their pain was often misdiagnosed or ignored by their doctors (Owens, 2021). These stories also reminded me of how my mother's and grandmother's pain were not taken seriously by their doctors. And, I was wondering if my doctors did not meet my needs as a Black person with diabetes.

Or perhaps it is more than just my disability and also my race. As a Black person living in the U.S. with its very public history of racism and the experiences of so many Black people, and medical racism, I cannot help but wonder if I have been the victim of such a thing. Truthfully, I used to think that medical racism was something other Black people dealt with. It seems like it is always like that. We often underestimate the distance a major social problem is to our social location.

When I look at the diagnostic stories of primarily white people on YouTube, I see a common theme: sickness, fear, diagnosis, more fear, then medical assistance. It is the medical assistance that often catches my ear. They all say that their doctors placed them on both long-acting and rapid-acting insulin immediately. Also, they set them up with a diabetes educator to understand how to use these insulins correctly. Another thing I did not have was access to rapid-acting insulin and a diabetes educator. The internet was my educator.

Between my hometown doctor and my undergraduate university doctor, I found it odd that none of the doctors found it strange that I was operating on one type of insulin instead of the standard two that other (white) diabetics had. I wondered if these same doctors would understand the racialized nature of what happened to me. Considering medical racism constantly happens to people of color, they may employ colorblind understandings of why people of color receive inadequate care at disproportionate rates (Burgess et al., 2019).

I tried to look for the experiences of other Black type one diabetics but could only find experiences from Black type two diabetics. Not to say that their experiences don't matter, but I needed to hear from Black type one diabetics. Unfortunately, finding those stories during those days was often like finding a unicorn. As such, I could not truly understand whether my situation was unique or not. However, I still find it odd that I was denied the standard insulin regimen that so many other type one diabetics begin with on day one.

COMMUNICATION, DISABILITY, AND FUTURE DIRECTIONS

What is fascinating about communication and disability is their co-constitutive nature. At the core of humans' experiences with disability is how our communication not only attempts to represent a reality around disability but also how it constitutes disability via interpersonal communication and communication within social institutions. Though there is a physical aspect to disability, humans can communicate disability by creating realities that are oppressive to people who think, speak, and move differently from the presumed majority. Additionally, social identities such as race, gender, and class also affect our perception and experience of disability. In other words, disability is not a category separated into an isolative silo but is fully present in the social construction of other identities (Annamma, Connor, & Ferri, 2013).

In the stories I presented, I showed how understandings of disability can be intersected by perceptions of race, gender, and class. What this means is that understanding disability, for some people, is fundamental in understanding other social identities and vice versa. Scholars need to continue communicating disability in an intersectional way that is cognizant about how disability and other social identities co-constitute one another. By doing so, we avoid the assumption that everyone with disabilities shares identical struggles. We can highlight more experiences with disability that don't always get told.

It is also within this potential that we see a critical part of disability and communication: the balancing of the material and the conceptual experience with disability. For example, as diabetics, the focus is often on numbers: how high and low we are. To be considered healthy, we have to have the numbers in a "happy" medium at least for 80% of a three-month time period. We also have to purchase expensive equipment to get these numbers. Though the focus on numbers is medically justifiable, I do believe there is a need to investigate how medical establishments encourage certain people with disabilities to relate to themselves more in the abstract than in a corporeal manner. An example of this contrast is a person who focuses on test results so much that they ignore their body's signs that something is wrong. Additionally, as a future path for further inquiry, it would also be a good idea to investigate what we lose in such an abstract identification with our disability and how we can communicate disability in a way that promotes a material focus on it.

CONCLUSION

In this essay, I sought to describe how issues of race, class, and disability merge together in my life through stories of events I found critical to understanding myself at those intersections. I have narrated stories that describe how my racial, gender, and class identity, and the social constructions thereof, also inform my perception of my disability and how others perceived it and its cause. The social construction of my identity as a Black man who was raised in a lower-income household affected my understanding of what was possible for life post-diagnosis. It also affected my fears and frustrations that could not have existed if I resided at other intersections of identity. Selecting the stories was difficult because there are so many. Some stories involved a deep conversation with an aunt about how things are going to change, convincing another aunt that I will not suffer as my mother had, to stories about why I resisted the disability label for such a long time. However, these were also stories that had an immense emotional load that I physically could not write. I hope you, dear reader, learned something about how the intersections of race, class, and disability can occur in the life of someone who has diabetes.

REFERENCES

Annamma, S. A., Connor, D., & Ferri, B. (2013). Dis/ability critical race studies (DisCrit): Theorizing at the intersections of race and dis/ability. *Race Ethnicity and Ethnicity, 16*(1), 1–31. https://doi.org/10.1080/13613324.2012.730511

Bennett, J. A. (2018). Containing Sotomayor: Rhetorics of personal restraint, judicial prudence, and diabetes management. *Quarterly Journal of Speech, 104*(3), 257–278. https://doi.org/10.1080/00335630.2018.1486033

Burgess, D. J., Bokhour, B. G., Cunningham, B. A., Do, T., Gordon, H. S., Jones, D. M., Pope, C., Saha, S., & Gollust, S. E. (2019). Healthcare providers' responses to narrative communication about racial healthcare disparities. *Health Communication, 34*(2), 149–161. https://doi.org/10.1080/10410236.2017.1389049

Cameron, N. O., Muldrow, A. F., & Stefani, W. (2018). The weight of things: Understanding African American women's perceptions of health, body image, and attractiveness. *Qualitative Health Research, 28*(8), 1242–1254. https://doi.org/10.1177/1049732317753588

George, A. M., Jacob, A. G., & Fogelfeld, L. (2015). Lean diabetes mellitus: An emerging entity in the era of obesity. *World Journal of Diabetes, 6*(4), 613–620. https://doi.org/10.4239/wjd.v6.i4.613

Goad, K. (2018, November 2). What's race got to do with it? *AARP*. Retrieved May 20, 2021, from https://www.aarp.org/health/healthy-living/info-2018/role-of-race-in-diabetes.html

Hardy, O. T., Czech, M. P., & Corvera, S. (2012). What causes the insulin resistance underlying obesity? *Current Opinion in Endocrinology, Diabetes, and Obesity, 19*(2), 81–87. https://doi.org/10.1097/MED.0b013e3283514e13

Healthwise Staff. (2021, July 28). Types of insulin. *The Children's Hospital of Montefiore*. Retrieved February 14, 2022, from https://www.cham.org/HealthwiseArticle.aspx?id=aa122570

Mayer-Davis, E. J., Bell, R. A., Dabelea, D., D'Agostino, R., Imperatore, G., Lawrence, J. M., Liu, L., & Marcovina, S. (2009). The many faces of diabetes in American youth: Type 1 and type 2 diabetes in five race and ethnic populations: The search for diabetes in youth study. *Diabetes Care, 32*(2), S99–S101.

Mulvey, A. (2020, December 9). Aha! An autoimmune disease. *Juvenile Diabetes Research Foundation*. Retrieved February 16, 2022, from https://www.jdrf.org/blog/2020/12/09/aha-autoimmune-disease/

Owens, D. C. (2021). Listening to Black women saves Black lives. *The Lancet, 397*(10276), 788–789. https://doi.org/10.1016/S0140-6736(21)00367-6

Spanakis, E. K., & Golden, S. H. (2013). Race/ethnic difference in diabetes and diabetic complications. *Current Diabetes Reports, 13*(6), 1–18. https://doi.org/10.1007/s11892-013-0421-9

Yan, K. (2021, January 25). Diabetes stigma is everywhere, but you can do something about it. *diaTribe*. Retrieved February 14, 2022, from https://diatribe.org/diabetes-stigma-everywhere-you-can-do-something-about-it

CHAPTER 11

Physical Disability in Interabled Romantic Relationships: Exploring How Women with Visible, Physical Disabilities Navigate and Internalize Conversations About Their Identity with Male Romantic Partners

Lisa J. DeWeert and Aimee E. Miller-Ott

Disability is not always visible to the outsider's eye (Zitzelsberger, 2005). Individuals can conceal and make choices about when to disclose to others about an invisible physical disability (i.e., one not apparently noticeable by physical appearance) (Horan et al., 2009; Matthews & Harrington, 2000). A visible disability, however, is typically readily apparent to others, meaning the person does not always have a choice whether to disclose their disability to others (Horan et al., 2009). Individuals who have a visible, physical disability may be faced with the burden of talking about their disability, especially during the beginning stages of a new relationship (Braithwaite, 1990; Braithwaite & Eckstein, 2003). Because of the visible disability, outsiders may view the individual with a physical disability as "abnormal," which quickly categorizes them into a stigmatized group identity (Byrd et al., 2019). Further, research indicates that people with visible and/or more severe disabilities often face a host of romantic challenges including meeting new people, dating, and marrying

L. J. DeWeert
Naperville, IL, USA
e-mail: ldeweer@ilstu.edu

A. E. Miller-Ott (✉)
Illinois State University, Normal, IL, USA

© The Author(s), under exclusive license to Springer Nature Switzerland AG 2023
M. S. Jeffress et al. (eds.), *The Palgrave Handbook of Disability and Communication*, https://doi.org/10.1007/978-3-031-14447-9_11

when compared to their able-bodied counterparts, often because of stereotypes of people with disabilities as dependent and asexual (Collisson et al., 2020).

Although talk about disability may help relational partners bond (Blockmans, 2015), there exists a risk that partners will respond to talk about disability in ways common among people who identify as able-bodied, including over-accommodating, over-helping, over-nurturing (Ryan et al., 2006), communicating with a condescending tone or message, or providing an exaggerated amount of sympathy that conveys pity (e.g., Duggan et al., 2010). Within the context of a romantic relationship in which partners may feel particularly vulnerable, talking for the first time about the disability and following conversations about the disability may be risky (Boucher, 2015) and profoundly impact people's experiences in the relationship and as they relate to the partner. We focused on initial interactions about the disability between women with visible physical disabilities and their male romantic partners and on the sense-making process that women voice in their talk about their romantic partners and relationships. Our aim as communication scholars was to position communication at the heart of women's experiences in their relationships.

We chose to focus on women with disabilities in interabled relationships (i.e., a relationship in which one person has a disability and the other partner does not) for a few reasons. Physical attractiveness is a highly valued component in the selection and maintenance of romantic relationships (Meltzer et al., 2014), particularly for heterosexual men, who tend to place a higher value on women's physical attractiveness than women do of men's (Li et al., 2002). Evolutionary theories indicate that men and women have grown to value different characteristics in their potential cross sex romantic partners; specifically, men are attracted to women who have traits associated with youth and vibrance (e.g., fertility), and women are attracted to men with traits of providing and protection (e.g., Weeden & Sabini, 2005). These studies suggest that a woman's visible physical disability may affect the degree to which male romantic partners perceive women as attractive and as potential partners, and women's perceptions of their own physical attractiveness to potential and current male partners. Also, scripts guiding early dating interactions (e.g., self-disclosures, behaviors on first dates) are often gender-specific, with men expected to be direct and dominant and women reactive (Romaniuk & Terán, 2022). Because we were interested in studying early dating interactions and disclosures to see if and how gender and disability intersected, it was important to us to focus on heterosexual women and their male dating partners.

Women's Disclosure of a Visible, Physical Disability

Compared to men with disabilities, women with disabilities often report having a more difficult time finding a romantic partner (Retznik et al., 2017). Further, people with a visible disability report more difficulty getting to know a potential romantic partner compared to those with an invisible disability (Retznik et al., 2017). Having a romantic partner without a disability may place added value to the communication surrounding the disability (Blockmans, 2015), as those with visible, physical disabilities report feeling like outsiders and fear social rejection (Schreiner et al., 2018), yet simultaneously experience a heightened desire for a romantic partner's love and acceptance (Blair & Hoskin, 2019). In addition, people often adapt their communication differently when interacting with someone with a physical disability compared to those without one (e.g., Duggan et al., 2010). Blockmans (2015) and Baker et al. (2011) found that people tend to over-accommodate, such as over-helping or communicating condescendingly, which, in result, threatens the autonomy of the individual with a disability. Other individuals tend to also show an exaggerated amount of sympathy, which results in a high level of frustration for the individual (Blockmans, 2015; Duggan et al., 2010) and thus, enforces a negative stereotype.

The often immediate disclosure of a visual disability, and the inability to easily avoid conversations about the disability, can have noteworthy implications for romantic relationships (Boucher, 2015). Many relationship and communication scholars have explored the level of openness during disclosures and the level of closeness following disclosures (e.g., Goldsmith & Domann-Scholz, 2013). Most people participate in selective disclosing when revealing sensitive information to someone with whom they are in a relationship, meaning they regulate the amount of information shared and rely heavily on the recipient's response for cues (Afifi et al., 2007; Petronio, 2002). Donovan et al. (2017) confirmed that engaging in some sort of disclosure within a relationship will increase relational quality and level of closeness. Agne et al. (2000) also pointed out that self-disclosing about a particularly stigmatized identity can present a whole new set of challenges, potential rewards, and uncertainty. In fact, St. Lawrence et al. (1990) highlighted that people can have difficulty sharing about their specific identity due to a fear of being stigmatized.

(Non)mutual membership within a stigmatized group, such as people with a physical disability, along with others' interactions of people within the same group, may impact the amount of communication regarding the disability within a romantic relationship (Jung & Hecht, 2004). However, anticipated reactions could be related to past conversations surrounding the identity as a whole, in addition to the couple's relational quality (Greene & Serovich, 1996). Greene and Serovich (1996) found that past discussions surrounding a difficult topic increased the likelihood that individuals would feel comfortable disclosing. They also discovered that when individuals claimed their relational quality was high with their partner, they were more likely to disclose. The nature of these conversations also tends to reinforce intimacy (Petronio, 2002). Stereotypes about individuals with disabilities may impact how people communicate with someone with a physical disability (Blockmans, 2015), communication that people with visible disabilities may wish to avoid but cannot because of the visual nature of their disability. As Zitzelsberger (2005) posited, disability is not always visible to the outsider's eye. However, a visible disability is typically readily apparent to others, meaning the person does not always choose to disclose their disability to others (Horan et al., 2009). Because the physical disability is noticeable to the eye, they lose the choice to disclose.

Outsiders may view women with a physical visible disability as "abnormal," which quickly categorizes them into a stigmatized identity (Byrd et al., 2019). How women will talk about their disability is influenced, in part, by the extent to which they see themselves as being different and their perceptions of what others think about their disability (Meisenbach, 2010). Thus, if a woman with a disability in an interabled relationship believes that their romantic partner sees the disability and will communicate differently with her, she may try to avoid conversations about the disability or limit situations that may draw attention to their disability (Meisenbach, 2010). We were interested in understanding how disability is first addressed in an interabled heterosexual romantic relationship, in which the woman has a visible physical disability. When the disability is obvious, but partners do not discuss it, the disability becomes stigmatized. Thus, our first research question was:

RQ1 : How are first conversations between women who have a visible, physical disability, and their male romantic partners who do not have a visible, physical disability, initiated?

INTERSECTION OF WOMEN'S VIEWS TOWARD DISABILITY AND COMMUNICATION WITH MALE PARTNERS

A focus on women in heterosexual romantic relationships allowed us to explore the intersection of femininity and disability for women in the relationship and expectations of beauty and identity that heterosexual men may have for their romantic partners. Further, Scott (2015) found that women's disclosure of their disability can affect their interpretations of their own feminine identity. In addition, through stereotypical perceptions of women with disabilities, people infer that women cannot meet their partners' needs, need a caretaker, and are asexual in their relationships (Collisson et al., 2020). These views toward the female body impact how women identify with their own bodies. Gaining the experiences of women with disabilities contributes to a discussion about "appearance politics, which identifies staring and spectatorship as central to the discussion of gender and disability" (Hammer, 2016, p. 413), and looking at their talk about experiences with able-bodied male partners helps uncover how they make sense of their identities and disabilities, and the intersection of both.

Many mediated Westernized discourses frame the idealized female body as a sexualized being with specific beauty standards that do not include disability (Nemeth, 2000; Vandenbosch et al., 2013). Never would an idealized feminine body have any signs of disability (Nemeth, 2000). Further, women living in Westernized cultures often view themselves from the perspective of others (Hammer, 2016). Garland-Thomson's (2002) piece on the "Politics of Staring" posits four visual rhetorics of the disabled body being on display:

wondrous (i.e., body is amazing or admired), sentimental (i.e., body is helpless, sympathetic, or pitiful), exotic (i.e., body is alien, entertaining, or sensationalized), and realistic (i.e., body differences are minimized or normalized). Staring and gazing is central in the lives of people with a disability, enforcing the idea that disability is different or uncomfortable (Hammer, 2016), or from Garland-Thomson's framework, *sentimental,* and a woman's visible disability may increase feelings of being on display and being ostracized or judged by potential or current romantic partners. Thus, our second research question was:

RQ2 : How does women's talk about dating reflect their views toward and intersection of disability, identity, and relationships with male partners?

METHOD

After obtaining university IRB approval, we recruited participants through a communication research board, emails to campus members, social media posts, and contacts with community groups. Nineteen adult women, ages 23 to 48 (with the average age of 31), who identified as having a physical difference or disability and who had been in a past heterosexual relationship, participated in our study. In Zitzelsberger's (2005) interviews of women with a physical disability, they found that many participants preferred the term "difference" instead of "disability." As we present the findings, we follow the lead of the participants in the terms used. We refer to each participant as having a "difference" or "disability" according to the terminology that each woman used to identify themselves. Fourteen were Caucasian, three were Mexican/Latina, and two identified as Eastern European. Seven participants were in a committed dating relationship, five were single, five were married, and two were engaged. All women explained their disability as visible and clearly noticeable to others. Regarding their disabilities, eight participants lack a full or partial upper extremity (e.g., arm); four reported a motor disability that affects movement and appearance of various body parts (e.g., difficulty walking or limited function in limbs); and three participants have a difference significantly impacting their hands and/or arms. Two participants have a bone disease in which visible tumors develop and cause stunted bone growth. One participant has a skin condition that causes her skin to tighten and visually appear different, and one participant has a lower extremity difference that impacts the appearance and function of her leg and foot. Three of the participants use a wheelchair. Sixteen participants have congenital disabilities, and three women acquired their disability.

One of the researchers conducted all of the in-depth qualitative telephone interviews individually with each participant that averaged 60 minutes. The data were collected prior to the COVID-19 pandemic, when people were not regularly using Zoom to conduct video interviews. Telephone interviews allowed the researchers to spread a wider net for recruiting and not focus solely on our immediate physical location. We also felt that participants may have been more comfortable talking to the researcher without physically showing their disability during the interview (thus, a reason why we chose to avoid video interviews like via Skype or FaceTime).

After gaining consent from each participant, the researcher conducting the interviews used an interview guide to ask participants the same set of questions. First, participants answered a series of demographic questions. They were asked to tell stories about any of their romantic partners (e.g., "How did you meet?"). Next, they explained their physical disability and the relationship between their disability and personal identity (e.g., "How much of your physical disability or difference is a part of your identity?"). Participants were then asked questions about communication about disability within the romantic relationship (e.g., "When did conversations start about your physical disability/difference?"). To end, participants were asked to give advice to other women with a physical disability/difference to help navigate romantic relationships. The researcher transcribed each interview, resulting in a total of 362 single-spaced typed pages. Each participant was assigned a pseudonym.

We used Braun and Clarke's (2006) process of thematic analysis to analyze interview data. First, both researchers familiarized themselves with the data by reading the transcripts. Second, the first author generated initial codes from the transcripts, by rereading the transcripts and marking specific sentences or stories that stood out as noteworthy. Both researchers then met to discuss the initial set of codes and made edits based on their interpretations of the data. The researchers then used the initial set of codes to identify specific themes related to the two research questions. When coding for RQ1, the researchers aimed to understand, from the data and in their conversations about the data, ways that the disability was first addressed in the relationship, including who first talked about the disability (if someone verbally addressed it) and how it was first addressed. For RQ2, the researchers aimed to understand, from the data and in their conversations about the data, women's talk that illuminated their views toward and the intersection of disability, identity, and relationship with male partners. Both researchers then met to determine specific wording for each theme and locate excerpts to best illustrate each theme.

FINDINGS

First Conversations about Women's Disability

We first wanted to know how women's disability was initially addressed in their romantic relationships. We learned that despite their difference being visible, the first conversation or acknowledgment about the disability is a significant one, often perceived by women as a turning point. As Hallie recalled, "It was a pivotal moment. It was my 32nd birthday ... I really made it a huge moment for me."

First Conversations Initiated by the Woman

Most often women were the first to bring up the topic. They viewed information about their disability as private, something they owned and about which they wanted to be in control, even though their disability was visible. They chose to initiate these first conversations because they often saw their disabilities as what Annie referred to as the "elephant in the room." Typically, these conversations happened when the relationship started to become serious or exclusive. Annie explained:

> When it's been like, kind of more serious, yeah, I'm kind of the one to be like "Okay, so you probably noticed but I'm just gonna get this out of the way and like explain what's going on just so it's not the elephant in the room." I feel like a lot of the time people are too scared to say anything because they don't want to offend me or, you know, they really don't know what to say. So, I'll be the one to be like "Okay, so here's the thing." But I'll only ever be the one to sit down and have a conversation about it when it feels a little more serious. You know, someone who I have some pretty serious feelings for and I want something long term with.

First conversations often took place during a time when women felt vulnerable but in a safe environment. As Gabriella explained, "It was just the night that we were just like talking a lot just about, you know, deeper things and I just— I felt more and more comfortable with him to talk about like anything."

Fear of judgment was the common reason that women sometimes delayed or tried to avoid these conversations. Jess had a really hard time bringing up her disability to new partners. She admitted, "I just—I don't want to be judged for it. I don't want to be pitied." They often also talked about not having the communication skills to have a comfortable conversation about their disability. For instance, Daisy said, "I didn't really feel comfortable in being able to explain everything, because I didn't feel that I had the confidence to go ahead and do so." This fear of judgment seemed to be more salient for women whose identities were strongly tied to their differences.

A common strategy that women used to start these conversations was to ask partners about their past experiences with people with disabilities. Annie explained:

> The way I sorta bring it up is, be like, "So do you know what cerebral palsy is? Or have you ever heard of it?" That'll be how I open the conversation. And if he's like, "No," or "Yeah, I've heard of that," it's pretty telling to me. It's like, at least you're aware versus not, ya know … But he did tell me that he's never seen it before and never really like interacted with it before. That was actually pretty interesting to me. I was like, "Wow, you've never met anyone who had any kind of disability?" Like, cerebral palsy is a pretty common. I mean, there's a lot of people who can have it.

She kept the conversation broad and asked about his general experience with people with disabilities. After understanding his exposure to disability, she then addressed her difference. Through this method of initiating conversations, participants gained important insights into their partners' experiences. Sometimes they learned that family background contributed to partners' views toward people with disabilities. For instance, Annie realized that her boyfriend's upbringing contributed to his lack of diverse experiences. She explained, "I think he was brought up so much more sheltered. Yeah, he was just not exposed to a ton … That's just how he was raised and didn't come across a lot of things outside of the norm." Daisy's boyfriend knew other people with differences. She said, "Luke is in the military and also he's seen a lot of things as far as like people missing one limb. He wasn't fazed by me." Asking about their partners' past experiences seems to be less face-threatening and simply a way to ease into the conversation, rather than jumping in and acknowledging their own disabilities first.

Women talked about the anticipation of these first conversations as stressful, although many recalled receiving anticlimactic responses from their partners. For instance, when Annie asked her boyfriend if he had noticed that she does things differently physically, his reaction was, "Yeah, I mean, I noticed it. I didn't really register it because I didn't really care." These nonchalant responses may suggest that men are uncomfortable talking about women's disabilities and do not want to focus on the difference, or the men may not view the difference as a significant part of the women and/or their relationships.

Sometimes women relied on a physical task or activity to address disability for the first time. For instance, Annie recalled having to ask her boyfriend for help putting her hair in a ponytail before they had a first conversation about her disability. She explained, "I really did not want to ask him and I was definitely embarrassed. But I did ask him, 'Can you help me, like I can't get this rubber band like around my hair?' And he totally did." This was the first time her disability had been addressed in the relationship, which seemed to open the door for more conversations. Rebecca recalled how holding hands prompted a conversation: "I was uncomfortable holding his hand for a little while, but I do remember specifically one time. I like kind of brought it up for the first time. He was like, 'No, I like that about you.'"

First Conversations Initiated by the Male Partner
Although women often broached the subject, men at times were the ones who initiated conversations. Participants reported that men often started the conversation by asking, "Can I ask you a personal question?" Men's initiation of these conversations tended to occur earlier in the relationship than when women started them. The participants always responded "yes" to this question, as they typically knew what question or topic was going to follow. Laura recalled this experience after matching with a man on an online dating website:

And before we met, he was like "Hey, so I have a question for you." He was like being super awkward about it and I knew exactly what he was gonna ask me. He was like "Oh, I don't wanna offend you, but I noticed in your pictures. Is there something wrong with your arms?" And I just said, "Oh, I was just born like this and can't raise both my arms but can still do everything."

Starting the conversation with this question appears to be direct, but prefacing the direct question with a type of "pre-question" lessens the intensity of the question, thus indicating that men understood the seriousness of the topic for women. These opening questions also allowed men to gauge women's openness talking about their disabilities.

Sometimes, men addressed the disability by not making it a big deal and instead talking about making an accommodation for the disability that women considered supportive and normalizing of their disability. For example, Nora had never brought up her physical difference to her boyfriend, and he decided they should play pool. This brought up a lot of anxiety for Nora, as she was nervous how she was going to play pool with one hand. She told me how his actions spoke volumes to her:

He automatically showed me like, "Hey, this is how you can do it with one hand." And it was just so normal. … He was the first guy that didn't treat me like there was something wrong with me. He didn't address it at all. He was just like, "this is how you do it." You know, like, coming from like a helping way and not like, making me feel less than. I feel like that was the first experience I had with that.

Interestingly, Nora believed that her boyfriend never addressing the disability signified that he thought she was "normal." When he automatically demonstrated how to play pool using one hand, she felt immediately comfortable and empowered.

First Sharing Disability Online

Eleven of the participants met significant others through an online dating app or website. Women were often strategic in how they presented themselves online and to what extent they revealed their disability through their profile before having conversations with men on- and off-line. Their presentation of disability online provided women an opportunity to share their disability for the first time. However, it was not an easy task for women to decide what to share online, and some women chose to conceal their disability until they got to know a potential partner first or until the male partner asked about photos that showed their disability. Veronica explained, "I purposefully did not put pictures like that on there. I didn't want people judging me before they got to know me." Hallie did not show her disability on her profile, but she struggled with the moral aspect of it:

No, it wasn't [on my profile]. It caused a lot of anxiety for sure. It felt a little deceptive ... And I'm like "Am I catfishing by not disclosing my hand?"... But at the same time, I also felt like, lots of people have things and when they're not obvious, you don't have to lead with them until you have a connection.

These decisions to conceal their disability until getting to know someone better supports the earlier finding that women wanted to wait until a relationship became more serious before talking about their disability.

Some women became more comfortable posting information about their disability over time. Peyton explained:

My trajectory of online dating was like when I first did it, I did barely any pictures that showed my bone disease ... By the time I ended app dating, I was more open and vulnerable on my dating app than I was on any social media. I would post a full body picture just to be like "Here you go."

Some women were consistent in what they shared online. CeCe said, "My profile was fully filled out in detail. I've always been very transparent about my one leg and all that, you know, and that was on there."

Thus, whether and how to share their disability when online dating seems to be a very personal choice and may be influenced by women's views of their difference and their desire to avoid judgment. As Kelsey pointed out, online dating allows individuals to "control their own narrative" and be in control of people's first impressions of them. When the power is placed in these women's hands, it seems to become an ongoing struggle of knowing the right decision to make.

After deciding how to create their profile, the women had to figure out what to say, if anything, about the disability prior to meeting with their matches. Laura spoke a lot about this in her interview:

So, at this point, it's just hard because I'm like "Do I need to be checking in with guys?" Like when we're gonna meet, should I be like "Hey, just you know, just wanted to make sure you looked at my pictures." Sometimes I feel like I should, but other times, I'm like "No!" That's on them and I'm hoping for the best that they did see and they don't care.

When it is time to meet the man in person, there are also unique struggles that the participants expressed about preparing for the date. When Peyton would prepare to meet an online match in person, she said:

I had it down to a science. I would wear the same outfit. I was like "I don't want to feel like insecure about having to pick out something that I'm comfortable in." So, I had the exact same outfit picked out for every single date.

Choosing clothes for the date seemed to be a significant decision for the women, as their disability was more or less visible based on clothing. Hallie also said: "I'm also really good at hiding my hand, 100%, really good. Yeah, I get away with it. I think I get away with it because I have my wrist and palm. So, if I wear long sleeves, it's easy." Similar to deciding what photos to post on their profiles, the decision of what to wear became a large step in this online dating process. Because online dating allows people to control how others see them for the first time, this presents a unique option for women with physical disabilities.

Talk about Disability, Identity, and Romantic Relationships with Male Partners

In the second research question, we aimed to understand how women's talk indicated their views toward and intersection of disability, identity, and relationships with male partners. In their talk during interviews, women seemed to grapple with how their views of themselves impacted their male romantic partners and their relationships with the male partners. We outline three themes related to their sense-making of their disability, identity, and romantic relationships.

View of Self-Impacting Reactions to Disability Talk in a Romantic Relationship

Almost every single participant spoke about the value they placed on their partner's talk about their disability. It appeared that women's view of self, which includes their level of acceptance and pride in their disability, directly impacted how they responded to their partners when they discussed the disability. It became increasingly noteworthy how different each participant spoke of their partner's reactions, however, this view of self often fluctuated. Factors such as their surroundings, events, or conversations that had happened prior to their talk, and their overall attitude impacted the way the women made sense of their own reactions to talk with partners about disability. Some women, at times, appreciated the men's awareness of their potential daily hurdles, willingness to help, and sensitivity to their limitations. Other women, at times, were offended when their partners would say or do something that acknowledged the disability. These perceptions varied greatly among participants, and upon further analysis, it became more evident that the women's perceptions of men's talk about disability seemed to stem from the women's own attitude toward their disability.

Women seemed to interpret their partners' reactions more positively when they were more confident in their own disabilities. For example, CeCe, who talked about loving her physical difference, recalled:

> I totally twisted my other ankle … And this man, we had been dating maybe a month, and he just scooped me up and carried me down the stairs and took me to the hospital … He just immediately—like it was not like, "Wow, this is what I have to look forward to." He just cared about me and made sure that I was okay.

And was just like right in it, you know, like he didn't skip a beat. He just assumed the caretaker. And that to me kind of showed that I didn't really need to, like educate. Like he was just kind of like—he was just there. He was in it, and he definitely had the ability to adapt and wanted to.

When CeCe twisted her "good" ankle, her partner reacted swiftly and confidently. As CeCe discussed, his instincts guided him to do what would be the most helpful for her. Similar to CeCe's experience, Stephanie also appreciated when her husband acknowledged her limitations: "He looks for little things that's too much for me. He's not gonna say 'Oh you can't do this.' It's more of 'Let me help you in a nonchalant way where you won't know I'm helping you.'" When I asked Stephanie if she liked when her husband does those little things for her, such as opening a jar before she needs it, she mentioned how she feels extremely cared for during those interactions. She said, "He's always been a silent observer." She interprets his ability to notice potentially difficult tasks to be a sign of support.

On the other hand, Kelsey, who said, "It's so hard for me to see myself, like past the disability … I think about what my life would be like if I didn't have it," also recalled a memorable situation with her boyfriend:

This was probably a month in. And then, as we dated, he would say—we'd be walking somewhere and he'd say, "I see that everyone's like staring at you." Like you're an idiot, like why would you bring that up? Just keep that to yourself. Just pretend—I know everybody's staring at me, but you don't have to say that.

Kelsey's response to that comment showed her frustration with her boyfriend acknowledging what was happening around them. As Kelsey stated, it is difficult for her to consider her identity to be anything except her disability. Perhaps when she is in a committed romantic relationship, her identity of that relationship starts to overshadow her identity of being a person with a disability.

When partners make their disability salient in an interaction, women seem to be reminded abruptly of their insecurities and low comfort levels with their disability. For example, Felicity talked about what happens when her husband offers to help her: "There are times where he's been like 'I can help you' but then I'm like 'I got this. You can help me because I'm your wife but not because you think I'm handicapped.'" Women's talk in interviews revealed two main themes, or views toward how their disability, gender, and relationships all intertwine, which we discuss next.

Men as Ideal Partners Compared to Women

A theme that consistently emerged throughout the interviews that seemed to reflect women's views toward dating, disability, and gender was the women's attitude of men's sacrifice and physical perfection. Women often seemed to look up to their partners as ideal.

First, some women believed that the men must be making huge sacrifice to stay in a relationship with someone with a disability. Because the women seemed to talk about themselves as less valuable, they had an extra appreciation for their partners for choosing to be with them. Thus, the women often spoke of their partners with exorbitant, positive language. For example, Daisy stated this when asked about her long-term boyfriend:

> I find him to be, what I would consider, a perfect individual. He doesn't have flaws that are noticeable. I think I uphold myself as being a perfect individual for him, but I knew I was holding something back because I wasn't as unflawed as what I thought he was.

Because she was tired of feeling judged about her insecurity, Daisy always tried to hide her one arm. It appears that she focused a lot on her flaws and shortcomings in the way she talked about herself. Therefore, it seems that her self-identity came a lot from having one arm, and that was not a positive or proud side of her identity. Her overall perception of her boyfriend was that, compared to her, he was perfect. Because he chose her despite her disability, she carried an attitude of being thankful and overly appreciative of him, which shows itself in the words she uses to describe him. Her overly positive attitude about her partner seems to be stemming from her negative view of herself.

Some women seemed surprised that men would date them. For example, Kelsey struggled with believing that a man would willingly pick her. Her moment of frustration sheds light on the issue:

> Whenever we would like bring up my disability, I would get really upset. I'd be like, "Why don't you just go back to your ex? Go back to her. She doesn't have what I have and it'd be so much easier." Like I always—I always compare myself to like the able-bodied woman because, to me, that's what beauty is. And he kept saying "No, I want to be with you" … That's just always been what it is. Whenever I would get upset or whenever something like that would happen, I would compare myself to his past relationship or someone able-bodied because that's my biggest insecurity, obviously.

From the way that Kelsey told her boyfriend that his former partner would be easier to date, it is evident that her view of self is not strong. By claiming that his ex would be easier to date simply because she does not have a physical difference reveals that she is "less than ideal." Kelsey admitted to always comparing herself to the able-bodied women because, in her mind, that is the most ideal body type. Her perception crossed into her communication with her male partner. Daisy and Kelsey view their bodies as flawed.

Second, when the women talked about their romantic partners, they tended to use overwhelming positive language, particularly about their physical characteristics. For example, Elsa laughed when she spoke how perfect her fiancé is for her:

He jumps in. He's like a golden retriever. He is like smiling, like tail wagging. He's like the most helpful, thoughtful person. He's the type that he's happy for making other people happy. So, the thought of like, helping somebody just speaks so well to his like, you know, what he needs. He's like ideal for somebody with physical limitations. Like he wants to help.

In the words that Elsa used to describe him, she pointed out how perfect he is for someone who may need additional help.

Because of the women's physical limitations, some of the men's physical qualities seemed to stand out to them more than others did. Annie explained:

I tend to go for—I think I've noticed like, guys that are physically are usually, like taller than me, bigger than me. I feel like—it sounds stereotypical, but protects me and helps me lift heavy things and stuff like that. I'm sure that's totally subconscious, like "Oh, he's six foot [sic.], he can totally reach things for me!"

Relationship as Source of Self-Worth and Confidence

It became evident in the interviews that for many women, the largest source of their confidence and self-worth stemmed from their romantic relationships. Nora articulated this perfectly when she vulnerably stated, "A lot of my self-worth stuff is based on a loving relationship and having someone else prove to me that they can love me with a disability." Kelsey's words below shed light on the complexity of disability and identity:

I have so much trouble loving myself. So, I feel like the only reason I'm comfortable with my arm is because I'm in a relationship with him ... I definitely love myself because he loves me and like, I love my arm. Well, I don't love my arm. I like it because he's okay with it.

In one part of this quote, Kelsey expressed that she loved her arm. That aspect of her identity came to the forefront. However, after realizing what she said, she corrected herself and realized that she only loved her arm because of her boyfriend's acceptance of it. It seems as though her identity is strongly based in her relationship and knowing whether her partner accepts her.

The notion of beauty and appearance standards emerged when women discussed the challenges of dating with a disability. Participants' feelings of self-worth were often impacted by husband's talk about the women's appearance. Felicity spoke frequently about how much she felt beautiful around her husband when they were dating:

He gave me this self-esteem. He doesn't stop complimenting me. He doesn't stop saying how beautiful I am, how sexy I am, how much I turn him on. And now I'm like "Yes, I believe him," whereas before him, I was like "I'm never gonna get married. Nobody's gonna like me. Nobody's gonna ever notice me."

Felicity, along with several other participants, voiced their struggle with feeling beautiful. However, once they entered a supportive relationship, their confidence in their appearance seemed to dramatically increase, particularly when perceiving that their partners viewed them as beautiful.

Because many of the participants seemed to place a lot of their self-worth, confidence, and perceptions of beauty in the hands of their partners and relationships, they were fearful of those relationships ending. Their talk indicated a fear that they would not find another relationship in the future. For example, Peyton explained:

> It was the worst breakup of my life because I wanted to stay together ... I'm like, "How am I ever gonna find someone who loves me as much as you do and loves me so well? He moved out, and within 3 months, he met someone else and now he's married ... And she weirdly looks like me. For my confidence, it was like—you were so in love with me and all of a sudden not, and you found someone else who resembles me and doesn't have a bone disease."

For Peyton and others who talked about dissolved relationships, it became evident that the process of making sense of ended relationships often overlapped and intertwined with their perceptions of self, their partners, and their relationships. They feared that they were unlovable and that their difference would interfere with their chance to find love again, particularly when former boyfriends started new relationships with women who did not have a visible disability.

DISCUSSION

In our study, we aimed to understand how women's disability was first addressed in interabled relationships with male dating partners who do not have a visible physical disability. We also wanted to understand how women's talk about their interabled romantic relationships reflected their views and possible intersection of identity, disability, and romantic relationships.

We learned that the first conversation in a romantic relationship about a woman's visible physical disability is a significant turning point for the woman and her relationship. Although the disability was visible, participants felt that the disability needed to be addressed directly at least once with male partners. In some relationships, they discussed the disability in the early stages of the relationship, at times before the relationship began (e.g., when first meeting someone online). In other relationships, this conversation happened much later. In addition to the timing of the conversation, the reason for initiation also impacted the conversation. Some women believed that their disability was the stigma that needed to be discussed.

The women found the first conversation to be often times uncomfortable but still an important step in the relationship. There appeared to be some strategies utilized to perhaps lessen the discomfort addressing the disability. Some women chose to initiate the conversation by asking about their partners' past experiences with individuals with disabilities, explicitly telling their partner about their disability, or asking if the partner had ever heard of a specific disability. In these cases, the women had control over their narrative and were able to control how and when the conversation happened.

Other times, the male romantic partner was the one to first address the disability, sometimes by directly bringing up the disability but first by asking "Can I ask you a question?" or by offering help during a shared activity. If a woman perceived that her partner was offering or asking because he saw her as incapable, she grew more uncomfortable or even upset that it was addressed this way. However, if the woman perceived that curiosity or a desire to understand her better was the impetus for addressing the disability, she responded positively and felt more open to further talk about the disability. It seemed as though women lost some autonomy in choosing when and how to disclose when they found themselves in a situation where the disability became more salient (e.g., when engaging in a shared task that was not easy for them), much as Goffman (1963) explained that the salience of a stigmatized identity fluctuates depending on the setting and can change in different environments.

Choosing to self-disclose about a specific stigmatized identity can present a heavy amount of uncertainty and new set of communicative challenges, such as knowing when to have the conversation and what words to use (Agne et al., 2000). However, individuals with a visible, physical disability must manage their communication surrounding their disability even though they may not always need to disclose that the disability exists (Duggan et al., 2010; Horan et al., 2009). In the present study, first conversations surrounding the disability are noteworthy moments in the relationship and often do include talk about the disability. Similar to the findings of Blockmans (2015), women desire to have a conversation about their disability, at least once to address the presence of the disability. These first conversations for women in this study often included topics such as women's feelings about their differences, their physical capabilities, impacts of the disability in women's pasts, and appropriate ways to offer help when necessary. Considering that people tend to rely heavily on the recipient's cues when self-disclosing (e.g., Afifi et al., 2007), participants recalled that the male romantic partners' reactions and willingness to have these conversations played a significant role in how the conversation unfolded.

Additionally, women's talk during interviews revealed an intertwining of identity, relationships, and disability, in that women often made sense of their disability and their views toward their disability in relation to the partner and the relationship. Many women voiced comparisons to other women without disabilities, particularly as they made sense of why their partners would date them and why their relationships ended. The ways that they talked about their identities seemed to fluctuate based on what their partners thought of them, even to the point of placing an immense amount of personal value on their partners' perceptions of them, their attractiveness, and their worth. This aligns with previous work on romantic relationships of women with disabilities, such as Retznik et al. (2017) who concluded that "female interviewees also described feeling that their appearance and capacity were less than that of women without disability... women are more susceptible to beauty ideals with regards to sexuality than men and are more harshly judged in terms of physical beauty and attractiveness" (p. 426). They claimed that women's view of self in relation to their disability was comprised of feedback from others and observation. It may be that women with visible physical disabilities tie their self-worth to partners because, as existing research suggests, they know that they may be less likely to attract potential partners if this relationship ends compared to their able-bodied female peers. While acknowledging that influence from a partner can indicate closeness, we challenge women to avoid placing the value of their identity in others. When self and identity are so directly connected to others' feedback, then their sense of self appeared to be inconsistent. Specifically, in a romantic relationship, feelings of support and closeness fluctuate over the span of the relationship. Particularly in a romantic relationship in which one partner does not share the physical disability, it is important for women to develop their sense of self and worth before developing, or at least apart from developing their romantic relationship.

The internalization of the stigma of disability (Byrd et al., 2019; Ryan et al., 2005) can lead to feelings of shame and inadequacy (Brandhorst, 2020). This idea of self-stigma, coined by Corrigan et al., (2011), tends to develop over time. In the present study, participants' talk often revealed what we saw as self-stigma, particularly as they discussed internalizing outsiders' messages about disability. Most of the participants felt that their disability had directly impacted their dating experiences. From the conversations during interviews, we understood that some women struggle with comparing themselves to other women without disabilities. It did not seem to be in an envious manner; but instead, they started to vocalize that men may not select them as a first choice. Some participants vocalized that it is difficult to consider themselves a sexual or attractive woman, which seems to stem from outside messages that make them feel inadequate and also from stereotypes of women with disabilities as asexual or needy (Collisson et al., 2020). Because women based their views of self on others' perspectives, the ways they talked about their identities fluctuated based on how they perceived others to see them and their disability. When the participants started to put their identity and self-worth solely in their partners' or relationships' hands, their sense of self seemed to undoubtedly fluctuate.

For most participants in the study, the interview itself was a monumental step forward for them, as they appeared quite apprehensive talking openly about how their disability has impacted dating. They expressed how anxious yet excited they were to talk about dating. Many women said that nobody had ever asked them these questions before. Considering that social lives are often left out of the scholarly conversations about disability (Hammer, 2016), researchers should continue to gather stories about the dating lives of people with disabilities. Zitzelsberger (2005) argues that there is a need to understand everyday social interactions especially in relationships among people with differences in ability. Without the shared identity as people with disabilities, partners may struggle with the appropriate ways to talk about the difference in their everyday interactions, which may have negative implications for relational outcomes like satisfaction and closeness.

Individuals who do not identify as having a disability may not always know what questions to ask about the disability, or whether certain talk about disability is appropriate or welcome. In future work, we suggest that scholars utilize focus groups to collect data, as the groups may provide catharsis for participants as well as help women to feel comfortable sharing their experiences with others who share this identity. Regarding the male partners, because reactions can be so impactful to the women, we recommend they work hard to listen to the women as they are disclosing their disability and enact a heightened awareness of their responses and provision of support and understanding. As scholars continue to study talk about disability within personal relationships, they should aim to understand which communication strategies, such as face-saving and humor, women may use to increase their comfort in talking about their disability with romantic partners.

We were able to illuminate the importance of communication within a romantic relationship when parties do not share a particular identity, in this case, visible, physical disability. We hope that this research encourages women with visible, physical disabilities and differences to embrace their stories and use their differences as their greatest strengths when navigating romantic relationships.

REFERENCES

Afifi, T. D., Caughlin, J. P., & Afifi, W. A. (2007). The dark side (and light side) of avoidance and secrets. In B. H. Spitzberg & W. R. Cupach (Eds.), *The dark side of interpersonal communication* (2nd ed., pp. 61–92). Lawrence Erlbaum Associates. https://doi.org/10.4324/9780203936849

Agne, R. R., Thompson, T. L., & Cusella, L. P. (2000). Stigma in the line of face: Self-disclosure of patients' HIV status to health care providers. *Journal of Applied Communication Research, 28*(3), 235–261. https://doi.org/10.1080/00909880009365573

Baker, S., Gallois, C., Driedger, S. M., & Santesso, N. (2011). Communication accommodation and managing musculoskeletal disorders: Doctors' and patients' perspectives. *Health Communication, 26*(4), 379–388. https://doi.org/10.1080/1041023 6.2010.551583

Blair, K. L., & Hoskin, R. A. (2019). Transgender exclusion from the world of dating: Patterns of acceptance and rejection of hypothetical trans dating partners as a function of sexual and gender identity. *Journal of Social & Personal Relationships, 36*(7), 2074–2095. https://doi.org/10.1177/0265407518779139

Blockmans, I. G. E. (2015). "Not wishing to be the white rhino in the crowd": Disability-disclosure at university. *Journal of Language & Social Psychology, 34*(2), 158–180. https://doi.org/10.1177/0261927X14548071

Boucher, E. M. (2015). Doubt begets doubt: Causal uncertainty as a predictor of relational uncertainty in romantic relationships. *Communication Reports, 28*(1), 12–23. https://doi.org/10.1080/08934215.2014.902487

Braithwaite, D. O. (1990). From majority to minority: An analysis of cultural change from ablebodied to disabled. *International Journal of Intercultural Relations, 14*(4), 465–483. https://doi.org/10.1016/0147-1767(90)90031-Q

Braithwaite, D. O., & Eckstein, N. J. (2003). How people with disabilities communicatively manage assistance: Helping as instrumental social support. *Journal of Applied Communication Research,31*(1),1–26.https://doi.org/10.1080/00909880305374

Brandhorst, J. K. (2020). Combatting mental health stigma on college campuses. *Spectra, 56*(2), 24–27. https://www.natcom.org/Spectra

Braun, V., & Clarke, V. (2006). Using thematic analysis in psychology. *Qualitative Research in Psychology, 3*(2), 77–101. https://doi.org/10.1191/1478088706qp063oa

Byrd, G. A., Zhang, Y. B., Gist-Mackey, A. N., & Pitts, M. J. (2019). Interability contact and the reduction of interability prejudice: Communication accommodation, intergroup anxiety, and relational solidarity. *Journal of Language & Social Psychology, 38*(4), 441–458. https://doi.org/10.1177/0261927X19865578

Collisson, B., Edwards, J. M., Chakrian, L., Mendoza, J., Anduiza, A., & Corona, A. (2020). Perceived satisfaction and inequity: A survey of potential romantic partners of people with a disability. *Sexuality and Disability, 38*, 405–420. https://doi.org/10.1007/s11195-019-09601-7

Corrigan, P. W., Rafacz, J., & Rüsch, N. (2011). Examining a progressive model of self-stigma and its impact on people with serious mental illness. *Psychiatry Research, 189*(3), 339–343. https://doi.org/10.1016/j.psychres.2011.05.024

Donovan, E. E., Thompson, C. M., LeFebvre, L., & Tollison, A. C. (2017). Emerging adult confidants' judgments of parental openness: Disclosure quality and post-disclosure relational closeness. *Communication Monographs, 84*(2), 179–199. https://doi.org/10.1080/03637751.2015.1119867

Duggan, A., Bradshaw, Y., & Altman, W. (2010). How do I ask about your disability? An examination of interpersonal communication processes between medical students and patients with disabilities. *Journal of Health Communication, 15*(3), 334–350. https://doi.org/10.1080/10810731003686630

Garland-Thomson, R. (2002). The politics of staring: Visual representations of disabled people in popular culture. In S. L. Snyder, B. J. Brueggemann, & R. Garland-Thomson (Eds.), *Disability studies: Enabling the humanities* (pp. 56–75). Modern Language Association.

Goffman, E. (1963). *Stigma: Notes on the management of spoiled identity*. Prentice-Hall.

Goldsmith, D. J., & Domann-Scholz, K. (2013). The meanings of "open communication" among couples coping with a cardiac event. *Journal of Communication, 63*(2), 266–286. https://doi.org/10.1111/jcom.12021

Greene, K. L., & Serovich, J. M. (1996). Appropriateness of disclosure of HIV-testing information: The perspective of PWLAs. *Journal of Applied Communication Research, 24*(1), 50–65. https://doi.org/10.1080/00909889609365439

Hammer, G. (2016). "If they're going to stare, at least I'll give them a good reason to": Blind women's visibility, invisibility, and encounters with the gaze. *Signs: Journal of Women in Culture & Society, 41*(2), 409–432. https://doi.org/10.1086/682924

Horan, S., Martin, M., Smith, N., Schoo, M., Eidsness, M., & Johnson, A. (2009). Can we talk? How learning of an invisible illness impacts forecasted relational outcomes. *Communication Studies, 60*(1), 66–81. https://doi.org/10.1080/10510970802623625

Jung, E., & Hecht, M. L. (2004). Elaborating on the communication theory of identity: Identity gaps and communication outcomes. *Communication Quarterly, 52*(3), 265–283. https://doi.org/10.1080/03637759309376297

Li, N. P., Bailey, J. M., Kenrick, D. T., & Linsenmeier, J. A. (2002). The necessities and luxuries of mate preferences: Testing the tradeoffs. *Journal of Personality and Social Psychology, 82*(6), 947–955. https://doi.org/10.1037/0022-3514.82.6.947

Matthews, C. K., & Harrington, N. G. (2000). Invisible disability. In D. O. Braithwaite & T. L. Thompson (Eds.), *Handbook of communication and people with disabilities: Research and application* (pp. 405–422). Lawrence Erlbaum.

Meisenbach, R. (2010). Stigma management communication: A theory and agenda for applied research on how individuals manage moments of stigmatized identity. *Journal of Applied Communication Research, 38*(3), 268–292. https://doi.org/1 0.1080/00909882.2010.490841

Meltzer, A. L., McNulty, J. K., Jackson, G., & Karney, B. R. (2014). Sex differences in the implications of partner physical attractiveness for the trajectory of marital satisfaction. *Journal of Personality and Social Psychology, 106*(3), 418–428. https://doi.org/10.1037/a0034424

Nemeth, S. (2000). Society, sexuality, and disabled/ablebodied romantic relationships. In D. O. Braithwaite & T. L. Thompson (Eds.), *Handbook of communication and people with disabilities* (pp. 37–65). Lawrence Erlbaum.

Petronio, S. S. (2002). *Boundaries of privacy: Dialectics of disclosure*. State University of New York Press.

Retznik, L., Wienholz, S., Seidel, A., Pantenburg, B., Conrad, I., Michel, M., & Riedel-Heller, S. (2017). Relationship status: Single? Young adults with visual, hearing, or physical disability and their experiences with partnership and sexuality. *Sexuality & Disability, 35*(4), 415–432. https://doi.org/10.1007/s11195-017-9497-5

Romaniuk, O., & Terán, L. (2022). First impression sexual scripts of romantic encounters: Effect of gender on verbal and non verbal immediacy behaviors in American media dating culture. *Journal of Social and Personal Relationships, 39*(2), 107–131. https://doi.org/10.1177/02654075211033036

Ryan, E. B., Anas, A. P., & Gruneir, A. J. S. (2006). Evaluations of overhelping and underhelping communication: Do old Age and physical disability matter? *Journal of Language & Social Psychology, 25*(1), 97–107. https://doi.org/10.117 7/0261927X05284485

Ryan, E. B., Bajorek, S., Beaman, A., & Anas, A. P. (2005). "I just want you to know that 'them' is me": Intergroup perspectives on communication and disability. In J. Harwood & H. Giles (Eds.), *Intergroup communication: Multiple perspectives* (pp. 117–140). Peter Lang. https://doi.org/10.1177/0261927X05284485

Schreiner, N., Pick, D., & Kenning, P. (2018). To share or not to share? Explaining willingness to share in the context of social distance. *Journal of Consumer Behaviour, 17*(4), 366–378. https://doi.org/10.1002/cb.1717

Scott, J.-A. (2015). Almost passing: A performance analysis of personal narratives of physically disabled femininity. *Women's Studies in Communication, 38*(2), 227–249. https://doi.org/10.1080/07491409.2015.1027023

St. Lawrence, J. S., Husfeldt, B. A., Kelly, J. A., Hood, H. V., & Smith, S. (1990). The stigma of AIDS: Fear of disease and prejudice toward gay men. *Journal of Homosexuality, 19*(3), 85–99. https://doi.org/10.1300/J082v19n03_05

Vandenbosch, L., Vervloessem, D., & Eggermont, S. (2013). "I might get your heart racing in my skin-tight jeans": Sexualization on music entertainment television. *Communication Studies, 64*(2), 178–194. https://doi.org/10.1080/1051097 4.2012.755640

Weeden, J., & Sabini, J. (2005). Physical attractiveness and health in Western societies: A review. *Psychological Bulletin, 131*(5), 635–653. https://doi. org/10.1037/0033-2909.131.5.635

Zitzelsberger, H. (2005). (In)visibility: Accounts of embodiment of women with physical disabilities and differences. *Disability and Society, 20*(4), 389–403. https://doi. org/10.1080/09687590500086492

CHAPTER 12

Disposable Masks, Disposable Lives: Aggrievement Politics and the Weaponization of Disabled Identity

Brian Grewe and Craig R. Weathers

On November 24, 2015, the world watched as the future 45th President of the United States mocked a reporter with a visible physical disability. At a campaign event in Myrtle Beach, Trump jerked his hands in spastic, disjointed movements, while creating an open-mouthed facial expression imitating Serge Kovaleski, an American investigative reporter for *The New York Times*. Kovaleski has a visible physical disability that stems from a congenital joint condition (Carmon, 2015). In this moment, America witnessed an act that communicated a message devaluing people with disabilities. The disabled community has long been the victim of inappropriate, derogatory, and hate-filled representations. Public discourses position disability as undesirable, and the people with disabilities as being less valuable and less capable than those who live without an identified disability (Snyder & Mitchell, 2006).

Television and movie tropes similarly perpetuate stigmatic views of disability. Common representations of disabled folx in popular media center on their inability to perform tasks, the willingness of characters to do anything to be rid of their disability, and that death is more desirable than disability (e.g., *Million Dollar Baby*). Though inaccurate and genuinely offensive, these tropes shape

B. Grewe (✉)
Arapahoe Community College, Littleton, CO, USA
e-mail: brian.grewe@arapahoe.edu

C. R. Weathers
University of Denver, Denver, CO, USA

© The Author(s), under exclusive license to Springer Nature Switzerland AG 2023
M. S. Jeffress et al. (eds.), *The Palgrave Handbook of Disability and Communication*, https://doi.org/10.1007/978-3-031-14447-9_12

185

audience members' perceptions of disability and contribute to the cultural understanding of what life with disability is like. Another common trope is characters who fake a disability to further an agenda or to achieve a personal advantage. Medical and legal procedurals show people faking serious injuries, wearing neck braces, and using wheelchairs to win court cases and subsequent financial benefits. Similarly, we see characters who fake amnesia, insanity, or other mental health conditions to receive reduced punishments, preferred prison placements, and other benefits. These tropes are extremely common, and unlike the stigmatic representations of disabled characters, are far more indicative of an unfortunate reality: disabled identities and related accommodations are co-opted for their perceived advantages, with deleterious impacts on the disabled community.

How disability is portrayed impacts how people, disabled or able-bodied, view themselves (Haller & Zhang, 2010; Jeffress, 2021). Identity scholars note that disability is socially constructed as a defining characteristic for an individual (Braithwaite, 1990). Other scholars argue that disabled identity is experience-based and that disability shapes how a person is perceived, influencing their relationships and interactions with others (Putnam, 2005). Much of the identity research on disabled people has been framed through a model of deviancy, through which disabled people are viewed differently from abled people (Braithwaite & Braithwaite, 1988; Braithwaite, 1990) and from the majority of society (Lindemann, 2010). In the past decade, disabled identity has been explored from an internalized perspective. Identity scholarship has utilized research methodologies that privilege the individual voice and lived experience (Garland-Thomson, 2014); explored embodiment/performance of disability (Scott, 2013); and employed an intersectional lens to the experience of stigma and representation (Chaudoir & Quinn, 2010; Siebers, 2004).

Utilizing a critical rhetorical approach, this chapter extends on these lines of inquiry to explore how disabled identity has been co-opted and weaponized to materialize a self-aggrieved status that provides access to physical spaces and services that are generally reserved for disabled people. Specifically, we consider how nondisabled people deploy the trope of victimhood to weaponize cultural beliefs surrounding disability to minimize perceived inconvenience, gain advantages in relation to accessible parking, acquire preferred seating at specific concert venues, skip lines at theme parks, represent pets as service animals, and circumvent masking ordinances during the COVID-19 pandemic.

CRITICAL RHETORIC: THEORIES OF VICTIMHOOD

Critical rhetoric is an approach to critique developed by McKerrow (1989) with an aim "to understand the integration of power/knowledge in society" and which "intervention strategies might be considered appropriate to effect social change" (p. 91). Importantly, critical rhetoric is not a method for critique one should follow but is an "orientation to critique" (p. 92). Rather than selecting a particular speech, media text, or other singular artifact, critical rhetoric constructs texts for analysis from cultural fragments and is attentive to the flows of power in and around the seemingly disparate elements that comprise constructed texts. This project approaches the construction of the text through what DeLuca (1999) called a theory of articulation.

Reality, as a site of struggle, is comprised of people, institutions, physical locations, and other "nodes," and the shape of our reality is a product of the links between each of those component parts. Selecting which nodes factor into a particular text is akin to a cartography that is "contingent and particular and is the result of a political and historical struggle" (p. 335). One particular articulation that is useful to this project is Protevi's (2009) notion of "thanatography" or "representations of violence provoking physiological changes" (p. 159). According to Protevi, analysis of thanatography should be "differential and population based: there are no simple linear functions [but] there are patterns, thresholds, and triggers distributed in a population" (p. 159). Representations need not be unidirectionally causal to be noteworthy. We are not concerned so much with proving media effects as we are with how each factor discussed in this chapter shapes our "affective cognition" (p. 143). To that end, we focus on how media representations and popular discourses, mutually constituted, shape our identities and create the frames upon which aggrievement and victimhood circulate rhetorically.

Specifically, we explore how aggrievement, situated within a victim frame, can be used to leverage existing power relations at the expense of marginalized groups. For DeLuca, antagonisms "point to the limit of a discourse" and "make possible the investigation, disarticulation, and rearticulation of a hegemonic discourse" (p. 336). The antagonism for this project is the disabled body, as it both challenges and creates hegemonic discourses around safety. Ultimately, our identities-in-relation shows us to what degree certain bodies are valued and cared for, and which bodies are not. This chapter is an attempt to trace those relationships to identify the most fruitful points for intervention. We begin this process by examining victimhood-as-identity as one point for analysis.

Victimhood-as-Identity

Victimhood-as-identity in a territorial sense (as opposed to religious[1]) emerged in the modern U.S. cultural imaginary out of the culture wars of the early 1900s. Industrialization created needs within urban spaces that quickly conflicted with the day-to-day operations, values, and practices of rural communities (Dionne, 2008). This conflict positioned people against each other because of physical location, living environment and differing needs, entrenching a binary "us" vs. "them" cultural frame. Victimhood cannot exist without a privileged oppositional identity as foil for the victimized: in some cases, nationalism is the driving force (Bergmann, 2008). During the early 1900s, this identity was born from living within an urban or rural community. Rural individuals claimed an aggrieved status through the illustration of urban people having more influence over governance, which negatively impacts rural communities. This divide persists to the present day.

The victim identity is co-constructed and constituted through communication between individuals who have experienced trauma, material or perceptual, in relation to a perpetrator who enacted some form of violence or wrongdoing. Victimhood can circulate outside of traditional structures of power, relying more on moral or ethical norms to ground claims of aggrievement. According to Jacoby (2015), these positions are constructed through self-referential discourses that cast some individuals as either perpetrators or victims of trauma; in other words, political identities that force a distinction between victimization (an act of harm or transgression against an individual or group) and victimhood (a collective identity formed as a result of the harm or transgression). Jacoby identifies a sequence of five stages that illustrate this process: (1) structural conduciveness, (2) political consciousness, (3) ideological concurrence, (4) political mobilization, and (5) political recognition (p. 513).

Structural conduciveness is the context in which the grievance occurs. This includes, but is not limited to: cultural and societal expectations in behavior, dominant definitional discourses, state and federal legislation, access to economic support-based resources, and civic engagement and participation. Understanding the context behind the victimization allows us to better understand the creation of the victim identity. Each act of misrepresentation of disabled identity creates the space for structural conduciveness. When a person pretends to be disabled and then is discovered not to be disabled, it challenges our cultural expectations. Dominant discourses of disability, specifically on one's ability, provide context for how we understand and engage with disabled identity and further perpetuate a negative representation of the actual lived experiences that people with disabilities have on a day-to-day basis.

Political consciousness is the level of self-awareness that an individual or group has within their own political system. By understanding one's own positionality within the system, an identity can fall under a politic of grievance. The degree to which one can voice their grievance is directly related to how much influence one has over our collective political consciousness. What channels exist for community members and others who might also be subject to consequences of victimization to share their grievances? What is considered normative and non-normative in behavior, communication, and action between interlocutors is also relevant here. Utilizing disabled identity falsely as a plot device or trope is an intentional act that shifts the lived experience of disability and creates a figurative or metaphorical meaning, laying the foundation for harm to disabled people.

Ideological concurrence is couched in the recognition that norms were violated and that the grievance is situated within a larger political context. This stage is where the grievance, or act of victimization, transitions from an act of harm to an act of wrongdoing. The distinction between the two is that an act of harm is a transgression against one's interests, while an act of wrongdoing violates social norms. More accurately, the act of wrongdoing operates outside of the expectations of normalcy and creates space for a collective outcry. This violation does not exclude actual harm, and is operationalized through the connection between past history and the current state of being. This is also when victimhood is no longer solely an individual experience, as it transforms into a collective identity. While collective identities typically draw on the past, victimhood can also draw on the present. Jacoby (2015) argues:

> This forging of the past into the present is particularly salient in identities that are grounded in grievance. Feelings of trauma, for example, may not necessarily be based on the actual experience of victimization; it may not even have occurred in the same historical epoch but nonetheless links people across space and time. The process of victimization to victimhood is cyclical and can perpetuate itself through the perception of experiencing a transgression that ultimately causes harm, even if the victims are not directly tied to that historical moment. (p. 523)

An example of this could be how the common television trope of a person faking a disability to get out of a punishment or other negative consequence is considered a transgression. People faking disabilities, even if only in media representations, create legitimacy issues surrounding actual disabilities. This can also be viewed as an act of wrongdoing because harm is created in how audiences internalize what they think disability is, specifically in cases of invisible disabilities. A person claiming insanity as a defense within a courtroom, or news coverage of mass shooting events that scapegoat mental illness, creates actual harm: people with mental illness are far more likely to be victims of violence than perpetrators, and people with mental illness are no more likely to commit acts of violence than people without mental illness (Metzl et al., 2021). Within our current political landscape, mental health is often scapegoated as the reason for school or mass shootings, and these tropes reinforce that belief.

Political mobilization is a person's ability to create change. This can occur through the establishment of a social movement through existing political structures or by the recruitment of others who have shared experience or ideology. The future 45th President of the United States experienced backlash via media outlets and activist groups after mocking Serge Kovaleski (Arkin, 2015). While well deserved, the limits of political mobilization became apparent when the act of imitating and mocking a disabled reporter was drowned out by multiple other vulgar acts within a short time span, and the inability of the outcry (or the act itself), to alter the outcome of the forthcoming elections. Relatedly, when a person who is not otherwise noteworthy fakes a disability, the ability to hold them accountable is even more limited. Most people risk very little when co-opting a disabled identity.

Political recognition occurs when people in power recognize and acknowledge the aggrieved status that victimhood creates. Recognition is relationally based on how the victim, perpetrator and audience are connected and the power held in relation. If a person co-opts disabled identity for personal gain (perpetrator), the people immediately impacted (victims) are often unable to act as the audience consists of only the people present and the people who are potentially exposed to the act afterwards (audience). Another way to think about this is the degree to which an interlocutor (individual, or group) can hold a perpetrator accountable. In this sense, victimhood is constituted within structures of communication, belief, and action. In praxis, victimhood within the construction of a victim-identity can only exist in relation to a transgression or act of harm. When a person co-opts a disabled identity, there is collective harm to the disabled community. This harm creates a sense of resentment within the community as they already exist within a marginalized space, and because the medical model of disability is so dominant within the discourses of disability, any outcry that is recognized is often met with pity, sometimes sympathy, but rarely justice.

Victimhood and the Politics of Aggrievement

Weaponizing victimhood via a politics of aggrievement is a common tactic in politics that can be traced throughout history, often as an important component of aggrievement politics. We define aggrievement politics as any instance where an advantaged, dominant individual or group perceives a wrongdoing and adopts a victim-identity to defend or justify an action against a marginalized individual or group. A recurring trope we see throughout history is when an outside group is cast as a threat to inspire fear in a dominant in-group. One example would be when Henry Ford claimed that the presence of Jewish students would "abolish… Christmas and Easter out of schools," (Denvir, 2013). In this instance, Ford casts himself as the victim in service of his antisemitism. This tactic was echoed some 80 years later when Bill O'Reilly started reporting on the "War on Christmas." Trump parroted O'Reilly's claims during the 2016 election, and repeatedly cast himself as the victim throughout his campaign in relation to other events (Holmes, 2018).

In addition to the xenophobia, nationalism, and racism undergirding those earlier attempts, Giroux (2017) notes that Trump weaponized victimhood by creating a culture of cruelty that eschewed cooperation (i.e., building bridges, being generous and showing compassion), and instead focused on divisiveness, alienation, and a fear of inadequacy. In this frame, compassion and empathy are a weakness, and anyone displaying those traits should be treated with contempt. This rhetoric, explicitly derived from libertarian conservative ideals, inhibits collective identity by promoting hyper-masculinized individual responsibility and a survival-of-the-fittest mentality. In this perverse Darwinian frame, it is not the disadvantaged, marginalized, or oppressed who have a claim to aggrievement, but the "fittest" among us who are held back or otherwise disadvantaged by everyone else's existence. Any state of need becomes an attack on our society.

The deployment of aggrievement politics was evident when Trump mocked Serge Kovaleski. In essence, he exploited an already existing system (ableism) to bolster his claims of aggrievement. This is a problem in and of itself, but

Trump's rhetoric, deployed among an electorate already primed to accept social Darwinian notions of inferiority, poses an even greater danger. Hurley (2004) notes that humans have an "automatic and unconscious tendency to imitate" each other, something social psychologists have dubbed the "chameleon effect" (p. 171). Trump framed himself as the victim of attacks from a vengeful and vindictive reporter and deployed an ad hominem attack aimed at Kovaleski's disability. This triggered a chameleon effect in the audience (evident while watching back a video of the rally), essentially encouraging people to do likewise. When confronted, Trump denied, lied and defended his actions, depending on the source of the challenge (Kessler, 2016). By situating himself as the "real victim," he shifted blame away from himself, directed it toward Kovaleski and the press, and preemptively dismissed anyone who was critical of his actions. Thanatography in relation to disability is not only evident in overt public attacks against disabled folx, but also in everyday encounters with ableism.

Playing the "Disability Card": Examples of Co-optation

A disability can be visible and/or invisible and is positioned structurally in a world that does not already plan or provide access. While these viewpoints align with well-established work in both the social and medical model of disability, a disconnect occurs when accommodations or adjustments to access are introduced. We argue that accommodations served as a key articulation that allows for the co-opting and weaponization of disabled identity to emerge at this historical conjuncture.

The purpose of accommodations is to provide equitable access for qualified persons with a disability, as the Americans with Disabilities Act (ADA) defines disability as a physical or mental impairment that substantially limits one or more major life activities (ADA National Network, 2021). The various sections (Titles) under the ADA detail the right to accommodations that provide access spaces, activities, or services that the general public has access to. As many disability services offices within institutions of higher education can attest, there is a strong belief or perception among nondisabled people that accommodations are advantages granted to the individual with a disability (Student Disability Services, 2021). This perception is false, as the purpose accommodations is not success, but access to it. In public spaces, accommodations can range from access to elevators, escalators, or curb cuts. They can also include braille signs, sounds that identify entrance and exit points at crosswalks, or textured walkways and streets for people partaking in cane travel. Folx with invisible disabilities are also accommodated with interpreters, quiet spaces, and rest points. While these accommodations are practical, not all accommodations provide an advantage when they are co-opted. Most people would never think twice about adding braille signage or installing textured walkways and curb cuts. They do, however, arise when people see accessible parking as "rockstar" parking. This perception is what provides the fuel to establish an aggrieved status and ultimately provides the opportunity for weaponizing disability to achieve a specific goal or outcome. The following examples demonstrate how individuals have co-opted and weaponized disability.

Co-opting Disabled Identity at an Iconic Music Venue

Red Rocks Amphitheater is an iconic music venue located in Morrison, Colorado. It was originally purchased by the city of Denver in 1936 and the construction of the amphitheater was completed in 1941. Set within a 200-million-year-old formation of red rocks, this amphitheater has become an iconic music and performance venue for musicians, comedians, and other performers (Colorado Music Hall of Fame, 2019). Due to being built within a naturally formed rock structure, seating and access has always been a challenge. Seating is organized in a series of 70 rows. The accessible seating is in Row 1 (directly in front of the stage) and row 70 (at the very top of the amphitheater). Initially, scalpers were purchasing all the tickets in rows 1 and 2 to resell them. In 2015, Red Rocks Amphitheater came under fire for their ticket-selling practices (Blasius, 2015). Two years later, following a very large and public lawsuit, Red Rocks shifted their ticket sale process to curb the scalping of accessible seating so that people with disabilities could get tickets (Walker, 2017). While the solution is not perfect, the shift did make it more possible for disabled people to attend events at the venue.

In this example, we can see how disabled identity is both co-opted and weaponized against the disabled community to gain access to highly desirable and extremely limited seats. As a venue, Red Rocks can seat approximately 9500 people, while only 78 seats are wheelchair accessible and just under 200 are reserved for disabled patrons. This makes the front row, the one specifically reserved for disabled people, some of the best seats at the venue. For years, people would purchase tickets for the "best seats" in the front row, actively ignoring the disclaimers that this row was reserved for wheelchair users, even going so far as to claim disability status to obtain their seats. This still works to this day, as inquiring into a person's disability status is prohibited due to the stipulation of protection written into the ADA. By co-opting disabled identity, nondisabled people weaponize disability against actual disabled people, exacerbating exclusion at an inherently exclusionary venue.

Abusing Accessible Parking Spots

Passage of the ADA in 1991 established standards to provide a minimum number of accessible spaces in parking lots across the country. Nearly 20 years later, standards for parking lots were updated, mandating one accessible space for every 25 parking spaces within a lot (U.S. Department of Justice, Civil Rights Division, 2010). Anyone who regularly utilizes accessible parking spaces can tell you that finding parking can be a challenge. For instance, it is more difficult to find accessible parking in strip malls and private lots than at larger department and grocery stores. People who need accessible parking spend more time waiting for spaces to become available or finding alternate options further from their destination. In addition, many people who use these spaces can attest to how often these spaces are taken by people who do not display the appropriate placard or license plate. While not unique, nor the only example, in March 2021, the Portsmouth Ohio Police Department took to their social media and the news to warn people from buying and using fake ADA placards for parking in accessible spots (Newman, 2021). Even with warnings of penalties including felony charges and loss of vehicle, people continue to buy and sell "handicap" placards because they provide access to more convenient parking spots.

The perceived grievance that allows for the co-opted identity stems from the desirability and limited availability of parking spaces closer to building entrances. The rise of sales in fake placards to access accessible parking spaces is a clear indicator of ongoing harm to disabled people who rely on accessible parking. Many people within the disabled community have taken to complaining about folx who appear to be able-bodied parking and walking away from accessible parking spots. With so many people abusing fake placards, this becomes the first thought, rather than considering that the person walking away from the accessible parking may have an invisible disability. Not only does the practice cause harm in a direct sense, but it also changes the way people perceive each other—people are more likely to be seen as abusing the system rather than having a legitimate need if they are using an accessible spot without a visible disability.

Weaponizing Disability at THE HAPPIEST PLACE ON EARTH™

While Disneyland has historically been active in serving disabled visitors, it was not until the establishment of Disability Access Services that Disney provided explicit support for disabled patrons. The Disability Access Services program at Disney provides access to all services, rides, and programs within the boundaries of the park. A common accommodation provided to people who qualify for the "disability pass" is the ability to wait virtually in line for all rides. Further, they are provided earlier access to the entrance and can access other amenities without having to wait (Dufresne, 2021). The challenge to this program is that it operates on the honor system, and almost since its inception, nondisabled people have been taking advantage of it to streamline their experience. Like most entertainment venues, resources dedicated to serving disabled people are limited, and the sheer number of individuals who abuse the "disability pass" has created problems for disabled guests. In 2013, the original method of serving guests with disabilities changed because patrons were hiring folx with disabilities to purchase tickets and accompany groups to gain unlimited front-of-the-line access to rides and attractions (Bell, 2020). The new system allows anyone to join a queue that will announce when and how they can join a ride or an attraction without physically waiting in line. Experienced visitors streamline their visits by queuing rides in a specific order, while inexperienced visitors still end up waiting for every single ride or attraction.

In this example, the co-opted disabled identity was weaponized to provide nondisabled guests an efficient experience. This ultimately creates a barrier to access for disabled people. For example, a person who needs to visit rides or attractions in a specific order cannot always do so due to the number of guests present on a specific day. This was the basis for a lawsuit in 2014 against the 70-year-old park (Bell, 2020). This shift in practice has significantly and disproportionately impacted specific people within the disabled community and could have been avoided had people not co-opted and weaponized disability in the first place.

Emotional Support, Service, and Pet Animals

The legitimacy of service animals in assisting members of the disabled community in their day-to-day activities was also established by the ADA. A service animal is defined as a dog that is specifically trained to do work or perform tasks for an individual with a disability (U.S. Department of Justice, Civil Rights Division, 2015). Originally established in the early 1900s, service animals have served people with disabilities for over 100 years.

Service animals are different from emotional support animals (ESA) in that a service animal is protected in virtually every space, while ESAs have very few rights. ESAs were originally meant to support people with emotion-based disabilities and mental health conditions. The training of an ESA is functionally different, as an ESA is trained to recognize and respond to a person's emotional state. Untrained animals pose a danger to people, can distract and/or attack legitimate service animals, and their untrained behaviors can erode trust in the legitimacy of trained service animals needed by disabled people in their day-to-day life (Tilbury, 2018). Online marketplaces are full of unauthorized and unofficial vests and clothing to disguise pets as service animals. Those articles of clothing are generally enough to deceive, as the only two questions an owner can be asked are, "is the dog a service animal required because of a disability" and "what work or tasks has the dog been trained to perform" (U.S. Department of Justice, Civil Rights Division, 2015). On January 1, 2022, California passed a law to curb a dramatic rise in untrained animals being presented in public spaces as service animals (Daugherty, 2021), but there is currently no effective, equitable method for determining between service animals and household pets that are misrepresented as service animals.

This problem extends to media representations as well. In a recent movie, *Dog* (Carolin & Tatum, 2022), Channing Tatum portrays a military veteran who is attempting to make it to a fellow soldier's funeral. Throughout the film, Tatum's character pretends to be blind and presents a military working dog as a guide dog. The film also explores how Tatum's character manages post-traumatic stress disorder that was acquired during his military service. This movie demonstrates how easy it is to pass off a non-service animal as a service animal, as well as being an inaccurate and offensive portrayal of the abilities of blind people in practice.

Circumventing Mask Ordinances During the COVID-19 Pandemic

As of January 1, 2022, the COVID-19 virus had infected 289,659,230 people and claimed the lives of more than 5,456,867 individuals worldwide. The U.S. accounts for 55,846,519 (19.2%) of these cases and 847,162 (15.5%) of the total deaths thus far (Worldometer, 2022). According to claims data analysis by FAIR Health (2020) COVID-19 patients with "development disorders" had the highest odds of dying from COVID across all age groups (p. 2). People with intellectual disabilities and related conditions had the third highest risk of death. A study from the Office for National Statistics found that nearly six out of every ten people who died with COVID in England last year were disabled (BBC, 2021). Another study of 547 U.S. health care organizations found that "having an intellectual disability was the strongest independent risk factor for presenting with a COVID-19 diagnosis and the strongest independent risk factor other than age for mortality" (Gleason et al., 2021). All of this research demonstrates how the disabled community as a whole is at significantly higher risk than other groups of people.

During the pandemic, mask mandates emerged everywhere. Outside of lockdown and shelter-in-place orders, many spaces require individuals to properly wear a mask to interrupt transmission. Due to this practice, people have co-opted disabled identity by presenting an ADA mask exemption card to circumvent mask ordinances. These cards consistently contain information linking the Department of Justice and the ADA national telephone number with language that claims exemption from wearing a face covering/mask. From the late spring through the summer of 2020, a rise in usage of ADA mask exemption cards forced the Department of Justice to issue a press release debunking the practice (U.S. Department of Justice, Office of Public Affairs, 2020). Similar messaging came from local and national news agencies and disability activist groups (Pucket et al., 2020; Gibson, 2020; Angel, 2020; Heasley, 2020).

In the act of buying and using these cards, individuals co-opted and weaponized disability through the justification of victimhood. The analysis that follows will explore the relationship between identity and the medical model of disability; discuss the sociopolitical function of victimization in relation to disability; and identify how disabled identity became weaponized in the attempted use of fake ADA mask exemption cards.

IMPLICATING THE MEDICAL MODEL OF DISABILITY

The disabled community has struggled with the concept of disabled identity. To activists and academics, it is obvious that disabled identity exists and plays an important role in daily life. At the same time, for many disabled people, models and understanding of disability are bound within their own experience and those that surround them. Garland-Thomson (2014) writes:

...most disabled people are understood as foreigners within their own families, as an interruption in the continuity of sameness upon which familial solidarity is founded. The narrative of likeness crucial to group unity fractures critically with the arrival of disability to a family or circle. (n.p.)

This commentary illustrates the breadth of how disability is understood within the community, but also the variance of depth. Similarly, people who do not have a close connection to the disabled community are far less likely to carry positive or accurate understandings of the lived experiences of disabled people (Phillips, 1990).

As communication scholars, we understand that like all identities, disabled identity is constituted through communication (Bergen & Braithwaite, 2009; Darling, 2013). We also understand that disabled identity carries within it an unremovable stain that marks all actions, achievements, and acts that a person has done and will do (Grewe, 2022; Mitchell & Snyder, 2013). This identity framework positions disability as a negative attribute. A major disconnect within disability identity scholarship is a lack of identifying and accounting for how culture relates to and is constitutive of identity, especially at a pre-personal level. Specifically, we see a deficit in identifying the role of ascribed and avowed identity (Collier, 1997). An *ascribed disabled identity* occurs when a disability is visibly written on the body and recognized by others. This could be identified through a physical characteristic that is deemed non-normative by able-bodied standards, recognized through observation of body movement (i.e., gait, a limp, or manual manipulation), or through the presence of mobility equipment (i.e., wheelchair, crutches, prosthetic limb). An *avowed disabled identity* may or may not be obvious and may or may not be visible to others. This identity stems from the group affiliations that an individual feels connected to. An avowed identity may significantly differ from ascribed identities.

Disabled identity is also viewed as vulnerable. From the perspective of the ascribed identity, the disabled person is viewed as less-than or otherwise unable to perform specific tasks. For wheelchair users, stairs and steep hills seem impossible, while students with dyslexia or ADHD are seen as less capable in educational spaces. The avowed perspective is also seen as vulnerable; the disabled identity becomes salient as people are forced to confront actual or perceived limitations that they have. Unlike other visible, marginalized identities (such as race, gender, or age), a physical disability is rarely seen as a fear-inducing threat, though some invisible disabilities and mental health conditions can (e.g., when mental illness is scapegoated as the reason perpetrators commit acts of violence).

When disabled identity is co-opted, it is most often done through a non-threatening or a vulnerable lens. This co-opting discards disability-as-identity and instead relies on the structure and tenets of the medical model of disability. The perpetrators exploit how disability makes others uncomfortable, capitalize on legislation that prevents people from asking for private information, and reinforces the idea that disability is an unwanted and undesirable condition. In other words, the medical model is an essential component of framing disability within a victim frame.

Co-opting Disabled Identity and the Weaponization of Disability

From buying concert tickets to circumventing lines, able-bodied people have a history of adopting disabled identity and gaining the perceived advantages that come along with accommodations. Users of the card perceived mask ordinances as violations of their bodily autonomy, fabricating an aggrievement that allowed them to justify the co-opting of disabled identity. Looking back at Jacoby's (2015) five stages (specifically victimhood through ideological concurrence) demonstrates that delineating between harm and wrongdoing requires ignoring intention and impact, as the aggrieved status operates outside of the consequences to the co-opted identity. In every example of co-opting disabled identity presented in this chapter, it is difficult to imagine that the individuals who did so understood the impact their actions had on disabled people. Regardless, these ongoing practices create immediate and long-term impacts to the disabled community. While not getting front row tickets or having to park further from a building entrance may seem like an inconvenience, exploiting these accommodations communicates a lack of care and understanding and perpetuates social beliefs and behaviors which further marginalize disabled folx. In the case of mask exemption cards, those impacts were extremely dangerous.

As stated previously, the disabled community has been disproportionately impacted by COVID-19, making up an estimated 60% of all COVID-19-related deaths. One study suggested that people with "severe" physical disabilities were three times more likely to die from COVID-19 (BBC News, 2021). In another study, individuals with developmental and intellectual disabilities carried a mortality rate that was eight times higher than the general population (Gleason et al., 2021). Many states did not update triage procedures, leaving guidance in place that privileged nondisabled individuals with access to supply-limited life-saving care like ventilators (Ne'eman et al., 2021). Death is also not the only negative outcome the disabled community faced during the COVID-19 pandemic. The response to COVID-19 created a number of barriers that affected disabled people's access to safety in congregate living and health facilities, food delivery, internet service, COVID-19 testing, and other health care services (Shakespeare et al., 2021). Co-opting disabled identity for the purposes of using a fake ADA mask exemption card weaponizes disability by embracing the deficit orientation inherent to the medical model and created a more dangerous environment for disabled people.

Conclusion

Throughout this chapter, we traced some of the factors that impact our affective cognition, ranging from the seemingly innocuous acts of paying for rock-star parking, to the future 45th President's open mocking of a disabled reporter. Through each example, we can clearly see that disabled people are not seen as important or valuable. Further, by mapping the different acts that situate disabled bodies as both being undesirable, but also in need of desirable accommodations, we can begin to understand the harm that disabled folx experience on a day-to-day basis—even when the actions that cause harm were meant to be helpful. This is reflected by CDC Director, Rochelle Walensky, on January 7, 2022, in her comments on *Good Morning America*:

> The overwhelming number of deaths, over 75%, occurred in people who had at least four comorbidities, so really these are people who were unwell to begin with, and yes, really encouraging news in the context of omicron…We're really encouraged by these results. (Good Morning America, 2022)

Coming back to Protevi's (2009) notion of thanatography, these comments, along with Trump mocking Kovaleski, and all the examples of co-opting and weaponizing disability, are acts of communicative violence that create, provoke, and reinscribe ableism.

The co-optation and weaponization of disability are not new, nor would we predict that this will ever stop completely. The difficulty in creating change is that the offending party who is co-opting and weaponizing disability does so to sidestep public health orders, like the ADA, that exist to protect the most vulnerable. Disability, and the juridical structures designed in service of disability, have been weaponized as a tool in an ideological battle, and the disabled community is once again cast to the side to be bystanders and casualties. This results in the despondent effort of arguing about mask mandates and other health orders and instead pulls focus away from how dangerous misrepresenting an ADA mask exemption card is to the disabled community. The terms for engagement around the issue are defined by a group of individuals who do not believe, accept, or even understand how their actions are harmful.

Unlike other examples of co-opting and weaponizing disability, the COVID-19 pandemic provided us with immediate saliency, where the practice played out and functioned with near immediate consequence on a massive scale. This was enabled by every instance, experience, and misrepresentation of disability; with every instance in which a disabled identity was co-opted for advantage, benefit, or profit—the COVID-19 pandemic increased the violent outcomes of this behavior. By removing COVID-19 precautions and promoting a return to "normalcy" disabled lives become acceptable and understandable losses. There was a perfect storm of events ranging from the proliferation of access to goods and services via online ordering and concierge shoppers to the almost overnight shift of workplaces, classrooms, and personal relationships to an entirely digitally mediated environment.

This chapter represents a number of current articulations and their effects, but it is important to recognize that this isn't how things have to be—we can all work together to change these perceptions through our social interactions and the spaces we create together. We must shift the conversation around disability away from the medical model. Helping people understand themselves, and the world we all inhabit, as a vast network of social relationships that come together to construct our shared reality.

Note

1. A detailed accounting of the roots of the victimhood identity in Christianity can be found in Moss (2013).

References

ADA National Network. (2021, December 30). *What is the definition of disability under the ADA?* ADATA. https://adata.org/faq/what-definition-disability-under-ada

Angel, J. (2020, August 5). A warning about fake face mask exemption cards. *New England ADA Center Blog.* https://www.newenglandada.org/blog/warning-about-fake-face-mask-exemption-cards

Arkin, D. (2015, November 26). Donald Trump criticized after he appears to mock reporter Serge Kovaleski. *NBC News.* https://www.nbcnews.com/politics/2016-election/new-york-times-slams-donald-trump-after-he-appears-mock-n470016

BBC News. (2021, February 11). Covid: Disabled people account for six in 10 deaths in England last year—ONS. https://www.bbc.com/news/uk-56033813

Bell, T. (2020, July 1). Lawsuit over disability access policy decided in Disney's favor. *Disney Information Station.* https://www.wdwinfo.com/news-stories/lawsuit-over-disability-access-policy-decided-in-disneys-favor/

Bergen, K. M., & Braithwaite, D. O. (2009). Identity as constituted in communication. In W. F. Eadie (Ed.), *21st century communication: A reference handbook* (pp. 165–173). Sage. http://www.credoreference.com.bianca.penlib.du.edu/entry/sagetfccomm/identity_as_constituted_in_communication

Bergmann, W. (2008). Anti-Semitic attitudes in Europe: A comparative perspective. *Journal of Social Issues, 64*(2), 343–362. https://doi.org/10.1111/j.1540-4560.2008.00565.x

Blasius, M. (2015, October 19). Some fans ignore disability seating rules at Red Rocks. *Coloradoan.* https://www.coloradoan.com/story/news/local/colorado/2015/10/19/fans-ignore-disability-seating-rules-red-rocks/74208662/

Braithwaite, D. O. (1990). From majority to minority: An analysis of cultural change from ablebodied to disabled. *International Journal of Intercultural Relations, 14*(4), 465–483. https://doi.org/10.1016/0147-1767(90)90031-Q

Braithwaite, D. O., & Braithwaite, C. (1988). Viewing persons with disabilities as a culture. In L. A. Samovar & R. E. Porter (Eds.), *Intercultural communication: A reader* (pp. 147–153). Wadsworth.

Carmon, I. (2015, August 11). Donald Trump's worst offense? Mocking disabled reporter, poll finds. *NBC News.* https://www.nbcnews.com/politics/2016-election/trump-s-worst-offense-mocking-disabled-reporter-poll-finds-n627736

Carolin, R., & Tatum, C. (Directors). (2022). *Dog* [Film]. Metro-Goldwyn-Mayer.

Chaudoir, S., & Quinn, D. (2010). Revealing concealable stigmatized identities: The impact of disclosure motivations and positive first-disclosure experiences on fear of disclosure and well-being. *Journal of Social Issues, 66*(3), 570–584. https://doi.org/10.1111/j.1540-4560.2010.01663.x

Collier, M. J. (1997). Cultural identity and intercultural communication. In L. A. Samovar & R. E. Porter (Eds.), *Intercultural communication: A reader* (8th ed., pp. 36–44). Wadsworth Press.

Colorado Music Hall of Fame. (2019, March 22). History and future of Red Rocks Ampitheatre. https://cmhof.org/red-rocks-amphitheatre-kicks-off-another-season/

Darling, R. B. (2013). *Disability and identity: Negotiating self in a changing society.* Lynne Rienner Publishers.

Daugherty, P. (2021, December 13). New California law cracks down on emotional support animal (ESA) fraud. *City Watch LA.* https://www.citywatchla.com/index.php/cw/animal-watch/23296-new-california-law-cracks-down-on-emotional-support-animal-esa-fraud

DeLuca, K. (1999). Articulation theory: A discursive grounding for rhetorical practice. *Philosophy and Rhetoric, 32*(4), 334–348. https://www.jstor.org/stable/40238046

Denvir, D. (2013, December 16). A short history of the war on Christmas: How everyone from Bill O'Reilly to Jon Stewart became a co-conspirator in an annual farce. *Politico.* https://www.politico.com/magazine/story/2013/12/war-on-christmas-short-history-101222/

Dionne, E. J. (2008, March 1). Culture wars? How 2004. *Real Clear Politics.* https://www.realclearpolitics.com/articles/2008/03/reclaiming_faith_and_politics.html

Dufresne, A. (2021, December 13). Disney guests speak out on others abusing free disability service. *Inside the Magic.* https://insidethemagic.net/2021/12/disney-guests-speak-out-das-ad1/

FAIR Health. (2020). *Risk Factors for COVID-19 Mortality among Privately Insured Patients: A Claims Data Analysis.* [White paper, in collaboration with the West Health Institute and Marty Makary, MD, MPH, from Johns Hopkins University School of Medicine]. https://s3.amazonaws.com/media2.fairhealth.org/whitepaper/asset/Risk%20Factors%20for%20COVID-19%20Mortality%20among%20Privately%20Insured%20Patients%20-%20A%20Claims%20Data%20Analysis%20-%20A%20FAIR%20Health%20White%20Paper.pdf

Gibson, K. (2020, June 30). Face mask 'exemption' cards are fakes, feds warn. *CBS News.* https://www.cbsnews.com/news/face-mask-exemption-card-freedom-to-breathe-agency-fraudulent/

Giroux, H. (2017, March 22). The culture of cruelty in Trump's America. *Truthout.* https://truthout.org/articles/the-culture-of-cruelty-in-trump-s-america/

Gleason, J., Ross, W., Fossi, A., Blonsky, H., Tobias, J., & Stephens, M. (2021). The devastating impact of covid-19 on individuals with intellectual disabilities in the United States. *NEJM Catalyst..* https://catalyst.nejm.org/doi/full/10.1056/CAT.21.0051

Good Morning America. (2022). *CDC director responds to criticisms on COVID-19 guidance* [Video]. YouTube. https://www.youtube.com/watch?v=gxZT7ra-oxs

Grewe, B. (2022). On marking disability using language: A stain on the soul. *Listening: Journal of Communication Ethics, Religion, and Culture, 57*(2).

Haller, B., & Zhang, L. (2010). Survey of disabled people about media representations. *Media & Disability Resources.* Retrieved December 3, 2019, from https://mediadisability.wordpress.com/survey/

Heasley, S. (2020, July 7). Face mask exempt cards citing ADA are fake, Justice Department says. *Disability Scoop.* https://www.disabilityscoop.com/2020/07/07/face-mask-exempt-cards-ada-fake/28559/

Holmes, J. (2018, December 18). Trump is milking the war on Christmas for every last penny. *Esquire.* https://www.esquire.com/news-politics/a25615175/donald-trump-war-on-christmas-fundraising-email/

Hurley, S. (2004). Imitation, media violence, and freedom of speech. *Philosophical Studies: An International Journal for Philosophy in the Analytic Tradition, 117*(1/2), 165–218. http://www.jstor.org/stable/4321442

Jacoby, T. A. (2015). A theory of victimhood: Politics, conflict and the construction of victim-based identity. *Millennium, 43*(2), 511–530. https://doi.org/10.1177/0305829814550258

Jeffress, M. S. (Ed.). (2021). *Disability representation in film, TV, and print media.* Routledge.

Kessler, G. (2016, August 2). Donald Trump's revisionist history of mocking a disabled reporter. *Washington Post.* https://www.washingtonpost.com/news/fact-checker/wp/2016/08/02/donald-trumps-revisionist-history-of-mocking-a-disabled-reporter/

Lindemann, K. (2010). Cleaning up my (father's) mess: Narrative containments of "leaky" masculinities. *Qualitative Inquiry, 16*(1), 29–38. https://doi.org/10.1177/1077800409350060

McKerrow, R. (1989). Critical rhetoric: Theory and praxis. *Communication Monographs, 56*, 91–111.

Metzl, J., Piemonte, J., & McKay, T. (2021). Mental illness, mass shootings, and the future of psychiatric research into American gun violence. *Harvard Review of Psychiatry, 29*(1), 81–89. https://doi.org/10.1097/HRP.0000000000000280

Mitchell, D., & Snyder, S. (2013). Introduction: Disability studies and the double bind of representation. In D. T. Mitchell & S. Snyder (Eds.), *The body and physical difference: Discourses of disability* (pp. 1–31). University of Michigan.

Moss, C. (2013). *The myth of persecution.* HarperCollins.

Ne'eman, A. Stein, M. A., Berger, Z. D., & Dorfman, D. (2021). The treatment of disability under crisis standards of care: An empirical and normative analysis of change over time during COVID-19. *Journal of Health Politics, Policy and Law, 46*(5), 831–860. https://doi.org/10.1215/03616878-9156005

Newman, J. (2021). Southern Ohio Police Department warns of fake handicap placards selling on marketplace. *SCIOTO Post.* (May 26). https://www.sciotopost.com/southern-ohio-police-department-warns-of-fake-handicap-placards-selling-on-marketplace/

Phillips, M. J. (1990). Damaged goods: Oral narratives of the experience of disability in American culture. *Social Science & Medicine, 30*(8), 849–857.

Protevi, J. (2009). *Political affect: Connecting the social and the somatic.* University of Minnesota Press.

Pucket, J., Tregde, D., Spry Jr., T. (2020, June 25). VERIFY: Face mask exemption cards are fake. *9news.* https://www.9news.com/article/news/verify/verify-fraudulent-face-mask-exempt-card-doesnt-actually-do-anything/

Putnam, M. (2005). Conceptualizing disability developing a framework for political disability identity. *Journal of Disability Policy Studies, 16*(3), 188–198. https://doi.org/10.1177/10442073050160030601

Scott, J.-A. (2013). Problematizing a researcher's performance of "insider status": An autoethnography of "designer disabled" identity. *Qualitative Inquiry, 19*(2), 101–115. https://doi.org/10.1177/1077800412462990

Shakespeare, T., Ndagire, F., & Seketi, Q. E. (2021). Triple jeopardy: Disabled people and the COVID-19 pandemic. *The Lancet, 397*(10282), 1331–1333. https://doi.org/10.1016/S0140-6736(21)00625-5

Siebers, T. (2004). Disability as masquerade. *Literature and medicine, 23*(1), 1–22. https://doi.org/10.1353/lm.2004.0010

Snyder, S. L., & Mitchell, D. T. (2006). *Cultural locations of disability.* University of Chicago Press.

Student Disability Services. (2021, December 30). *The myth of the unfair advantage.* University of Mississippi. https://sds.olemiss.edu/the-myth-of-the-unfair-advantage/

Garland-Thomson, R. (2014). The story of my work: How I became disabled. *Disability Studies Quarterly, 34*(2). http://dsq-sds.org/article/view/4254/3594

Tilbury, K. (2018, May 16). Fake service dogs, real problems. *Associated Press.* https://apnews.com/article/1a28f8e528424fdca2040ea8139e3014

U.S. Department of Justice, Civil Rights Division. (2010). Americans with Disabilities Act ADA Compliance BRIEF: Restriping Parking Spaces. https://www.denvergov.org/content/dam/denvergov/Portals/643/documents/Offices/Disability/DPEP/ADA%20Parking%20Lot%20Requirements.pdf

U.S. Department of Justice, Civil Rights Division. (2015). Frequently asked questions about service animals and the ADA. https://www.ada.gov/regs2010/service_animal_qa.html

U.S. Department of Justice, Office of Public Affairs. (2020, June 30). *The Department of Justice warns of inaccurate flyers and postings regarding the use of face masks and the Americans with Disabilities Act.* [Press Release]. https://www.justice.gov/opa/pr/department-justice-warns-inaccurate-flyers-and-postings-regarding-use-face-masks-and

Walker, C. (2017, November 16). Following lawsuit, Red Rocks trying new ticketing system for accessible seats. *Westword.* https://www.westword.com/music/red-rocks-to-implement-new-ticketing-system-following-disability-lawsuit-9700315

Worldometer. (2022). COVID-19 Coronavirus pandemic. https://www.worldometers.info/coronavirus/

PART III

Cultural Artifacts and Disability

CHAPTER 13

Communicating AI and Disability

Gerard Goggin, Andrew Prahl, and Kuansong Victor Zhuang

In recent years, technology has moved center-stage in how societies work, in how they seek to improve the lot of people, and how they envision and plan for the future. A great deal of contemporary conversations and discourse, especially on official levels, feature technology—not least artificial intelligence (AI).

AI has been many decades in the making, but the most recent phase of AI—machine learning, data, automation, and other associated technologies—has captured the imagination of many worldwide. There is good reason for this, because AI and machine learning have become widely embedded in technology systems and are utilized across a wide range of things we do in everyday life (Elliott, 2019; Katz et al., 2021), as well as in workplaces and a wide range of institutions, economic settings, and civil society (Roberge & Castelle, 2021).

Increasingly around the world we communicate with machines, gain information, undertake interpretation, query, discuss, and gain support for our decision-making and actions via machine learning, AI, and datasets. The International Telecommunications Union (ITU) estimated that approximately 4.9 billion people (some 63 percent of the world's population) were using the Internet in 2021 (ITU, 2021b). A great proportion of these users access the Internet via mobile Internet and mobile broadband devices, especially in low- and middle-income settings where mobile Internet is often the default mode of

G. Goggin (✉)
Discipline of Media and Communications, University of Sydney, Sydney, Australia
e-mail: gerard.goggin@sydney.edu.au

A. Prahl • K. V. Zhuang
Wee Kim Wee School of Communication and Information, Nanyang Technological University, Singapore, Singapore

© The Author(s), under exclusive license to Springer Nature Switzerland AG 2023
M. S. Jeffress et al. (eds.), *The Palgrave Handbook of Disability and Communication*, https://doi.org/10.1007/978-3-031-14447-9_13

Internet access (Donner, 2015; ITU, 2021b, pp. 10-12). Billions of people rely upon apps on their smartphones or feature-phones, which in turn are powered by software, digital infrastructures, databases, computational capacities, and algorithms that have significant and rapidly improving capability to analyze written, spoken, visual, haptic, and other forms of multi-modal communication (Goggin, 2021).

When we inquire about our finances, or a travel booking, or check our social media feeds, or answer an email via Google, or participate in a video call with automatically generated captioning, we are often encountering AI. The continuing development of digital, social, mobile, computational, locational, software and app media, and intelligent systems relies increasingly on AI—in ways that have become taken-for-granted (Lanzara, 2016; Ling, 2012). These things also constitute our contemporary technologies of communication.

A further dimension to the salience of AI is how it has become pivotal in conversations about societies and their futures. As it turns out, such talk relies upon, plays with, and communicates powerful ideas about disability. There are at least two major ways that social relations and innovations in disability are entwined in the rise of AI and associated technologies.

DISABILITY IN THE RISE OF AI

First, many people with disabilities use, or even rely upon, specific technologies for communication. The area of augmentative, alternative, and assistive technologies has seen significant change with the rise of mobile, personal, and mainstream devices such as smartphones and iPads, and the social practices associated with these (Alper, 2015, p. 12). Alper's work, especially her 2017 book *Giving Voice*, has shown the social contexts and dynamics of the shaping of these technologies, especially their influence in social inequalities; in how children with disabilities negotiate access; and the knowledge of, expertise in, and use of such technologies for communication (Alper, 2017).

Second, across a range of areas, AI and machine-learning are being deployed to underpin a wide range of communication technologies; machines, as part of their data training sets, are "learning" about disability and users with impairments and disabilities. This is a new phase of the developments over the past three or so decades where digital communication has become a major part of overall communication.

How we discuss, depict, represent, and tell stories about our machines also has striking and constitutive relationships to disability. The topic of AI and disability has thus been paid increasing attention by disability scholars and activists, policymakers, companies, governments, designers and engineers, and citizens and publics alike.

A common starting point is the potential of AI and machine learning to advance the cause of accessibility and digital inclusion for people with disabilities—and via innovative, universal and inclusive design philosophies and practices, to extend access, usability, inclusion, and indeed democratization of technologies for all. What is striking, however, are the various ways that discourses about AI and disability go well beyond traditional emphases of accessibility and inclusion to engage large registers of human development, empowerment, and life enhancement.

In this chapter, we wish to reflect upon the state-of-the-art of such talk that yokes together disability and AI—and what this examination reveals about the broader role technology plays in the visions and plans of societies.

IMAGINING TECHNOLOGY AND DISABILITY

Theoretical Background

Humans have always been optimistic about new technologies, regardless of the domain, be it education, health care, work, and so on. Such optimism has flowed into a particular fascination with technology and disability, which has deep roots. In the second half of the twentieth century, explicit development of technology and disability saw development of areas such as assistive technology, rehabilitation science and engineering, and other areas. A longstanding and central scholar in the area, Roulstone (2016) notes that even up to the 1980s and 1990s it was still the case that "[m]uch rehabilitation, clinical practice and computer science of the time continued to focus on disabled people's deficits and the fixative qualities of technologies" (p. 91). Roulstone points to the salience of "narratives of technology," centering on "a number of themes, principally rescue" (p. 91). Such narratives were often underpinned by "deficit" models of disability, especially the idea of disability as "tragedy" (Roulstone, 2016, p. 91). A key way such "techno-optimistic" accounts of disability vary from other accounts is the assumption that technology makes possible what was not possible (rather than technology making better or easier what was already possible—as in discourses of automation of work).

Against such accounts, Roulstone (2016) points to work through the 1990s and 2000s that questioned and complicated such dominant framing, suggesting that the "reframing of technology by disability studies as an aid to a more enabling society represented a paradigm shift in moving beyond the individual, fixative and body-focused paradigm" (p. 101).

Roulstone notes the various debates on the enabling versus disabling role of technology, the innovation in socio-technical development even among those working with narrower notions of disability, the benefits of technology, and the issues about technologies being shaped by economic, social, and political forces (not least dynamics of social inequality and exclusion). He notes from disability studies especially the growing view about the fluidity and flexibility of relationships between disability and technology: "Technology clearly has potential for some disabled people sometimes...At other times technology is clearly often a means to a variety of ends ...." (Roulstone, 2016, p. 114). This assessment is borne out by the many studies in the area of disability and technology that have emerged during the past two decades, evidence that the field is clearly in ferment (Hamraie & Fritsch, 2019; Hendren, 2020; Mills, 2022; Pullin, 2009; Sterne, 2021; Tkaczyk et al., 2020; Williamson, 2019). This energy is captured in Hamraie and Fritsch's bold (2019) "Crip Technoscience Manifesto." Hamraie and Fritsch call for "technoscientific activism and critical design practices" to be "rooted in disability justice, collective access, and collective transformation toward more socially just disability relations"—in order to "expand possible futures for disabled people" (2019, p. 22).

Disability in Technology Communication

The theoretical background just outlined is important to understand the dominant ways disability is conceived, framed, and discussed in relation to technology. Noting Roulstone's caveats, as well as the shifts in conceptualization and discourse in recent years, it is striking to observe the ways that disability figures regularly and prominently in the dominant discourses on these technological changes and visions. Consider, for instance, passages on disability in three widely popular discourses on technology in the past few decades.

First, we see disability figuring in futurist and inventor Ray Kurzweil's highly influential account of the potential of technological advancement in areas of genetics, nanotech, and robotics:

> The compelling benefits of overcoming profound diseases and disabilities will keep these technologies on a rapid course, but medical applications represent only the early-adoption phase. As the technologies become established, there will be no barriers to using them for vast expansion of human potential. (Kurzweil, 2005, p. 563)

Kurzweil, of course, had long been interested in disability. As well as his pioneering role in optical character recognition, he developed text-to-speech and synthetic speech technologies as "reading machines" for "people who are blind" and offered them as "tiny devices you put in your pocket" (Kurzweil, 2003, p. 583). Second, disability crops up in the discourses on the "new second machine age." Consider the way that new technologies are presented as something miraculous in this key text:

> Digital technologies are also restoring hearing to the deaf via cochlear implants and will probably bring sight back to the fully blind .... Considered objectively, these advances are something close to miracles—and they're still in their infancy. (Brynjolfsson & McAfee, 2014, p. 114)

Third, disability figures in the much vaunted "Fourth Industrial Revolution," often framed in this kind of way:

> Technological developments in this new era, such as the integration of ultrasonic sensors with computer vision techniques for those with visual impairment, and integration of electroencephalography-based brain-controlled lower-limb exoskeletons for those with paraplegia, bring unprecedented hope for persons with disabilities. (Delgado, 2019, p. 993).

Here Delgado, a specialist in child neurology, declares: "In this new world, in which technology bridges the gaps between performance and participation in more efficient ways, the concept of 'disability' will have to be revised" (Delgado, 2019, p. 993). Potentially this puts on the agenda the need to think about disability in new ways. However, a radical rethinking of disability—as discussed in the second half of this chapter—is rarely on the agenda in these dominant ways of knowing and presenting technology.

Imaginaries

Developed by various thinkers, imaginaries have been a way to grasp and analyze the powerful role of ideas, signs and meanings, discourses, practices, material arrangements, and so on, that form dominant ways of seeing and orienting societies (French & Corker, 1999; Grue, 2015). Titchkosky (2019), for instance, has drawn attention to "disability imaginaries" in media, showing that while shape-shifting these imaginaries play important social functions. Other disability scholars have also discussed the ways how disability imaginaries play a crucial role in the shaping of general communication (Bostad & Hanisch, 2016; Bunch et al., 2021; Ginsburg & Rapp, 2019; Shuttleworth & Meekosha, 2013).

When it comes to technology, a fertile move is to look at the cross-over between disability imaginaries and what Jasanoff (2015) has called "sociotechnical imaginaries":

> Sociotechnical imaginaries, in our view, are "collectively held, institutionally stabilized, and publicly performed visions of desirable futures, animated by shared understandings of forms of social life and social order attainable through, and supportive of, advances in science and technology." (p. 322)

Jasanoff (2015) further notes: "Science and technology have been involved in efforts to reimagine and reinvent human societies for close to two hundred years" (p. 321). Hence, she contends that sociotechnical imaginaries are helpful to grasp such efforts. Such imaginaries are not rigid or simple to appreciate because they "take shape in varied social and cultural contexts and … in turn help reorient the evolution of those contexts" (p. 322). However, such imaginaries do achieve "mass and solidity" and play an important role in practice as they fuse "imagination, objects, and social norms" (p. 322).

Mansell (2015) has delineated "contending social imaginaries" associated with the evolution of the Internet. She points to a dominant imaginary that is consistent with a "notion of autonomous technology and it privileges increasing quantities of information over the messy world of situated meaning construction ... how society adjusts to the shock of rapid technological innovation" (p. 25). Thus a "prevailing social imaginary is of machines that can 'think' and make 'choices' on behalf of human beings" (p. 25). We can see social imaginaries as a mode of "perceiving the future" through technologies (Katz et al., 2021). This is apparent in Alper's (2019) work on "future talk" as a way to describe "everyday imaginaries of the future that exist in relation to other future discourses" in the lives of young people with disabilities (p. 729).

With these considerations noted, attention now turns to the function of disability in AI imaginaries.

Imagining AI and Disability: Can AI Be a Game Changer?

The prevailing narratives of AI and machine learning revolve around the considerable benefits that technology will bring—with disability figuring as a key area, such as the contribution of Dengel et al. (2021) to a 2021 academic volume on AI and humanity.

Disability has been addressed in the touchstone notion of "AI for Good" (Floridi et al., 2020; Tomašev et al., 2020). Like other technology "for good" discourses, linking disability with AI for Good helps companies to advance their reputations for corporate social responsibility (CSR), as well as offering fodder for public relations and marketing.

Corporate Initiatives

Microsoft is one company with a long record of engagement and controversy in relation to accessibility (Goggin & Newell, 2003; Lazar et al., 2015; Morris et al., 2019). More recently it became known for its *Seeing AI* app, featured in a 2016 keynote by CEO Satya Nadella (Microsoft, n.d.). In 2018, Microsoft launched an *AI for Accessibility* program (Smith, 2018). "AI can be a game changer for people with disabilities," Microsoft President Brad Smith avers, noting that: "Already we're witnessing this as people with disabilities expand their use of computers to hear, see and reason with impressive accuracy" (Smith, 2018). He lauds "real-time speech-to-text transcription, visual recognition services, and predictive text functionality..." that "offer enormous potential..." for people with disabilities "...to do more in three specific scenarios: employment, modern life and human connection" (Smith, 2018).

For its part, Intel's *AI for Social Good* program has the tagline "Enriching Lives Around the World" (Intel, n.d.). Intel has three signature AI for Good initiatives for addressing "Global Challenges"; one is "Perceiving the World with AI," which includes a smart backpack with voice activation (Intel, n.d.).

Google is another prominent company that has adopted various strategies in the area of AI, accessibility, and disability. Disability also is prominent in Google's framing of its larger claims to align its technology design, policy, and business for aims of societal benefit via AI for Social Good initiatives. Among the list of ways that AI can "meaningfully improve people's lives" is to "dramatically improve the lives of people with disabilities" (Google, n.d.-a, para. 1). A signature effort is Google's *Project Euphonia*:

> … a research initiative focused on helping people with atypical speech be better understood. The approach is centered on analyzing speech recordings to better train speech recognition models. (Google, n.d.-b)

Project Euphonia invites people who "have a voice that may be considered difficult to understand (but not because of an accent)" to record a set of phrases (Google, n.d.-b). explains that "the algorithms have not heard nearly as many examples from people with impaired speech" (Google, n.d.-b).

As well as these three programs, there are many other initiatives underway around the globe. Pioneering efforts have been made in East Asia especially, in particular, Japan, Korea, and China (Digital Asia Hub, 2017; Goggin et al., 2019; Nakada et al., 2021; Samsung, 2021). The discourse and framing of such organizations can take on an agenda-setting role for other organizations, and sometimes academic researchers, to follow. Another view is that, especially in relation to disability, many such corporations have been reactive and often only acted in relation to legal obligations as has been evident in research on technology and the Americans with Disabilities Act (Blanck, 2021; Lazar & Stein, 2017). Such discussion raises the broader issues of law and regulation, and how a range of policy actors and agencies are approaching AI and disability (Pathakji, 2018).

Global Media Policy

In the area of global media and technology policy (Mansell & Raboy, 2011), the United Nations (UN) has developed policy using the rubric of AI for Good. One lead UN agency has been the International Telecommunications Union (ITU), which initiated a global forum on AI for Social Good in 2017 and then an AI for Good platform ([https://aiforgood.itu.int/programme/]). The ITU has a particular focus on digital inclusion, and those unconnected or less connected: "The AI for Good platform focuses on uses of AI to help fulfil the essential needs of humanity, including achieving the 17 SDGs [Sustainable Development Goals] set out by the UN to be achieved by 2030 …." (ITU, 2021a). The ITU notes "AI has extraordinary potential to act as a force for good. However, considerable challenges persist" (ITU, 2021a). Disability is mentioned explicitly in relation to the key challenge of bias (ITU, 2021a). The

ITU also notes overarching issues of "equitable uses of AI," notably: "Unequal access to computing power and to data deepens the divide between a few companies and elite universities which do have resources, and the rest of the world which does not" (ITU, 2021a).

There is a great deal more to be discussed in relation to the ways in which societal benefit, the good life, and so on, figure prominently in the dominant social imaginaries of AI. In this section, we have pointed to three examples from tech companies. We have also highlighted a leading initiative from the UN, which though having waned in the past two decades still plays a surprisingly significant role in shaping discourses, regulation, and policy in areas of inequality, justice, and inclusion in information and communication technologies (ICTs) and media (Couldry et al., 2018). What we have aimed to sketch out is the function that disability plays in such imaginaries. In the penultimate section of the paper, we will turn to alternative imaginaries that are emerging.

Alternative Imaginaries of Disability and AI

Critiques and New Research

Disability was a relatively late arrival on the scene of critical interrogations of AI. One of the foremost scholars of emerging technologies and disability has been Wolbring, who has undertaken pioneering work on narratives, imagery, and representations in areas such as robots (Wolbring, 2016; Wolbring & Yumakulov, 2014; Yumakulov et al., 2012), brain-computer interfaces (Kögel & Wolbring, 2020). Lillywhite and Wolbring have contributed two studies of the coverage of disability and AI (Lillywhite & Wolbring, 2020, 2021). Specifically in relation to an examination of AI in academic literature, Canadian newspapers, and tweets, they found the term "patient" was overused compared to terms "disabled people" or "people with disabilities" and the "tone of coverage was mostly techno-optimistic" (Lillywhite & Wolbring, 2020, p. 12). Strikingly, they also found that "content related to AI/ML causing social problems for disabled people was nearly absent," as were "discussions around disabled people being involved in, or impacted by, AI/ML ethics and governance discourses" (Lillywhite & Wolbring, 2020, p. 12). Their final major finding was an "absen(ce) of content around 'AI for good' and 'AI for social good' in relation to disabled people" (Lillywhite & Wolbring, 2020, p. 12). As we have seen, efforts have been made across AI for Good initiatives to create such content—both in acknowledging issues and potential innovations focused on people with disabilities. Fair to say, however, that while the discourse on AI for Good has shifted to be more inclusive people with disabilities, there remains a fair way to go.

A 2019 workshop organized jointly by AI Now Institute and Microsoft captured the rising discontent. It brought together a range of participants to discuss where disability fits into the growing concerns associated with AI systems (Whittaker et al., 2019). The workshop identified a major problem being that "much of the AI targeted at disabled people implicitly promises to make them more like non-disabled people, based on an implied understanding that non-disabled is the norm" (Whittaker et al., 2019, p. 13).

Encouragingly, since 2019, a growing body of research has explored the shaping of AI technologies and disability and the implications of developing the former through the lens of the latter for both communication and society. Various scholars have explored the contours of these issues in relation to disability (Bennett & Keyes, 2020; Hofmann et al., 2020; Morris, 2020).

Various scholars have argued that there are limitations in the narrow notions of bias (Fazelpour & Danks, 2021) and fairness as default ways of approaching the topic, pointing out that these can obscure and detract from the large contexts and dynamics of power, inequality, and injustice which require urgent attention (Crawford, 2021; Pasquale, 2015, 2020; Zajko, 2021).

Data is a major issue when it comes to the complex diversity of disability. If it is true that people with disabilities are under-represented in important areas of society such as education and workforce (Chennat, 2019; Danforth & Gabel, 2016; Fielden et al., 2020; Turner et al., 2017), then it might be said that they are under-represented in traditional datasets and new kinds of digital data collections (Deitz et al., 2021). There is also the issue that different kinds of data classification, gathering, and coding struggle to include and adequately represent people with disabilities (Park & Humphry, 2019), and indeed many others, as Crawford has shown (Crawford, 2021). Thus, Nakamura has pointed out: "Many facial recognition training datasets pre-code values of trinary 'race' and binary 'gender' which reify shifting social categories, and they omit faces that are not 'normal,' such as those of people who are disabled, ill, or disfigured" (Nakamura, 2019, 2).

Informed by a growing recognition and awareness of issues of privacy, data subjectivity, protection, and sovereignty in relation to disability, researchers are giving greater scrutiny to AI systems' use of personal and user data. Researchers are exploring the complex and specific nature of data when it comes to the diversity of people with disability, their personal information and data, and the societies and markets in which they live. Wald (2020) brings up a key argument for consideration by noting that people with disabilities include those whose experience and requirements for AI do not fit into the majority conceptions of much digital data: "Classification using big data struggles to cope with the individual uniqueness of disabled people, and whereas developers tend to design for the majority so ignoring outliers, designing for edge cases would be a more inclusive approach" (p. 1). So, the idea that there is a major opportunity in inclusion by "designing for edge cases" has attracted considerable support (Treviranus, 2016, 2019).

Global Media Policy Response

The groundswell of research, advocacy, activism, and intervention has led to international, regional, and national legislators and policymakers acknowledging the profound issues in AI and disability—and the ways that these are not well captured in dominant imaginaries. Disability is included in some of the most ambitious and comprehensive efforts to tackle the glaring issues raised by AI. We can see this registered, for instance, in the encompassing effort of the United Nations Educational, Scientific and Cultural Organization (UNESCO)'s *Recommendation on the Ethics of Artificial Intelligence* adopted in November 2021 (UNESCO, 2021). Disability is mentioned in important provisions that offer a holistic account of both AI and its relationships with people, the environment, and ecosystems. Stipulation number 15, for instance, addresses AI for those in receipt of assistance and care (UNESCO, 2021, p. 6). Obviously, the implementation of the UNESCO Ethics & AI Recommendation will be a work-in-progress. At the least, the UNESCO Recommendation is a landmark articulation of everyone's stake in and rights concerning AI, including people with disability (Lazar & Stein, 2017). As a statement of values, it adds further to the benchmark of the UN Convention on the Rights of Persons with Disabilities (CRPD), ratified by 177 countries. Of course, such UN treaties and policies are not a "magic wand," especially given the CRPD treaty has not been signed by some countries (notably the U.S.), and that enforcement is notoriously difficult (Lazar & Stein, 2017). Add to which, for its part, UNESCO has often been criticized for seeking to advance communication equality—infamously in the response to the MacBride report—and faces issues of enforcement (Goggin, 2017). Nonetheless, both the CRPD and UNESCO's Recommendation do offer us widely shared international framework and vocabulary for reimagining disability and AI.

Common Elements in Alternative Imaginaries

A growing number of other critiques, alternative perspectives, and innovations in disability and AI are providing some common elements in alternative imaginaries. These elements include:

- critiques of "normalcy," drawing attention to the wide diversity of human bodies, experiences, identities, and contexts (Nakamura, 2019; Treviranus, 2016; Whittaker et al., 2019);
- proposing the concept of "interdependence" as way to reimagine the needs, desires, and dwelling in society of all, including people with disabilities (Bostad & Hanisch, 2016; Kittay, 2011; Sandry, 2020);
- the specificities and dynamics of data when it comes to people with disabilities (Treviranus, 2016, 2019);
- calls for more radical, foundational change in the area of design, mapped out in a range of recent work on disability, design, and innovation (Hendren, 2020);
- the constitutive role of people with disabilities in shaping AI technologies (Morris, 2020; Wald, 2020);

- the need to reframe AI in terms of power, justice, human rights, democracy, and equalities (Crawford, 2021; Hamraie & Fritsch, 2019; Whittaker et al., 2019).

These elements are worth bringing together and noting here, because they represent the conceptual assumptions and values—the "building blocks"—that take us well beyond the dominant imaginaries as well as the efforts by policy-makers, such as UNESCO, to offer frameworks.

CONCLUSION

In this chapter, we have looked at a relatively new area of disability and communication: AI. As outlined, the discourses, language, and representation of disability in relation to AI need to be understood against the backdrop of evolving ideas of disability and technology—which for some time have been at a crossroads. Despite fundamental changes to the bedrock social relations and realities of disability, despite hopes inspired by the repeated promises of the benefits of new technologies, disabling accounts, social and digital exclusions, injustice, and inequalities persist, and indeed take new forms through technological "progress."

To gain insight into why change remains slow, we turn to the concept of social imaginaries. While very much a generalization, we have argued the case that there are dominant social imaginaries of AI and disability, which are limiting. These imaginaries obscure the flaws in the mainstream ways that autonomous intelligent systems such as AI are constituted and being developed.

Set aside these, there are alternative imaginaries—which can no longer be ignored or downplayed. These alternative imaginaries are new avenues opening up for AI and machine learning; intelligent systems, and other technologies can be reimagined and remade as sustainable, just, and genuinely meeting the goals of extending accessibility, inclusion, participation, and rights for people with disabilities (Sætra, 2021). AI and its dominant social imaginaries are in the throes of a severe crisis of legitimacy. New ways of imagining and communicating about AI and disability are essential, and they will help us in the urgent, broader project of rethinking technology and social futures.

Acknowledgments Research for this chapter has been supported by a 2019–2021 NTU Start-Up Grant for the project *Smart Equalities*, as well as a Micron-NTU Institute of Technology for Humanity (NISTH) Responsible AI grant for the project *Designing AI to Stop Disability Bias*. Thanks to Jocelyn Tay for her research assistance on disability and AI.

REFERENCES

Alper, M. (2015). Augmentative, alternative, and assistive: Reimagining the history of mobile computing and disability. *IEEE Annals of the History of Computing, 37*(1), 96. https://doi.org/10.1109/MAHC.2015.3

Alper, M. (2017). *Giving voice: Mobile communication, disability, and inequality.* MIT Press.

Alper, M. (2019). Future talk: Accounting for the technological and other future discourses in daily life. *International Journal of Communication, 13,* 715–735. https://ijoc.org/index.php/ijoc/article/view/9678

Bennett, C., & Keyes, O. (2020). What is the point of fairness?: Disability, AI and the complexity of justice. *ACM SIGACCESS: Accessibility and Computing, 125*(article 5), 1–5. https://doi.org/10.1145/3386296.3386301

Blanck, P. (2021). On the importance of the *Americans with Disabilities Act* at 30. *Journal of Disability Policy Studies.* Advance online publication. https://doi.org/10.1177/10442073211036900

Bostad, I., & Hanisch, H. (2016). Freedom and disability rights: Dependence, independence, and interdependence. *Metaphilosophy, 47*(3), 71–384. https://doi.org/10.1111/meta.12192

Brynjolfsson, E., & McAfee, A. (2014). *The second machine age: Work, progress, and prosperity in a time of brilliant technologies.* Norton & Company.

Bunch, M., Johnson, M., Moro, S.S., Adams, M.S., & Sergio, L. (2021). Virtual reality hope machines in a curative imaginary: Recommendations for neurorehabilitation research from a critical disability studies perspective. *Disability and Rehabilitation.* Advance online publication. https://doi.org/10.1080/09638288.2021.1982024

Chennat, S. (Ed.). (2019). *Disability inclusion and inclusive education.* Springer.

Couldry, N., Rodriguez, C., Bolin, G., Cohen, J., Volkmer, I., Goggin, G., Kraidy, M., Iwabuchi, K., Qiu, J. L., Wasserman, H., Zhao, Y., Rincón, O., Magallanes-Blanco, C., Thomas, P. N., Koltsova, O., Rakhmani, I., & Lee, K.-S. (2018). Media, communication and the struggle for social progress. *Global Media and Communication, 14*(2), 173–191. https://doi.org/10.1177/1742766518776679

Crawford, K. (2021). *The atlas of AI: Power, politics, and the planetary costs of artificial intelligence.* Yale University Press.

Danforth, S., & Gabel, S. L. (Eds.). (2016). *Vital questions facing disability studies in education* (2nd ed.). Peter Lang.

Deitz, S., Lobben, A., & Alferez, A. (2021). Squeaky wheels: Missing data, disability, and power in the smart city. *Big Data & Society, 8*(2), 1–16. https://doi.org/10.1177/20539517211047735

Delgado, M. R. (2019). Disability in the fourth industrial revolution. *Developmental Medicine and Child Neurology, 61*(9), 993. https://doi.org/10.1111/dmcn.14296

Dengel, A., Devillers, L., & Schaal, L. M. (2021). Augmented human and human-machine co-evolution: Efficiency and ethics. In B. Braunschweig & M. Ghallab (Eds.), *Reflections on Artificial Intelligence for humanity* (pp. 203–227). Springer.

Digital Asia Hub. (2017). *AI in Asia: AI for Social Good.* Conference, March 6–7, Waseda University. https://www.digitalasiahub.org/2017/02/27/ai-in-asia-ai-for-social-good/

Donner, J. (2015). *After access: Inclusion, development, and a more mobile Internet.* MIT Press.

Elliott, A. (2019). *The culture of AI: Everyday life and the digital revolution.* Routledge.

Fazelpour, S., & Danks, D. (2021). Algorithmic bias: Senses, sources, solutions. *Philosophy Compass, 16*(8), e12760. 1–16. https://doi.org/10.1111/phc3.12760

Fielden, S. L., Moore, M. E., & Bend, G. L. (Eds.). (2020). *Palgrave handbook of disability at work*. Palgrave.

Floridi, L., Cowls, J., King, T. C., & Taddeo, M. (2020). How to design AI for social good: Seven essential factors. *Science and Engineering Ethics, 26*, 1771–1796. https://doi.org/10.1007/s11948-020-00213-5

French, S., & Corker, M. (Eds.). (1999). *Disability discourse*. Open University Press.

Ginsburg, F., & Rapp, R. (2019). "Not dead yet": Changing disability imaginaries in the twenty-first century. In V. Das & C. Han (Eds.), *Living and dying in the contemporary world* (pp. 525–541). University of California Press.

Goggin, G. (2017). Communications rights, disability, and law: The Convention on the Rights of Persons with Disabilities in national perspective. *Law in Context, 35*(2), 129–149. https://doi.org/10.26826/law-in-context.v35i2.21

Goggin, G. (2021). *Apps: From mobile phones to digital lives*. Polity.

Goggin, G., & Newell, C. (2003). *Digital disability: The social construction of disability in new media*. Rowman & Littlefield.

Goggin, G., Yu, H., Fisher, K. R., & Li, B. (2019). Disability, technology innovation and social development in China and Australia. *Journal of Asian Public Policy, 12*(1), 34–50. https://doi.org/10.1080/17516234.2018.1492067

Google. (n.d.-a). AI for Social Good. Retrieved February 25, 2022, from https://ai.google/social-good/

Google. (n.d.-b). Project Euphonia. Retrieved March 22, 2022, from https://sites.research.google/euphonia/about/.

Grue, J. (2015). *Disability and discourse analysis*. Routledge.

Hamraie, A., & Fritsch, K. (2019). Crip technoscience manifesto. *Catalyst, 5*(1), 1–33. https://doi.org/10.28968/cftt.v5i1.29607

Hendren, S. (2020). *What can a body do?* Riverhead Books.

Hofmann, M., Kasnitz, D., Mankoff, J., & Bennett, C.L. (2020). Living disability theory: Reflections on access, research, and design. In T. Guerreiro, H. Nicolau, & K. Moffatt (Eds.), *22nd International ACM SIGACCESS Conference on Computers and Accessibility* (pp. 1-13). ACM. https://doi.org/10.1145/3373625.3416996

Intel. (n.d.). AI for Good. Retrieved March 22, 2022, from https://www.intel.com/content/www/us/en/artificial-intelligence/ai4socialgood.html

ITU. (2021a). Artificial Intelligence for good. Retrieved March 22, 2022, from https://www.itu.int/en/mediacentre/backgrounders/Pages/artificial-intelligence-for-good.aspx

ITU. (2021b). Measuring digital development: Facts and figures 2021. Retrieved March 22, 2022, from https://www.itu.int/itu-d/reports/statistics/facts-figures-2021/

Jasanoff, S. (2015). Imagined and invented worlds. In S. Jasanoff & S.-H. Kim (Eds.), *Dreamscapes of modernity: Sociotechnical imaginaries and the fabrication of power* (pp. 321–341). University of Chicago Press.

Katz, J., Floyd, J., & Schiepers, K. (Eds.). (2021). *Perceiving the future through new communication technologies: Robots, AI and everyday life*. Springer

Kittay, E. F. (2011). The ethics of care, dependence, and disability. *Ratio Juris, 24*(1), 49–58. https://doi.org/10.1111/j.1467-9337.2010.00473.x

Kögel, J., & Wolbring, G. (2020). What it takes to be a pioneer: Ability expectations from brain-computer interface users. *Nanoethics, 14*, 227–239. https://doi.org/10.1007/s11569-020-00378-0

Kurzweil, R. (2003). The future of intelligent technology and its impact on disabilities. *Journal of Visual Impairment & Blindness., 97*(10), 582–584. https://doi.org/10.1177/0145482X0309701002

Kurzweil, R. (2005). *The singularity is near: When humans transcend biology.* Penguin.

Lanzara, G. F. (2016). *Shifting practices: Reflections on technology, practices, and innovation.* MIT Press.

Lazar, J., & Stein, M.A. (Eds.) (2017). *Disability, human rights, and information technology.* University of Pennsylvania Press.

Lazar, J., Goldstein, D., & Taylor, A. (2015). *Ensuring digital accessibility through process and policy.* Morgan Kaufmann.

Lillywhite, A., & Wolbring, G. (2020). Coverage of artificial intelligence and machine learning within academic literature, Canadian newspapers, and Twitter tweets: The case of disabled people. *Societies, 10*(1), 23. https://doi.org/10.3390/soc10010023

Lillywhite, A., & Wolbring, G. (2021). Coverage of ethics within the artificial intelligence and machine learning academic literature: The case of disabled people. *Assistive Technology, 33*(3), 129–135. https://doi.org/10.1080/10400435.2019.1593259

Ling, R. S. (2012). *Taken for grantedness: The embedding of mobile communication into society.* MIT Press.

Mansell, R. (2015). Imaginaries, values, and trajectories: A critical reflection on the Internet. In G. Goggin & M. McLelland (Eds.), *Routledge companion to global Internet histories* (pp. 23–33). Routledge.

Mansell, R., & Raboy, M. (Eds.). (2011). *Handbook of global media policy.* Wiley-Blackwell.

Microsoft. (n.d.). Seeing AI: An app for visually impaired people that narrates world around you. Retrieved March 22, 2022, from https://www.microsoft.com/en-us/garage/wall-of-fame/seeing-ai/

Mills, M. (2022). *Hearing loss and the history of information theory.* Duke University Press.

Morris, J., Thompson, N., Lippincott, B., & Lawrence, M. (2019). Accessibility User Research Collective: Engaging consumers in ongoing technology evaluation. *Assistive Technology Outcomes and Benefits, 13*(1), 38–56.

Morris, M. R. (2020). AI and accessibility. *Communications of the ACM, 63*(6), 35–37. https://doi.org/10.1145/3356727

Nakada, M., Kavathatzopoulos, I., & Asai, R. (2021). Robots and AI artifacts in plural perspective(s) of Japan and the West: The cultural–ethical traditions behind people's views on robots and AI artifacts in the information era. *Review of Socionetwork Strategies, 15*, 143–168. https://doi.org/10.1007/s12626-021-00067-8

Nakamura, K. (2019). My algorithms have determined you're not human: AI-ML, Reverse Turing Tests, and the disability experience. In J. P. Bigham (Ed.), *ASSETS '19: The 21st International ACM SIGACCESS Conference on Computers and Accessibility* (pp. 1–2). https://doi.org/10.1145/3308561.3353812

Park, S., & Humphry, J. (2019). Exclusion by design: Intersections of social, digital and data exclusion. *Information, Communication & Society, 22*(7), 934–953. https://doi.org/10.1080/1369118X.2019.1606266

Pasquale, F. (2015). *The black box society: The secret algorithms that control money and information.* Harvard University Press.

Pasquale, F. (2020). *New laws of robotics.* Harvard University Press.

Pathakji, N. (2018). *Corporations and disability rights: Bridging the digital divide.* Oxford University Press.

Pullin, G. (2009). *Design meets disability.* MIT.

Roberge, J., & Castelle, M., Eds. (2021). *The cultural life of machine learning: An incursion into critical AI studies.* Springer.

Roulstone, A. (2016). *Disability and technology: An interdisciplinary and international approach.* Palgrave Macmillan.

Sætra, H. S. (2021). AI in context and the Sustainable Development Goals: Factoring in the unsustainability of the sociotechnical system. *Sustainability, 13*(4), 1738. https://doi.org/10.3390/su13041738

Samsung. (2021). Accessibility for everyone. Retrieved March 22, 2022, from https://www.design.samsung.com/global/contents/accessibility_design/

Sandry, E. (2020). Interdependence in collaboration with robots. In K. Ellis, G. Goggin, B. Haller, & R. Curtis (Eds.), *Routledge companion to disability and media* (pp. 316–326). Routledge.

Shuttleworth, R., & Meekosha, H. (2013). The sociological imaginary and disability enquiry in late modernity. *Critical Sociology, 39*(3), 349–367. https://doi.org/10.1177/0896920511435709

Smith, B. (2018, May 7). Using AI to empower people with disabilities. *Microsoft on the Issues blog.* Retrieved March 22, 2022, from https://blogs.microsoft.com/on-the-issues/2018/05/07/using-ai-to-empower-people-with-disabilities/

Sterne, J. (2021). *Diminished faculties: A political phenomenology of impairment.* Duke University Press.

Titchkosky, T. (2019). Disability imaginaries in the news. In K. Ellis, G. Goggin, B. Haller, & R. Curtis (Eds.), *Routledge companion to disability and media* (pp. 13–22). Routledge.

Tkaczyk, V., Mills, M., & Hui, A. (Eds.). (2020). *Testing hearing: The making of modern aurality.* Oxford University Press.

Tomašev, C. J., Hutter, F., Mohamed, S., Picciariello, A., Connelly, B., Belgrave, D. C. M., Ezer, D., van der Haert, F. C., Mugisha, F., Abila, G., Arai, H., Almiraat, H., Proskurnia, J., Snyder, K., Otake-Matsuura, M., Othman, M., Glasmachers, T., de Wever, W., et al. (2020). AI for social good: Unlocking the opportunity for positive impact. *Nature Communications, 11*(1), 2468. https://doi.org/10.1038/s41467-020-15871-z

Treviranus, J. (2016). The future challenge of the ADA: Shaping humanity's transformation. *Inclusion, 4*(1), 30–38. https://doi.org/10.1352/2326-6988-4.1.30

Treviranus, J. (2019). The value of being different. In A. Hurst & C. Duartes (Eds.), *W4A '19: Proceedings of the 16th International Web for All Conference* (pp. 1–7). https://doi.org/10.1145/3315002.3332429

Turner, D. M., Bohata, K., & Thompson, S. (2017). Introduction. Special issue. Disability, work and representation: New perspectives. *Disability Studies Quarterly, 37*(4). https://doi.org/10.18061/dsq.v37i4.6101

UNESCO. (2021). *Recommendation on the Ethics of Artificial Intelligence.* UNESCO. Document code: SHS/BIO/REC-AIETHICS/2021. UNESCO. Retrieved March 22, 2022, from https://unesdoc.unesco.org/ark:/48223/pf0000380455

Wald, M. (2020). AI data-driven personalisation and disability inclusion. *Frontiers in Artificial Intelligence, 5*(571955), 1–7. https://doi.org/10.3389/frai.2020.571955

Whittaker, M., Alper, M., Bennett, C.L., Hendren, S., Kaziunas, L., Mills, M., Morris, M. R., Rankin, J., Rogers, E., Salas, M., & West, S. M. (2019). *Disability, bias, and AI*. AI Now Institute, New York University. Retrieved March 22, 2022, from https://ainowinstitute.org/disabilitybiasai-2019.pdf

Williamson, B. (2019). *Accessible America: A history of disability and design*. New York University Press.

Wolbring, G. (2016). Employment, disabled people and robots: What is the narrative in the academic literature and Canadian newspapers? *Societies, 6*(15), 1–16. https://doi.org/10.3390/soc6020015

Wolbring, G., & Yumakulov, S. (2014). Social robots: Views of staff of a disability service organization. *International Journal of Social Robotics, 6*, 457–468. https://doi.org/10.1007/s12369-014-0229-z

Yumakulov, S., Yergens, D., & Wolbring, G. (2012). Imagery of disabled people within social robotics research. In S. S. Ge, O. Khatib, J.-J. Cabibihan, R. Simmons, & M.-A. Williams (Eds.), *Social robotics. Proceedings of the 4th International Conference, ICSR 2012, Chengdu, China, October 29–31, 2012* (pp. 168–177). Springer.

Zajko, M. (2021). Conservative AI and social inequality: Conceptualizing alternatives to bias through social theory. *AI & Society, 36*, 1047–1056. https://doi.org/10.1007/s00146-021-01153-9

CHAPTER 14

Thinking Inclusiveness, Diversity, and Cultural Equity Based on Game Mechanics and Accessibility Features in Popular Video Games

Alexandra Dumont and Maude Bonenfant

Over the past few decades, video games have taken a prominent place in our cultural and social landscape. From profits exceeding the US box office to being showcased on national television, video games are hardly a niche hobby. For 2020 alone, the global video game industry generated an estimated $177.8 billion, indicating a 23.1 percent increase over 2019 (Newzoo, 2021). With an estimated 2.81 billion players, gamers now represent more than a third of the world's population (Newzoo, 2021).

The newfound interest in video games has turned what was once a participatory pastime into a spectatorial one. The enthusiasm for video game streaming has led to eSports' growing importance and frequent coverage in traditional media platforms such as ABC and ESPN (Bogage, 2019). In this context, some gamers gain such recognition that they become household names. Professional gamers (N0tail, Faker, S1mple), Twitch[1] personalities (Ninja, Pokimane, Shroud), and YouTubers (PewDiePie, Markiplier, Jacksepticeye) have all become prominent icons within their respective games or platforms. Their notoriety has earned them opportunities in adjacent industries unrelated to video games, strengthening gaming's footing within popular culture. For

---

A. Dumont (✉) • M. Bonenfant
Université du Québec à Montréal, Montréal, QC, Canada
e-mail: dumont.alexandra.3@courrier.uqam.ca; bonenfant.maude@uqam.ca

© The Author(s), under exclusive license to Springer Nature
Switzerland AG 2023
M. S. Jeffress et al. (eds.), *The Palgrave Handbook of Disability and Communication*, https://doi.org/10.1007/978-3-031-14447-9_14

221

instance, in 2019, Ninja appeared on *Celebrity Family Feud*, *The Tonight Show Starring Jimmy Fallon*, *The Masked Singer*, and was also invited for the Times Square Ball Drop in 2018. Inversely, politicians and musicians joined famous streamers to play video games. For example, Drake and Ninja played *Fortnite* (Epic Games, 2017), whereas Alexandria Ocasio-Cortez and Pokimane played *Among Us* (InnerSloth, 2018).

This permeability between video games and popular culture accompanies a change of discourse in the media. Long described as a vector of violence and sexism and a danger to children and society, video games are now a legitimate form of entertainment (Shaw, 2010; ESA, 2018), art (Isbister, 2016; Antonelli, 2012), and a tool for socialization (Steinkuehler & Williams, 2006; Pitaru, 2008). Furthermore, as video games become a more significant part of the cultural landscape, they are gradually receiving recognition for their aesthetic and creative aspects from various mainstream media outlets (Bogage, 2019; The Guardian, n.d.). Therefore, this change in the media's discourse contributes to the video game industry's cultural legitimization.

Recognizing the popularity of video games and their growing cultural, social, and economic importance, all who desire must have access to this media in a way that fits their unique capabilities and needs. However, despite the industry's recent efforts to offer more inclusive features such as color blindness mode and closed captioning, video games remain inaccessible for many players with motor, visual, hearing and/or cognitive disabilities (Aguado-Delgado et al., 2020; Porter & Kientz, 2013; Grammenos et al., 2009). This inaccessibility, caused by poor design choices and a lack of knowledge from the developers (Heron, 2012; Ellis & Kao, 2019), excludes a significant portion of the population from participating in this cultural, artistic, and social phenomenon.

According to the Centers for Disease Control and Prevention (CDC), one out of every four American adults, or 26 percent of the population, has some type of disability (CDC, 2020). This figure, together with the fact that 67 percent of the American adult population plays video games, may indicate that the number of disabled gamers is not insignificant (ESA, 2021). A 2008 study estimated that gamers with permanent or temporary disabilities constituted 20 percent of the gaming population; 92 percent of them pursued their play session even though they encountered inaccessible designs (Chin, 2015). Despite these data being several years old, it remains one of the few statistical sources addressing this topic. Consequently, the development of accessible video games is not a marginal issue: it is a matter of cultural equity, that is, having access to all video games regardless of players' capabilities. Inclusive video game design not only promotes access to a diverse range of players, but it also communicates, promotes, and normalizes a specific perception of what disability represents in society.

For this reason, the present chapter aims to analyze the discourse conveyed on disabilities through accessibility features and game mechanics of popular video games. Like any other media, video games are vectors of social representations whose analysis provides insight into a society's worldviews and values

(Hall, 1973; Hall, 1997; Pérez-Latorre et al., 2017). While visual representations (avatars with disabilities), design, and narrative elements are predominant in the video game experience, they are not the only way to convey discourses. Adopting the approach of sociosemiotics and disability media studies, we aim to highlight how game mechanics implemented and playability options contribute, by their discursive components, to the social construction of disabilities. For this purpose, we identified the following research questions: (1) How do developers of popular video games conceive inclusiveness, diversity of practices, and cultural equity through the design of game mechanics and accessibility options? (2) What do these games tell us about the discursive and social context from which they originate?

In order to address these main questions, we have divided this chapter into four sections. The first section focuses on defining accessibility and cultural equity in the context of video games. The second section describes the research process and technique, while the third section presents the analysis results of the selected titles. Finally, the last portion of this chapter relates to the discussion of our findings and concluding remarks.

Cultural Equity and Accessibility in the Video Game Context

Contrary to equality, which implies that everyone receives the same resources, equity relies intrinsically on notions of justice and fairness by allocating resources based on present conditions, which vary depending on each individual's circumstances (George Washington University's Online Public Health, 2020). Hence, equity is about acknowledging that not everyone has the same range of capabilities and providing resources specific to everyone's needs, allowing them to engage in equal and shared experiences. Directly related, cultural equity seeks to ensure that everyone has access to the cultural sphere and the social benefits it can provide (Lomax, 1980). In the context of video games, cultural equity aims to create accessible video games that support an equitable gameplay experience through their flexible design. Game Accessibility Guidelines (n.d.) define accessibility as "avoiding unnecessary barriers that prevent people with a range of impairments from accessing or enjoying your output." Through their design choices, some video games represent a greater level of challenge for many players with disabilities, if not downright inaccessible (Heron, 2012).

Developing video games that consider different players' agency achieves cultural equity. Janet Murray, a game studies pioneer, explains that "Agency is the satisfying power to take meaningful action and see the results of our decisions and choices" (1998, p. 123). When analyzing the video game experience, the notion of agency is typically associated with the concept of affordance. Generally speaking, "An affordance is a relationship between the properties of an object and the capabilities of the agent that determine just how the object could possibly be used" (Norman, 2013, p. 11). From a game studies standpoint, affordances refer to the possibilities of interaction offered by the game environment according to the player's capabilities. The articulation of the game's affordances and the player's agency determine how the game can be played (Norman, 2013, p. 11). While the concept of agency empowered players, affordances nonetheless constrain what can be actualized: "Agency is best understood as the socially and biochemically constructed capacity to act, where nobody is free in the sense of undetermined" (Barker, 2002, p. 92). Therefore, to ensure an equitable gaming experience, games' affordance must respect their players' various agencies without modifying its general objectives. The dilemma then becomes how to retain the game's essence while displaying multiple interaction possibilities.

While everyone encounters video games differently, Csikszentmihalyi's concept of flow can help shed light on one's experience. Understood as "the state in which people are so involved in an activity that nothing else seems to matter; the experience itself is so enjoyable that people will do it even at great cost, for the sheer sake of doing it," this notion can help better understand a player's interactions with a video game (Csikszentmihalyi, 1990, p. 4). Since "games are one of the best kinds of activities to produce flow" (Salen & Zimmerman, 2004, p. 420), this concept has been widely used in game studies since video game structure seeks to fulfill the three primary flow state conditions: (1) The game's goals are usually always clear, (2) the player receives immediate feedback on his actions, and (3) there is a balance between the challenges offered by the game and the capabilities of the players (Csikszentmihalyi, 1997, pp. 29–30). "Optimal experiences usually involve a fine balance between one's ability to act, and the available opportunities for action" (Csikszentmihalyi, 1997, p. 30). Accordingly, too much of a challenge causes players anxiety: the game's objectives are not sufficiently accessible to the range of capabilities of the players (Csikszentmihalyi, 1997, p. 31). Conversely, a lack of challenge leads to boredom: the game's goals are too easily attainable compared to the players' capabilities (Csikszentmihalyi, 1997, p. 31). Both instances drive players to abandon the game.

The question then becomes how to keep players with varying capabilities engaged in a flow state while playing the same game. Designing game features and settings that meet players' varying capabilities can help achieve this particularity. Hence, producing a video game following the principles of cultural equity requires an early commitment to accessibility in the development process (Neely, 2017, p. 17). Therefore, we define accessibility and cultural equity in the video game environment as providing all players, regardless of their capabilities, with an equitable gaming experience by removing unnecessary barriers and allowing them to tailor games to meet their agency. We believe that a fair gaming experience relies on a game system's versatility to adjust to every play style to achieve a flow state.

Methodology

In order to address our research questions, we first identified our research corpus through a fixed set of criteria. Therefore, titles selected for this research must: (1) have been released between 2017 and 2020 to report on the most recent advances in game design, (2) represent both major gaming companies and independent studios, (3) have received some recognition from the media and player communities as a result of their accessibility, either through award nominations or extensive coverage, and (4) be from North America in order to fit the researchers' discursive context.

Accordingly, the titles selected for this research are *Celeste* (Matt Makes Games, 2018a), *Marvel's Spider-Man: Miles Morales* (Insomniac Games, 2020a), and *The Last Of Us Part II* (Naughty Dog, 2020). In addition to the selected game's interfaces, our corpus also includes promotional materials, official websites, press kits, and interviews with respective developers. The use of external documents related to these productions allows us to provide a faithful portrayal of the developers' discourse and additional signs that can infer their worldviews and values.

Our analysis employs a sociosemiotic approach to study the signs and meaning produced by the discursive context from which the cultural objects emerge. In turn, these objects contribute to the discourse's construction. Consequently, sociosemiotics examines the production of meaning from a discursive macro-system rather than the meaning produced on an individual's level. Distinguishing discursive systems enables the identification of social organization: "Socio-semiotic analysis is configured as an analysis of social discourses, understood as discourses through which a society presents itself, thinks itself and, thereby, builds itself" (Semprini, 1995, p. 165). Sociosemiotics, and by extension discourse analysis, may be used to infer one's understanding of the world and its social institutions. Accordingly, examining the selected games and their related paratexts may provide insight into the developers' perspectives and beliefs regarding accessibility and cultural equity.

Through this approach, we were able to infer the discursive and social context from which the selected games originate and how they participate in constructing this discursive macro-system. Discourse, according to Michel Foucault, is a coherent set of more or less abstract statements (*énoncés*) transmitted not just through what is "spoken," but also by the meaning conveyed by the objects (Foucault, 1972; Véron, 1987). Thus, we identified signs from the game's interface, including menus, game screen appearances, features implemented, and mechanics, as statements to reconstruct the discursive context that made their enunciation possible. Subsequently, the game's promotional materials study allows us to complete this analysis by inferring the discursive context from which the developers evolve. While not constitutive of the selected productions, these aspects are an extension of them (Genette, 1997, p. 1). In his book *Paratexts: Thresholds of Interpretation* (1997), Gérard Genette describes the different texts surrounding a production, such as title, prologue, or interviews, as paratexts whose purpose is to "ensure the text's presence in the world" (p. 2). Constituted of an "a heterogeneous group of practices and discourses of all kinds and dating from all periods [...]," the study of paratextual messages can inform us about a text's production conditions (Genette, 1997, p. 2). Ultimately, the discourse and sociosemiotic analysis of the three selected games and their paratexts informed us of the developers' perception of inclusivity, diversity of practices, and cultural equity.

Inclusivity, Diversity of Practices, and Cultural Equity Through Game Designs and Accessibility Options

Presentation of Celeste and Its Accessibility Options

The first game discussed in our study is the independent game *Celeste*. This title, which has received critical acclaim for the difficulty of its gameplay and the vast range of options provided by its Assist Mode,[2] demonstrates that independent studios can create innovative accessibility measures with limited resources. Created by Matt Makes Games and released in 2018, this platform game follows the story of Madeline, who confronts her inner demons while ascending the Celeste mountain.

Accessible through the game's title screen, the Assist Mode includes options such as adjusting the game speed, offering infinite stamina, increasing the number of air dashes available, activating a dash assist, and granting the player invincibility. These features, described by various gaming media as granular, offer a significant degree of flexibility, allowing players to tailor their experience to fit their capabilities (Klepek, 2019; Klepek, 2018; Frank, 2018). Individuals can then finely adjust the game's components to ensure a pleasant experience free of frustration and boredom, encouraging *Celeste* players to reach the flow state that is specific to them. By avoiding the pejorative use of difficulty levels and providing all players with the same content without sacrificing any material, the Assist Mode keeps the game's essence and intended experience intact.

Although the studio behind *Celeste* created a particularly innovative Assist Mode, these settings are absent from the options menu. Individuals interested in these features must activate them prior to their gaming sessions; otherwise, they must exit the game, return to the title screen, and enable its Assist Mode. The clear separation between the options menu and the Assist Mode emphasizes any disparities between players while underlining the foreign status of these options. Moreover, by opting for such a structure, developers require additional efforts from players to gain access to these accessibility features.

These particularities are all the more reinforced by the preamble accompanying the Assist Mode. This description, which appears every time players activate these features, may dissuade some from using them. When first published, the preamble was as follows:

Assist Mode allows you to modify the game's rules to reduce its difficulty. This includes options such as slowing the game speed, granting yourself invincibility or infinite stamina, and skipping chapters entirely.

Celeste was designed to be a challenging, but accessible game. We believe that its difficulty is essential to the experience. We recommend playing without Assist Mode your first time.

However, we understand that every player is different. If *Celeste* is inaccessible to you due to its difficulty, we hope that Assist Mode will allow you to still enjoy it. (Matt Makes Games, 2018a)

The Assist Mode's initial description suggested that its development was to compensate for the difficult nature of the game and that its use would be at the expense of the production's essence. Thus, the creators dismissed the idea that the game's affordance, which does not reflect its users' range of agency, could be responsible for the obstacles faced by players with disabilities. Accessibility consultant, Clinton Lexa, criticized then subsequently helped rectify this clumsy and othering introduction: "[…] Celeste overall handles it [game accessibility] well! However, I feel obligated to mention that the Celeste Assist Mode preamble felt othering for many individuals when it mentioned 'intended' gameplay, leaving folks feeling insulted for needing the assists at all" (Clinton "Halfcoordinated" Lexa, 2019). The current preamble is as follows:

Assist mode allows you to modify the game's rules to fit your specific needs.

This includes options such as slowing the game speed, granting yourself invincibility or infinite stamina, and skipping chapters entirely.

Celeste is intended to be a challenging and rewarding experience. If the default game proves inaccessible to you, we hope you can still find that experience with Assist Mode. (Matt Makes Games, 2018a)

Notwithstanding this considerable improvement, we question the use of the term "default" to describe the game production. Accordingly, the activation of the Assist Mode would then oppose the player to the "standard" experience predetermined by the developers. Thus, the "good" or the "real" game experience does not appear to be accessible to all players. This perspective is also reinforced by the invitation to skip entire chapters. Moreover, the term "mode," referring to the various configurations or methods of interaction, denotes a distinction between two or more elements, which can connote the irregularity and abnormality of the accessibility features.

Celeste's Paratext and Its Many Perils

The consultation of external documents relating to *Celeste*'s production, such as the official website, the press kit, and the developers' interviews, supports these observations as they remain evasive on the game characteristics and accessibility. For instance, the game's website contains no mentions of *Celeste*'s

Assist Mode (Celeste, n.d). As a result, individuals seeking to know if the game is suitable for them remain unanswered. Furthermore, the press release only references the game accessibility in terms of controls: "The controls are simple and accessible—simply jump, air-dash, and climb—but with layers of expressive depth to master, where every death is a lesson" (Matt Makes Games, 2018b). Hence, the developers associate the low number of buttons to press as an accessibility feature, regardless of the combination and the precise timing they required. While appreciated, this particularity is not sufficient to ensure the game's accessibility.

The failure to mention accessibility measures, added to the many references made to the difficulty of *Celeste* ("super-tight, hand-crafted platformer"; "600+ screens of hardcore platforming challenges and devious secrets"; "bravest mountaineers"), leads us to believe that there is some confusion between the concepts of accessibility and approachability and/or usability. As a result, when discussing their accessibility measures in their various promotional materials, *Celeste* developers emphasize their user-friendliness rather than their ability to provide a flexible and accessible gaming experience. However, when asked about their vision as a game designer, Maddy Thorson's answer suggests that the implementation of accessibility measures was likely the result of compromises:

> "From my perspective as the game's designer," Thorson said, "Assist Mode breaks the game. I spent many hours fine-tuning the difficulty of *Celeste*, so it's easy for me to feel precious about my designs. But ultimately, we want to empower the player and give them a good experience, and sometimes that means letting go." (Klepek, 2018)

An interview published later that year with the same developer confirms this element: "I was originally against the idea, but I think it was Noel, Amora, and Gabby from the team who workshopped the idea and it started making sense late in development" (Castruita, 2018). Moreover, the addition of an Assist Mode in the game's final month of development demonstrates the studio's secondary concerns in their video game's accessibility. Resistance from the lead developer could then explain the contradictions and clumsiness regarding *Celeste*'s accessibility features.

Neely (2017) highlights the ethical consequences of such an approach: "In this case, the player with disabilities is clearly regarded as less important than other players since something that is required for one group to participate in the game is being sacrificed for something that is desired by another group" (p. 12). While "sacrificing something that one group requires for something that another group simply desires, however, is much more questionable," it also testifies to the developers' discursive context and their perception of disabled players (Neely, 2017, p.12).

Presentation of *Marvel's Spider-Man: Miles Morales* and Its Accessibility Options

Released as a PlayStation 5 launch title in November 2020, *Marvel's Spider-Man: Miles Morales* centers on Peter Parker's trainee, Miles Morales, who recently acquired spider-like abilities. This latest title of the Insomniac Games' *Marvel's Spider-Man* series follows the adventures of this newly formed Spider-Man who tries to defend New York City and his new neighborhood, Harlem, from the war raging between an energy corporation and high-tech criminals.

This game offers a relatively impressive number of accessibility settings. Mainly focused on visual, hearing and motor accessibility, these features meet numerous recommendations suggested by the Game Accessibility Guidelines (n.d). Furthermore, the integration of settings described as "advanced" by the association, such as Quick Time Event Auto-Complete, Look at Waypoint, and Mission Waypoint Display, informs us about the game's development process and the studio's concerns about the game's accessibility, as their implementation necessitated early coordination among the studio's various departments.

Following these guidelines, many settings provided by *Miles Morales* aim to convey the game's feedback and contextual cues in various formats so that players are "able to receive stimuli, determine an appropriate response, and finally provide input back to the game to action their response to the stimuli" (Yuan et al., 2011, pp. 83–84). Accordingly, options such as Accessibility Vibration, Vibration Intensity, Adaptive Triggers, Crime Notifications, and High Visibility Spider-Sense, inform individuals of actions that could escape them if they were only visual, auditory, or haptic.

Further accessibility settings offer additional support to players by adapting the game system in circumscribed ways. For example, the Chase Assist option slows down enemies, the Web Shooter Burst shoots three webs at once, etc. While not significantly altering the game's meaning, these options enable disabled players to tailor its affordances to their agentivity. Therefore, individuals with disabilities can enjoy the game in its entirety without being excluded from some portion of it.

While *Miles Morales* includes various difficulty levels, it mitigates the negative connotations associated with their use by employing non-pejorative language. The implementation of difficulty settings is often the subject of debate, mainly due to the derogatory terms some games use and the exclusion they create among players (Brown & Anderson, 2020, p. 712). Levels such as Easy, Medium, Hard, Can I play, Daddy? (*Wolfenstein II: The New Colossus*, 2017) or I'm Too Young to Die (*Doom franchise*, 1993–2019) are examples of titles deliberately chosen to generate embarrassment to the players using them. Hence, the difficulties included in this game are titled: Friendly Neighborhood; Friendly; Amazing; Spectacular. *Marvel's Spider-Man: Miles Morales* prevents from imposing judgment based on the difficulty level selected by their players through the use of a neutral or even positive vocabulary.

In addition to including a wide range of accessibility settings, *Miles Morales* seamlessly integrates them without significant discrimination or moralizing explanations. This peculiarity is further noticeable from the first opening of the game. During players' initial gaming sessions, a menu neutrally named "Before you start" greets them, placing them all on an equal footing, without discrimination. This menu allows players to make adjustments before beginning the game, including various options such as listening mode, mono audio, graphic mode, subtitles, and accessibility. While a more detailed menu is available once in the game, this addition of early accessibility options underlines their importance to the developers. Furthermore, using the game's accessibility measures does not necessitate any additional steps, nor does it penalize its users. Players can then modify the game's settings and difficulty to match their current agency level and thus maintain an enjoyable degree of challenge while ensuring their flow states.

Importance of the Game's Paratext in Players' Buying Decisions

The accessibility and cultural equity of a video game are determined not only by its design, but also by how its developer and publisher advertise it. Insomniac Games claims on their FAQ website to have their games' accessibility at heart: "Accessibility is something that is very important to Insomniac Games and PlayStation and we are committed to offering accessibility options in each of our games" (Insomniac Games, 2020b). Noticeable from a gameplay standpoint, this intention, however, seems absent from their promotional discourse. Rather than informing players of its accessibility, *Miles Morales*'s marketing strategy focused only on the characters' social representation and diversity.

Accordingly, neither the PlayStation nor Insomniac Games official websites provide information about accessibility features in a clear and easily discernible manner. This information is only available on the Insomniac Game website's FAQ page and an official studio Twitter account. Considering that the average cost of a video game is $60USD, players must know if the product they are interested in is accessible to them. This lack of transparency is even more concerning given that these publications are imprecise and difficult to access, especially for players using screen-reading software. Developers' official communications have a significant weight as several media outlets subsequently relay them. Therefore, discourse expressed by developers is crucial as it directly shapes how the media reports the information.

Presentation of the The Last of Us Part II and Its Accessibility Options

Our third game, *The Last of Us Part II* (TLOU2), released in 2020 on PlayStation consoles, is an adventure game set in a post-apocalyptic US, where its inhabitants must survive in a threatening environment occupied by infected and hostile survivors. This title, developed by Naughty Dog, is an exemplary case of game accessibility, with 60 accessibility settings organized around the key categories of the Game Accessibility Guidelines (n.d). Players may then customize various game components based on their capabilities and agency, including controls, controller's orientation, input mode of the buttons (hold, press, toggles), navigation assistance, and various visual or auditory indicators relaying environmental cues. This flexibility not only makes TLOU2 accessible but also enjoyable insofar as all players may achieve a state of flow.

These characteristics, introduced in a "simplified" menu following the game's first opening, offer Text-to-speech, Language, Brightness and Adjustments options, including Subtitles, Audio, and Accessibility Settings. Naughty Dog prefaces these options with the following message: "Here are some common features you may want to adjust before playing. A comprehensive list of adjustments is available from the Options menu." The inclusion of accessibility measures in this opening menu, combined with the phrases "common features" and "adjustments," which connote something "usual" or "standard" and "fine-tuning," contributes to the normalization and exploration of the settings available to all players.

Following this initial menu, players access the game's main title screen. Although individuals are free to begin their journeys, the game's cursor is immediately placed on the Options tab, inviting them to interact with the game settings. This detailed and illustrated menu includes various options such as Controls, Heads-Up Display (HUD), Subtitles, Display, Audio, Language, and Accessibility. Furthermore, accessibility settings are not restricted to a dedicated menu, as some of them appear on multiple locations related to their pertinence, thus increasing their accessibility while also making them commonplace. While informing us on the developers' attitude, these design choices may shift players' perception of video games' accessibility by reducing the reluctance and stigmas surrounding their uses.

From a technical standpoint, TLOU2 accessibility features primarily translate into aesthetic modifications, therefore preserving the game's essence. For example, the traversal cue option displays an arrow on the ground, indicating players the direction to follow to progress in their quest. Alternatively, enhancing pre-existing mechanics, such as the Listen Mode, can benefit players with visual, auditory, or cognitive disabilities. Initially introduced to scan the game audio environment to locate enemies or objects via audio and visual cues, players can use the game settings to adjust the distance covered by the scan and the time necessary to reach its maximum distance.

Despite its impressive accessibility, TLOU2 nonetheless uses difficulty levels and pejorative vocabulary. Naming its challenge options Very Light, Light, Moderate, Hard, and Grounded, the game employs a connoted language that is further discernible in the descriptions that follow the game's challenge level.

Moderate: "Provides a balanced experience. Resources are limited."

Grounded: "The most challenging and realistic experience. Listen Mode, HUD, and other gameplay elements are altered in this game mode. For veteran

The Last of Us fans, Grounded difficulty represents the ultimate test of skill. [...]" (Naughty Dog, 2020.)

The word "balance" might imply that prior difficulty levels favored their users unjustly, resulting in an inequitable experience and an unsatisfying flow state. Similarly, the Grounded mode's framing, based on the concept of "veteran fans," presupposes that all series enthusiasts have equivalent ability levels, and thus those who cannot complete these challenges are not "real fans of the series," hence resulting in their discrimination.

These vocabulary choices are, at first glance, contradictory to Naughty Dog's general discourse. Nonetheless, TLOU2's difficulty options allow players to tailor the game's affordances to their agency by letting them modulate specific game components such as character profile, enemies, allies, stealth, and resource elements. As a result, players have greater control over the game's challenges and ultimately over their flow state experience.

TLOU2's Paratext as a Source of Information and Advocacy

TLOU2's paratext and the developers' interviews reflect Naughty Dog's concerns surrounding their game's accessibility. This aspect is first identifiable through the game's official website. Using a quickly identifiable tab on the page header, players can easily access information relating to the game's accessibility without significant research or effort. Furthermore, Naughty Dog provides extensive descriptions in various formats, including pictures or videos. The developers, through this dedicated tab and its contextualization, explicitly state their intentions regarding their game experience:

> Naughty Dog's goal has been to ensure that as many fans as possible have an opportunity to experience the game through their most robust accessibility feature set to-date. [...] Naughty Dog encourages everyone to take advantage of these features to create a gameplay experience that's right for them. (PlayStation, 2020)

Furthermore, numerous accessibility descriptions demonstrate developers' basic understanding of the frustrations faced by disabled players when confronted by inaccessible designs.

Text, UI, and gameplay elements that are too small or difficult to read can be frustrating. To address these issues, you can fine-tune the HUD size, color, and contrast.

> Any information that is only represented visually is unavailable to a blind player. To address this discrepancy, Naughty Dog created several options to convey this information through sound and controller vibration instead. (PlayStation, 2020)

The developers' acknowledgment of the barriers imposed by inaccessible video games suggests that the TLOU2's production directly addressed such issues.

Thus, Naughty Dog demonstrates an understanding of disabled players' realities while fostering a sense of trust. The recognition attributed to the seven accessibility consultants who assisted in creating these features supports this specificity (PlayStation, 2020).

Media coverage and interviews with Emilia Schatz (co-lead designer), Matthew Gallant (lead system designer), and Anthony Newman (co-director) reaffirm the studio's commitment to game accessibility.

> "We absolutely had to plan these features early in production," Matthew Gallant says. "It was absolutely critical." There were three features in particular—text-to-speech, fully remappable controls, and the high-contrast mode—that required large technical resources, and they wouldn't have been possible without so much time. (Webster, 2020)

Naughty Dog conceptualized its accessibility settings alongside the game's development rather than incorporating them at the end of the design process. This method required several departments, some of whom were unfamiliar with game accessibility, to collaborate in developing cohesive game designs (Webster, 2020). From this perspective, Naughty Dog could anticipate, identify, and resolve their production's shortcomings preemptively. By positioning accessibility as an essential component of the game's development, developers indicate that equitable access to video games is not an afterthought but fundamental.

Developers indicate in interviews that they perceive accessibility in terms of player "experience," "enjoyment," "comfort," and playability rather than the simple access to a game title (Webster, 2020). Moreover, when asked to describe their accessibility features, Schatz relies on notions specific to cultural equity: "Accessibility for us is about removing barriers that are keeping players from completing a game," she says. "It's not about dumbing down a game or making a game easy. What do our players need in order to play the game in parity with everyone else?" (Webster, 2020). Thus, the developers clearly position their process in accordance with the principles of cultural equity while addressing the common misconception surrounding video game's difficulty and accessibility. By emphasizing their design practices and the importance of equitable access to the gaming experience, developers contribute to the normalization and advocacy of game accessibility from the player standpoint, and also within the industry.

Moreover, Naughty Dog demonstrates the importance of knowledge transferability related to video game accessibility. By building on the groundwork laid down in *Uncharted 4: A Thief's End* (Naughty Dog, 2016), the developers were able to focus on optimizing their prior game's features to improve accessibility for players experiencing fine-motor, hearing, low vision, or blind disabilities (PlayStation, 2020). Naughty Dog proves that accessible game design is a crucial investment as it reduces the subsequent production time and cost while gaining specialized knowledge.

Discursive and Social Context of the Selected Games

Although the three games examined include accessibility measures praised by gamers, the industry, and the media alike, two of them nonetheless portray contradictory or incompatible discourses regarding their intentions. Whether through advertising campaigns, interviews, or official material, a mismatch between the developers' discourse and their actions is perceptible. Thus, by analyzing and inferring the discursive context of these games, we were able to determine the discourse conveyed by the developers, voluntarily or not, relating to the notions of inclusiveness, diversity of practices, and cultural equity. This approach also provided an overview of the different discourses circulating within the gaming industry, among players, and, more broadly, society. Identifying these discursive contexts is significant since it informs us about how symbolic and discursive representations are produced, transmitted, and reproduced by the cultural objects represented by video games.

Tyranny of Normality

From that perspective, *Celeste*'s analysis allowed us to highlight the developers' commitment to the inclusivity and accessibility of their product through the integration of innovative accessibility measures, the developers' willingness to improve their game in response to criticisms voiced by disabled players, as well as the vocabulary used during interviews. Despite these preoccupations, *Celeste* bears the traces of a sometimes awkward and conflicting discourse, showing a narrow understanding of the realities faced by players with disabilities. *Celeste*'s conception of cultural equity proves to be inconsistent through its use of the term "default" to describe the Assist Mode's absence, by keeping the accessibility features separate from the options menu, by enforcing the recurrence of the preamble and the blunders of the game's original release. These inconsistencies provide a contradictory message, which ultimately muddles the developers' initial good intentions.

The lead developer's resistance to the Assist Mode, as well as its last-minute developments, may be to blame for the ambiguity between functionalities and the game's discourse. Accordingly, Matt Makes Games perpetuates the dominant discourse in which able-bodies are viewed as the norm while disabled bodies are considered abnormal and less skilled. This discourse, which Lennard Davis refers to as the "hegemony of normalcy," expresses that any variation from the ideal or normal body is perceived as a "deviant body" (Davis, 1995, p. 34).

Based on the medical model of disabilities, *Celeste* was initially created for players deemed "normal" by the studio. Its accessibility was only considered afterward for individuals on the periphery of the "acceptable capabilities." As a result, accessibility is more of an addition to the game rather than an inherent part of the development process, reinforcing the distinction between "normal" and "abnormal" and perpetuating the "tyranny of normality" (Goodley, 2016,

p. 8). Thus, Assist Mode reinforces the perception that disabilities result from individual deficits that need fixing and whose presence makes disabled gamers helpless and stripped of agency (Goodley, 2016, p.8). From a social perspective, the developers' approach seems to reflect a division and exclusion between able-bodied and disabled individuals. By doing so, they oppose the concept of an inclusive society in which its social environment acknowledges every form of agency by including various affordances without apparent distinction.

Toxic Meritocracy

This discursive context reflects the numerous debates and resistance from the industry but also the gaming community surrounding the development and integration of accessibility measures. Opponents of game accessibility, commonly referred to as the "get gud" culture, will frequently invoke arguments related to the preservation of a game's artistic integrity, the decision of developers not to make a game available to everyone, or the "foolishness" of some players in requesting accessibility options. Ultimately, some think that the only barriers preventing players from accessing a game are their gaming skills (redhatGizmo, 2019). This discourse, prevalent among discussions related to games known for their difficulty, can be understood as gatekeeping (Barzilai-Nahon, 2009, p. 10). This strategy, defined by Barzilai-Nahon (2009) as "the process of controlling information as it moves through a gate or filter" in connection to the exercise of power (p. 10), may be used to preserve a culture.

The lead developers' resistance to implementing accessibility measures, the use of connoted language, and the emphasis on the game's difficulty are all signs of a control process aimed at maintaining the idea that video games are a niche activity requiring special skills and reserved for a select group of players. This "toxic meritocracy" (Paul, 2018) is *de facto* exclusionary and perpetuates the discourse according to which there are players with acceptable abilities and players who do not deserve access to video games. Through gatekeeping, players and the industry reiterate the discourse surrounding the hegemony of normalcy and participate in the invisibilization of disabled players and their realities (Porter & Kientz, 2013, p. 52). It is possible to argue that players could engage in gatekeeping to reaffirm the normality of their bodies in the face of social norms participating in defining disabled bodies as deficient or deviant (Siebers, 2001). Thus, despite having innovative accessibility features, *Celeste* expresses a discourse aimed at distinguishing good or real gamers from unsuitable ones. However, it is important to note that the developers' commitment to consistently update their Assist Mode more than three years after the game's release attests to the knowledge they have gained, the evolution of their opinion on accessibility and its potential implications for its current discursive context.

Imbalance Between Action and Discourse

Inversely, *Miles Morales* demonstrates an understanding and awareness of the importance of video games' accessibility. Accordingly, the developers focus the accessibility of their game on the design of a flexible environment in which several modes of interaction are possible. Made possible by the relatively fair treatment given to its accessibility options, *Marvel's Spider-Man: Miles Morales* allows players to flex the affordances of its narrative to their agency, thus ensuring the experience of flow. The fluid integration and simple access to these settings allow players with disabilities to fully experience the game without being excluded from certain portions, thus ensuring cultural equity.

However, despite the range of the accessibility features offered by Insomniac Games, the discourse surrounding the promotion of *Miles Morales* is sometimes inconsistent and constraining. The game's promotion and available information are more directed on its characters' social representation and diversity. Although it is not required to focus the advertising campaign on the game's accessibility, all information related to this aspect must be publicly available in a format compatible with assistive technology prior to the game's release (Ellis & Kao, 2019). This imbalance between action and discourse could be related to the importance given by the studio and its developer to these particularities. Hence, *Marvel's Spider-Man: Miles Morales* considers inclusiveness and cultural equity in broad terms that also include cultural context and social diversity.

It would be possible to infer that the game's discursive context primarily positions inclusivity and cultural diversity in a representational perspective, which by its nature does not need to be explicitly described for players to benefit from it. While representation plays a crucial role in inclusivity, this approach is unsuitable for communicating game features and providing clear and simple information about accessibility settings. The developers appear to recognize the structural roles of game design in the exclusion of players with disabilities but fail to communicate these specificities adequately with them. This discursive context, from which *Miles Morales* originated, is representative of the recent efforts of the industry to offer more inclusive and accessible titles. Nonetheless, various developers must make an educational effort to address and promote the accessibility of their games effectively.

TLOU2's excellent accessibility standing, on the other hand, is undeniable, which can be seen by its numerous awards (GOTY, Best Direction, Best Performance, Innovation and Accessibility) and praise received from disabled gamers. Through the seamless implementation of their features, the granular control provided to players, and its predominant neutral and positive language, except for its difficulty settings, Naughty Dog encourages all its players to participate in the video game activity the way they want and need. While the accessibility settings may cover a wide variety of capabilities and fix unnecessary obstacles, TLOU2 encourages individuals to modulate the game's affordances to fit their agency and ensure an optimal and challenging experience. By addressing all players without distinction, TLOU2 carries a discourse focused on inclusiveness and diversity of practices and not conferring any judgment toward the players using them.

The paratext surrounding TLOU2 allows us to observe a concordance between the discourse conveyed by the game and the studio's actions. The developers' interviews in which they clearly state their intentions to design accessible and comfortable experiences, the ease of access to information relating to accessibility features as well as their exhaustive descriptions on the game's website contribute to the notions of inclusivity and cultural equity. These interventions indicate a desire to normalize games' accessibility among players, but more importantly, on the industry level. By adopting and publicizing their position on cultural equity, inclusiveness, and diversity of practices, Naughty Dog participates in discussions between players and developers on video game's accessibility, their relevance, and their possible impact on artistic integrity. Naughty Dog seems to evolve in an environment that considers disability the product of social and cultural institutions rather than medical conditions requiring a cure. Therefore, the developers perceive disabilities according to their social and political dimensions and believe that society's moral obligation is to remove any barrier that may constrain and oppress disabled persons. Furthermore, based on the language used, the developers' insistence on detailing their accessibility measures, and their collaborations with consultants, it is reasonable to conclude that Naughty Dog engages in game accessibility advocacy.

More than creating one of the most accessible video games, Naughty Dog demystifies their development process and openly invites others to build on their work. TLOU2's success demonstrates how it is possible to develop accessible AAA games without sacrificing game mechanics or narrative components, and at the same time using these characteristics as a promotional strategy. Through their discourse, mainly focused on a positive vocabulary, the developers raise awareness of the reality and challenges encountered by players with disabilities and thereby contribute to the destigmatization of video game accessibility. Consequently, the discursive context in which Naughty Dog operates seems inclusive but also aimed at developing culturally equitable games while pushing the industry to follow in its footsteps.

CONCLUSION

At the beginning of this chapter, we demonstrated that video games are not a marginal medium but, on the contrary, are becoming a major cultural object and a "societal phenomenon of growing importance" (Miesenberger et al., 2008, p. 253). In recent years, accessibility in video games has become an increasingly discussed topic in the media, industry, and gaming communities. Nevertheless, most video games, whether mainstream or indie, remain designed for a specific user profile, leaving disabled gamers excluded. In the last years, three studios have made efforts to develop games accessible to a more significant number of people by allowing players to configure the game's affordances based on their agency.

Following the elaboration of a sociosemiotic methodological framework based on the Foucauldian concept of "discourse," we proceeded to the analysis of the mechanics and accessibility settings of the video games *Celeste, Marvel's Spider-Man: Miles Morales,* and *The Last Of Us Part 2,* as well as the paratexts surrounding their release (promotional materials, official websites, press kits, and interviews). While some games originate from a discursive context based on a precise image of video game activity that institutes exclusion, others aim to correct this prevalent prejudice. In this sense, the discursive contexts in which these games occur allowed us to provide an overview of the video game industry's various perspectives on inclusivity, accessibility, and cultural equity.

Thus, we observed that *Celeste* offers a modulation of its game's difficulty and various settings that allow greater accessibility. However, through its menu, information materials, and interviews, the company's discourse prioritizes a "difficult" challenge level that makes this experience the norm against which other types of gaming experiences get judged. This viewpoint of accessibility reflects a pejorative vision in which the norm, regarded as common and able, portrays disability as an abnormality that is inevitably less skilled. In this regard, *Celeste* exemplifies the industry's hesitancy to adopt equitable gaming experiences. From this perspective, accessibility is either an adaptation or a compromise.

On the other hand, *Miles Morales* demonstrates a genuine commitment to inclusivity by offering a variety of settings in a neutral tone and without promoting any particular game style. However, the studio's discourse does not reflect the game's great accessibility, making this aspect secondary in its promotional material. *Miles Morales* exemplifies studios' often insufficient or inadequate efforts to communicate accessibility features to players in a clear and accessible manner. This invisibilization may reflect a hegemonic view in which disability appears to be on the margins of the public discourse (Davis, 1995). Thus, despite developers' intentions to produce accessible gaming environments, certain pitfalls might remain.

Finally, TLOU2 presents a wide variety of settings that demonstrate the studio's strong desire for inclusion. Its remarkable accessibility originates from Naughty Dog' discourses and easily accessible information. The coherence between the game design and its implementation indicates a positive viewpoint where disability is not something that needs fixing but one of the ways of being in the world. Through this title, the studio underscores how acknowledging its players' diverse experiences can benefit everyone. Therefore, while focusing on the normalization of inclusivity and cultural equity, TLOU2 also actively advocates for the gaming industry to change its practices.

Whether managed by the industry artisans or by players, various associations celebrate and award prizes to games with innovative accessibility features. Although it is critical to acknowledge progress and engage in discussions about their roles or particularities, video game accessibility should not be considered a feature nor courtesy, but rather a fundamental necessity. The ability to experience a video game in a fair and unrestricted manner is essential in the perspective that everyone should be free to engage and participate in society's cultural sphere. Therefore, video game accessibility involves more than simply providing specific options to players or rearranging the video game production process; it entails correcting the prejudice and stigma associated with persons living with disabilities. Accordingly, we believe that video games are more than just a mere object or form of entertainment: they are a method of constructing and conveying discourses that may contribute to the inclusion of every citizen in all spheres of society.

Notes

1. Twitch is a video streaming website geared particularly toward video games. Individuals can use the website to broadcast their video games sessions, esports tournaments or other activities such as music or commentary. A chatbox allows viewers and content providers to engage in real-time (Twitch, n.d).
2. Assist Mode refers to a series of options related to game speed, stamina, the number of air dashes or invincibility. These settings are accessible via the game's main title.

References

Aguado-Delgado, J., Gutierrez-Martinez, J. M., Hilera, J. R., de Marcos, L., & Otón, S. (2020). Accessibility in video games: A systematic review. *Universal Access in the Information Society, 19*(1), 169–193. https://doi.org/10.1007/s10209-018-0628-2

Antonelli. (2012, November 29). *Video games: 14 in the collection, for starters.* Retrieved May 18, 2021, from https://www.moma.org/explore/inside_out/2012/11/29/video-games-14-in-the-collection-for-starters/

Barker, C. (2002). *Making sense of cultural studies: Central problems and critical debates.* Sage. https://doi.org/10.4135/9781446220368

Barzilai-Nahon, K. (2009). Gatekeeping: A critical review. *Annual Review of Information Science and Technology, 43*(1), 1–79. https://doi.org/10.1002/aris.2009.1440430117

Bogage, J. (2019, March 28). *Esports continue TV push with ESPN and Turner, sparking enthusiasm, ire.* Retrieved May 18, 2021, from https://www.washingtonpost.com/sports/2019/03/28/esports-continue-tv-push-with-espn-turner-sparking-enthusiasm-ire/

Brown, M., & Anderson, S. L. (2020). Designing for disability: Evaluating the state of accessibility design in video games. *Games and Culture, 16*(6), 702–718. https://doi.org/10.1177/1555412020971500

Castruita, B. (2018, November 16). *Celeste interview with Matt Thorson of Matt Makes Games.* Retrieved May 18, 2021, from https://web.archive.org/web/20201108165429/; https://chargedshot.com/blog/2018/11/16/celeste-interview; Celeste. (n.d.). *Celeste.* Retrieved May 18, 2021, from http://www.celestegame.com

Centers for Disease Control and Prevention. (2020, September 16). *Disability impacts all of us*. National Center on Birth Defects and Developmental Disabilities. Retrieved January 2, 2022, from https://www.cdc.gov/ncbddd/disabilityandhealth/infographic-disability-impacts-all.html

Chin, W. 2015. *Around 92% of people with impairments play games despite difficulties.*. Retrieved May 18, 2021, from https://www.game-accessibility.com/documentation/around-92-of-people-with-impairments-play-games-despite-difficulties/

Clinton "Halfcoordinated" Lexa [@Halfcoordinated]. (2019, April 4). These are good suggestions and yes, Celeste overall handles it well! However, I feel obligated to mention that the Celeste assist mode preamble felt othering for many individuals when it mentioned "intended" gameplay, leaving folks feeling insulted for needing the assists at all. [Tweet]. Twitter. Retrieved May 18, 2021. https://twitter.com/halfcoordinated/status/1113880862121242624?s=20

Csikszentmihalyi, M. (1990). *Flow: The psychology of optimal experience*. Harper & Row.

Csikszentmihalyi, M. (1997). *Finding flow: The psychology of engagement with everyday life*. Basic Books.

Davis, L. J. (1995). *Enforcing normalcy: Disability, deafness and the body*. Verso.

Ellis, K., & Kao, K.-T. (2019). Who gets to play? Disability, open literacy, gaming. *Cultural Science Journal, 11*(1), 111–125. https://doi.org/10.5334/csci.128

Entertainment Software Association [ESA]. (2018, April). *2018 essential facts about the computer and video game industry*. Retrieved May 18, 2021, from https://www.theesa.com/esa-research/2018-essential-facts-about-the-computer-and-video-game-industry/

Entertainment Software Association [ESA]. (2021, February). *2021 essential facts about the video game industry*. Retrieved January 2, 2022, from https://www.theesa.com/resource/2021-essential-facts-about-the-video-game-industry/

Epic Games. (2017). *Fortnite*. [Video game, PC, Nintendo Switch, PlayStation 4, PlayStation 5, Xbox One, Xbox Series X/S, iOS, Android]. Cary, North Carolina: Epic Games.

Foucault, M. (1972). *The archaeology of knowledge and the discourse on language (A. Sheridan Smith, Trans.)*. Pantheon Books. (Original work published in 1969).

Frank, A. (2018, January 26). *Celeste is hard, but its creators are smart about difficulty*. Retrieved January 3, 2022, from https://www.polygon.com/2018/1/26/16935964/celeste-difficulty-assist-mode

Game Accessibility Guidelines. (n.d.). *Game accessibility guidelines: Full list*. Retrieved May 18, 2021, from http://gameaccessibilityguidelines.com/full-list/

Genette, G. (1997). *Paratexts: Thresholds of interpretation*. Cambridge University Press.

George Washington University Online Public Health. (2020, November 5). *Equity vs. equality: What's the difference?* Retrieved May 18, 2021, from https://onlinepublichealth.gwu.edu/resources/equity-vs-equality/

Goodley, D. (2016). *Disability studies: An interdisciplinary introduction*. Sage.

Grammenos, D., Savidis, A., & Stephanidis, C. (2009). Designing universally accessible games. *Computers in Entertainment, 7*(1), Article 8, 1–29. https://doi.org/10.1145/1486508.1486516

Hall, S. (1973) *Encoding and Decoding in the television discourse*. Discussion Paper. University of Birmingham.

Hall, S. (1997). The work of representation. In S. Hall (Ed.), *Representation: Cultural representations and signifying practices* (2nd ed., pp. 13–74). Sage.

Heron, M. (2012). Inaccessible through oversight: The need for inclusive game design. *The Computer Games Journal, 1*(1), 29–38. https://doi.org/10.1007/BF03392326

InnerSloth. (2018). *Among Us.* [Video Game, PC, Nintendo Switch, PlayStation 4, PlayStation 5, Xbox One, Xbox Series X/S, iOS, Android]. InnerSloth.

Insomniac Games. (2020a). *Spider-Man: Miles Morales.* [Video game, PlayStation 4, PlayStation 5]. Sony Interactive Studio.

Insomniac Games. (2020b). *What Accessibility options does Marvel's Spider-Man: Miles Morales feature?* Retrieved May 18, 2021, from https://support.insomniac.games/hc/en-us/articles/360052412831-What-Accessibility-options-does-Marvel-s-Spider-Man-Miles-Morales-feature-

Isbister, K. (2016). *How games move us: Emotion by design.* MIT Press. https://doi.org/10.7551/mitpress/9267.001.0001

Klepek, P. (2018, February 7). *Why the very hard 'Celeste' is perfectly fine with you breaking its rules.* Retrieved January 3, 2022, from https://www.vice.com/en/article/d3w887/celeste-difficulty-assist-mode

Klepek, P. (2019, September 16). *The small but important change 'Celeste' made to its celebrated assist mode.* Retrieved January 3, 2022, from https://www.vice.com/en/article/43kadm/celeste-assist-mode-change-and-accessibility

Lomax, A. (1980). Appeal for cultural equity. *African Music: Journal of the International Library of African Music, 6*(1), 22–31. https://doi.org/10.21504/amj.v6i1.1092

Matt Makes Games. (2018a). *Celeste.* [Video game, Windows, macOS, Linux, Nintendo Switch, PlayStation 4, Xbox One, Stadia]. Matt Makes Games.

Matt Makes Games. (2018b). *Celeste press kit* [Press release]. Retrieved May 18, 2021, from https://www.dropbox.com/sh/87lycjzncb0o9ns/AACcA3s5Uyzkeicn3-26qLBWa?dl=0

Miesenberger, K., Ossmann, R., Archambault, D., Searle, G., & Holzinger, A. (2008). More than just a game: Accessibility in computer games. In A. Holzinger (Ed.), *HCI and Usability for Education and Work* (pp. 247–260). Springer.

Murray, J. H. (1998). *Hamlet on the holodeck. The future of narrative in cyberspace.* MIT Press.

Naughty Dog. (2016). *Uncharted 4: A Thief's End.* [Video game, PlayStation 4]. Sony Interactive Studio.

Naughty Dog. (2020). *The Last of Us 2.* [Video game, PlayStation 4]. Sony Interactive Studio.

Neely, E. L. (2017). No player is ideal: Why video game designers cannot ethically ignore players' real-world identities. *ACM SIGCAS Computers and Society, 47*(3), 98–111. https://doi.org/10.1145/3144592.3144602

Newzoo. (2021, July 1). *Newzoo Global Games Market Report 2021.* Retrieved January 2, 2022, from https://newzoo.com/insights/trend-reports/newzoo-global-games-market-report-2021-free-version/

Norman, D. (2013). *The design of everyday things.* Basic Books.

Paul, C. A. (2018). *The toxic meritocracy of video games: Why gaming culture is the worst. University of Minnesota Press.* https://doi.org/10.5749/j.ctt2204rbz

Pérez-Latorre, Ó., Oliva, M., & Besalú, R. (2017). Videogame analysis: A social-semiotic approach. *Social Semiotics, 27*(5), 586–603. https://doi.org/10.1080/10350330.2016.1191146

Pitaru, A. (2008). E is for everyone: The case for inclusive game design. In K. Salen (Ed.), *The Ecology of Games: Connecting Youth, Games, and Learning* (pp. 67–86). MIT Press. https://doi.org/10.1162/dmal.9780262693646.06

PlayStation. (2020). *The Last of Us Part II.* Retrieved May 18, 2021, from https://www.playstation.com/en-ca/games/the-last-of-us-part-ii/

Porter, J. R., & Kientz, J. A. (2013). An empirical study of issues and barriers to mainstream video game accessibility. *Proceedings of the 15th International ACM SIGACCESS Conference on Computers and Accessibility—ASSETS '13*, 1–8. https://doi.org/10.1145/2513383.2513444

redhatGizmo. (2019, April 12). *Video game difficulty is an accessibility issue.* [Online forum post]. Reddit. Retrieved May 18, 2021, from https://www.reddit.com/r/gaming/comments/bcbg1g/video_game_difficulty_is_an_accessibility_issue/

Salen, K., & Zimmerman, E. (2004). *Rules of play: Game design fundamentals.* MIT Press.

Semprini, A. (1995). *L'objet comme procès et comme action: De la nature et de l'usage des objets dans la vie quotidienne* [The Object as Process and as Action: On the Nature and Use of Objects in Everyday Life]. L'Harmattan.

Shaw, A. (2010). What is video game culture? Cultural studies and game studies. *Games and Culture, 5*(4), 403–424. https://doi.org/10.1177/1555412009360414

Siebers, T. (2001). Disability in theory: From social constructionism to the new realism of the body. *American Literary History, 13*(4), 737–754. https://doi.org/10.1093/alh/13.4.737

Steinkuehler, C. A., & Williams, D. (2006). Where everybody knows your (screen) name: Online games as "third places." *Journal of Computer-Mediated Communication, 11*(4), 885–909. https://doi.org/10.1111/j.1083-6101.2006.00300.x

The Guardian. (n.d.). Culture: Games. Retrieved May 18, 2021, from https://www.theguardian.com/games

Véron. E. (1987). *La sémiosis sociale: Fragments d'une théorie de la discursivité* [Social Semiosis: Fragments of a Theory of Discursivity]. Presses Universitaires de Vincennes.

Webster, A. (2020, June 1). *The Last of Us Part II isn't just Naughty Dog's most ambitious game—it's the most accessible, too.* Retrieved May 18, 2021, from https://www.theverge.com/21274923/the-last-of-us-part-2-accessibility-features-naughty-dog-interview-ps4

Yuan, B., Folmer, E., & Harris, F. C. (2011). Game accessibility: A survey. *Universal Access in the Information Society, 10*(1), 81–100. https://doi.org/10.1007/s10209-010-0189-5

CHAPTER 15

Posthuman Critical Theory and the Body on *Sports Night*

Peter J. Gloviczki

BACKGROUND AND POSITIONALITY

As theorist Rosi Braidotti writes: "Posthuman critical theory proposes to resist any foregone conclusion about the transition that the 'human' and 'humanity' is going through and to focus instead on the ongoing processes of transformation" (2017, p. 21). How does *Sports Night* engage posthuman critical theory in its coverage of the body? This chapter will work to answer that question. Aaron Sorkin's short-lived but critically acclaimed sitcom *Sports Night* showcases an inclusive assemblage of bodies in a way that is (perhaps) forward thinking for its 1990s popular American moment. This analysis is relevant now because the intersection of disability and communication benefits from recent historical understandings of representation in popular culture. Braiding autoethnography into new media technology history, this chapter uses Braidotti's "Posthuman Critical Theory" to explore the role of the physical body on the sitcom, including how bodies reflect, reinforce, and challenge conceptions of dis/ability, through an examination of what the characters on the show may have to teach us about success, failure, times of crisis, and everyday life. Autoethnography (Ellis, 1999) is a writing-based research method (Richardson, 1994) that explores the dynamics between personal world and cultural world (Reed-Danahay, 1997). Employing this method as part of the research toolkit helps this work move beyond media analysis to its broader communication and

P. J. Gloviczki (✉)
Western Illinois University, Macomb, IL, USA
e-mail: PJ-Gloviczki@wiu.edu

© The Author(s), under exclusive license to Springer Nature
Switzerland AG 2023
M. S. Jeffress et al. (eds.), *The Palgrave Handbook of Disability and Communication*, https://doi.org/10.1007/978-3-031-14447-9_15

243

sociological implications. The chapter will focus on the episode "Dear Louise," (S1, E7) with an emphasis on dialogues through the middle of the episode, where the program broadcasts a graphic remembering the life of Archibald "A.K." Russell, a Negro Leagues baseball player who pitched for the Kansas City Monarchs baseball team. The chapter will study the dialogue in relevant scenes to examine whether and to what extent those scenes rise to the level of critical humanism, as articulated by Braidotti. It is the modest hope of this chapter to better understand how the critical body exists in *Sports Night* in particular and throughout popular culture in general. There is a need to better understand how the body is portrayed in media because mediation may reflect one of the primary ways that audiences learn about the opportunities and challenges associated with living with and through life in bodies that may be outside the mainstream of Western culture. I recognize the tradition of other disability studies scholars who are, and have long been, engaged in important work in this arena (see, for example, Zhang & Haller, 2013).

I am writing this book chapter as a qualitative researcher with a particular interest in representation in the digital age. My prior research (Gloviczki, 2015, 2021) utilizes the case study research strategy (Yin, 2003; Stake, 1995), auto-ethnography (Reed-Danahay, 1997; Ellis, 1999), and textual analysis (McKee, 2003) to offer a new media technology history that spans from 1991 through 2018. Mediated discourses particularly help audiences make meaning in those instances where audience members lack reliable, unmediated ways of knowing about the issues being represented. Another modest goal of this chapter is to trouble both the mainstream and the margins, challenging why what is central exists there and why what is peripheral exists there. Position should exist along a fluid, dialogic continuum rather than within any fixed, monologic space.

Understanding and employing posthuman critical theory is a relatively new challenge for me. I wish to apply new theoretical lenses to learn new ways of seeing the world around me and of understanding its particulars. In addition to posthuman critical theory, I have lately been influenced by the writings of post-structuralists including Jane Bennett (2010), Derek McCormack (2018), and Nidesh Lawtoo (2013). While my focus on this chapter is on Braidotti's posthuman critical theory, I come to that theory heavily influenced by each of these authors. I mention them here because having recently read their ideas, I certainly am under their counsel as I approach other texts, including the ones that I take up directly in this chapter. I go, always seeking dialogic and representational solutions for the future of media culture.

Sports Night is, in my view, the most realistic depiction of a journalistic newsroom in popular culture. Aaron Sorkin's short-lived program, which began in 1998, only ran for two seasons, but I feel fortunate to have watched it over and over again. First on DVDs and, today, via YouTube. Any scholarship that I produce about the body (mediated or otherwise) also benefits from and is read through the reality of my own physical body. As I have written about extensively in the past (Gloviczki, 2016, 2021), I was born with a physical disability, cerebral palsy, which impacts my balance, stamina, and coordination.

Though I walk unaided, I nonetheless do happily see the world as an outsider, walking with and through a body that is aware of its own particulars. While rewatching *Sports Night* to write this book chapter, I found myself wondering when or if there might be a character on a major sports program, a sitcom like this one, with cerebral palsy. I write about our technological future with a sense of optimism, with genuine and profound hope about what is to come for disabled representation and embodiment.

The Implications of Braidotti's Embrace

The way that bodies are represented across cultures matters, in large part, because representation helps make sense of and brings meaning to bodies as sites of/for inquiry. Braidotti, for her part, places the critical posthuman as a way of understanding our times and how we progress through/with/along them. Braidotti (2017) writes: "The present is both the record of what we are ceasing to be and the seed of what we are in the process of becoming: it is here and now, but also virtual" (p. 11). Braidotti, importantly, views such an undertaking as needing to be guided by a particular framework, noting: "The crucial ethical imperative is to refuse to conceal the power differentials that divide us" (2017, p. 22). To study the critical posthuman in a Braidottian way, therefore, is an ethical engagement that looks for, and works to make sense of, where and for whom lines of power are demarcated. I will work to take up this line of inquiry. In addition, a critical posthuman undertaking such as this one must and does wrestle with the self on the one hand and the social context through which the self is constructed on the other hand. Sociologist and autoethnographer Carol Rambo writes: "Self and society are intertwined in such a way that the boundaries of each idea are dialectically blurred into one" (2007, p. 538). Taking an optimistic view, I view this Ramboian "blurring" as an opportunity for self to positively impact social and social to positively impact self. As I have written elsewhere (see, for example, Gloviczki, 2021), mediation tells us in the audience about the potentials of/for bodies, including bodies that are represented in popular culture. Returning to Rambo on the self and the social, representations of the body may matter for another reason as well. As Rambo writes: "We derive formulas for how to act toward the world and ourselves based, in part, on the impressions left on us by society" (2007, p. 537). In this chapter, I assert that mediation of/for the body may influence how and if we conceptualize bodies (our own and others') in the present and the future.

The Virtues and Vices of "Dear Louise"

"You write letters?" … "I write to Louise." … "My sister can't hear."

—*Sports Night*, "Dear Louise." (S1, E7)*Sports Night* is to be praised for foregrounding the body through its consideration of Louise's deafness. To write plainly and elevate deafness in this context is to layer Louise's unseen body into the broader corporeal narrative of the show. *Sports Night* is a show about athletes, but *Sports Night* rarely visualizes the athletes themselves. Accordingly, Louise's status as a family member (Jeremy's sister) being written to (but never visualized) slides effectively into this overarching theme. Moreover, by emphasizing Louise's deafness in the natural flow of conversation, Jeremy works to normalize deafness in the human experience. Exploring autoethnographically, I appreciate how this scene foregrounds difference. Doing so normalizes disability, rather than bracketing othered bodies toward exceptionalism. Representing difference in this way allows a show about athletes to begin refashioning itself as a show about humans and their pluralities. Within the context of an after-work letter, the scene also allows the viewer to conceptualize Jeremy as a relational being: he is choosing to prioritize his relationship with his sister through this act of authorship. Jeremy's act also arguably builds his social capital among his colleagues because he has chosen to build and sustain a familial relationship in this particular manner. Principally, this act strongly suggests Jeremy as a dependable individual who follows through on his commitment to those individuals he cares about. As a relatively new employee on the show, Jeremy's dependability is arguably a trait that his colleagues will recognize as also transferable to his work environment. When disabled bodies are only or mostly used as props of virtue, they are elevated in ways that diminish their human fallibility. Jeremy's dependability, and his sister's dependability as his correspondent, is admirable precisely because humans are flawed beings, not often known for their interpersonal, professional, or relational dependability.

For each of these virtues, neither this scene nor subsequent scenes in the episode reveal any meaningful characteristics about Louise's humanity. We in the audience know her as Jeremy's sister, a college student, a deaf woman, but none of these descriptors allow the audience a truly full or layered portrayal of her particulars. The conversation about deafness that the scene admirably opens is left at least somewhat unfulfilled. The dialogue about deafness begins with promise and gestures toward normalization, but it is incomplete and ultimately unsatisfying. The scene could have, but does not, move deeper than its initial nominal descriptor about Louise. As a result, this scene does not appear to rise to a level of Braidottian critical posthumanism. Louise is still ensnared, corporeally categorized, by her seeming sensory lack. Crafting Louise's character using a more evocative sensorial portrait would allow her humanity to shine through in a novel and humane way.

Jeremy builds the backstory of his work life for both Louise and the viewing audience. He invites us into the emotional landscape of his labor, as he reveals both his apparent relief at the goodness of fit in his work environment and the blending between work and home in the Western cultural moment. On a microlevel, to write a letter at work—after work—is to choose to remain in a workspace as part of leisure time. Jeremy's body remains amid the conditions of its labor (at his desk) after his obligations to labor have concluded. On a macro level, Jeremy recognizes that his coworkers, through their invitation to him, are coming to see him as more than just a potential coworker, they are hoping to know him as a friend, too. Jeremy also suggests that he, too, is moving beyond seeing his coworkers as laborers, because he praises their ability to perform in stressful situations. Accordingly, in this scene, the first potential transition toward Braidottian critical posthumanism is revealed, because characters on the show are described as valuable beyond their nominal, instrumental qualities. The narrative in the scene foreshadows the more humane dialogues that are to come in the episode. Louise is an instrument to more fully appreciate others' humanity, but her own humanity is still underexplored in the episode. Exploring autoethnographically, this process feels dangerously close to the way that other people have sometimes told me that my corporeal feats are inspiring to them. Mining the disabled self for the sake of the improvement of the other, as an emotional buoy, is a discouraging theme. Louise is a vehicle to other characters without active representation.

Spotlighting the Story of Archibald "A.K." Russell

There are four rundown meetings a day. Noon, six o'clock, eight o'clock, and ten. I'm sure that in no time, I'll have forgotten about it. But, at the moment, I can't stop thinking about the noon rundown a few weeks ago, and a guy you've never heard of named Archibald Russell.
—Jeremy in *Sports Night*, "Dear Louise." (S1, E7)
Dana to Jeremy: "Jeremy, put together something on an old Negro Leagues pitcher named Archibald Russell."
—*Sports Night*, "Dear Louise." (S1, E7)
I felt terrible for suggesting that the story lacked the importance to be placed in an early segment. But as terrible as I felt then, it was nothing compared to what I was going to feel that night.
—Jeremy to Louise (in letter), *Sports Night*, "Dear Louise." (S1, E7)
Archibald "A.K." Russell is probably not a name you're familiar with, unless you were lucky enough to watch the Kansas City Monarchs play baseball the way it was meant to be played. He had three 20-win seasons, he's an associate pastor at the Barryhill Baptist Church, and oh yeah, taught himself how to read and write. He was driving the Cadillac Seville that his four sons had given him for his 80th birthday, when he stopped for a red light this morning. He was dragged from his car, beaten with sticks and bottles, and left at the side of the road. A.K. is in critical condition in Mercy Hospital in Kansas City and the thoughts and prayers of everyone here are with him.
—Casey on air, *Sports Night*, "Dear Louise." (S1, E7)
The Russell story smartly reveals the group's admiration for and deference to Isaac's wishes that his friend Russell be spotlighted in the evening broadcast. Their dialogue clearly suggests this wish to fulfill Isaac's stated desire. In this way, the show opens a conversation about racial injustice and, even more specifically, the problem of racist violence in America. *Sports Night* notably chooses to make the Russell story a national story, despite Jeremy's protest for it to be otherwise. That said, this scene misses an opportunity for Isaac to discuss any

of those issues directly, preferring instead to allow the coverage of the story "up front" to ostensibly speak for him or for itself. Like the unseen, unspoken-about body, the violence at the core of the story is not commented upon beyond a cursory mention of Russell being "in Mercy Hospital." The potential entry into a discussion about race in this scene is not further explored, just as was the reality with the potential entry into a conversation about deafness in the first scene studied in this chapter. Continual emphasis on Russell as Jaffee's friend provides an (unutilized) vehicle to discuss broader cultural issues, but it provides the reasoning that the rest of the staff use to tell the story. Accordingly, the staff can follow Jaffee's lead and address neither race nor social justice issues directly in their decision-making process. The story and the decision to run it are presented as spearheaded by friendship. Like the sibling bond that is fore-grounded in Jeremy's decision to write to Louise, the friendship bond (between Jaffee and Russell) is foregrounded in the staff's decision to prioritize the Russell story in the broadcast. In each instance, the bonding issues (family, friendship) stand in for the social issues. Each story is told such that it in no way disturbs, critiques, or even questions existing Western power dynamics. Jaffee was close to Russell and the staff is close to Jaffee. Unexamined closeness, and the staff's desire (admirable though it may be) to please their boss, leads to the story being placed early in the broadcast. As a result, this scene does not rise to the level of Braidottian critical posthumanism.

In this scene, Jeremy continues to reveal his vulnerability to his sister in his letter writing process. We in the audience learn that Jeremy ostensibly feels comfortable baring his emotional state to his sister, which suggests an especially strong familial bond between the two of them. The second short paragraph of this scene foreshadows that Jeremy's emotional pain is just beginning, and the writers and producers on *Sports Night* are to be celebrated for drawing Jeremy's character with this considerable degree of emotional depth. What is certainly missing in this scene, though, is a deeper dive about why exactly Jeremy felt "terrible." Principally, the unspoken, unexamined questions emerge: (1) Did he feel terrible because he was contradicting his boss? (a work-related reason) or (2) Did he feel terrible because of the underlying social issues in the story? (a sociocultural reason). Where Jaffee is at least willing to gesture toward the importance of making space for racial violence in the broadcast by requesting that the story be run "up front," Jeremy does not even make any mention of race in his letter to Louise. It is simply implied that race might be one of the reasons Jeremy's character might feel "terrible." No further consideration of any specific social issues is provided in this scene. Accordingly, this scene also does not engage in Braidottian critical posthumanism.

This scene is notable in the episode for several reasons. First, this scene reveals Dan and Casey doing the work for which they have been planning: hosting a cable television sports program and, more specifically, telling the story of Archibald "A.K." Russell per Isaac's request. Second, this scene reveals the staff doing the work that was requested of them by their boss: the power dynamic has indeed remained undisturbed. Third, the broadcast reveals that the entire group are offering well wishes, which is a socioculturally accepted, and relatively passive, form of expressing solidarity in Judeo-Christian culture (see, for example, Gloviczki, 2015). For all three of these reasons, this scene does not rise to the level of Braidottian critical posthumanism.

There are also at least two vague references that need to be addressed in this scene. First, it should be noted that there is a very vague gesture toward the past as something better than the present in this scene: "play baseball the way it was meant to be played" (*Sports Night*, "Dear Louise," (S1, E7)) but this vague gesture feels like an almost empty reference to the past as *better* (emphasis mine) without any explanation about why that may have been the case. It is possible that the story intended to reference the athletic skill of Russell and his teammates, but this possibility is muddled at best. Much like earlier scenes, this scene also leaves lingering questions. Principally, how was baseball meant to be played? And by whom? As it stands, the nature and trajectory of this reference is unclear. If a gesture toward social justice was intended, the lack of clarity about it strongly suggests it remains unfulfilled. Second, the Kansas City Monarchs, furthermore, are not even specified as a Negro Leagues baseball team. Their lack of contextualization suggests the viewing audience during the broadcast is simply expected to know who that team was and what they represented. Elsewhere in the episode, Isaac does mention how Russell played "with Gibson and Jackie," (*Sports Night*, "Dear Louise," (S1, E7)) referencing famous Black players Josh Gibson and Jackie Robinson, but this information may be unclear to non-sports fans of *Sports Night* and this connection was not made during the broadcast for viewers of the show. Accordingly, a connection between Russell and other Black athletes may require insider knowledge for anyone viewing the broadcast. For this reason, the episode misses yet another opportunity to delve more deeply into the subject of race specifically or social issues more generally. The fact that the broadcast does state Russell "taught himself to read and write" is a vague claim about social issues (literacy), but the narration does not go any further into any social issue in this scene. The audience is left, as it is throughout the episode, to infer any connections between what is broadcast and any broader cultural struggles. Put simply, power is never directly addressed. These two vague references may be seeking to disturb existing structures, but if that was the intent, neither one appears to have succeeded. The Russell storyline concludes in the episode when the group learns that he has died in the hospital. A graphic is broadcast on air, showing a picture of Archibald "A.K" Russell, ostensibly in his baseball uniform, with birth year and death year under his name.

250   P. J. GLOVICZKI

The Complicated Reality of "Kyle Whitaker's Got Two Sacks"

Sports Night provided some coverage of bodies that might be considered path-setting, even posthuman critical in its theoretical orientation, especially for its time. Consider, for example, the show's coverage in one episode of Kyle Whitaker, producer Dana Whitaker's brother, a professional football player who was part of a performance enhancing drug scandal. The frailty of the athletic body is on display in this episode, as a professional athlete willingly and knowingly turns to banned drugs to increase their performance on the field. Recognizing her brother's name is about to be broadcast in the scandal live on the air, a stunned Dana takes off her headset, says "I'm going to call my parents" and leaves the control room. On the phone, Whitaker says: "Hey, mom, it's me, turn off your television." (*Sports Night*, "Kyle Whitaker's Got Two Sacks," (S2, E7)). The cultural power of television is fully on display in this brief exchange. Dana, the leader in the control room, is unable to control the power of television, when the story being broadcast is regarding her brother's misuse of performance enhancers. Media culture is revealed to be an entity all its own. The opportunities for further inquiry here are manifold, and yet, the turn in the scene is to the familial, rather than the cultural. Again, as with Louise and Russell, the immediate turn is to the bond and the relationship—inward to self, rather than outward to culture. The posthuman critical opportunity is avoided.

Conclusion

As I have worked to make clear throughout this chapter, the scenes studied here often opened with plenty of critical posthuman promise, that promise was just never brought to ultimate fruition. Taking a charitable approach to the episodes studied, the scenes may have gone as comfortable as they felt going at the time. And perhaps they should be applauded, to an extent, for the way that they might have opened some dialogue about issues surrounding deafness, race, and even performance-enhancing drug use. The body is often the subject on display in *Sports Night*, which may well explain its enduring critical posthuman promise. The critical posthuman promise was never sustained in the way that it might have been, however. The sitcom usually retreats when it could, and as I assert throughout this chapter *should*, go deeper. This choice is what most often leaves the bodies on display underexamined.

I believe that the two episodes of *Sports Night* considered in this book chapter [(Dear Louise (S1, E7)) and Kyle Whitaker's Got Two Sacks (S2, E7)] represent a beginning in my study of the ways in which *Sports Night* portrayed athletic bodies, the working realities of the 1990s, and foretold about the future of sports media, journalism, and mass communication. I am both heartened and disappointed that the sitcom only lasted two seasons. I am heartened because it helps me recognize how much meaningful television can be produced in a short timeframe. I am disappointed because I wonder what insights *Sports Night* would have to offer, were it still on the air, about the changing sports media world of today. Just as NBC's *Law and Order* keeps adding to popular culture scholars' critical lexicon, I wonder what additions *Sports Night* would have to offer us as scholars and practitioners in the media world, if the sitcom had lasted longer than two seasons.

I am, through a Braidottian lens, rather convinced that *Sports Night*'s portrayals of the body did not reveal a posthuman critical turn. That said, I am keen to examine other ways in which the sitcom may have correctly foretold a more personalized future of and for mass culture. Having studied it, I believe I have opened a path for looking that will sustain some of my work going forward. I am especially interested in how and if networked communication technologies were represented on *Sports Night* and, if so, what that representation may mean for how the sitcom represented the future of journalism. I am keen to travel that research path in the future. I am also interested in how the characters on the sitcom (as employees at a TV show) interacted with other media entities on the show. Accordingly, I am planning to study how *Sports Night* personalities used and were used by media within the universe of the sitcom. My hope is that each of the directions for future research mentioned in this section will help me make sense of *Sports Night* and its impact within the landscape of its late 1990s critical/poststructuralist popular culture moment.

This chapter sought to answer the research question: How does *Sports Night* engage posthuman critical theory in its coverage of the body? Analysis of a key episode in the series, "Dear Louise," which featured numerous opportunities to closely examine both deafness and racial violence in the African American community, did neither in sufficient ways to rise to the level of critical posthuman theory. While the episode opened promising dialogues on each topic, through consideration of Jeremy's sister Louise and Isaac's friend Archibald "A. K." Russell, neither one ultimately carried posthuman critical thought forward in significant ways. Analysis of the program in general and the episode in particular does yield a meaningful model for moments in popular culture where critical posthuman thought was promising but ultimately stalled.

Finally, of particular note in the sitcom is the way bodies usually outside of the mainstream media (Louise's body as a deaf woman and A.K. Russell's body as a Negro Leagues baseball pitcher) are given a hearing, made space for, in prominent ways. Jeremy is not at all perfect and I have taken care to detail some of his (and the show's) missteps. But Aaron Sorkin's Jeremy and Isaac, respectively, might each be considered as bonafide advocates, people somewhat ahead of their time. More than 20 years after *Sports Night* wrapped, the murders of George Floyd and Daunte Wright remind us how the racism Isaac was fighting remains a major problem in American society. My white skin affords me unearned privilege; I cannot know their fear nor fully understand their lived experiences. Sorkin's Kyle Whitaker, too, points toward potential frailties among professional athletes, reassuring audiences that there are no superhumans on the playing field. Gesturing toward complex corporeal realities while revealing sociocultural terrain seems *Sports Night*'s most enduring contribution. In doing so, the sitcom suggests some worthwhile strides toward diversity, equity, inclusion, and belonging in media culture.

REFERENCES

Bennett, J. (2010). *Vibrant matter: A political ecology of things*. Duke University Press.

Braidotti, R. (2017). Posthuman critical theory. *Journal of Posthuman Studies, 1*(1), 9–25. https://doi.org/10.5325/jpoststud.1.1.0009

Ellis, C. (1999). Heartful autoethnography. *Qualitative Health Research, 9*(5), 669–683. https://doi.org/10.1177/104973299129122153

Gloviczki, P. J. (2015). *Journalism and memorialization in the age of social media*. Palgrave Macmillan.

Gloviczki, P. J. (2016). Leaving London: Three autoethnographic sketches. *Journal of Loss and Trauma, 21*(4), 286–289. https://doi.org/10.1080/1532502 4.2015.1067093

Gloviczki, P. J. (2021). *Mediated narration in the digital age: Storying the media world*. University of Nebraska Press.

Lawtoo, N. (2013). *The phantom of the ego: Modernism and the mimetic unconscious*. Michigan State University Press.

McCormack, D. P. (2018). *Atmospheric things: On the allure of elemental envelopment*. Duke University Press.

McKee, A. (2003). *Textual analysis: A beginner's guide*. Sage.

Rambo, C. (2007). Sketching as autoethnographic practice. *Symbolic Interaction, 30*(4), 531–542. https://doi.org/10.1525/si.2007.30.4.531

Reed-Danahay, D. (1997). *Auto/ethnography: Rewriting the self and the social*. Berg.

Richardson, L. (1994). Writing as a method of inquiry. In N. K. Denzin & Y. S. Lincoln (Eds.), *Handbook of Qualitative Research* (pp. 516–529). Sage.

Stake, R. E. (1995). *The art of case study research*. Sage.

Yin, R. K. (2003). *Case study research design and methods* (3rd ed.). Sage.

Zhang, L., & Haller, B. (2013). Consuming image: How mass media impact the identity of people with disabilities. *Communication Quarterly, 61*(3), 319–334. https://doi.org/10.1080/01463373.2013.776988

CHAPTER 16

Never Go Full Potato: Discourses of Ableism and Sexism in "I Can Count to Potato" Memes

Jeff Preston

In 2012, Heidi Crowter, a young woman with Down syndrome from the United Kingdom, made a simple public appeal: stop using her image as part of an ableist meme. Years earlier, Internet users had accessed a childhood picture of Crowter and converted it into a stock character meme with "I can count to potato" written in iconic black and white text. Seeded by a line from the Johnny Knoxville film *The Ringer* (2005), the "I Can Count to Potato" memetic cluster deploys variations of the term "potato" in online communities to sardonically imply people or objects are silly, dumb, or otherwise unworthy of serious consideration. An evolution of the vernacular use of "retarded," a catachresis that leverages the symbolic meaning of intellectual and developmental disabilities to denote objects or people as "dumb" or "bad," the Potato meme evokes the same symbolic weight of cognitive impairment while sidestepping the overt usage of the "r-word." But as we heard clearly from Crowter, the Potato memes, and the r-word before it, present a fantasy of cognitive impairment, a funhouse mirror version replicating stereotypes generated from past representation as opposed to accurately describing the lived experience (and value) of people with cognitive impairments.

Confronted with this cognitive dissonance, meme creators bristled at Crowter's plea to relinquish control of her image, initiating a new flurry of memetic generation that reasserted ableist imaginations of cognitive impairment—the simulacra of cognitive impairment was simply truer to reality than

---

J. Preston (✉)
King's University College, London, ON, Canada
e-mail: jeff.preston@uwo.ca

© The Author(s), under exclusive license to Springer Nature
Switzerland AG 2023
M. S. Jeffress et al. (eds.), *The Palgrave Handbook of Disability and Communication*, https://doi.org/10.1007/978-3-031-14447-9_16

253

Crowter's dissimulation. Where Crowter embodied an example of those with Down syndrome being meaningful and astute people, both valuable and loved, memetic creators saw only another Potato, devoid of nuance or intelligibility. Not only did the new memes double down on the connection between the invalid subject position of disability, Crowter's appearance and femininity became indicative of a collision with another stigmatized identity: Crowter was now not just disabled but also a woman. Just like people with Down syndrome, female minds are imagined as dysfunctional and fall outside the demands of compulsory able-bodiedness. The meaning of the Potato meme was rooted in a fervently believed fact of cognitive impairment not reflected by Crowter—the meme now precedes the reality of Heidi Crowter and her very personhood must realign with the truth of the representation.

Situated at the intersection of discourse analysis and Internet archeology, the objective of this chapter is two-fold: first, to consider a memetic analysis augmented by Baudrillard's simulacra (1994) and second, to apply this lens in unpacking the underlying ableist beliefs propagated and validated through the Potato memetic cluster. The chapter begins by considering the collision of current research on digital memetic culture and the work of French postmodernist Jean Baudrillard. From this perspective, the chapter considers the ways Internet memes subjugate symbolic identities, as people become transformed into useful objects (re)inscribed with hyperreal meaning once entering the symbolic refractory of memetic cultures. The chapter concludes by considering what happens when memes speak back, using the Crowter example to explore how other experiences of oppression can become entangled with disability in disputes about language, culture, and identity.

This chapter contains overt and implied reference to offensive and hurtful language and memes that seek to delegitimize and dehumanize those with intellectual and developmental disability. Where possible, memes have been reproduced in this chapter in an editorialized fashion, to limit the use of offensive language, while retaining links to the original content for those wishing to engage directly with the content. Some memes, however, are presented without alteration to ensure there is no ambiguity of their discursive intent.

On Memes, Simulacra, and Ableism

Rooted in the work of Richard Dawkins, as described in *The Selfish Gene* (Dawkins, 1989), "meme" is used to describe "contagious patterns of 'cultural information' that get passed from mind to mind and directly generate and shape the mindsets and significant forms of behavior and actions of a social group" (Knobel & Lankshear, 2007, p. 199). This original definition, considering idea clusters spreading virally from person-to-person and driven by Darwin's natural selection, has found new life in the social media age to describe the digital content deployed by users to give nuance to otherwise textual speech online. At the same time, as Yasmin Ibrahim so eloquently points out, Dawkins' original conception of "meme" is perhaps too simplistic to capture the true weight and function of memetic culture online:

> Memes remain as part of a popular genre often articulated through their virality as a form of contagion or through Dawkins' discussions of evolutionary genetics collapsing them through modes of uncontrollable transmission while somewhat downplaying the agentic role of audiences as relays of information and the individual preference, and communal endorsements in enabling their success. (Ibrahim, 2021, p. 11)

Grant Kien shares a similar opinion on the benefits (and consequences) of social media that serves as an important disconnect between the original person-to-person communication connected to Dawkins' concept of "meme" and the one-to-many transmission capabilities enabled by social media (2019). Namely, Kien critiques the notion that ideas survive or die based on their quality, noting:

> The mass mediation capabilities social media puts in the hands of the audience have the potential to accelerate and amplify feedback loops in the global media system: within, across, and between platforms. The exponential amplification of even little pieces of communication in our media ecosystem highlight what Godwin (1994) explained as an "obligation to improve our informational environment," since any piece of information, whether true, false, good, evil, or benign, is subject to rapid and disproportional outcomes. (Kien, 2019, p. 14)

This evolution of Dawkins' original definition, bringing the "meme" into the digital context, suggests we must focus not just on the ways memes are rooted in mimicry, or repeating that which has already been done, but also in the ways memes open up the potential to be "remixed," creating our own intertextual versions as part of the Internet's fabled participatory culture (Shifman, 2013, Chap. 1).

Building off the work of Ryan Milner (Milner, 2012, 2016) to investigate groups of meme "genres" based on the memes' content, form, and/or stance, Shifman goes on to denote genre categories of the popular digital memes at the time (Shifman, 2013). One of those "genres" of meme, the stock character macro, or what Kien simplifies to "image macro" (Kien, 2019, p. 6), plays a central role in the Potato memetic cluster. In a typical image macro, the image itself is the vehicle (form) that structures the meme, allowing users to modify/remix the text (content) that gains symbolic meaning in relation to the image. However, sometimes it is the text itself, the content of the original image macro, that extends beyond the original image to become connected to other memetic vehicles.

While these simple combinations of image and text may seem superfluous or insignificant, Shifman argues that stock character macros are of particular importance to academic inquiry as

> This array of stock character macros provides a glimpse into the drama of morality of the First World of the twenty-first century: it is a conceptual map of types that represent exaggerated forms of behavior … these extreme forms tend to focus on success and failure in the social life of a particular group. (Shifman, 2013, Chap. 7)

In this way, analysis of image macros provides a glimpse into the common ideological discourses circulating within and animating the cultural practice of these digital affinity groups (citing James Paul Gee in Knobel & Lankshear, 2007, p. 200). Shifman urges us to consider memes not as mundane or arbitrary cultural artifacts, but instead to honor how "[memes] actually reflect deep social and cultural structures. In many senses, Internet memes can be treated as (post)modern folklore, in which shared norms and values are constructed through cultural artifacts such as Photoshopped images or urban legends" (Shifman, 2013, Chap. 3). Gal, Shifman, and Kampf go on to say we must "conceptualize memes as performative acts, applied both for persuasive purposes (preventing gay teen suicide) and for the construction of collective identity and norms" and note the importance of "determining who was included in and excluded from the discourse, as well as which narratives, conventions, and behaviors were embraced and legitimized" (Gal et al., 2016, p. 1710).

But how does one approach analyzing or interpreting these cultural artifacts: ostensibly pithy comments shouted out anonymously into the digital abyss? Knodel and Lankshear's early study of digital memes proposes a typology of memes based on their intended purpose, noting that memes in their sample tended to either be used for social commentary, absurdist humor, otaku/manga fandom or hoaxes (Knobel & Lankshear, 2007). Aligning with Shifman's work, Wiggins and Bowers support the use of genre to understanding memes, noting that "the meme, viewed as a genre, is not simply a formula followed by humans to communicate, but is a complex system of social motivations and cultural activity that is both a result of communication and impetus for that communication" (Wiggins & Bowers, 2015, p. 1893). Segev et al. evolve this concept to explore the ways "that (a) higher cohesiveness of meme families is associated with a greater uniqueness of their generic attributes; and (b) the concreteness of meme quiddities is associated with cohesiveness and uniqueness" (Segev et al., 2015). For Grant Kien, we need to turn to the field of cybernetics to best understand the complex ecosystem of online discourse to better grasp how "[i]nterlocked and interrelated systems all work in a sophisticated, ever-shifting, and changing network to correct for fluctuations and maintain a relative state of equilibrium" (Kien, 2019, p. 19).

For this chapter, however, we turn to an emerging methodology centered on conceiving digital memes not as stand-alone or simplistic semiotic units but as Baudrillardian simulacra: hyperreal representations that no longer represent reality but precede it. To understand digital memes as simulacra, we must consider the ways they are not just copied or imitated cultural ephemera but symbolic representations that point back to a referent that does not necessarily exist. It is the way memes claim reality, posing as a captured authentic emotive experience that speaks to a sense of reality the viewer finds meaningful to their own experience, that contributes to the liking or sharing of the meme onward.

Baudrillard's concept of simulacra picks up, in part, where Walter Benjamin left off in discussing the aura destroying powers of mechanically reproduced art and the ways mass replications untether artistic work from any sense of authentic origin (Benjamin, 1982). As Bill Nichols puts it, "Mechanical reproduction makes copies of visible objects, like paintings, mountain ranges, even human beings, which until then had been thought of as unique and irreplaceable. It brings the upheavals of the industrial revolution to a culmination" (Nichols, 1988, p. 24). The ever-expanding representational systems, spurred on by globalizing capital and telecommunications, leave Baudrillard to lament,

> It is no longer a question of imitation, nor duplication, nor even parody. It is a question of substituting the signs of the real for the real, that is to say of an operation of deterring every real process via its operational double, a programmatic, metastable, perfectly descriptive machine that offers all the signs of the real and short-circuits all its vicissitudes. (Baudrillard, 1994, p. 2)

Baudrillard here deploys the term "simulacra," or copy of a copy, to describe the ways spectacular images no longer reflect or denature a "profound reality," nor even necessarily hide the outright absence of a "real" reality, but are now wholly realized simulation that, like a repeatedly photocopied image, has lost any sort of fidelity with the original referent (Baudrillard, 1994, p. 6). Ibrahim sums up Baudrillard's crisis of representation, considering "simulation as castrated from territory, referentiality or substance produces the notion of the real without origin or reality. Simulacra as signs become transacted and interlocked with other elements instead of the real for Baudrillard" (Ibrahim, 2021, p. 19).

From this understanding of simulacrum, the analyst is not uncovering a sense of "true" reality but exploring the representational reality offered by the simulation. This reflects what Scott Durham refers to as the dystopian figure of the simulation, which "interprets repetition in terms of its distance from a founding identity" (Durham, 1998, p. 15). Durham explains,

> To the extent to which the concrete time and space of the consumer (with all his or her desires, memories, and narratives) are unassimilable or unregularizable within the framework of this dominant code, they appear, in cybernetic terms, as mere noise—as useless, irrecuperable, and inexpressible. This is Baudrillard's grim version of that now-familiar postmodern topos, "the death of the subject": the spectating subject appears as a mere monitor or terminal, as the screen on which all these codes and images intersect. (Durham, 1998, p. 21)

Here we, the viewer, are conceived as but vessels for the symbolic code, able only to consume and digest but not produce: cogs in the symbolic system as opposed to agentic creators.

Baudrillard's dystopic view of the simulacra is contrasted by another French postmodernist, Gilles Deleuze, who considers simulacra and the potential for resistance to dominant ideology. For Deleuze, the simulacra is not to be considered a hollow or empty copy of a copy, but rather "an image without resemblance" with the capacity to "reveal a truth beyond the apparent" (Deleuze, 1994, p. 106). This utopian construction of the simulacra does not worry about its *lack* of resemblance but considers how it may "appear as at once the mask and the creation of subversive powers of the false, which through their theatrical repetitions of 'names and images and legends', appropriate and transform them in their turn" (Durham, 1998, p. 9). As Ibrahim explains, this inversion of the simulacrum's trickery shifts from pejorative to possibility:

> In Deleuzian philosophy the simulacrum becomes renewed through its difference, acquires a purity and a means to examine its cultural signification and formulate new ideas through its intrinsic qualities, this being the central spine of the conceptualization, enabling one to look beyond the surface resemblance or identity. (Ibrahim, 2021, p. 18)

Through repetition, simulacra become untethered and "formless," open to new possibilities and meaning. For Ibrahim, this shift from concerning one's self with the lack of resemblance with the original, and the logics of capitalism and consumerism seen through Baudrillard, provides an opportunity to investigate memetic content to "reveal human vulnerabilities and affectivities" (Ibrahim, 2021, p. 19). For Deleuze, the analyst must focus not just on how the copy fails to capture the authenticity of the original but on the animating differences and repetitions that tap into deeper human desire and understanding.

While Durham sets up these two different definitions of the simulacra as opposites, one rooted in a dystopian fear and the other built on a utopian dream, he also believes that we should not consider the simulacra as one or the other: in fact, we must consider them both at once. For Durham, simulacrum's "true nature" is ultimately "inseparable from the potential for variation and displacement that haunts it, and from the effects that we—in appropriating and repeating it in our turn—are apt to draw from its repetitions in our lives and thought" (Durham, 1998, p. 15). It is for this reason I argue that digital memes, seen as hyperreal simulacrum, should be considered in two distinct but interconnected ways: first, as pure simulacra not referring to a sense of reality but preceding it, demanding the real to assimilate to the representation; and second, the differences between digital memes and reality, and that which is repeated, to reveal where the material world ends and the symbolic begins. Put another way, through cycles of repetition, what changes and what remains the same? Which ideas, notions, or perspectives are carried forward and which are left behind, deemed too different to remain part of this ideological cluster?

Finally, this chapter is firmly situated within the academic field of critical disability studies, seeking to destabilize biomedical dominance in discussions and interventions in the lives of disabled people. Within disability studies, hegemonic understanding of disability as rooted in bodily impairment, solidified by the birth of modern medicine and the expanding medical gaze (Foucault, 1975), are drawn into question by disability studies scholars seeking to explore and critique the binary opposition of dis/ability (Goodley, 2014) to think critically about how disabled people are imagined as subaltern to the nondisabled "normate" (Garland-Thomson, 1997, p. 8).

Memetic Catachresis: Tracking *I Can Count to Potato*'s Memetic Evolution

While some digital memes appear serendipitously, without any clear inciting moment, most digital memes are but new links in longer semiotic chains that exist well before the meme itself. In Shifman's terminology, these "founder-based" memes (Shifman, 2013, Chap. 5) gain their structure from the "seed" that sprouts memetic content through important intertextual relationships of difference and repetition. The source of a meme does not have control over the ways the meme will later be used, a point of particular importance when considering the *Potato* meme, but understanding the cultural milieu from which the meme emerges does help in understanding what makes a meme meaningful. The origin of a meme also provides some explanation of the underlying logics informing both the content and form of a digital meme cluster, contrary to some strands of simulacra theorizing that would argue the origin is meaningless. For the *Potato* meme, I propose three important seeds that inform its formation: (1) the vernacular use of the word "retarded," (2) the film *The Ringer*, and (3) the "Spread the Word to End the Word" campaign and its connection to the film *Tropic Thunder*.

The first important seed for the Potato meme is the pejorative use of the word "retarded." The term, henceforth referred to as the "r-word," like other terms before it used to describe cognitive limitation, has shifted out of the biomedical world to become an invective slang term to describe objects or people deemed to be silly, unfit, or otherwise bad (Siperstein et al., 2010, pp. 127–128). Similar to the derogatory use of the word "gay," as explored by Mary Louise Rasmussen (2004), the r-word became a useful catachresis or words "used as descriptors applied to existing terms in situations where a proper term does not exist" (Payne, 2010, p. 53). The term itself is thought to have become untethered from those with intellectual impairments, mirroring Judith Butler's apt description of catachresis as "the use of a proper name to describe that which does not properly belong to it" (cited in Rasmussen, 2004, p. 301). The linguistic function of this catachresis is simple: "When the r-word is used toward an individual or object, it is meant to express disapproval, and to transfer the negativity associated with individuals with ID onto this individual or object" (Albert et al., 2016, p. 391).

The use of the r-word in offline spaces has seamlessly transitioned into the online world as well. For example, in the early 2000s a variant of the digital axiom "Danth's Law," which quips about lack of value in arguing with people online (Amanda & shevyrolet, 2012), features a young man with Down syndrome running on a track with the text "Arguing on the internet is like running in the Special Olympics. Even if you win, you're still retarded" (Wolfdash94, 2010). Here the notion that the Special Olympics is not a serious form of athletic competition is tethered to the stigmatized identity of cognitive impairment, marking the accused as having failed to live up to the intellectual demands of ableism. It is from this catachresis usage of the r-word that the Potato meme will eventually sprout.

The second important seed for the Potato meme is the 2005 film *The Ringer*. In the comedy, Johnny Knoxville plays Steve Baker, a down-on-his-luck actor who attempts to rig the Special Olympics to resolve the consequences of a gambling debt (Blaustein, 2005). To do this, Baker simulates an intellectual disability, assuming the name "Jeffy," in order to cheat at and win the competition. In order to passably simulate his disability, Baker learns about intellectual impairment by reviewing a series of films, including *Rain Man*, *Forrest Gump*, *I Am Sam*, and "The Best of Chevy Chase," and practicing/imitating various lines from the films (Blaustein, 2005, 00:14:26). Baker proceeds to perfect his simulation by dressing up in mismatching clothing, wearing thick glasses that make his eyes bulge, and saying several lines including "My name is Arthel, and I can count to potato" (Blaustein, 2005, 00:15:30).

Within this scene, we see repetitions of representations—a fictional character performing a pantomime of intellectual disability based on popular representations of disability which are the mediated interpretations of intellectual disability as written and performed by other nondisabled writers and actors. Stripped away is the biological or medical presence of intellectual impairment and what remains is the simulacra of impairment: irregular or sloppy clothing, bulging eyes, and nonsensical speech, all used to denote a dysfunctional mind. While this scene is likely intended as satire, the symbols of intellectual impairment rang true for some viewers, leading to the phrase being lifted out of the context of the film and repeated in a digital meme designed to label others as similarly impaired.

I argue, though, that the third and perhaps most important seed for the Potato meme, the impetus for the shifting of the symbolic weight of the r-word to become re-embodied within the term "potato" is the forming and (arguable) success of the "Spread the Word to End the Word" campaign orchestrated by the Special Olympics in the United States. Three years after the release of *The Ringer*, another film would cause ripples in its usage of the r-word and spawn yet another popular Internet meme: Ben Stiller's *Tropic Thunder* (Stiller, 2008). While the Special Olympics endorsed *The Ringer*, despite its flagrant use of the r-word (Elder, 2005), the organization would call for national protests against *Tropic Thunder* because of the offensive "Simple Jack" character and the excessive use of the r-word in a tirade by character Kirk Lazarus (Special Olympics, 2008). As head of Special Olympics Timothy Shriver stated at the time,

The degrading use of the word "retard" together with the broader humiliation of people with intellectual disabilities in the film goes way too far. When the R-word is bandied about and when bumbling, clueless caricatures designed to mimic the behavior of people with intellectual disabilities are on screen, they have an unmistakable outcome: they mock, directly or indirectly, people with intellectual disabilities. (Shriver, 2008)

While the infamous "full retard" scene is an attempt to satirize and critique the glorifying of these very caricatures Shriver mentions, with the thrust of the monologue being that Hollywood will not reward genuine representation of cognitive impairment but only super crip representations, Shriver was quite right about the potential danger.

Shortly after the film was released, a screenshot featuring the Lazarus character with the text "Never go full retard" began circulating online, used as Shifman's discursive weapon (Gilson & andcallmeshirley, 2011). Once again, a representation of cognitive impairment referring to other representations of cognitive impairment is removed from its original context and used to articulate deeply held beliefs about intellectual and developmental disabilities. Following the momentum of the *Tropic Thunder* protests, and in response to calls from youth advocates, the first annual "Spread the Word to End The Word" campaign was launched in March 2009 (Wee, 2015, p. 185). Building off the original "Stop the R-Word" campaign launched in 2004, the campaign aimed to "combat the inappropriate use of the R-word in common usage" (cited in Wee, 2015, p. 185).

Continuing over a decade later, I argue the "Spread the Word" campaign serves an important role in the seeding and expansion of the Potato meme in part because of its success—as the r-word became increasingly stigmatized, Potato became a convenient catachresis that retains all the same linguistic functions of the r-word without explicitly using the offending term and risking ostracization. As it turns out, one of the earliest Potato meme images featuring a man with Down syndrome emerges on *The Chive* mere days before the official launch of the "Spread the Word" campaign in 2009 (M5000 & Y F, 2011).

I Can Count to Potato: A Memetic Analysis

The precise origin story of the Potato meme is difficult to determine, a central challenge when investigating memes (Kien, 2019, Introduction). For the Potato memetic cluster, it is also difficult to discern author intent: are these genuine beliefs or intentionally offensive? There is some indication that the Potato meme was a part of an elaborate prank orchestrated by social media site 4chan to target rival Internet community 9gag by posing as members and being as offensive as possible (Venom123, 2012). Conversely, as Angela Nagle explores in *Kill All Normies*, this could be yet another example of the de Sadian "culture of transgression" popular on chan sites and, more recently, within the Alt-Right (Nagle, 2017, pp. 38–39). The question for this chapter, however, is not *why* these specific memes were created, but what are the discursive and symbolic elements animating individual and clusters of Potato memes?

Following the methodology outlined by Shifman (2013), the Potato meme can be broken down into three main sites of inquiry: the meme's form, content, and stance. Like other image macros, the form of the Potato meme predominantly affixes the line from *The Ringer*, either in full or simplified to just "potato" to various images to denote the individual featured as being silly, foolish, or stupid. There appear two dominant constellations of Potato memes that, like celestial bodies, are meaningful both individually and in the bigger picture composed by their interrelationship. The first cluster of memes focuses on people or objects thought to be bad, inappropriate, or dumb. While this is typically presented as an image macro, the phrase itself has also been used to ridicule low or bad quality photography or video online as well (biffcollins, 2015). The second cluster, as we will see in the Crowter example, is animated by images of people with facial features or differences that imply disability, including but not limited to Down syndrome.

An early example of the meme being used to criticize nondisabled people is based on a photo of Heidi Montag (*Image—128477*, 2011), a much maligned reality television star (Shrayber, 2019). In this image, Montag is shown strutting on the beach in a bikini with mouth agape. This image connects with one of the primary uses of the phrase—ridiculing celebrities, athletes, or politicians. Celebrities like Charlie Sheen, with eyes edited to be looking in different directions, can count to potato (k.johnson10, 2016). So can hockey player, Dustin Brown, smiling happily while struggling to drink from a water bottle (Image—*251362*, 2012). Barack Obama, with eyes askew and mouth agape, is thought to struggle with understanding the national debt because of his potato-based numeracy (Image—*254453*, 2012). Former Toronto mayor Rob Ford is said to be unable to count to potato because he can only count to crack (Trippity, 2013), a reference to the viral extortion video of Ford smoking the narcotic (Raw video, 2016).

Another cluster of Potato memes is directly connected to disability itself, featuring various images of people with facial differences, especially those associated with Down syndrome. Whereas the first cluster discussed deploys Potato in a comparable way to the colloquial and ambiguous use of the r-word, this cluster directly tethers nonsensical speech to disabled people. An early example, posted to the website *The Chive*, has been photoshopped into a demotivational poster of a young man with Down syndrome holding a piece of paper with the quote, adding "because counting to turnip would be silly" (Image—*128748*, 2011). Another example sits at the intersection of racism and ableism, depicting an Asian man with Down syndrome in tuxedo, directing an opera with the text "and-a one, and-a four, and a ching chong potato" (Image—*128745*, 2011). Some images break from Down syndrome specifically, using people with facial deformity (And I Can Count to Potato, n.d.) or animals (I Can Count To Potato, n.d.). Finally, and perhaps most important to this chapter, is the image of a young Heidi Crowter, photoshopped in front of a colorful pinwheel background, featuring a variety of phrases including "I can count to potato" (Image—*128749*, 2011). Here the meme is used to insert discontiguous responses to preparatory questions or assertions (Favorite Color of the Alphabet, n.d.), deploy puns using reference to the word down(s) or the r-word (Syndrome of a Down, n.d.), or make jokes refer to stereotypical behavior of people with intellectual and developmental disabilities (We Ride the Same Bus, n.d.). All of these memes develop a cohesive, if not extreme, picture of the cognitively impaired subject: silly or nonsensical people tethered to institutional regimes and disconnected from the rational world, fully imbued with disability to the point of being able to only speak or see through the diagnosis.

But within these webs of simulation and repetition there is little connection to the original referent. In most of these memes we see critique of *human* activities or behaviors informed by the simulacra of cognitive impairment, not to the lived experiences or realities of those with medical diagnosis. Heidi Crowter's attempt to reclaim her image is so important because it helps reveal the ways the meme built upon her appearance is just that: an appearance. Within the Potato meme, we do not see any sort of truth or reality of intellectual disability, but as Baudrillard predicted in the 1980s, Crowter's symbolic Down syndrome would precede the reality of her disability.

WHEN MEMES TALK BACK: THE CROWTER CASE STUDY

In 2012, several years after the initial flurry of Potato memes, something rather miraculous happened—a meme began speaking back. The young woman, now teenager, whose childhood image was used in the Potato image macro did not want her image being used to make ableist jokes. In speaking to the press, we learned that Heidi Crowter's childhood image had been lifted from a Facebook support group for parents created by her mother Liz years earlier ("Web Trolls," 2012). Additional reporting indicates the photo may not have been taken from Facebook but, instead, was copied from Liz & Steve Crowter's autobiography *Surprise Package* (Zimmerman, 2012). In an interview with the BBC, we learned that Heidi was distraught to hear her image had been used to make offensive jokes on the Internet, with content that ran contrary to her own sense of self. In the segment, Heidi's sister comments that the Internet trolls creating these memes think Heidi is "stupid or something" whereas she believes Heidi to be quite intelligent, to which Heidi confidently replies "Aww I know" (Anonymax, 2012, 2:45).

While news stories on Heidi becoming a meme are focused on the family's fight to reclaim the image, stop the reproduction of the meme, and protect others from having their photos stolen, more interesting to this chapter is how Heidi's representation of self so dramatically differs from that of the memetic generation. Heidi and her sister in the BBC interview are not wrong—Heidi *has* lived a productive and interesting life outside the discourses of ineptitude that animate the memetic cluster. Heidi has graduated from school, worked in a hair salon, cheered on the local football team, and gotten married (Woods,

2021). She has also become politically active, advocating against cuts to employment services for people with disabilities (Clarke, 2015) and campaigning in the United Kingdom and abroad, speaking eloquently against genetic screening and disability-selective abortion (Woman Alive, 2020). Throughout her work and life, Crowter appears aligned with a social model of disability perspective, reflecting on the ways the external world has disabled her, whether it is the attitudes of people on and off the Internet or the programs and services that fail to enable quality lives for people with Down syndrome.

Despite Deleuze's hope for the simulacra to untether from past representation to reveal unspoken truths, the memetic construction of intellectual and developmental disability appears more as repetition of past representation than difference. Considering the content and stance of Potato memes in juxtaposition to the lived reality of Heidi Crowter, several key features become readily apparent. The meme itself relies upon the belief that people with intellectual disabilities are unable to comprehend numeracy or mathematics with humor being generated by the substitution of "potato" for a number. Here the simulacra of cognitive impairment acts as narrative prosthesis for those who have acted in a foolish or silly manner. As first identified by David Mitchell and Sharon Snyder, narrative prosthesis is a term used to describe the ways in which disability is used in representational forms like a crutch to assist in characterization of characters (Mitchell & Snyder, 2001, p. 63). In the case of the potato meme, intellectual disability is prostheticized to make manifest these inadequate or inappropriate choices or behaviors. Poor decisions, temporary or isolated, are presented as dangerously close to the spoiled identity of cognitive impairment. Conversely, behaving poorly or making bad choices is conceived as a natural outcome of intellectual disability. So too do socially annoying behaviors become collapsed into medical deficiency, connecting intellectual impairment with social ineptitude.

Numeracy then becomes an important part of the Potato story, representing those who can count to potato not just as children who cannot count large numbers but someone with a complete misunderstanding of numbers in general. Numeracy here is tethered with the concept of cognitive ability while at the same time implying that this ability is simple or taken for granted, designating anyone who is *un*able to perform these tasks as worthy of ridicule. The meme also naturalizes intellectual pursuit under the auspices of formalized education, using skills typically developed in grade school as being indicative of (adequate) intelligence in general. Underlying this ideology is what Robert McRuer has dubbed "compulsory able-bodiedness," or the ways that the deficiency of disabled bodies and minds is simply taken for granted—we should all desire a return to "normal" ability (McRuer, 2006, p. 8). In the assertion that those with intellectual or developmental impairments are substandard or deficient, we normalize certain kinds of intelligence while valorizing function above the standard—being "smart" becomes tethered to success and happiness while being "dumb" is deterministically imagined to result in failure and sadness.

The inability to count is not the only way cognitive inability is materialized, as the simulacra of cognitive impairment similarly looks to physical actions and appearance as symbolic of intellectual inadequacy. Of particular interest is the focus on the eyes, photoshopped or naturally appearing bulging, crossed or otherwise out of alignment. The focus on unruly eyes to represent dysfunctional minds becomes clearer, though, when considered through the work of Lennard Davis who discusses how philosophy and literature rely upon metaphors of sight and hearing as emblematic of intelligence or insight (Davis, 1995, p. 103). For the Potato meme, we find yet more repetition of representational copies of copies that rhetorically ask, "If one cannot see or hear, how could they possibly *know*?" just as *The Ringer* deployed thick-rimmed glasses to simulate the appearance of intellectual impairment.

Whether an example of the Streisand Effect (Masnick, 2005), an elaborate prank orchestrated by 4chan to get revenge on 9gag (etan_causale, 2012; kunoburesu, 2012), or an example of Nissenbaum and Shifman's "discursive weapon" used "to justify judgment, condemnation, and exclusion of others" (Nissenbaum & Shifman, 2017, p. 495), the potato meme shifts slightly after the Crowter family went public, leading to a new wave of memes that ridicule the complaint itself, mock the seeming impotence of Liz Crowter to stop the "trolls" and reaffirm Heidi Crowter as a "potato," now with an added layer of sexism. Regardless of the intention, either to make jokes about Down syndrome or to be as offensive as possible to drive animosity, the created memes continue to reveal a specific discursive imagination of intellectual and developmental disabilities rooted not in lived experience but the preceding simulacra of cognitive impairment.

In some ways, the new wave of memetic discourse complies with earlier incarnations of the Potato meme, centered on injecting the word incorrectly into sentences to denote stupidity or dysfunction (Show and Tell Tomorrow?, n.d.). Crowter is again marked as a body of dysfunction, with one meme remixing the Limes Guy meme (scwizard & Sophie, 2010) to joke about her inability to carry potatoes (WHY CANT I HOLD ALL THESE POTATOES, n.d.). Some new memes acknowledge that Crowter has gotten older and is perhaps wiser, scoffing that now she can surely count to firetruck (Count to Potato Now *16*, n.d.). Other meme creators opine that we should not be surprised Crowter is upset about the memes because "taters gonna tate" (Taters Gonna Tate, n.d.). At the end of the day, another meme jokes, all of these Potato memes have got Crowter feeling "downs" (Potato Girl—Quickmeme, n.d.). Throughout these memes, Crowter is seen not as a person but as a vehicle to repeat the original meme, unable to transcend the boundaries of the simulacrum.

Central to the memetic generation is the notion that the Crowter's complaint itself is foolish and ignorant of how the Internet functions. The Crowters are labeled as being "butt hurt" (U Mad Bro?, n.d.) or having their "jimmies" rustled (YOU RUSTLED MY DAUGHTERS JIMMIES, n.d.), a common memetic phrase denoting those upset by the actions of trolls (Chris & andcallmeshirley, 2012). Another meme critiqued the Crowters' focus on getting groups removed from Facebook, suggesting they will sue Facebook for "potato dollars" (I Sued Facebook, 2017). Liz Crowter, Heidi's mom, becomes a particular focus of the meme, whether it is questioning why it took two years before she started to care about the original meme (Been a Meme since *2010*, n.d.). There is also an indication that Liz may have ulterior motives, with one meme questioning why she would go to the press if her intention was to minimize the ridicule her daughter was facing (Daughter's Wellbeing, 2019). The new focus on Liz may suggest a belief that Heidi is not an agentic actor in the plea, but rather is just a tool being used by her mother.

One significant difference from the original Potato meme comes with the injection of gender to the memetic discourse. While the original Potato meme featuring Crowter was focused almost exclusively on cognitive ability and function, the response to Crowter's request began openly addressing her presence as a teenage woman. One meme states Crowter's "bitching" on national television provoked this response (Redmon Bray, 2012). Using a screenshot from Katy Perry's girl power anthem *Roar* (Hall & Kudsi, 2013), the empowering chorus lyric which proclaims we will all hear Perry roar is subverted, denied to Crowter, who we will only hear say "#potato" (Kalle69, 2013). Crowter's appearance and style are also targeted, deploying the famous Maybelline make-up company slogan (Maybe She's Born with It, n.d.). While Maybelline models may be born with natural beauty, Crowter's deficient appearance is a direct result of being born "potato." And just as women who experienced disproportionate threats of violence during #GamerGate (Mortensen, 2018; Salter, 2018), one meme ominously states: "I hope you can count to 9-1-1" (You Can Count to Potato?, n.d.).

Comparing the original deployment of the "I can count to potato" meme with the response to Crowter's request, there are both important differences and similarities. The word "potato" is perhaps even more directly deployed as catachresis for Down syndrome, a vernacular similarly evoking the symbolic weight of intellectual disability as an invalid or bad subjectivity. Crowter does not just have a disability but becomes completely subsumed under its logic—she does not *have* Down syndrome, she is nothing *but* Down syndrome. As the disability becomes fully universalized, Crowter is then seen as having nothing useful to say: both Heidi and her complaints are potato. Or worse, Crowter may be speaking but those words become neutralized through the filter of simulacra. Femininity, and proximity to feminine things, is then deployed to add further validation to the core message of these memes—the Crowters are emotionally overreacting. The memes suggest there is no reason to be upset about a silly meme online. Those who feel otherwise are then pathologized as having some form of cognitive impairment as well, as any rational and intelligent (male) individual would get the joke. Liz and Heidi Crowter's status as woman, and Heidi's identity as a disabled woman specifically, only further prove that their feelings on the matter are excessive, misplaced, or otherwise dismissible.

Concluding Thoughts

Internet user "Mr_Brett" famously shared an animated gif of a cat featuring the text "The Internet is Serious Business" (Tomberry & Don., 2009). Sarcastic in nature, this catchphrase reflects an all-too-common perspective—cyberspace is not inherently *real* and, as such, we should not take the happenings online too seriously. Years later it is difficult to distinguish where the "real world" ends and the cyber space begins. Both spaces are, of course, intertwined because they are mere manifestations of the broader cultural production of the people who occupy both spaces. What happens online is informed by the offline world just as the activities of online users can have very real impacts on the offline world. Heidi Crowter is but one exemplar of this reality—a real person drawn into the memetic refractory, reinscribed with meaning far beyond her context and near powerless to reclaim the image she calls self. While utopian imaginations of the simulacra dreamt of a liberation of symbolic meaning from culture industries, the Crowter example reveals a repetition of representation past. Considering the memetic construction of intellectual and developmental disability, in general, and Down syndrome, specifically, we find not a wholly disconnected symbolic system but rather the rhizomatic repetition of past stereotypes, tropes, and mediations of intellectual and developmental disability from elsewhere in popular culture. What we are left with is a simulacra of cognitive impairment, a hyperreality that does not just precede but supersedes all. Thankfully Crowter herself lives far beyond the simulacra of cognitive impairment, defying it, even if her own story is unable to disrupt the dominant imagination of cognitive impairment. Having said that, Crowter's sin was perhaps not that she spoke out against the use of her image in the creation of memes but that her life, her actual existence, is only seen as a faulty copy of the true hyperreality. The only way she could become meaningful again in this symbolic system, then, was to be silenced through resignification—she had to be brought into realignment with the hyperreality that preceded her, subjugated through a new wave of memetic generation.

To begin the chapter, we considered definitions and methods of exploring digital memes, thinking of them not as frivolous cultural ephemera but reflective of deeper discourses of power and identity manifested through the remixing and remaking of images, text, video, and audio and spread through social media platforms online. I argue that digital memes, above all, should be considered through the lens of Baudrillard's simulacra, copies of copies so far down the semiotic chain that they no longer have any significant connection to that which they claim to signify. Instead, they are of their own hyperreality, images and icons that precede material reality and become a reality in and of itself. To watch this simulacra in action we turned to one specific memetic cluster, the "I can count to potato" meme, to consider how through repetition and difference we have come to hold a purely symbolic understanding of intellectual disability, converting lived experience and diagnosis into useful discursive catachresis, unleashing the destructive power of stigma upon whatever person or object to which it becomes affixed. In deploying intellectual and developmental disability in this way we do not just disparage that which it describes but further validate the binary opposition of ability and its subaltern, *dis*ability. We are led to believe that being labeled as disabled is a bad thing because, of course, it is not good to be "disabled"—those who cannot hear or see or speak cannot think and that which cannot think is not a person at all. At the same time, we acknowledge the potential for disability to contaminate—it is not a label we are safe from incurring and therefore must be vigilant to avoid falling to its logics through injury, illness, or reproduction. Proximity to intellectual disability then risks a total collapse of the subject, to become erased and seen more as object, a potato, than an agentic human being. This is the cold eugenic underbelly of discourse passed off as simple joke or jest.

In this way, the story of Heidi Crowter began long before her and her family's intervention. The Crowters were merely entering into a deeper discursive debate around the appropriateness of disability metaphor, or the use of the symbolic stigma of disability to criticize, satirize, or dismiss others. I argue the appearance of the potato meme stands as evidence of the success of the Special Olympics campaign to eliminate the r-word, with memetic creators agreeing to leave behind the offensive signifier while at the same time refusing to give up the ever important signified. Rather than using the r-word, users have simply transferred the symbolic weight to a new signifier: the term "potato." Driven by the line from *The Ringer*, potato becomes the perfect mediation of all that is wrong with dysfunctional minds. For the past decade, as the "Spread the Word to End the Word" campaign has expanded, so too has the usage of "potato" to mean the same thing, indicating that we may change the term but, in this case, that has done little to deactivate the symbolic stigma attached to the medical diagnosis.

References

Albert, A. B., Jacobs, H. E., & Siperstein, G. N. (2016). Sticks, stones, and stigma: Student bystander behavior in response to hearing the word "retard." *Intellectual and Developmental Disabilities, 54*(6), 391–401. https://doi.org/10.1352/1934-9556-54.6.391

Amanda, B., & Shevyrolet. (2012, June 13). *Danth's law.* Know Your Meme. Retrieved April 4, 2021, from https://knowyourmeme.com/memes/danths-law

And I can count to potato. (n.d.). Meme Maker. Retrieved May 30, 2021, from https://www.mememaker.net/meme/and-i-can-count-to-potato/

Anonymax. (2012, April 13). *Heidi Crowter ("I can count to potato" girl)—Midlands Today 12/04/12 (Internet Trollers).* Retrieved April 4, 2021, from https://www.youtube.com/watch?v=BYowYqNOjUQ

Baudrillard, J. (1994). *Simulacra and simulation* (S. F. Glaser, Trans.). University of Michigan Press.

Been a meme since 2010. (n.d.). Retrieved June 1, 2021, from http://memegenerator.net/instance/19515463/i-can-count-to-potato-been-a-meme-since-2010-mom-gives-a-shit-in-2012

Benjamin, W. (1982). The work of art in the age of mechanical reproduction. In *Modern art and modernism: A critical anthology* (1st ed., pp. 217–220). Harper & Row.

biffcollins. (2015, December 31). *Where did the term "potato quality" come from?* [Social media]. Reddit. Retrieved June 1, 2021, from https://www.reddit.com/r/OutOfTheLoop/comments/3yzgku/where_did_the_term_potato_quality_come_from/

Blaustein, B. W. (2005). *The Ringer* [Comedy; DVD]. 20th Century Fox Home Entertainment.

Chris, & and callmeshirley. (2012, February 13). *That really rustled my jimmies.* Know Your Meme. Retrieved June 1, 2021, from https://knowyourmeme.com/memes/that-really-rustled-my-jimmies

Clarke, L. (2015, August 27). Disabled Coventry woman thanks threatened employment support service for first job. *Coventry Observer.* Retrieved June 1, 2021, from https://coventryobserver.co.uk/news/disabled-coventry-woman-thanks-threatened-employment-support-service-for-first-job-9308/

Count to potato now 16. (n.d.). Me.Me. Retrieved June 1, 2021, from https://me.me/i/count-to-potato-now-16-girl-can-count-to-firetruck

Daughter's wellbeing. (2019, May 10). esmemes.com. Retrieved June 4, 2021, from https://esmemes.com/i/isconcerned-for-her-daughters-wellbeing-draws-attention-to-her-on

Davis, L. J. (1995). *Enforcing normalcy: Disability, deafness and the body.* Verso.

Dawkins, R. (1989). *The selfish gene* (2nd ed.). Oxford Paperbacks.

Deleuze, G. (1994). *Difference and repetition (P. Patton, Trans.).* Columbia University Press.

Durham, S. (1998). *Phantom communities: The simulacrum and the limits of postmodernism.* Stanford University Press.

Elder, R. K. (2005, December 23). *'Ringer' endorsements don't patch its problems* [Newspaper]. *The Chicago Tribune.* Retrieved June 4, 2021, from https://www.chicagotribune.com/news/ct-xpm-2005-12-23-0512230148-story.html

etan_causale. (2012, May 30). *When 4Chan attacks 9GAG* [Reddit Comment]. R/Funny. Retrieved June 4, 2021, from www.reddit.com/r/funny/comments/ucbx6/when_4chan_attacks_9gag/c4u8ugt/

Favorite color of the alphabet. (n.d.). Memegenerator.Net. Retrieved June 4, 2021, from https://memegenerator.net/instance/25179076/i-can-count-to-potato-potato-is-my-favorite-color-of-the-alphabet

Foucault, M. (1975). *The birth of the clinic: An archaeology of medical perception.* (A. Sheridan Smith, Trans.). Vintage Books. (Original work published in 1973).

Gal, N., Shifman, L., & Kampf, Z. (2016). "It gets better": Internet memes and the construction of collective identity. *New Media & Society, 18*(8), 1698–1714. https://doi.org/10.1177/1461444814568784

Garland-Thomson, R. (1997). *Extraordinary bodies: Figuring physical disability in American culture and literature.* Columbia University Press.

Gilson, C., & andcallmeshirley. (2011, May 9). *Full retard.* Know Your Meme. Retrieved June 4, 2021, from https://knowyourmeme.com/memes/full-retard

Goodley, D. (2014). *Dis/ability studies: Theorising disablism and ableism.* Routledge.

Hall, G., & Kudsi, M. (2013, September 5). *Roar* [YouTube]. Retrieved June 4, 2021, from https://www.youtube.com/watch?v=CevxZvSJLk8

I can count to potato. (n.d.). Funny Captions. Retrieved May 30, 2021, from http://www.funnycaptions.com/img/110633/i-can-count-to-potato/

270   J. PRESTON

I sued facebook. (2017). Meme Generator. Retrieved May 30, 2021, from http://memegenerator.net/instance/19446224/i-can-count-to-potato-i-sued-facebook-for-potato-dollars

Ibrahim, Y. (2021). *Digital icons: Memes, martyrs and avatars.* Routledge.

Image—128745. (2011, May 31). Know Your Meme. Retrieved May 30, 2021, from https://knowyourmeme.com/photos/128745-i-can-count-to-potato

Image—128748. (2011, May 31). Know Your Meme. Retrieved May 30, 2021, from https://knowyourmeme.com/photos/128748-i-can-count-to-potato

Image—128749. (2011, May 31). Know Your Meme. Retrieved May 30, 2021, from https://knowyourmeme.com/photos/128749-i-can-count-to-potato

Image—251362. (2012, February 15). Know Your Meme. Retrieved May 30, 2021, from https://knowyourmeme.com/photos/251362-i-can-count-to-potato

Image—254453. (2012, February 19). Know Your Meme. Retrieved May 30, 2021, from https://knowyourmeme.com/photos/254453-i-can-count-to-potato

k.johnson10. (2016). *Charlie Sheen DERP.* Imgflip. Retrieved May 30, 2021, from https://i.imgflip.com/11dvyf.jpg

Kalle69. (2013, October 21). *#Potato.* Know Your Meme. Retrieved May 30, 2021, from https://knowyourmeme.com/photos/627395-i-can-count-to-potato

Kien, G. (2019). *Communicating with memes: Consequences in post-truth civilization.* Lexington Books.

Knobel, M., & Lankshear, C. (2007). Online memes, affinities, and cultural production. In M. Knobel & C. Lankshear (Eds.), *A new literacies sampler* (pp. 199–227). Peter Lang.

kunoburesu. (2012, April 25). *4chan is putting all the blame on 9gag* [Social media]. Reddit. Retrieved May 30, 2021, from https://www.reddit.com/r/AdviceAnimals/comments/ssn0w/guess_who_just_found_out_she_was_a_meme/c4gpf9w/?utm_source=reddit&utm_medium=web2x&context=3

M5000, & Y F. (2011, May 31). *I can count to potato.* Know Your Meme. Retrieved May 30, 2021, from https://knowyourmeme.com/memes/i-can-count-to-potato

Masnick, M. (2005, January 5). *Since when is it illegal to just mention a trademark online?* Techdirt. Retrieved May 30, 2021, from https://www.techdirt.com/articles/20050105/0132239.shtml

Maybe she's born with it. (n.d.). Quickmeme. Retrieved June 1, 2021, from http://www.quickmeme.com/meme/3qrcpc

McRuer, R. (2006). *Crip theory: Cultural signs of queerness and disability.* New York University Press.

Milner, R. M. (2012). *The world made meme: Discourse and identity in participatory media* [Dissertation]. University of Kansas.

Milner, R. M. (2016). *The world made meme: Public conversations and participatory media.* The MIT Press.

Mitchell, D. T., & Snyder, S. L. (2001). *Narrative prosthesis: Disability and the dependencies of discourse.* University of Michigan Press.

Mortensen, T. E. (2018). Anger, fear, and games: The long event of #GamerGate. *Games and Culture, 13*(8), 787–806. https://doi.org/10.1177/1555412016640408

Nagle, A. (2017). *Kill all normies: The online culture wars from Tumblr and 4chan to the alt-right and Trump.* Zero Books.

Nichols, B. (1988). The work of culture in the age of cybernetic systems. *Screen (London), 29*(1), 22–47. https://doi.org/10.1093/screen/29.1.22

Nissenbaum, A., & Shifman, L. (2017). Internet memes as contested cultural capital: The case of 4chan's /b/ board. *New Media & Society, 19*(4), 483–501. https://doi.org/10.1177/1461444815609313

Payne, B. M. (2010). Your art is gay and retarded: Eliminating discriminating speech against homosexual and intellectually disabled students in the secondary arts education classroom. *Art Education, 63*(5), 52–55. https://doi.org/10.1080/00043125.2010.11519088

Potato girl—Quickmeme. (n.d.). Me.Me. Retrieved June 1, 2021, from https://me.me/i/all-these-memes-ace-got-me-feeling-downs-quickmeme-com-all

Rasmussen, M. L. (2004). "That's so gay!": A study of the deployment of signifiers of sexual and gender identity in secondary school settings in Australia and the United States. *Social Semiotics, 14*(3), 289–308. https://doi.org/10.1080/10350330408629681

Raw video released of Rob Ford smoking crack. (2016, August 11). The Globe and Mail. Retrieved May 30, 2021, from https://www.theglobeandmail.com/canada/toronto/video-video-raw-video-released-of-rob-ford-smoking-crack/

Redmon Bray. (2012, April 25). *Round 2.* Know Your Meme. Retrieved May 30, 2021, from https://knowyourmeme.com/photos/291683-i-can-count-to-potato

Salter, M. (2018). From geek masculinity to gamergate: The technological rationality of online abuse. *Crime, Media, Culture, 14*(2), 247–264. https://doi.org/10.1177/1741659017690893

scwizard, & Sophie. (2010, September 27). *Limes guy / Why can't I hold all these limes?* Know Your Meme. Retrieved May 30, 2021, from https://knowyourmeme.com/memes/limes-guy-why-cant-i-hold-all-these-limes

Segev, E., Nissenbaum, A., Stolero, N., & Shifman, L. (2015). Families and networks of Internet memes: The relationship between cohesiveness, uniqueness, and quiddity concreteness. *Journal of Computer-Mediated Communication, 20*(4), 417–433. https://doi.org/10.1111/jcc4.12120

Shifman, L. (2013). *Memes in digital culture.* The MIT Press.

Show and tell tomorrow? Potato. (n.d.). Quickmeme. Retrieved June 1, 2021, from http://www.quickmeme.com/meme/3p931v

Shrayber, M. (2019, July 9). *Exclusive: Spencer Pratt opened up about Heidi Montag's plastic surgery and it's actually heartbreaking.* Cosmopolitan. Retrieved June 1, 2021, from https://www.cosmopolitan.com/entertainment/tv/a28339096/the-hills-new-beginnings-episode-2-recap-spencer-pratt-heidi-plastic-surgery/

Shriver, T. (2008, August 12). *Special Olympics chairman Timothy Shriver's remarks at "Tropic Thunder" protest.* Special Olympics. Retrieved June 4, 2021, from http://www.specialolympics.org/Special+Olympics+Public+Website/English/Press_Room/Global_news/Tropic+Thunder/Shriver+Protest+Remarks.htm

Siperstein, G. N., Pociask, S. E., & Collins, M. A. (2010). Sticks, stones, and stigma: A Study of students' use of the derogatory term retard. *Intellectual and Developmental Disabilities, 48*(2), 126–134. https://doi.org/10.1352/1934-9556-48.2.126

Special Olympics. (2008, August 14). *Special Olympics and coalition of disability organizations protest DreamWorks' "Tropic Thunder."* Special Olympics. Retrieved February 10, 2022, from https://www.specialolympics.org/Special+Olympics+Public+Website/English/Press_Room/Global_news/R-Word-Tropic+Thunder.htm

Stiller, B. (2008, August 13). *Tropic thunder.* . Retrieved June 4, 2021, from https://www.imdb.com/title/tt0942385/

Syndrome of a down. (n.d.). Memegenerator.Net. Retrieved June 4, 2021, from https://memegenerator.net/instance/25176266/i-can-count-to-potato-my-favorite-band-is-syndrome-of-a-down

Taters gonna tate. (n.d.). Quickmeme. Retrieved June 1, 2021, from http://www.quickmeme.com/meme/3p11lv

Tomberry, & Don. (2009, August 19). *The Internet is serious business.* Know Your Meme. Retrieved June 1, 2021, from https://knowyourmeme.com/memes/the-internet-is-serious-business

Trippity, F. (2013, December 15). Toronto mayor Rob Ford can't count to potato. *Funny Meme-Mories.* Retrieved June 1, 2021, from http://funnymeme-mories.blogspot.com/2013/12/toronto-mayor-rob-ford-cant-count-to.html

U mad bro? (n.d.). Quickmeme. Retrieved June 1, 2021, from http://www.quickmeme.com/meme/3qcfzx

Venom123. (2012, April 25). *"I can count to potato" girl finally realizes she's a meme!— Off-Topic.* Comic Vine. Retrieved June 1, 2021, from https://comicvine.gamespot.com/forums/off-topic-5/i-can-count-to-potato-girl-finally-realizes-shes-a-664306/

We ride the same bus. (n.d.). Memegenerator.Net. Retrieved June 4, 2021, from https://memegenerator.net/instance/25176748/i-can-count-to-potato-hey-i-know-you-we-ride-the-same-bus

Web trolls: Mum's horror over abuse of down's syndrome daughter. (2012, April 12). *BBC News.* Retrieved June 4, 2021, from. https://www.bbc.com/news/uk-england-coventry-warwickshire-17676553

Wee, L. (2015). Mobilizing affect in the linguistic cyberlandscape: The R-word campaign. In R. Rubdy & S. Ben Said (Eds.), *Conflict, exclusion and dissent in the linguistic landscape* (pp. 185–203). Palgrave Macmillan UK. https://doi.org/10.1057/9781137426284

WHY CANT I HOLD ALL THESE POTATOES. (n.d.). Me.Me. Retrieved June 1, 2021, from https://me.me/i/why-cant-i-hold-all-these-potatoes-none

Wiggins, B. E., & Bowers, G. B. (2015). Memes as genre: A structurational analysis of the memescape. *New Media & Society, 17*(11), 1886–1906. https://doi.org/10.1177/1461444814535194

Wolfdash94. (2010). *Arguing on the internet is like running in the Special Olympics* [Photo]. https://www.flickr.com/photos/57149147@N08/5264741674/

Woman Alive. (2020, December 15). There's more to me than just having down's syndrome. *Woman Alive.* https://www.womanalive.co.uk/stories/view?articleid=3335

Woods, R. (2021, May 16). Down's syndrome campaigner Heidi Crowter on marriage and loving life. *BBC News.* https://www.bbc.com/news/uk-england-coventry-warwickshire-57089602

You can count to potato? (n.d.). Quickmeme. Retrieved June 1, 2021, from http://www.quickmeme.com/meme/3ozguz

YOU RUSTLED MY DAUGHTERS JIMMIES. (n.d.). Me.Me. Retrieved June 1, 2021, from https://me.me/i/yourustled-mydaughters-jimmies-o-myonerator-ne-none

Zimmerman, N. (2012, April 26). *Girl with down's is unwitting subject of mean internet meme.* Gawker. http://gawker.com/5905373/girl-with-downs-is-unwitting-subject-of-mean-internet-meme

CHAPTER 17

#DisabilityTikTok

Jordan Foster and David Pettinicchio

"Hello beautiful people of the internet," says Lacey Richcreek to her 80.3 thousand (and counting) followers on TikTok—a web-based and mobile social media application. "Today is March 1st which is the start of cerebral palsy awareness month." Lacey continues by sharing her own experience as one of the over 17 million people with cerebral palsy (CP) around the globe (World CP Day, 2020). She is not alone. Like other young people on TikTok, Lacey creates videos about disability, sharing information and personal life stories alongside hashtags like #disabled, #disability, and #disabilitytiktok. To date, these hashtags have generated more than 1 billion views, with everyday users tuning in to share their stories, learning more online about disability than they would otherwise.

Introduced in the fall of 2017, TikTok is among the fastest growing and most widely used social media applications, with some 800 million monthly visits (Abidin, 2020; Kennedy, 2020). Like other forms of social media, including Instagram and Snapchat, TikTok is a highly visual medium, centering the user's appearance in short video clips and digital assemblages. These videos range in length from 15 seconds to 3 minutes and can be set against music, sound effects, or other audio clips (Zulli & Zulli, 2020). While videos on TikTok tend to be less edited than their counterparts on Instagram (Leaver et al., 2020), the application does include options to filter or alter users' appearances with special effects and a built-in "beauty" tool.

TikTok content like that created by Lacey stands out against a mediascape that so often ignores or erases images of disability. People with disabilities are

J. Foster (✉) • D. Pettinicchio
University of Toronto, Toronto, ON, Canada
e-mail: jordann.foster@mail.utoronto.ca

© The Author(s), under exclusive license to Springer Nature Switzerland AG 2023
M. S. Jeffress et al. (eds.), *The Palgrave Handbook of Disability and Communication*, https://doi.org/10.1007/978-3-031-14447-9_17

273

vastly underrepresented in mainstream media and especially in media emphasizing appearance (Foster, 2021; Ganahl & Arbuckle, 2001; Heiss, 2011; Houston, 2019; Johanssen & Garrisi, 2020). In turn, TikTok has been praised as an inclusive and egalitarian space where anyone can become famous through viral videos and short clips on the app's *For You* page (see Abidin, 2020). Platforms like Instagram and YouTube are often celebrated for these same reasons (Cunningham & Craig, 2019)—as "democratizing" a field historically guarded by elite gatekeepers, as is the case with film and television (Ellis & Merchant, 2020). On these platforms, visibility and fame are, ostensibly at least, fair game for all.

Still, questions remain surrounding whether, and to what extent, platforms like TikTok have generated new opportunities for individuals otherwise excluded and marginalized by traditional content production. A cursory look at the social media landscape suggests that visibility is not only difficult to achieve, but also unevenly distributed, with a cast of conventionally attractive, largely White creators dominating the most widely used media applications (Phạm, 2015). With this in mind, we ask: how do TikTok videos intersect with creators' race, age, disability, and gender to inform their visibility and virality online? And, do these videos and their affordances—the in-application modalities and technical tools available to users—challenge or reinforce widely shared beliefs surrounding disability?

These questions arise as TikTok insiders report that the app suppressed creators of color, queer creators, and creators with disabilities (Botella, 2019), reifying existing inequalities around who is deemed worthy of visibility online. Rebecca Jennings (2021) recently called out the media platform whose biggest stars "are the popular kids...pretty people filming themselves being pretty." This phenomenon is not unique to TikTok. Rather, it is an example of ableist structures that inherently devalue certain appearances and promote others.

In this chapter, we shed light on the democratizing potential of TikTok's viral videos especially as they pertain to disability—a status significantly underrepresented in traditional media. We argue that many of these videos and the creators who post them challenge existing beliefs about disability, giving creators an opportunity to share their stories and experiences in ways that diverge from traditionally narrow disability media tropes and ableist stereotypes. Platform-based norms, however, appear to privilege only a select few creators and creators with disabilities are seldom among them. In part, this owes to a set of pervasive appearance norms that circulate within our visual and virtual culture, and algorithmic logics that favor a select number of "attractive" stars. With this in mind, we begin with a discussion of media representations—broadly defined—and their relationship to the production and reproduction of inequality. We then narrow in on the limitations of social media's democratic and inclusive affordances. Throughout, we illustrate how contemporary social media platforms like TikTok both facilitate and constrain opportunities for diversity and inclusion online.

Media Representations of Historically Marginalized Groups

The intersection of disability studies and media studies is indeed a fast-growing area of scholarship transcending interdisciplinary boundaries (Ellis et al., 2020). The particular focus on "inclusive technologies of mediation" (Ginsburg, 2020: xxiv) has inspired social scientists to innovate theory and method to better account for how the organization of media industries shapes cultural production.

Cultural products including advertisements, film, and television shows, communicate who is worthy of our attention. To borrow from Mears (2010, p. 24), they "do work," illustrating lives and lifestyles not as they are, but as they ought to be. This has important implications for marginalized groups who have historically been underrepresented in mainstream media (Baumann, 2008; Baumann & de Laat, 2012; Ellis et al., 2020; Garrisi & Johanssen, 2020; Houston, 2019; Jeffress, 2021).

In recent years, there has been a growing movement among mainstream media organizations and brands to include more people with disabilities in advertisements and on-screen productions. While these strides forward are, no doubt, important, "newfound visibility without informed and educated planning and portrayals could potentially be more damaging than no inclusion at all" (Loebner, 2020, p. 436). Even more recent representations of diversity tend to be quite narrow (Heiss, 2011; Loebner, 2020).

(Re)Producing Inequality

Representations of the body are especially limited (Duncan, 1994), excluding those who embody physical markers of difference based on gender, sexuality, and race. Well documented by scholars, industry gatekeepers like model scouts and talent agents rely on "safe bets" to guard against market ambiguities and production risks (Godart & Mears, 2009; Hoppe, 2019, 2020; Mears, 2010; Wohl, 2021). Representations of beauty do, for example, exclude women of color (Craig, 2002; Hoppe, 2021; Hunter, 2006; McMillan, 2019; Wissinger, 2015), or posture these women in narrow, often negative ways (Baumann, 2008; Mears, 2011). Images and advertisements on television are similarly narrow, favoring thin, young, White women while excluding or underrepresenting elderly women and women of color (Baumann & de Laat, 2012; Jerslev, 2017).

Media and feminist scholars alike alert us to social, political, and economic exclusion as important vehicles through which extant inequalities are reproduced and maintained (Baker-Sperry & Grauerholz, 2003; Banet-Weiser, 2012; Heiss, 2011; Houston, 2019; Mears, 2010; Widdows, 2019). As Hoppe (2021, p. 2) points out, exclusion of marginalized peoples from mainstream media representations reflects "a system of social closure and domination" in which some, but not all are invited to be seen.

Excluding Disability

People with disabilities are often missing from cultural products closely tied to appearance (Christensen-Stryno & Eriksen, 2020). Foster and Pettinicchio's (2021) recent analysis found weak representation of visible disability in fashion advertisements and images in *Vogue, Harper's Bazaar,* and *InStyle,* as well as campaigns by Nike, Aerie, and Tommy Hilfiger between 2014 and 2019. Cultural producers such as advertisers have often postured the disabled body in negative terms crafting content with young, non-disabled consumers in mind fearing that representations of disability will not resonate with a broad consumer base (Hughes et al., 2005, p. 5; see also Houston, 2019, on "risky" representation). Advertisers worry that inclusion of people with disabilities will result in a "no-win situation" and so ultimately decide against a cast of more diverse people (Ganahl & Arbuckle, 2001, p. 6). Even with more recent evidence suggesting that consumers respond favorably to advertisements featuring disability (Shelton & Waddell, 2021), people with disabilities remain underrepresented in popular media (Dorwart, 2019). Acting as gatekeepers (Foster et al., 2011), advertisers and industry tastemakers select what are thought to be more conventional figures and faces which almost always exclude people with disabilities.

When and if people with disabilities are included in mainstream media representations like advertisements, film, or television, they tend to be postured in ways that reproduce negative stereotypes surrounding the disability community. People with disabilities are, for example, sometimes included as "a source of amusement," invoking stereotypes related to "oddness" and difference (Haller & Becker, 2014, p. 4). Alternatively, disabled people may be featured to inspire pity (Shapiro, 1994; Pettinicchio, 2019; Timke, 2019) or to warm the hearts of readers with stories related to their triumph over disablement—a familiar media trope that has been referred to as "inspiration porn" (Liddiard, 2014; Cameron et al., 2021; Shelton & Waddell, 2021). These are common among athletes with disabilities who are championed for having "overcome" the limitations of their bodies' physicality (Hardin & Hardin, 2004; Hargreaves & Hardin, 2009; Loebner, 2020). Together, these representations reinforce a narrow set of beliefs about disability, perpetuating stereotypes that limit our understanding of the range of figures and faces available for view, and the fullness of their lives.

Challenging Production Dynamics

While existing representations of disability are especially infrequent and often naïvely construed (Heiss, 2011), several advertisers, brands, and tastemakers in film and fashion have cast a greater number of disabled people in images, advertisements, and big-budget sets in recent years. Disney, for example, introduced its first princess "designed with disability in mind" (Resene, 2017, p. 2), while major fashion and beauty retailers including Tommy Hilfiger and Sephora made efforts to include models with disabilities in their ad campaigns. Across television advertisements, representations of disability are on the rise too. Farnall and Lyons (2012), for example, reported a 200% increase in the number of disabled people when compared to advertisements a decade earlier. The Gay and Lesbian Alliance Against Defamation's (2020) report on representation and diversity showed a similar rise in the representation of characters with disabilities on television; the largest number of characters reported in 11 years. This is no less true online where social media applications and digital platforms increasingly provide the potential for greater representation and inclusion (Christensen-Stryno & Eriksen, 2020; Foster, 2021).

Social Media, Democratization, and Change

Social media represents a robust democratizing force that often (though not always) "disrupts traditional narratives" (Blevins et al., 2019, p. 1636) across a variety of fields by pushing past established media gatekeepers (see also Lewis, 2021; Powell et al., 2018). Indeed, social media including mobile and web-based applications have played an important role in providing users an opportunity to engage directly with industry figures, providing feedback, and making requests for greater diversity. Unlike their traditional counterparts, social media and their technical architecture offer users somewhat more autonomy to craft content and champion causes (Loebner, 2020). They allow people to be seen (Cunningham & Craig, 2019) as when, for example, social media platforms like Instagram spotlight body positive posts (Cohen et al., 2019), or champion fuller figured influencers and influencers of color (Lewis, 2021).

On TikTok, users can directly produce their own online content and share it with others. Content can quickly go viral turning young people into "stars" overnight (Grigoriadis, 2021). Among these stars, we find users with disabilities who share their personal stories aside hashtags and in-application edits—technological and platform-based affordances—that allow others to engage with and see people with disabilities in a new light.

Platform-based affordances include photo taking and sharing tools, as well as livestreaming (Caliandro & Anselmi, 2021; Hurley, 2019; Meisner & Ledbetter, 2020), personal storytelling (Cirucci, 2017), and the use of hashtags (Baker & Michael, 2018; Blevins et al., 2019). These provide several democratizing and inclusive potentials for everyday users and for creators online. Livestreaming, for example, allows social media creators to connect with their audiences in real-time, blurring the boundary between creators and their fans while producing a sense of intimacy between the two (Meisner & Ledbetter, 2020). Hashtags, meanwhile, can be used to share powerful stories and personal testimonies related to social justice causes, driving important conversations around these issues.

On TikTok, hashtags like #disability can be used to sort and organize videos to reach users who are part of the disability community and beyond. For example, Lacey Richcreek went viral during CP awareness month using TikTok specific hashtags including "fy" or "foryou." These hashtags allow users who might otherwise never be cast in mainstream media productions to gain a following and share their message online. These are just some among several "developments and trends" suggesting that social media may hold new opportunities for people with disabilities to be seen and heard (Christensen-Stryno & Eriksen, 2020, p. 37). In part, this is because TikTok's user-generated content faces fewer obstacles with respect to production and distribution than are common with traditional media. Absent a well-defined set of industry gatekeepers, social media applications like TikTok have given way to a cast of creators who challenge "the normative route through which media talent is filtered" (Cunningham & Craig, 2019, p. 11).

The Limits of TikTok

Despite these affordances, there are limits to the democratization potential of social media. Content creation through platforms like TikTok tends to mirror mainstream cultural production more broadly. Algorithmic suppression and "shadow bans" combine to narrow the range of figures and faces featured online (Cotter, 2019; O'Meara, 2019), while talent agents and brand representatives continue to channel resources to just a handful of social media stars. Many social media applications have been criticized for rewarding individuals and groups who embody the greatest share of social privilege especially where appearances are concerned. As Pham (2015, p. 50) observed in her work on influencers and super-bloggers, the "bodies and faces" of social media's most widely followed creators "generally reflect rather than challenge Western standards of beauty (including thinness, youthfulness, and cuteness)," reproducing existing norms surrounding appearance and its significance online.

On the one hand, TikTok, like Instagram and YouTube, shares affordances that can do much to challenge norms and conventions in large part because content is not curated by gatekeepers who make decisions about who consumers should see and emulate. They provide opportunities for consumers and users of media to create content that can be far more inclusive and diverse than that produced by industry gatekeepers (Cunningham & Craig, 2019). On the other hand, these cultural opportunities so closely tied to platform affordances reflect convergence around existing norms and mimetic appearances, highlighting the pervasiveness of widely recognizable beauty ideals and the "normative" bodies they tend to celebrate.

METHODOLOGY

To assess the ways in which social media applications like TikTok might challenge or reinforce existing beliefs surrounding disability, we look to a set of widely popular videos posted online. These videos have accrued hundreds of thousands—and in some cases—millions of views. For reference, the most watched video in our sample was viewed 18 million times, while the least watched video garnered 177,000 views. Importantly, these TikTok videos are publicly available and can be accessed on any web-browser without an account or login credentials.

To locate videos for inclusion we employed a keyword search using hashtags on TikTok. Specifically, the hashtags #disability, #disabled, #disabilitypride, #disabledtiktok, and #disabilitytiktok were used to locate relevant videos for our sample. Throughout, our search was guided by a modified version of Preferred Reporting Items for Systematic Reviews and Meta—Analyses (PRISMA) and followed a multi-step selection process (Moher et al., 2009). Using TikTok's own search tools, we refined our process further, analyzing videos that were sorted as the "top" most viewed for each hashtag search. From among these top-most viewed videos, we included content that featured a creator with a visible or non-visible disability or that reflected on disability or issues related to the disability community more broadly. Our units of analysis ultimately included 100 TikTok videos from 100 TikTok creators. These videos were posted between January of 2020 and November of 2021 and provide a window into the ways in which creators framed disability for their audiences.

Once located, we analyzed creators' videos with specific attention to creators' disability type and its visibility. We did this to determine which (if any) disabilities were more likely to appear online. Consistent with our research objectives, we also recorded each creator's race and gender to better understand how these status characteristics shape opportunities for visibility online. Because observations of race and gender can vary from an individual's own self-classification (Roth, 2016), we combined elements of digital netnography (Costello et al., 2017; Kozinets, 2015), with public searches to gather creators' self-classified race and gender where possible. Creators' disability(ies) was also verified through digital netnography. In practice, this meant searching for and viewing videos through search terms, reviewing creators' profiles and other videos, while taking notes on their public presentation and patterns of content production.

These viral creators may not always identify status characteristics like race within the actual content being analyzed. However, their virality lends itself to verifiability by locating public press stories, interviews, and other online reporting where creators often refer to their own race and gender. Additionally, press agencies like *Allure* and *Vox* have profiled multiple disabled creators including creators in our sample, providing additional details related to creators' race, gender, and disability (see also Lawson, 2021). Overall, 66% of the viral videos coded here were created by users who identify as women, and 34% by users who identify as men. Of these creators, 76% identify as having a visible disability including paraplegia, cerebral palsy, and Tourette syndrome, while 24% a non-visible disability including chronic pain. In our sample, 72% of all creators identify as White, 16% as Black, and 4% as East-Asian. Racial self-classifications were unavailable for 8% of the creators we sampled.

We examined how users framed disability for their audiences online. Drawing on a wide body of work related to media products and the representation of disability (e.g., Heiss, 2011; Jeffress, 2021; Resene, 2017), we used an iterative process, recording major themes and patterns as they emerged across our sample of videos (Zulli & Zulli, 2020). Consistent with existing studies of TikTok (Abidin, 2020), we assessed the captions creators used for their videos, as well as creators' principal activities, speech, and any added text they laid over their videos. Taken together, these elements help shape and communicate creators' messaging online.

Our analysis revealed three key frames: (1) challenging existing stereotypes related to disability, (2) personal stories and struggles among young people with disabilities, and (3) positioning people with disabilities as normatively beautiful. While these frames were not always mutually exclusive, creators did tend to emphasize one or another. As Table 1 shows, videos related to creators' personal stories and struggles were the most frequent among TikTok's viral disability content, followed by videos that challenged stereotypes related to disability, and finally, videos that focused on beauty and appearance. We describe each frame below and situate these within broader understandings of media portrayals of disability described by disability and media scholars. In line with the literature, we acknowledge that the frames we identify among TikTok users have broader significance beyond mobile applications and on-screen videos to shape how disability is generally perceived and understood.

Framing Disability

Challenging Stereotypes

TikTok provides creators an opportunity to address widely shared stereotypes related to disability. Much has been written by disability studies scholars about the prevalence of these negative attitudes and stigmas (Garland-Thomson, 1997; Oliver & Barnes, 2012). These include harmful stereotypes around mobility and athleticism (McGrail et al., 2020), sex and sexuality (Campbell, 2017), as well as dependence (Pettinicchio, 2019). Brenna Huckaby (@brennahuckaby), for example, challenges ableist notions of athleticism by documenting her physical fitness and weightlifting activities. In doing so, Brenna asserts her strength and physicality, undermining media narratives that cast people with disabilities as pitiful and necessarily dependent. Creator Hope Marie (@epohmp4) produced a similar video, challenging traditional media narratives that position disabled people as pitiful. In it, she explains to viewers that "most disabled people don't enjoy pity." Erin Novakowski (@wheelierin), a creator with spinal muscular atrophy, echoed this same sentiment, using captions to explain that she is not "inspirational," "extraordinary," or "innocent." She simply "exists."

Other creators adopt a similar approach, crafting video content that takes aim at widely shared misunderstandings and negative beliefs about disability. Toby Tremain (@Tobysmilesoffical) reminds his 875,000 followers that people with disabilities are every bit as intelligent as others around them, and that being disabled should not invite condescending or patronizing comments. Em (@happyinhoney), a TikTok creator who is paraplegic, puts it somewhat differently, reminding her audience that it is not okay to infantilize people with disabilities. She adds that invasive questions about their medical history are also not okay. Like other creators with disabilities, Toby and Em sought to raise awareness among TikTok users by providing helpful information and useful correctives related to their own lived experiences as disabled people. In doing so, these creators cast disability as far more complex than has mainstream media to date (Ganahl & Arbuckle, 2001; Haller & Becker, 2014).

In a similar fashion, creator Marcela Marañon asks her viewers to "stop saying these things to women in wheelchairs: 'you are too pretty to be in a wheelchair'," and "'since you're in a wheelchair you can't have sex right?'" This latter comment alludes to how women with disabilities are often perceived as violating traditional norms of sexuality particularly among those who already hold rigid beliefs around gender roles (Parsons et al., 2017; Foster, 2021). TikTok provides a space, however, where people with disabilities can challenge this narrative, shedding important light on topics like sex and sexuality. This is true when, for example, creators produce videos that address dating, take questions about sex or sexuality, and when creators share details of their romantic lives. Videos in this vein invite viewers to think more deeply about the "desires" and "pleasures" that they share with creators with disabilities so often missing from mainstream media coverage (Loeser et al., 2018, p. 257).

TikTok makes it possible for creators to respond to users' comments both with words and videos in turn allowing creators with disabilities to address users' questions (and criticisms) in real-time. Interaction with users can directly address negative stereotypes as creators provide more thoughtful information on theirs and others' lives. Consider, for example, Mya or @immarollwithit, a TikTok creator whose progressive physical disability has meant that Mya uses a chair to stabilize her body. One user, surprised by the extent of Mya's mobility, commented that she "is not actually disabled." Mya responded with a video informing this user and her audience that "not all wheelchair users are paralyzed" and that many conditions may require the use of a chair including CP and spina bifida. Her video caption reinforces the point, suggesting that "disability is a spectrum and is dynamic."

Still other creators structure their videos around frequently asked questions set to trending music on the application. James Sultiff (@james_sutliff) produced one such video, explaining to his 1.1 million followers that his disability—dystonia—was caused by an injury sustained while playing rugby. Puala Carozzo (@pauuzzoo) created a similar video, replying to questions like, "what happened to you?" and "does your leg hurt?" In replying to users' questions, creators like Puala and James provide a space where negative attitudes and misperceptions of disability can be dispelled. In crafting these videos, creators with disabilities take control of (and often re-write) dominant media narratives about disability, including narratives that posture disabled people simply as

282   J. FOSTER AND D. PETTINICCHIO

secondary to other focal persons or as "articles of adornment" used to dress-up a story (Billawalla & Wolbring, 2014).

Sharing Stories and Social Struggles

In addition to providing a space where creators can challenge disability stereotypes, TikTok allows people with disabilities to share personal stories. Creators with disabilities discuss what it is like to date, how they navigate spaces designed exclusively for non-disabled people, and moments in their lives where they felt defeated by disabling environments and social struggles.

Lucy Dawson (@ludawinthesky) produced one such viral video cued to the song, *It's The Hard Knock Life* (Charnin & Strouse, 1977). In this video, Lucy briefly captures what it is like to go "on dating apps as a young disabled woman." She motions back and forth as captions depict damaging comments men make to her like, for example, "does the stick [Lucy's cane] get involved in the bedroom." Accompanied by hashtags like #disabilityTikTok or #disabled, Lucy's video engages directly with other members of the disability community. This video and the hashtags that accompany it function as an avenue for receiving support or encouragement. At the same time, Lucy's video lends a voice to the very real experiences with persistent social and attitudinal barriers that are often ignored by mainstream media—even mainstream media that includes disabled characters and figures.

On TikTok, Chrissy (@chrissycanyouhearme) provides a somewhat different look at her day-to-day difficulties as a "profoundly deaf" young woman. In her video, Chrissy explains to viewers that others often assume she can hear because she can speak. She reminds viewers that being deaf and being mute constitute two different disabilities. In a similar style, Tatum Box (@tatumbx) reproduces a common conversation she has with those who misunderstand or doubt her disability—amplified musculoskeletal pain syndrome. As Tatum shows in her video, she is often in a position where she must justify her disability to others, some of whom tell Tatum that if they were in her shoes, "I'd kill myself." Both creators make it clear that these conversations are incredibly taxing, a feeling echoed by users in the comments that follow their videos.

In his viral video on TikTok, Louie (@notlewy) explains that being out in public is sometimes uncomfortable as young children tend to jeer and point at the visible markers of his disability. While Louie's video functions as a useful device for reminding users that this kind of behavior is not okay, it also communicates that the "disabled body" continues to be treated as "odd" or "unusual" and, in some cases, as a source for amusement (Haller & Becker, 2014). This kind of content brings the lived experiences of people with disabilities to a broad audience illustrating the dynamic relationship between disability and society and the widespread attitudinal barriers that continue to marginalize disabled people.

Hello Beautiful People: A Focus on Appearance

Some TikTok users with disabilities lean on the application's appearance norms and on broad appeals toward beauty to shape their message. When this is the case, users with disabilities stylize their content to align more closely with online trends and existing conventions shared among the application's most widely followed creators. They might, for instance, crop out visible markers of disability, pulling focus toward trending outfits, makeup, and facial features. Although these videos often overlap with others related to the stereotypes and personal stories shared above, they tend to perform especially well on TikTok, garnering hundreds of thousands, and in some cases, millions of views. Their success points to the centrality of appearance on TikTok, revealing both opportunities and obstacles for members of the disability community.

Alyssa (@alcequine_), for example, went viral by subverting beauty norms and users' expectations of appearance. At first in her video, she appears in frame wearing a black crop top and distressed denim jeans. Her blonde hair falls perfectly to the side of her face, as she lip-syncs to say, "You don't look disabled." Alyssa then steps back for the viewer, revealing that a prosthesis is supporting her right leg. In doing so, Alyssa challenges widely shared beliefs about disability, asking her viewers to understand that disability is not always visible. But Alyssa does something more too. In pulling focus to her normative good looks, Alyssa challenges users online to see her disability *as beautiful*.

Lucy (@ludawinthesky) provides a similar video for her viewers. In it, she recalls a moment in her life when a stranger assumed that she was not disabled because "she didn't look it"—presumably because Lucy embodies widely recognized norms surrounding appearance and attractiveness including light skin, and near perfect facial symmetry. She exclaims to viewers, "when will people realize that disability has no 'look' and that disability has no age." Creator Jiya Day (@bbjiya), a young woman of color with mild spastic quadriplegia cerebral palsy began her journey on TikTok with makeup and beauty videos—a popular genre of video online. Appearing for her viewers with brightly decorated eyelids and color treated hair, Jiya combines trending makeup looks with commentary on disability including videos on ableism and videos on her lived experience as a young person with cerebral palsy.

Taken together, the TikTok posts analyzed here serve as an important example of the continuing efforts of disabled people seeking to challenge beliefs that disability is incompatible with beauty and appearance norms so often touted in mainstream media. While these videos stand out in a virtual landscape that often privileges only a handful of typically White, thin, and non-disabled people, they should not be read uncritically (see Heiss, 2011 for an analogous example). Indeed, videos that emphasize the importance of beauty and attractiveness while obscuring or making-over markers of visible disability inevitably suggest that disability ought to be worked on, fashioned, and corrected if it is to connect with audiences online. What is more, not all TikTok users are able to marshal the language and conventions of beauty with much success. Rather, creators who embody forms of privilege related to their appearance including and especially White creators with non-visible disabilities appear best positioned to accrue likes and follows in response to their videos.

Consider Paige Layle's (@paigelayle) disability-related content. Paige, a young woman with autism, has 2.6 million followers on TikTok and has created several viral videos on the application. In one such video, Paige sings, "I don't have a perfect body, but sometimes I forget, I don't have a perfect body, cause I'm autistic and my body doesn't tell me when I need something." At the time of analysis, this video had amassed more than 1.2 million likes and some 6.4 million views, making it one of the most liked and viewed videos in our sample. In calling on the body, Paige shifts focus to her appearance. A young, slender, woman with blonde hair, Paige's admission of imperfection appears earnest and sincere. Still, Paige's body is conventionally attractive, and her disability is invisible to the average user. Her audience takes notice of appearance, commenting to say that Paige is "so cute" and, "ur seriously so so pretty."

Highly visible creators like Lucy and James (discussed above) are illustrative cases too. Each embodies widely shared norms related to beauty and appearance. And these norms, as news reports so often remind us, are especially important on TikTok (Jennings, 2021). James, a White, cis-gendered and obviously muscular man, embodies a set of widely shared ideals related to appearance, calling to mind images of the normatively attractive "man's man." Importantly, his disability is all but invisible in the static thumbnails that populate his page, suggesting perhaps that only those creators with less clearly visible disabilities are well positioned to find fame online.

While TikTok affords people with disabilities an opportunity to bypass traditional media gatekeepers and create content that might otherwise not make it on a billboard or big screen, the application sees far fewer viral videos on disability than it does videos on say, dance or lip-synch content. What is more, not a single creator with a visible disability makes it among the top 100 most followed creators on the application (Social Blade, 2022), raising important questions about who is (and is not) poised for virality online. A cursory look at this list suggests that the most widely followed creators are those who reflect conventional standards of beauty. They are, as Kennedy (2020, p. 1072) explains, "restricted to a narrow set of gendered, racialized, classed and sexualised ideals" and so, ultimately reinforce and reproduce existing privileges surrounding appearance online.

DISCUSSION

Social media applications like TikTok are often praised for their inclusive and democratic potential. Members of the press report on a cast of young people turned stars through carefully edited viral videos (Grigoriadis, 2021). Some comment on the rise of creators of color (Lorenz, 2020); others turn to important trends related to body diversity online (Yanagihara, 2021). While these press reports are not without merit, the stories that they tell are incomplete.

TikTok, like other social media applications, does indeed provide more inclusive opportunities for diverse creators. Bypassing industry gatekeepers like editors and media managers (Cunningham & Craig, 2019), these platforms present fewer obstacles to visibility and fame than more traditional media. Still, for all its democratizing potential, TikTok is not without issue. This platform, and others like it (Phạm, 2015), are dominated by a cast of uniformly attractive, largely White creators whose visibility owes in large part to the appearance-based privileges they embody (Foster & Baker, 2022).

Among these social media creators, we find a cast of young people with disabilities who have turned to TikTok to share their stories, dispel stereotypes surrounding the disability community, and educate other users online. As we have shown, TikTok provides an avenue through which creators with disabilities can craft and edit content that challenges existing beliefs and widely recognizable tropes related to disability, reaching a wide audience. TikTok also provides its creators a platform on which to share their personal struggles and stories about their lived experience with tens of thousands if not millions of followers. In this way, TikTok expands opportunities for visibility and storytelling beyond those available in the traditional media circuit and can push past narrow, often negative, stereotypes surrounding disability (Billawalla & Wolbring, 2014).

On TikTok, videos that help to dispel stereotypes or that center on the stories and struggles of young people with disabilities often intersected with content related to beauty and appearance. Videos that did so borrowed from the application's mimetic norms and conventions to center appearance and attractiveness in view. Importantly, videos that pair disability with appearance conventions and beauty ideals position disability in a new light, inviting viewers to see and understand those with disabilities as lying within conventional beauty norms. At the same time, videos emphasize users' conventionally attractive figures and faces while simultaneously obscuring markers of disability. By doing so, however subtly, they suggest that disability ought to be managed, worked-on and ultimately, sanitized for view. Like their mainstream media counterparts, these videos inadvertently reinforce "dominant beauty structures" when they erase or make over markers of disability (Heiss, 2011, p. 17).

For their part, creators with disabilities can engage more critically with discussions on beauty and appearance, and with the application's oft-cited emphasis on conventional "good looks" (Jennings, 2021). Owing to their exclusion from the traditional fashion and beauty landscape, creators with disabilities are uniquely positioned to comment on how appearance norms, broadly defined, shape our everyday experiences both online and off. Relatedly, creators with disabilities are encouraged to take aim at the algorithms, logics, and memetic trends that shape social media applications like TikTok, and narrow "content diversity" on the platform (Poell et al., 2022, p. 167). This is especially important now, as TikTok continues to grow in popularity.

SUGGESTIONS FOR FUTURE RESEARCH

Moving forward, scholars should attend more closely to media applications and their democratizing and inclusive potential for diverse users online. Specifically, we need to better understand what opportunities *and* obstacles these media might hold for marginalized peoples. Research in this vein would benefit from systematically analyzing users' comments in reply to TikTok videos and assess what these comments can tell us about production and consumption dynamics in a context of democratization.

While this chapter did not explicitly analyze users' comments across the sample, we allude to how these may function as a vehicle through which people with different disabilities connect with one another, sharing knowledge and experiences to produce a sense of community. Alternatively, public comments might be read to better understand how creators deal with criticism online. Creators with disabilities often report on or show their audiences the kinds of disparaging comments they receive on TikTok, raising important questions about the limitations (and risks) this mobile application presents for people with disabilities. To borrow from Johanssen and Garrisi (2020, p. 8), "while digital media may contribute to the self-empowerment of excluded and silenced bodies, they may equally open up spaces of discrimination, threats, hatred, trolling and silencing online."

Future research should also more systematically consider the algorithmic logics that shape social media platforms. Kelley Cotter (2019) and Victoria O'Meara (2019) provide a useful starting point for research of this kind, illustrating how algorithms shape visibility online. Still, more work is needed on TikTok—a relatively new and quickly growing social media application whose algorithms may act to constrain visibility for some individuals and groups.

CONCLUSION

Social media applications like TikTok provide opportunities for creators to achieve unprecedented visibility and, in some cases, fame. Among these creators are young people with disabilities who turn to TikTok to share their stories, triumphs, and struggles. Their videos stand out in a mediascape that has neglected and sometimes maligned disabled people. Their content represents an important stride toward greater diversity and inclusivity online with implications extending beyond the application and even the internet. Still, the app and its content are not without issue. Creators and viewers are encouraged to think critically about their use of TikTok and about the content they see and share, as it relates to direct and indirect messaging around inclusion, exclusion, and empowerment.

References

Abidin, C. (2020). Mapping internet celebrity on TikTok: Exploring attention economies and visibility labours. *Cultural Science Journal, 12*(1), 77–103. https://doi.org/10.5334/csci.140

Baker, S. A., & Michael, J. M. (2018). 'Good morning Fitfam': Top posts, hashtags and gender display on Instagram. *New Media & Society, 20*(12), 4553–4570. https://doi.org/10.1177/1461444818777514

Baker-Sperry, L., & Grauerholz, L. (2003). The pervasiveness and persistence of the feminine beauty ideal in children's fairy tales. *Gender & Society, 17*(5), 711–726. https://doi.org/10.1177/0891243203255605

Banet-Weiser, S. (2012). *Authentic™: The politics of ambivalence in a brand culture.* New York University Press.

Baumann, S. (2008). The moral underpinnings of beauty: A meaning-based explanation for light and dark complexions in advertising. *Poetics, 36*(1), 2–23. https://doi.org/10.1016/j.poetic.2007.11.002

Baumann, S., & de Laat, K. (2012). Socially defunct: A comparative analysis of the underrepresentation of older women in advertising. *Poetics, 40*(6), 514–541. https://doi.org/10.1016/j.poetic.2012.08.002

Billawalla, A., & Wolbring, G. (2014). Analyzing the discourse surrounding Autism in the *New York Times* using an ableism lens. *Disability Studies Quarterly, 34*(1), 1–25. https://doi.org/10.18061/dsq.v34i1.3348

Blevins, J. L., Lee, J. J., McCabe, E. E., & Edgerton, E. (2019). Tweeting for social justice in #Ferguson: Affective discourse in Twitter hashtags. *New Media & Society, 21*(7), 1636–1653. https://doi.org/10.1177/1461444819827030

Botella, E. (2019, December 4). Tiktok admits it suppressed videos by disabled, queer, and fat creators. *Slate Magazine.* Retrieved November 15, 2021, from https://slate.com/technology/2019/12/tiktok-disabled-users-videos-suppressed.html

Caliandro, A., & Anselmi, G. (2021). Affordances-based brand relations: An inquire on memetic brands on Instagram. *Social Media + Society, 7*(2), 1–18. https://doi.org/10.1177/20563051211021367

Cameron, L., Knezevic, I., & Hanes, R. (2021). Inspiring people or perpetuating stereotypes? The complicated case of disability as inspiration. In M. S. Jeffress (Ed.), *Disability representation in film, TV, and print media* (pp. 108–127). Routledge.

Campbell, M. (2017). Disabilities and sexual expression: A review of the literature. *Sociology Compass, 11*(9), 1–19. https://doi.org/10.1111/soc4.12508

Charnin, M., & Strouse, E. (1977). "It's the hard knock life." [Song recorded by Annie and the Orphans]. On Columbia Records.

Christensen-Stryno, M. B., & Eriksen, C. B. (2020). Madeline Stuart as disability advocate and brand: Exploring the affective economies of social media. In J. Johanssen & D. Garrisi (Eds.), *Disability, media, and representations* (pp. 35–50). Routledge.

Cirucci, A. M. (2017). Normative interfaces: Affordances, gender, and race in Facebook. *Social Media + Society, 3*(2), 1–10. https://doi.org/10.1177/2056305117717905

Cohen, R., Fardouly, J., Newton-John, T., & Slater, A. (2019). #BoPo on Instagram: An experimental investigation of the effects of viewing body positive content on young women's mood and body image. *New Media & Society, 21*(7), 1546–1564. https://doi.org/10.1177/1461444819826530

Costello, L., McDermott, M. L., & Wallace, R. (2017). Netnography: Range of practices, misperceptions, and missed opportunities. *International Journal of Qualitative Methods, 16*, 1–12. https://doi.org/10.1177/1609406917700647

Cotter, K. (2019). Playing the visibility game: How digital influencers and algorithms negotiate influence on Instagram. *New Media & Society, 21*(4), 895–913. https://doi.org/10.1177/1461444818815684

Craig, M. (2002). *Ain't I a beauty Queen?: Culture, social movements, and the rearticulation of race.* Oxford University Press.

Cunningham, S., & Craig, D. R. (2019). *Social media entertainment: The new intersection of Hollywood and Silicon Valley.* New York University Press.

Dorwart, L. (2019, July 25). What a new report says about disability representation in children's TV shows. *Forbes.* Retrieved March 7, 2021, from https://www.forbes.com/sites/lauradorwart/2019/07/25/what-a-new-report-says-about-disability-representation-in-childrens-tv-shows/#4039adb173c7

Duncan, M. C. (1994). The politics of women's body images and practices: Foucault, the panopticon, and Shape Magazine. *Journal of Sport and Social Issues, 18*(1), 48–65. https://doi.org/10.1177/019372394018001004

Ellis, K., & Merchant, M. (2020). Disability media work. In K. Ellis, G. Goggin, B. Haller, & R. Curtis (Eds.), *The Routledge companion to disability and media* (pp. 387–399). Routledge.

Ellis, K., Goggin, G., Haller, B., Curtis, R., & (Eds.). (2020). *The Routledge companion to disability and media.* Routledge.

Farnall, O. F., & Lyons, K. (2012). Are we there yet? A content analysis of ability integrated advertising on prime-time TV. *Disability Studies Quarterly, 32*(1). https://doi.org/10.18061/dsq.v32i1.1625

Foster, J. 2021. Framing disability in fashion. In R. L. Brown, M. Maroto, & D. Pettinicchio (Eds.), *The Oxford handbook of the sociology of disability* (online publication, n.p.). https://doi.org/10.1093/oxfordhb/9780190093167.013.15

Foster, J., & Baker, J. (2022). Muscles, Makeup, and Femboys: Analyzing TikTok's "Radical" Masculinities. Social Media + Society. https://doi.org/10.1177/20563051221126040.

Foster, J., & Pettinicchio, D. (2021). A model who looks like me: Communicating and consuming representations of disability. *Journal of Consumer Culture.* https://doi.org/10.1177/14695405211022074

Foster, P., Borgatti, S. P., & Jones, C. (2011). Gatekeeper search and selection strategies: Relational and network governance in a cultural market. *Poetics, 39*(4), 247–265. https://doi.org/10.1016/J.POETIC.2011.05.004

Ganahl, D., & Arbuckle, M. (2001). The exclusion of persons with physical disabilities from prime time television advertising: A two-year quantitative analysis. *Disability Studies Quarterly, 21*(2), 1–8. https://doi.org/10.18061/DSQ.V21I2.278

Garland-Thomson, R. (1997). *Extraordinary bodies: Figuring physical disability in American culture and literature.* Columbia University Press.

Garrisi, D., & Johanssen, J. (2020). Introduction. In J. Johanssen & D. Garrisi (Eds.), *Disability, media, and representations* (pp. 1–18). Routledge.

Gay & Lesbian Alliance Against Defamation. (2020). *Where we are on TV 2020-2021.* Retrieved November 15, 2021, from https://www.glaad.org/sites/default/files/GLAAD%20-%20202021%20WHERE%20WE%20ARE%20ON%20TV.pdf

Ginsburg, F. (2020). Foreword. In K. Ellis, G. Goggin, B. Haller & R. Curtis. (Eds.), *The Routledge companion to disability and media* (pp. xxii–xxvi). Routledge.

Godart, F. C., & Mears, A. (2009). How do cultural producers make creative decisions? Lessons from the catwalk. *Social Forces, 88*(2), 671–692. https://doi.org/10.1353/sof.0.0266

Grigoriadis, V. (2021, March 23). The beauty of 78.5 million followers. *The New York Times.* Retrieved November 15, 2021, from https://www.nytimes.com/2021/03/23/magazine/addison-rae-beauty-industry.html

Haller, B., & Becker, A. B. (2014). Stepping backwards with disability humor? The case of NY Gov. David Paterson's representation on "Saturday Night Live." *Disability Studies Quarterly, 34*(1), 1-21. doi:https://doi.org/10.18061/dsq.v34i1.3459.

Hardin, M., & Hardin, B. (2004). Performance or participation...pluralism or hegemony? Images of disability & gender in Sports 'n Spokes Magazine. *Disability Studies Quarterly, 25*(4). https://doi.org/10.18061/dsq.v25i4.606

Hargreaves, J., & Hardin, B. (2009). Women wheelchair athletes: Competing against media stereotypes. *Disability Studies Quarterly, 29*(2). https://doi.org/10.18061/dsq.v29i2.920

Heiss, S. (2011). Locating the bodies of women and disability in definitions of beauty: An analysis of Dove's campaign for real beauty. *Disability Studies Quarterly, 31*(1). https://doi.org/10.18061/dsq.v31i1.1367

Hoppe, A. D. (2019). License to tweak: Artistic license at first-tier Indian apparel suppliers. *Poetics, 76.* https://doi.org/10.1016/j.poetic.2019.05.001

Hoppe, A. D. (2020). Strategic balance or imperfect imitation? Style and legitimation challenges in a semi-peripheral city. In G. Cattani, S. Ferriani, F. Godart, & S. V. Sgourev (Eds.), *Aesthetics and style in strategy* (pp. 227–253). Emerald.

Hoppe, A. D. (2021). The microsociology of aesthetic evaluation: Selecting runway fashion models. *Qualitative Sociology.* https://doi.org/10.1007/s11133-021-09496-x

Houston, E. (2019). 'Risky' representation: The portrayal of women with mobility impairment in twenty-first-century advertising. *Disability & Society, 34*(5), 704–725. https://doi.org/10.1080/09687599.2019.1576505. https://www.cbpp.org/research/health/policy-basics-introduction-to-medicaid

Hughes, B., Russell, R., & Paterson, K. (2005). Nothing to be had 'off the peg': Consumption, identity and the immobilization of young disabled people. *Disability & Society, 20*(1), 3–17. https://doi.org/10.1080/0968759042000283601

Hunter, M. L. (2006). *Race, gender, and the politics of skin tone.* Routledge.

Hurley, Z. (2019). Imagined affordances of Instagram and the fantastical authenticity of female Gulf-Arab social media influencers. *Social Media & Society, 5*(1), 1–16. https://doi.org/10.1177/2056305118819241

Jeffress, M. S. (Ed.). (2021). *Disability representation in film, TV, and print media.* Routledge.

Jennings, R. (2021, May 18). The blandness of TikTok's biggest stars. *Vox.* Retrieved November 15, 2021, from https://www.vox.com/the-goods/2021/5/18/22440937/tiktok-addison-rae-bella-poarch-build-a-bitch-charli-damelio-mediocrity

Jerslev, A. (2017). The elderly female face in beauty and fashion ads: Joan Didion for Céline. *European Journal of Cultural Studies, 21*(3), 349–362. https://doi.org/10.1177/1367549417708436

Johanssen, J., & Garrisi, D. (Eds.). (2020). *Disability, media, and representations: Other bodies.* Routledge.

Kennedy, M. (2020). "If the rise of the TikTok dance and e-girl aesthetic has taught us anything, it's that teenage girls rule the internet right now": TikTok celebrity, girls and the Coronavirus crisis. *European Journal of Cultural Studies, 23*(6), 1069–1076. https://doi.org/10.1177/1367549420945341

Kozinets, R. (2015). *Netnography: Doing ethnographic research online.* Sage Press.

Lawson, M. (2021, January). How disabled creators on TikTok are going beyond "inspiration porn." *Allure.* Retrieved November 15, 2021, from https://www.allure.com/story/disabled-creators-on-tiktok

Leaver, T., Abidin, C., & Highfield, T. (2020). *Instagram: Visual social media cultures.* Polity Press.

Lewis, J. (2021, February 2). 11 Black, body-positive influencers you should be following right now. *POPSUGAR Fitness.* Retrieved November 15, 2021, from https://www.popsugar.com/fitness/black-body-positive-influencers-to-follow-on-instagram-48140604

Liddiard, K. (2014). Liking for like's sake—The commodification of disability on Facebook. *Journal of Developmental Disabilities, 20*(3), 94–101. https://oadd.org/wp-content/uploads/2014/01/41019_JoDD_94-101_v13f_Liddiard.pdf

Loebner, J. (2020). Advertising disability and the diversity directive. In K. Ellis, G. Goggin, B. Haller, & R. Curtis (Eds.), *The Routledge companion to disability and media* (pp. 341–355). Routledge.

Loeser, C., Pini, B., & Crowley, V. (2018). Disability and sexuality: Desires and pleasures. *Sexualities, 21*(3), 255–270. https://doi.org/10.1177/1363460716688682

Lorenz, T. (2020, December 11). The new influencer capital of America. *The New York Times.* Retrieved November 15, 2021, from https://www.nytimes.com/2020/12/11/style/atlanta-black-tiktok-creators.html

McGrail, E., McGrail, J. P., & Rieger, A. (2020). Friday night disability: The portrayal of youthful social interactions in television's Friday Night Lights. *Disability Studies Quarterly, 40*(4). https://doi.org/10.18061/dsq.v40i4.6801

McMillan, C. T. (2019). *Thick: And other essays.* The New Press.

Mears, A. (2010). Size zero high-end ethnic: Cultural production and the reproduction of culture in fashion modeling. *Poetics, 38*(1), 21–46. https://doi.org/10.1016/j.poetic.2009.10.002

Mears, A. (2011). *Pricing beauty: The making of a fashion model.* University of California Press.

Meisner, C., & Ledbetter, A. M. (2020). Participatory branding on social media: The affordances of live streaming for creative labor. *New Media & Society.* https://doi.org/10.1177/1461444820972392

Moher, D., Liberati, A., Tetzlaff, J., & Altman, D. (2009). Preferred reporting items for systematic reviews and meta-analyses: The prisma statement. *Annals of Internal Medicine, 151*(4), 264–269. https://doi.org/10.1136/bmj.b2535

O'Meara, V. (2019). Weapons of chic: Instagram influencer engagement pods as practices of resistance to Instagram platform labor. *Social Media & Society, 5*(4), 1–11. https://doi.org/10.1177/2056305119879671

Oliver, M., & Barnes, C. (2012). *The new politics of disablement.* Macmillan.

Parsons, A. L., Reichl, A. J., & Pedersen, C. L. (2017). Gendered ableism: Media representations and gender role beliefs' effect on perceptions of disability and sexuality. *Sexuality and Disability, 35*(2), 207–225. https://doi.org/10.1007/s11195-016-9464-6

Pettinicchio, D. (2019). *Politics of empowerment: Disability rights and the cycle of American policy reform*. Stanford University Press.

Pham, M. T. (2015). *Asians wear clothes on the internet: Race, gender, and the work of personal style blogging*. Duke University Press.

Poell, T., Nieborg, D., and Duffy, B. (2022). Platforms and Cultural Production. Wiley.

Powell, A., Overington, C., & Hamilton, G. (2018). Following #JillMeagher: Collective meaning-making in response to crime events via social media. *Crime, Media, Culture, 14*(3), 409–428. https://doi.org/10.1177/1741659017721276

Resene, M. (2017). From evil queen to disabled teen: Frozen introduces Disney's first disabled princess. *Disability Studies Quarterly, 37*(2). https://doi.org/10.18061/dsq.v37i2.5310

Roth, W. D. (2016). The multiple dimensions of race. *Ethnic and Racial Studies, 39*(8), 1310–1338. https://doi.org/10.1080/01419870.2016.1140793

Shapiro, J. P. (1994). *No pity: People with disabilities forging a new civil rights movement*. Three Rivers Press.

Shelton, S. S., & Waddell, T. F. (2021). Does 'inspiration porn' inspire? How disability and challenge impact attitudinal evaluations of advertising. *Journal of Current Issues and Research in Advertising, 42*(3), 258–276. https://doi.org/10.1080/10641734.2020.1808125

Social Blade. (2022, March 7). *Top 100 most followed TikTok accounts (sorted by followers count)*. Retrieved March 7, 2022, from https://socialblade.com/tiktok/top/100

Timke, E. (2019). Disability and advertising. *Advertising & Society Quarterly, 20*(3). https://doi.org/10.1353/asr.2019.0024

Widdows, H. (2019). *Perfect me: Beauty as an ethical ideal*. Princeton University Press.

Wissinger, E. (2015). *This year's model: Fashion, media, and the making of glamour*. New York University Press.

Wohl, H. (2021). Bound By Creativity. University of Chicago Press.

World CP Day. (2020, January 5). Millions of reasons. Retrieved March 7, 2021, from https://worldcpday.org/

Yanagihara, H. (2021, May 10). Who gets to be beautiful now? *The New York Times*. Retrieved November 15, 2021, from https://www.nytimes.com/2021/05/10/t-magazine/beauty-transforming-self.html

Zulli, D., & Zulli, D. J. (2020). Extending the internet meme: Conceptualizing technological mimesis and imitation publics on the TikTok platform. *New Media & Society*. https://doi.org/10.1177/1461444820983603

PART IV

Institutional Constructs and Constraints

CHAPTER 18

Communicating Vulnerability in Disasters: Media Coverage of People with Disabilities in Hurricane Katrina and the Tōhoku Earthquake and Tsunami

Liz Shek-Noble

As a country that experiences a disproportionate number of the world's annual earthquakes, Japan is arguably well-equipped to handle certain natural disasters. However, the large-scale destruction of Typhoon Hagibis, the most recent typhoon to have made landfall in Japan in 2019,[1] has raised concerns about the lack of accessible disaster information for non-Japanese-speaking people. These concerns were aggravated due to the influx of foreign travelers in the country for the 2019 Rugby World Cup. One feature for *The Japan Times* (Takahashi, 2019) reported on the difficulties experienced by fans in finding information about Typhoon Hagibis in languages other than Japanese. With respect to automatic evacuation notifications delivered to mobile phones, one fan commented that he "had no idea what they meant" (qtd. in Takahashi, 2019). He was also quoted saying that while there might be information available for foreign visitors, knowledge on where to locate such information was scant: "We know there's information out there for people like us, we just didn't know where to look" (qtd. in Takahashi, 2019).

I have started this chapter with reference to Typhoon Hagibis because doing so illuminates its central themes. Media reports in the wake of Typhoon Hagibis

L. Shek-Noble (✉)
University of Tokyo, Tokyo, Japan
e-mail: shek-noble@g.ecc.u-tokyo.ac.jp

© The Author(s), under exclusive license to Springer Nature Switzerland AG 2023
M. S. Jeffress et al. (eds.), *The Palgrave Handbook of Disability and Communication*, https://doi.org/10.1007/978-3-031-14447-9_18

295

highlight the urgent need to expand the scope of disaster communication to accommodate diverse groups (Alexander et al., 2012). Reference to Typhoon Hagibis also shows that media plays a crucial role in shaping how audiences understand or perceive groups in need of disaster relief and support. In the case of Typhoon Hagibis, much of the media coverage spoke to the inaccessibility of disaster information for foreign tourists based on language barriers. While this strategy may bring greater visibility to the distinct needs of one group, doing so may simultaneously obscure the needs of another, thereby limiting opportunities to improve existing social infrastructure, telecommunication systems, and evacuation facilities.

I would like to extend the anecdote further by including my personal experience of Typhoon Hagibis. As a resident of Tokyo, I, like many others, braced myself for what was anticipated to be the worst typhoon of 2019. The typhoon struck the city on October 12, 2019. While fierce winds and heavy rain assaulted my apartment, I received the following warning on my smartphone from the local government office. The message was also posted on the official Twitter account for Toshima City (@toshimabousai):

> こちらは豊島区です。 警戒レベル3 避難準備・高齢者等避難開始を発令 発令内容:避難時間にかかる人とその支援者は避難をしてください。 対象地域:豊島区全域 開設されている避難所 駒込小学校・目白小学校・巣鴨小学校・西部区民事務所・東部区民事務所・豊島区役所・椎名町小. (November 10, 2019)
> This is Toshima Ward. Alert Level 3. Evacuation preparations and evacuation of the elderly, etc., are in effect. Details of the announcement: Those who require evacuation time and their helpers should evacuate. Target Area: The entire Toshima Ward. Evacuation Centers: Komagome Elementary School, Mejiro Elementary School, Sugamo Elementary School, Toshima Ward Western Regional Office, Toshima Ward Eastern Regional Office, Toshima City Hall, Shiinamachi Elementary School. (Own translation)

This notification precipitated a fast-flowing accumulation of questions in my mind about the medium in which such critical information was communicated. I could not help but wonder whether this information was accessible not only to non-Japanese-speaking individuals, but also to a group that has been recognized as excessively disadvantaged in times of natural disaster: people with disabilities. Questions that immediately came to mind were: *Was this information available in a range of formats? As the message was advising people to evacuate their homes, how would people with disabilities be able to travel to temporary shelters? And even if they could make it to the shelters, would they be able to accommodate different impairments, some of which may require life-sustaining technologies and/or medicines?*

This chapter undertakes a comparative content analysis of news media coverage of Hurricane Katrina and the 2011 Tōhoku Earthquake and Tsunami in Japan. I focus on these disasters for a few reasons. First, both disasters are notable for the catastrophic damage they inflicted on natural and built environments. Second, Hurricane Katrina and the Tōhoku Earthquake and Tsunami resulted in extreme losses of human life, particularly people with disabilities. Third, problems with existing emergency management procedures and planning compounded the negative impact of these disasters on people with disabilities. I undertake an analysis of these disasters to highlight continuing problems associated with the communication of emergency warnings and protocols to people with disabilities as a result of inaccessible technologies and media formats, as well as subsequent challenges relating to expedient communication of disaster information and support once relocation to temporary shelters has occurred. This leads to people with disabilities being at an increased risk of harm and death in natural disasters (Twigg et al., 2018), but also being categorized as a "vulnerable" group whose suffering in disasters is perceived as a "natural" consequence of their impairments. Following on from Fjord (2007), Hemingway and Priestley (2006), and Abbott and Porter (2013), I argue that this categorization overlooks how the vulnerability of people with disabilities is exacerbated, or even "created" by Disaster Risk Reduction (DRR) and management initiatives that fail to incorporate voices from the community that can speak to their *own* specific concerns and needs.

The chapter will begin with a literature review on disaster theory and people with disabilities. I then provide an account of Hurricane Katrina and the Tōhoku Earthquake and Tsunami. Last, I undertake a comparative content analysis of English-language news sources from the United States of America and Japan to consider how people with disabilities were framed in these crises. I utilize content analysis to show that media coverage about people with disabilities relied upon existing stereotypical "frames" emphasizing their vulnerability. These frames ultimately reinforced medical and social pathological models of disability (Haller, 2000, p. 61), which perpetuate ableist[2] perceptions of people with disabilities as being dependent on non-disabled people for physical, medical, economic, and emotional support both during disasters and in daily life.

Literature Review on Disability and Disaster Communication

Literature about the effects of disasters on people with disabilities has been limited to a few studies. However, what unifies these studies is the strong conclusion that people with disabilities are negatively and differentially affected by natural disasters (Stough & Kelman, 2017). Furthermore, literature at the intersection of disaster research and disability studies argues that one reason for this inequality is that the needs of people with disabilities in emergencies are "overlooked" (Rouhban, 2014, p. 76) or not of "priority concern" in DRR planning (Wisner, 2002). The consequences of being overlooked are grave; Article 20 of the United Nations' "Addressing the Vulnerability and Exclusion of Persons with Disabilities: The Situation of Women and Girls, Children's

Right to Education, Disasters and Humanitarian Crises" (2015) identifies that the mortality rate for people with disabilities is typically "two to four times higher than that of the population without disabilities" during disaster situations. The Note cites two reasons why people with disabilities are "more vulnerable and disproportionately affected" than non-disabled people in disasters: "lack of awareness and inaccessible evacuation, response and recovery efforts" ("Addressing the vulnerability," 2015). Both reasons identify the current status of crisis communication for people with disabilities as being poorly arranged and unequipped to deal with their needs in treating the community as a "homogeneous demographic group" (Stough & Kelman, 2017).

Scholars working at the intersection of disability studies and disaster studies have also noted that existing models of crisis communication have ignored or sidelined the needs of people with disabilities during disasters because it is assumed that the normative individual is able-bodied. For Battle (2015), insufficient prioritization of the functional, access, and communication needs of people with disabilities can have deadly consequences in an emergency or a disaster; if people with disabilities do not have accessible evacuation routes, have difficulty understanding warning messages due to inappropriate media formats, or have reduced ability to communicate and respond to others, then "they are more likely to be left behind or abandoned" (2015, p. 232).

Hansson et al. (2020) also view communication as a variable that may positively or negatively affect one's level of vulnerability during a crisis. The "vulnerability" of people with disabilities is often enhanced because of challenges relating to communication including reduced ability to send, receive, or understand information (Hansson et al., 2020, p. 2). Delays when it comes to sending and receiving information may result in the untimely evacuation of people with disabilities from their homes, whereas the communication of information in an inaccessible format might mean disabled individuals are unaware that evacuation may have occurred at all.

Meanwhile, in their article about the Sendai Framework for Disaster Risk Reduction (2015–2030), Calgaro and scholars (2021) have found that communication barriers "are one of the greatest inhibitors to disaster preparedness and effective response" (p. 5). Drawing on a longitudinal assessment of d/ Deaf people in the Australian state of New South Wales, the authors noted that individuals within this community "felt greatly disadvantaged" in being unable to access vital information about emergencies and disasters quickly. The participants also highlighted that the media in which information was communicated, along with uneven access to such media, led to feelings of social disconnection and marginalization and a reduction of trust in government and emergency services (Calgaro et al., 2021, p. 5).

In order to raise awareness and reduce the disproportionate impact of disasters on people with disabilities, Twigg et al. (2018) call for a "disability-inclusive disaster management" procedure that attends to the "heightened vulnerability" of people with disabilities based on a larger pattern of intersecting inequalities. Specifically, they identify that people with disabilities "are more likely to be poor or unemployed, socially marginalised, excluded from decision-making processes and living in hazardous locations" (Twigg et al., 2018, p. 3). Alexander et al. (2012) make a similar point in their observation that economic inequality and lack of communication contribute to the inability of people with disabilities to react "effectively to crisis situations and stop them from using the facilities and assistance made available to [non-disabled people]" (p. 384). For them and other scholars, disability all too often intersects with social and economic disadvantage (Rouhban, 2014; White, 2006; Walsh-Warder, 2016), leading not only to a disproportionate fatality rate but ongoing systemic *and* systematic discrimination in the aftermath of a disaster.

The alarming low survival rate of people with disabilities in disaster-affected areas indicates that progress must be made to create accessible response procedures and facilities that account for a range of impairments. By way of example, Rouhban (2014) notes that while the "hazard-prone country," Bangladesh, has efficient warning systems, they are ultimately inaccessible to d/Deaf and hard of hearing people (hereafter DHH people) as the information is inaudible (p. 82). Furthermore, the timeliness of disaster evacuation information is paramount, given some people with disabilities require additional time (Stough & Kelman, 2017) and services in order to relocate. Alexander et al. (2012) observe that "none of the 700 people with post-polio paralysis on an island of the Andaman archipelago in India were able to survive the [December 2004] tsunami as they were unable to run to the top of surrounding hills" (p. 385).

Scholars have not only identified the disproportionately negative consequences for people with disabilities in disasters; they have also commented on the role that new technologies, specifically social media, can play in either improving or impeding the ability for people with disabilities to receive communication that enables them to act appropriately in crises. Consequently, the literature calls for technologies to become accessible for people with disabilities at all stages of the management cycle: mitigation, preparation, response, and recovery (Rouhban, 2014, p. 77). In particular, Ellis and Kent (2011) and Goggin and Newell (2003) have written about the phenomenon of "digital disability," that is, when technologies fail to be accessible to people with disabilities because sensorial and cognitive differences are not taken into account during their design (Kent & Ellis, 2015, p. 420). The reason this phenomenon occurs is partly attributable to the fact that social media consists of a "mash-up of overlapping platforms," which means that when a disabled person cannot access one type of social media, they are by default barred from the whole system (Kent & Ellis, 2015).

Current scholarship also suggests that social media is becoming an increasingly useful and commonly used tool for government offices to communicate with the public in disasters. Hjorth and Kim (2011) and Cho et al. (2013) discuss how social media, in particular Twitter, is changing the nature of crisis communication by multiplying the number of actors who may distribute information, as well as shifting the balance of communicative agency from government organizations to members of the general public. Cho et al. (2013) focus on how Twitter became an invaluable platform for communication immediately after the Tōhoku Earthquake and Tsunami. They discuss how peer-to-peer communication became invaluable during the earthquake, and note that the multimodal aspect of social media, whereby posts can include hashtags, images, and hyperlinked content (Cho et al., 2013, p. 29), create a dense network in which members of the public can receive up-to-date and real-time information about a disaster. For them (Cho et al., 2013), social media is an increasingly common and trusted means to receive information during crises among social media users (p. 30).

Although these studies point to the democratizing force of social media in allowing so-called ordinary members of the public to claim authority over the messages that are disseminated in crises, they also demonstrate an omission in the current literature on the inaccessibility of social media as a communication tool for people with disabilities. The inaccessibility of social media for people with disabilities speaks to two larger and interrelated problems this group experiences in disaster situations. The first problem is that people with disabilities are prevented from receiving life-saving information and services that are often available to non-disabled individuals due to inaccessible forms of communication. As Njelesani et al. (2014) observe, societal ableism manifests itself in the failure for governments to recognize that "persons with disabilities may have some specific needs" (p. 84) that diverge from the general population.

The second problem is that people with disabilities are all too easily typecast as helpless "victims" by current disaster management literature, which engenders "ableist assumptions" in its categorization of people with disabilities as "vulnerable" or "at risk" (Njelesani et al., 2014, p. 843). This construction overlooks the "obvious flaw" of disaster management discourse which uses an "able-bodied 'one size fits all' model" instead of models that utilize the knowledge of people with disabilities who already experience environmental and access barriers in their daily lives (Fjord, 2007, p. 22).

Indeed, these existing challenges might be precisely why people with disabilities *should* be included in the creation and evaluation of DRR policies; many people with disabilities are already equipped with important attributes necessary to cope with uncertain and potentially calamitous situations: resilience and adaptability (Abbott & Porter, 2013; Gerber, 2009; Ivey et al., 2014; Nakamura, 2009). Wisner (2002) and Stough and Kelman (2017) share this sentiment and argue that the inclusion of people with disabilities in disaster management policy ultimately benefits a greater number of individuals by accounting for variability in evacuation behaviors, disaster preparedness, and recovery rates following a disaster. While Njelesani et al. (2014) do note that "persons with disabilities may have some specific needs" (p. 84) that diverge from the general population, current nomenclature ultimately disempowers this group and overlooks the possibility that people with disabilities may be valuable and agential contributors to DRR planning (p. 79).

The following analysis will discuss the negative consequences that occurred during Hurricane Katrina and the Tōhoku Earthquake and Tsunami because emergency personnel and government organizations failed to integrate people with disabilities and their needs within their disaster preparation and intervention strategies. I will focus my attention on the problems of miscommunication and lack of accessible communication for people with disabilities during these disasters. This chapter follows Ivey et al.'s (2014) contention that it is imperative to involve people with disabilities in DRR discourse and emergency management.

Disability-inclusive emergency preparedness, response, and recovery procedures are crucial to the goal of eliminating disparities in the mortality rate between people with disabilities and non-disabled people. Indeed, as Kelman and Stough (2014) have observed, hazards do not necessarily have to become disasters leading to losses in human life; for these scholars, disasters "are actively designed by societies that fail to include the needs of all people" (p. 5). In other words, disaster, like disability, is a social construct that can further entrench inequality between "vulnerable" and non-vulnerable populations by creating barriers to effective, timely, and accessible communication. A shift toward using communication modes and technologies that are rooted in universal or inclusive design principles is vital to ensuring equitable treatment between disabled and non-disabled populations during disasters, as well as increasing the likelihood of survival for *all* individuals by enabling information to be diversified and repeated across various formats, as opposed to being "undifferentiated in content and placement" (Burke et al., 2010, p. 28).

Hurricane Katrina

Between August 23, 2005, and August 31, 2005, Hurricane Katrina struck the Gulf Coast of the United States of America. The category three storm strengthened into a category five hurricane on August 25, making landfall at Aventura and Hallandale Beach in Florida and then onto Louisiana and Mississippi on August 29. Katrina is notorious for being one of the deadliest hurricanes in the United States (Knabb et al., 2005; Brunkard et al., 2008), having caused an extreme number of casualties, damage and loss of property, and mass relocation of victims. The New Orleans metropolitan area and Mississippi coastline were greatly affected by storm surges, flooding, and strong winds, leading to the obliteration of entire communities (Knabb et al., 2005). Official estimates place the death toll of Hurricane Katrina at 1833 and property damage at around $175 billion USD (United States Census Bureau, 2015). This makes Hurricane Katrina the costliest hurricane in the recorded history of the United States. Among the populations hardest hit by the disaster were African-Americans, people with disabilities, and older adults. Brunkard et al.'s (2008) report on Katrina determined that the mortality rate for Black people in Louisiana who were 18 years or older was between 1.7 and four times higher than white people (p. 217). The number of deaths among older adults and people with disabilities was also significantly higher than the general population. Markwell and Ratard's (2014) study reported that people aged 75 years and above amounted to 47% of the total number of deaths among Louisiana residents (p. 538).

In much of the academic literature pertaining to Hurricane Katrina, people with disabilities are commonly believed to have been "disproportionately affected" by this disaster as compared to their able-bodied counterparts (Abbott & Porter, 2013; Hemingway & Priestley, 2006; Zoraster, 2012). While the National Council on Disability (NCD, 2006) concedes that "it is difficult to determine precisely what percentage of hurricane-related deaths were people with disabilities," statistics from Biloxi, Mississippi; Mobile, Alabama; and New Orleans, Louisiana, indicate that a significant number of individuals living in the three cities hit hardest by Katrina were disabled (around 155,000 individuals or about 25 percent of these cities' populations). Moreover, White et al. (2006) point to the 2000 census for the states of Mississippi, Alabama, and Louisiana, which claimed that there was at least one person with a disability living in over one million households in these three states.

Meanwhile, the National Organization on Disability (NOD) published the Report on Special Needs Assessment for Katrina Evacuees (SNAKE) Project (2005) to evaluate the impact of Hurricane Katrina on "disability and aging specific" populations. In their finding that "traditional response and recovery systems are often not able to successfully satisfy" the service and humans needs of people with disabilities and older adults, the SNAKE report drew attention to the already large percentage of people with disabilities living in hard-hit cities including New Orleans (23.2 percent) and St. Bernard Parish (23.4 percent). The report used these statistics to expose problems relating to traditional practices in emergency planning, preparedness, response, and recovery procedures, but also to assert that people with disabilities have "refined skill-sets and expertise" that can be leveraged during disasters so as to minimize loss of life across *all* demographics. A corresponding aim of the project was to recommend short and long-term actions to improve the way emergency professionals and response organizations attend to the "needs, geography, demographics and resources of individuals within their local areas" (SNAKE Project, 2006, p. 3). The next section will provide an overview of the 2011 Tōhoku Earthquake and Tsunami, providing details about the events leading to the nuclear accident at the Fukushima Daiichi Nuclear Power Plant and the mortality rate among disabled populations in the areas hardest hit by the tsunami.

The 2011 Tōhoku Earthquake and Tsunami

On March 11, 2011, an earthquake registering a magnitude of 9.0 struck at approximately 2:46 p.m. (JST) off the northeast coast of Honshu, the most populous island in Japan. The earthquake resulted in the production of tsunami waves as high as 40.5 meters (Takayama, 2017, p. 248), which subsequently caused extreme destruction in the Tōhoku region, particularly the prefectures of Miyagi, Iwate, and Fukushima. An unexpected and severe by-product of the earthquake and tsunami was the nuclear accident at the

Fukushima Daiichi Nuclear Power Plant in Ōkuma, Fukushima Prefecture. The nuclear accident led not only to the contamination of several units in the plant, but also to the release of radiation into the surrounding area and the subsequent evacuation of residents. There are parts of Fukushima that are still "off-limits" even after a decade, though the Japanese government reopened some areas prior to the torch procession for the Tokyo 2020 Summer Olympics (Yamaguchi, 2020).

According to the National Police Agency of Japan, the total number of deaths related directly and indirectly to the disaster, as well as those presumed dead, is 22,131 ("Japan marks 8th anniversary," 2019). In addition to its significant death toll, the Tōhoku Earthquake and Tsunami is notorious for being the strongest earthquake in the country's recorded history. In September 2012, the national broadcasting service of Japan (*Nippon Hōsō Kyōkai*, otherwise referred to as NHK or the Japan Broadcasting Corporation) conducted a survey in 31 municipalities in Iwate, Miyagi, and Fukushima. The survey determined that the mortality rate among people with disabilities was 1.43 percent, a significant rise from the general population which had a mortality rate of 0.78 percent (Osamu, 2014, p. 143). Other surveys indicated that the rate of mortality for people with disabilities was even higher than these percentages. Ono (2013) stated that the mortality rate was 2.5 times higher for people with disabilities than their non-disabled counterparts. According to an official survey from the Miyagi prefectural government (March 29, 2012), the total number of deaths within the disabled population was about 3.5 percent (Osamu, 2014, p. 143). A report by Fujii (2012) for the Japan Disability Forum found that people with disabilities had a mortality rate that was twice as high as non-disabled people (cited in Takayama, 2017, p. 249).

There are a number of reasons why people with disabilities were among the groups hardest hit by the Tōhoku Earthquake and Tsunami. In April 2011, the Japan National Assembly of Disabled Peoples' International (DPI-Japan) submitted the Petition against Countermeasures against East Japan Great Earthquake and Tsunami Disaster (Misawa, 2011). This document identified some of the major impediments faced by people with disabilities in the disaster, including a lack of closed captioning on disaster-related programming and news, as well as insufficient access to home helpers following temporary relocation.

DPI-Japan stated that some people with disabilities who needed to evacuate their hometowns could not receive assistance from daytime helpers in their temporary location, since "bureaucrats at the city office would say 'it was your decision to evacuate' and could not reach conclusions" (Misawa, 2011; cf. Abbott & Porter, 2013, p. 850). Yet studies have shown that individuals within the disability community are not affected equally during disasters. One alarming finding for Takayama (2017) was that DHH people had the highest mortality rate among all disability categories, with a total of 2.00 percent across the three prefectures of Iwate, Miyagi, and Fukushima (p. 250). According to Takayama (2017), an inadequate number of sign language interpreters to assist social workers in relocating DHH people to evacuation shelters is one way to account for this statistic, since certain members of the DHH community "decided to stay in their damaged homes" rather than follow the advice of the social workers to evacuate (p. 250).

Moving from specific to more general literature about the unique communication challenges experienced by DHH people during disasters, Ivey et al. (2014) mention that the community "fail[s] to receive the necessary information [to enable survival] in accessible and culturally appropriate forms and distribution channels" (p. 149). Problems relating to inaccessible or inappropriate formats for conveying information, the quality of information that is presented in such formats, and communicating with first responders and emergency personnel who are not proficient in the cultural and linguistic specificities of various disability groups all contribute to a reduced chance of survival for this population.

The following section will begin the task of understanding the particular problems faced by the disability community that entrench the social construction of this group as a "vulnerable" population during disasters. A comparative analysis of media content relating to Hurricane Katrina and the Tōhoku Earthquake and Tsunami will reveal the importance of including the voices of people with disabilities in DRR policy and practice.

COMPARATIVE ANALYSIS OF MEDIA CONTENT ABOUT HURRICANE KATRINA AND THE TŌHOKU EARTHQUAKE AND TSUNAMI

Methodology

This study involved collecting online news media stories from the database NewsBank and searching online archives for major English-language newspapers in Japan. NewsBank was used in order to obtain articles relating to Hurricane Katrina. NewsBank was chosen due to its wide-ranging access to internationally established and recognized news sources. For the Tōhoku Earthquake and Tsunami, individual searches of the online archives of *The Japan Times* and *The Mainichi* were conducted. *The Japan Times* was chosen as it has "the largest circulation of all domestic English-language newspapers" and is read by the largest number of non-Japanese readers within the country ("120-year history of The Japan Times"). Meanwhile, *The Mainichi* was chosen because it is connected with one of the four national newspapers of Japan, *The Mainichi Shimbun*. *The Mainichi*, established in 1922, has a long history of publishing articles for a non-Japanese readership in Japan ("The History of the Mainichi Shimbun"), first as a daily newspaper and then later as a news website.

The primary search terms used to retrieve articles from NewsBank relating to Hurricane Katrina were "Hurricane Katrina," "communication," "disabilities," "Deaf people," and "blind people." The primary search terms for stories about the Tōhoku Earthquake and Tsunami were "earthquake," "disabilities," "Tōhoku Earthquake and Tsunami," "Deaf people," and "blind people." The reason that the impairments of deafness and blindness were included in the search terms was due to existing scholarly literature having suggested that the particular communication needs of these groups are often insufficiently met or ignored during emergency preparedness and response stages. Problems experienced by these groups include but are not limited to: the absence of or insufficient number of sign language interpreters at evacuation shelters, lack of closed captioning on television programs, and lack of audio description of visual content contained in emergency news reports (Calgaro et al., 2020; Gerber, 2009; White, 2006).

The date range for the search was not limited. Following the retrieval of the articles, a manual review of their content led to the selection and omission of articles that did not contain explicit reference to problems relating to inaccessible or inappropriate modes of communication for people with disabilities in the disasters. A manual review of the articles meant that some were not excluded even if certain key terms did not appear in their headline. Thirteen articles retrieved via NewsBank have been included in the current study, based on their fulfillment of one or more of the following criteria: direct reference to accessibility problems and/or recommendations relating to Hurricane Katrina; reports from independent federal agencies or disability organizations recommending the inclusion of people with disabilities in emergency communication activities; or comparisons of disabled and non-disabled populations' experiences of Hurricane Katrina. Seven and three articles from *The Japan Times* and *The Mainichi* respectively were chosen based on their fulfillment of at least one of the three criteria mentioned above, albeit in relation to the Tōhoku Earthquake and Tsunami rather than Hurricane Katrina.

The unit of analysis for the searches was "people with disabilities," since this chapter focuses on a minoritized group deemed to be negatively and differentially impacted upon during natural disasters as a result of the group's alleged "vulnerability." It became important to consider whether such articles followed a traditional ableist model in discounting the role of societal barriers in amplifying the "vulnerability" of this group, rather than a social construction model of disability that views vulnerabilities as "pre-exist[ing] in society as chronic, ongoing conditions [...that] are only unmasked by hazard, thus making vulnerabilities visible as the disaster emerges" (Kelman & Stough, 2014, p. 8).

FRAMING THEORY AND CONSTRUCTIONS OF DISABILITY AND PEOPLE WITH DISABILITIES IN NEWS MEDIA

A comparative analysis of media content about Hurricane Katrina and the Tōhoku Earthquake and Tsunami elucidates the current inadequacies of emergency management planning and procedures for people with disabilities. The analysis also indicates that news media is consistent in representing people with disabilities as an especially vulnerable group that requires additional and unique forms of support during natural crises.

Framing theory contends that the media shapes an audience's understanding of a story or phenomenon through deliberate choices in language, visuals, tone, and information. Following on from the work of Goffman (1986 [1974]), media disability scholars including Haller and Zhang (2010), Haller (2000), and Clogston (1990) argue that the way the media typically packages its stories about disability and people with disabilities fall within a limited set of predictable, and often stereotypical, frames. These scholars have typically called out such frames as being stigmatizing and regressive in their representation. Content analysis of stories about Hurricane Katrina and the Tōhoku Earthquake and Tsunami suggests that both American and Japanese English-language news sources oscillate between representing people with disabilities as the tragic and inevitable victims of large-scale disasters (Hemingway & Priestley, 2006), and as individuals capable of resourcefulness and quick thinking in the immediate response period.

The following section identifies three frames that predominate in news media content about Hurricane Katrina and the Tōhoku Earthquake and Tsunami:

1. Evacuation procedures are inadequate and poorly arranged for people with disabilities;
2. Existing evacuation response procedures impede accessible and timely communication of information for people with disabilities; and
3. People with disabilities are a "vulnerable group" whose vulnerability increases due to lack of consideration in disaster preparedness.

Discussion of these frames yields important insight into the role that media plays in not only directing audience attention toward the considerable difficulties some people with disabilities experience in natural disasters, but also the systemic barriers that prevent emergency management policies from becoming more inclusive *and* applicable to a greater number of individuals. These frames continue to construct people with disabilities as a group whose needs must be better served by policymakers, governments, and medical services in the event of an emergency, rather than individuals who can make a vital contribution to such planning themselves.

Frame One: Inadequate and Poorly Arranged Evacuation Procedures

Newspaper articles indicated that the hardship people with disabilities experienced during Hurricane Katrina was exacerbated as a result of evacuation procedures that failed to take into account their impairments and use of different assistive technologies. Singer's (2006) feature revealed that people with disabilities were forced to abandon their assistive devices during the evacuation process. US Fed News (USA) ("Government accountability office," 2017) reported on mistakes that were made during the response and relief efforts of Hurricane Katrina, noting that the disaster functioned as a catalyst for state and municipal governments to re-evaluate existing procedures in emergencies. The article referred to initiatives that were established in the wake of the disaster, including the Post-Katrina Emergency Management Reform Act (2006). Quoting from this act, the article indicated that people with disabilities, those with limited English proficiency, and families were among the most disadvantaged by the disaster. Furthermore, it used specific images of people with disabilities within the disaster to highlight the inadequate and hazardous nature of evacuation attempts, for example, that after abandoning their wheelchairs, some wheelchair users could not evacuate because they could not "wait in long lines for evacuation buses" ("Government accountability office," 2017).

News sources about the Tōhoku Earthquake and Tsunami also raised concerns about the inadequacy of post-disaster infrastructure for people with disabilities. One feature for *The Japan Times* ("More barrier-free steps," 2012) commented that barrier-free design must be taken into account during post-evacuation planning. Shunsuke Abe, a wheelchair-using person, shared that his temporary housing in Miyagi prefecture only included a ramp outside. Although the inclusion of an outside ramp does demonstrate some architectural consideration toward the accessibility needs of those with mobility impairments, Abe criticized the lack of barrier-free design within the housing's interior. Yusuke Ishimori, another wheelchair-using person, had difficulty using temporary buses because they were not disability accessible. He was quoted as saying, "So people with disabilities in disaster-hit regions can't even go on an outing?" ("More barrier-free steps," 2012).

Frame Two: Existing Evacuation Response Procedures Impede Accessible and Timely Communication of Information to People with Disabilities

A tacit theme in media content about the disasters was the disproportionate challenges of the DHH community based on inappropriate crisis intervention and mobilization strategies. This theme connects with academic research that claims DHH people "are often the last group to receive emergency information" (Ivey et al., 2014, p. 149). As a result, out of all disability categories, DHH people are often hardest hit in disasters, both in terms of mortality and injury rate and perceived difficulties in responding to evacuation calls and communicating with non-DHH others at evacuation shelters. The thematic focus of newspaper articles on DHH people also supports existing scholarship that aims to particularize the experiences of people with disabilities and their impairments in order to enhance disaster preparedness and communication (Takayama, 2017, p. 248). The latter issue connects with Otake's (2013) article for *The Japan Times*, which focused on the experiences of deaf people in Miyagi Prefecture during the relief stage of the Tōhoku Earthquake and Tsunami. One elderly woman who is deaf, Nobuko Kikuchi, "breaks down" when describing her difficulties in living at the evacuation shelter one month after the earthquake: "she can't hear any of the announcements on food rationing and other assistance." Kikuchi's experience seems common among DHH people in this disaster, many of whom had trouble receiving adequate and appropriate support at evacuation shelters due to a "lack of cultural and linguistic crisis mobilization" (Takayama, 2017, p. 250).

News stories about Hurricane Katrina often highlighted how the American federal government had "failed dismally" (White, 2006) in its efforts to support DHH people in the disaster, many of whom lacked access to essential information due to loss of mobile technologies and inaccessible evacuation warnings. Media content, therefore, supports the findings of major disability organizations including the NOD's SNAKE Project that concluded the "most underserved group" (p. 8) at evacuation shelters were DHH people. The SNAKE Project determined that many DHH individuals "had no access to the vital flow of information" (p. 9) at shelters because the information was not accessible to them; for example, only 56 percent of shelters had areas where oral announcements had been transcribed, and 80 percent of shelters lacked TTY devices (SNAKE Project, 2005, pp. 8–9).

Doolittle's (2005) article noted the inadequacy of standard emergency preparedness campaigns for DHH people, which often told residents to "tune in to local TV and radio stations for instructions from your local government as to how to proceed." Another article in *USA Today* (Livadas, 2005) included the story of two deaf-blind brothers who were "oblivious to Katrina's danger" because telecommunications networks failed in the disaster. The brothers emerged from their home after the storm subsided to find their neighborhood totally abandoned. Shelters were portrayed as being inadequate in their accommodations for this group of people because of a reliance on auditory announcements (Singer, 2006). This is consistent with the findings of the National Council on Disability (NCD), which stated in its 2006 report on Hurricanes Katrina and Rita that information in the majority of evacuation shelters was inaccessible for those with sensory disabilities. Furthermore, the report (NCD, 2006) suggests that DHH people were not only disadvantaged at evacuation shelters because of inaccessible telecommunications (lack of closed-captioning televisions and TTY), but also in being unable to contact family and friends with the phones made available to them.

Articles in the wake of Hurricane Katrina also drew attention to the need for relief centers, planners at local and state levels, and telecommunications networks to reform existing practices to ensure future communication in disasters was accessible for DHH people. For instance, Johnson's (2005) feature for *Independent Record* describes how Montana state arranged a mass donation of text phones to DHH people in Louisiana, many of whom had lost their phones in the hurricane and thus their main way to receive information about recovery efforts. Johnson's article, like Jardine (2005) and Baker (2005), used Hurricane Katrina as a springboard for demonstrating how broadcasters, volunteer agencies, and state governments responded to criticisms about inequality between disabled and non-disabled people in both disasters and daily life. Baker's (2005) article for *The Washington Times* focused on how the National Court Reporters Association was "urging the House to pass an industry training bill" for closed-captioning services, arguing that more workers would be needed to meet a January 2006 deadline for all television programming to be accessible for DHH people. Hurricane Katrina is mentioned in passing in the article as a cautionary tale for what can happen if closed-captioning is not universally available in disasters: "it's not just an inconvenience, it puts them [DHH people] at risk" (Golden, qtd. in Baker, 2005).

By contrast, "Being deaf means he can really help" (Jardine, 2005) is initially a morale-boosting narrative about DeWayne Burger, a Red Cross volunteer who is deaf and who offered his assistance at the temporary shelter at the Houston Astrodome. Much of the article details Burger's life and family, including how he communicates with his hearing children. As a result, it misses an opportunity to raise concern over the often-insufficient number of emergency personnel who are trained to work with DHH people. According to the article, Burger at the time was "one of only two deaf people in the country trained to teach Red Cross CPR and first aid classes" (Jardine, 2005). The SNAKE report appears to corroborate Burger's concern about a lack of personnel available to assist this population; it concluded that "less than 30% of [evacuation] shelters had access to American Sign Language interpreters" (SNAKE project, 2005, p. 8).

Frame Three: People with Disabilities Are a "Vulnerable Group" Whose Vulnerability Increases Due to Lack of Consideration in Disaster Preparedness

Media content routinely described people with disabilities as being disproportionately affected during Hurricane Katrina and the Tōhoku Earthquake and Tsunami. In the case of Hurricane Katrina, an emphasis on the "vulnerability" of people with disabilities (often defined as this group having been disproportionately affected as a result of poor communication channels or inaccessible evacuation procedures) appeared in 10 out of 13 news features over a period of 11 years (2006–2011). When it came to news stories about the Tōhoku Earthquake and Tsunami, a similar pattern emerged; four out of seven articles and two out of three articles from *The Japan Times* and *The Mainichi* respectively referred to the unequal challenges faced by disabled and non-disabled populations in this disaster. The designation of people with disabilities as "vulnerable" in these stories belies how disaster paradigms rely on standardized, able-bodied approaches that by definition imagine death as the inevitable consequence of impairment for people with disabilities (Fjord, 2007, p. 14). Hudson (2009) described people with disabilities as "America's most vulnerable citizens," while Magee (2018), reporting on the United Nations for World Tsunami Awareness Day, claimed that "improving resilience" was of primary concern to ensure "those most vulnerable" are not abandoned during emergency situations.

The International Federation of Red Cross and Red Crescent Societies define "vulnerability" as "the diminished capacity of an individual or group to anticipate, cope with, resist and recover from the impact of a man-made hazard" ("What is vulnerability?"). This definition of vulnerability appears to have infiltrated news stories about the Tōhoku Earthquake and Tsunami, which focused on efforts made by the Japanese government to reduce the likelihood of fatalities for disabled and older people in future disaster situations. The main law that was revised to tackle the issue of people with disabilities being left behind in disaster-affected areas is The Basic Law on Disaster Control Measures;[3] this law allows municipal governments to share information about people with disabilities with community associations, fire departments, and welfare groups ("Upgrading anti-disaster measures," 2016). However, problems persist in implementing this law out of concerns for individual privacy ("Cities slow to submit info on people in need of special evacuation assistance," 2015) and "the burden in obtaining individual consent" ("Hyogo pref. to take steps," 2017).

The Mainichi also included a story about an emergency preparedness initiative launched by Sumida ward in Tokyo, in which people with disabilities are encouraged to fill out a "workbook" that includes information about their disability and medications ("Tokyo's Sumida ward spearheads project," 2016). Following an evacuation drill held at Sumida Fureai Center in October 2015, Sumida ward declared that a major way to increase the survival rate of people with disabilities in disasters is for their "information… to be swiftly transmitted to evacuation staff members and volunteers." While the "workbook" project and revisions to the Basic Law on Disaster Control Measures are two ways that emergency management planning takes into account the needs of people with disabilities in disasters, what is missing is the direct involvement of people with disabilities in this very process. Gerber (2009) writes, "successful planning and emergency preparedness must include first-hand expertise of disabled people themselves" (p. 73). Ivey et al. (2014) also stress that DHH people should be involved in preparedness research not only so that their needs are served, but so that society in general can benefit from their "capacity and resilience" (p. 154). The authors cite the "rapid uptake of new technologies" including smartphone use, video communications, and texting by this group, which could be taken up as effective modes of alternative communication for non-deaf people as well (Ivey et al., 2014).

Indeed, the undue focus on legislation and local government projects in these stories problematically reinforces the trope of people with disabilities as a protected group who must rely on non-disabled people to rescue them in disasters. As one senior official for the Hyogo prefectural government announced, "our utmost mission is to save the lives of those vulnerable to disasters" ("Hyogo pref. to take steps," 2017). That may be so; however, a glaring omission in news stories about Hurricane Katrina and the Tōhoku

Earthquake and Tsunami was a consideration of how people with disabilities may be empowered to help themselves in disaster situations if provided with adequate, relevant, and accessible emergency preparedness information. Moreover, these stories do not consider how people with disabilities negotiate environmental, architectural, and technological barriers in their everyday lives, and as such can provide valuable knowledge that can be used to enhance the effectiveness of accommodations during disasters for all populations.

CONCLUSION

This chapter undertook a comparative content analysis of media coverage about Hurricane Katrina and the Tōhoku Earthquake and Tsunami. It did so in order to identify how the "vulnerability" of people with disabilities in natural disasters is the result of failure within existing emergency management planning to take into account the need for alternative preparation, response, and relief strategies to safeguard this group against unnecessary risk. According to the Head of the UN Office for Disaster Risk Reduction (UNISDR) ("UN global survey explains," 2013), "The key reason why a disproportionate number of disabled persons suffer and die in disasters is because their needs are ignored and neglected by the official planning process." This statement goes against the prevailing ableist assumption that the "vulnerability" of people with disabilities and suffering in disasters are inevitable consequences of their impairments.

This chapter compared media content in the two disasters to single out examples in which emergency planning and response strategies failed to be accessible to people with disabilities. Yet the analysis also demonstrates that irrespective of geographical and climatic variations, people with disabilities are universally disadvantaged in disasters and that there is an urgent need for governments, aid groups, and volunteer organizations to include them in future emergency management planning.

In the words of the SNAKE Project, it is incumbent on emergency professionals to "seek out and utilize the expertise of disability and aging networks to… eliminate barriers to effective service delivery" (SNAKE Project, 2005). In so doing, they may not only minimize loss of life in disaster situations but work toward establishing emergency management procedures that promote social inclusion and collaboration.

NOTES

1. Since writing this chapter, Japan has experienced other destructive typhoons including Faxai (also known as Reiwa 1 Bōsō Peninsula Typhoon), the 15th typhoon of the 2019 Pacific typhoon season. However, in 2020, no typhoons made landfall in Japan.
2. The term "ableism" refers to discriminatory treatment of people with disabilities on the basis that being non-disabled is a superior form of embodiment. Ableism

has as one of its underlying assumptions that "disabled people require 'fixing'" (Eisenmenger, 2019).

3. This Act is also known in English as the Basic Act on Disaster Management, which was originally enacted on November 15, 1961 but later revised in June 1997.

REFERENCES

Abbott, D., & Porter, S. (2013). Environmental hazard and disabled people: From vulnerable to expert to interconnected. *Disability & Society, 28*(6), 839–852. https://doi.org/10.1080/09687599.2013.802222

Alexander, D., Gaillard, J. C., & Wisner, B. (2012). Disability and disaster. In B. Wisner, J. C. Gaillard, & I. Kelman (Eds.), *The Routledge handbook of hazards and disaster risk reduction* (pp. 413–423). Routledge. https://doi.org/10.4324/9780203844236.ch34

Baker, C. (2005, August 31). Caption writers push for training. *The Washington Times*, p. C10. Retrieved December 5, 2019, from https://infoweb-newsbank-com.proxy.library.nyu.edu/apps/news/document-view?p=WORLDNEWS&docref=news/10C579939EAF54D8

Battle, D. E. (2015). Persons with communication disabilities in natural disasters, war, and/or conflicts. *Communication Disorders Quarterly, 36*(4), 231–240. https://doi.org/10.1177/2F1525740114545980

Brunkard, J., Namulanda, G., & Ratard, R. (2008). Hurricane Katrina deaths, Louisiana, 2005. *Disaster Medicine and Public Health Preparedness, 2*(4), 215–223. https://doi.org/10.1097/DMP.0b013e31818aaf55

Burke, J., Spence, P. R., & Lachlan, K. A. (2010). Crisis preparation, media use, and information seeking during Hurricane Ike: Lessons learned for emergency communication. *Journal of Emergency Management, 8*(5), 27–37. https://doi.org/10.5055/jem.2010.0030

Calgaro, E., Craig, N., Craig, L., Dominey-Howes, D., & Allen, J. (2021). Silent no more: Identifying and breaking through the barriers that d/Deaf people face in responding to hazards and disasters. *International Journal of Disaster Risk Reduction, 57.* https://doi.org/10.1016/j.ijdrr.2021.102156

Calgaro, E., Villeneuve, M., & Roberts, G. (2020). Inclusion: Moving beyond resilience in the pursuit of transformative and just DRR practices for persons with disabilities. In A. Lukasiewicz & C. Baldwin (Eds.), *Natural hazards and disaster justice: Challenges for Australia and its neighbours* (pp. 319–348). Palgrave Macmillan. https://doi.org/10.1007/978-981-140466-2_17

Cho, S. E., Jung, K., & Park, H. W. (2013). Social media use during Japan's 2011 earthquake: How Twitter transforms the locus of crisis communication. *Media International Australia, 141*(1), 28–40. https://doi.org/10.1177/1329878X1314900105

Cities slow to submit info on people in need of special evacuation assistance. (2015, March 10). *The Japan Times.* Retrieved November 30, 2019, from https://www.japantimes.co.jp/news/2015/03/10/national/cities-slow-to-submit-info-on-people-in-need-of-special-evacuation-assistance/

Clogston, J. S. (1990). *Disability coverage in 16 newspapers.* Advocado Press.

Doolittle, A. (2005, October 6). Katrina reveals lack of resources to evacuate deaf. *The Washington Times*, p. B01. Retrieved December 5, 2019, from https://www.washingtontimes.com/news/2005/oct/5/20051005-095340-4787r/

Eisenmenger, A. (2019, December 12). Ableism 101: What it is, what it looks like, and what we can do to to [sic] fix it. *Access Living*. Retrieved December 21, 2019, from https://www.accessliving.org/newsroom/blog/ableism-101/

Ellis, K., & Kent, M. (2011). *Disability and new media*. Routledge. https://doi.org/10.4324/9780203831915

Fjord, L. (2007). Disasters, race, and disability: [Un]seen through the political lens on Katrina. *The Journal of Race and Policy, 3*(1), 7–27. Retrieved March 1, 2022, from https://web.p.ebscohost.com/ehost/pdfviewer/pdfviewer?vid=0&sid=a0c62260-1d00-47f9-823c-a475236ff536%40redis

Fujii, K. (2012, October 31). The Great East Japan Earthquake and disabled persons—Background to their high mortality rate. *DINF*. Retrieved December 5, 2019, from https://www.ding.ne.jp/doc/english/twg/escap_121031/fujii.html

Gerber, E. (2009). Describing tragedy: The information access needs of blind people in emergency-related circumstances. *Human Organization, 68*(1), 73–81. https://doi.org/10.17730/humo.68.1.tm17684j7u301668

Goffman, E. (1986). *Frame analysis: An essay on the organization of experience*. Northeastern University Press. (Original work published 1974).

Goggin, G., & Newell, C. (2003). *Digital disability: The social construction of disability in new media*. Rowman & Littlefield.

Government accountability office: Report. (2017, February 9). *US Fed News (USA)*. Retrieved December 5, 2019, from https://search-ebscohost-com.proxy.library.nyu.edu/login.aspx?direct=true&db=edsnbk&AN=1627092E3308BE38&site=eds-live

Haller, B. (2000). How the news frames disability: Print media coverage of the Americans with Disabilities Act. *Social Science and Disability, 1*, 55–83. https://doi.org/10.1016/S1479-3547(00)80005-6

Haller, B., & Zhang, L. (2010). Survey of disabled people about media representations. *Media & Disability Resources*. Retrieved December 3, 2019, from https://mediadisability.wordpress.com/survey/

Hansson, S., Orru, K., Siibak, A., Bäck, A., Krüger, M., Gabel, F., & Morsut, C. (2020). Communication-related vulnerability to disasters: A heuristic framework. *International Journal of Disaster Risk Reduction, 51*, 1–9. https://doi.org/10.1016/j.ijdrr.2020.101931

Hemingway, L., & Priestley, M. (2006). Natural hazards, human vulnerability and disabling societies: A disaster for disabled people? *Review of Disability Studies: An International Journal, 2*(3), 57–67. Retrieved March 2, 2022, from https://www.rdsjournal.org/index.php/journal/article/view/337/1037

Hjorth, K., & Kim, K.-H. Y. (2011). The mourning after: A case study of social media in the 3.11 earthquake disaster in Japan. *Television & New Media, 12*(6), 552–559. https://doi.org/10.1177/1527476411418351

Hudson, A. (2009, August 12). Disaster plans leave disabled behind—Report. *The Washington Times*, p. A01. Retrieved December 5, 2019, from https://www.washingtontimes.com/news/2009/aug/12/disaster-plans-leave-disabled-behind/

Hyogo pref. to take steps to boost disaster assistance measures for elderly, disabled. (2017, January 16). *The Mainichi*. Retrieved November 30, 2019, from https://mainichi.jp/english/articles/ 20170116/p2a/00m/0na/010000c

Ivey, S. L., Tseng, W., Dahrouge, D., Engelman, A., Neuhauser, L., Huang, D., & Gurung, S. (2014). Assessment of state- and territorial-level preparedness capacity for serving deaf and hard-of-hearing populations in disasters. *Public Health Reports, 129*(2), 148–155. https://doi.org/10.1177/003335491412900208

Japan marks 8th anniversary of 3/11 disaster in Tohoku region. (2019, March 11). *The Asahi Shimbun.* Retrieved November 30, 2019, from http://www.asahi.com/ajw/articles/AJ201903110021.html

Jardine, J. (2005, September 11). Being deaf means he can really help. *The Modesto Bee,* p. B1. Retrieved December 5, 2019, from https://search-ebscohost-com.proxy.library.nyu.edu/login.aspx?direct=true&db=edsnba&AN=10C9EBBAAF886948&site=eds-live

Johnson, C. S. (2005, September 19). State donates 118 text phones to Louisiana to help deaf. *Independent Record.* Retrieved December 5, 2019, from https://search-ebscohost-com.proxy.library.nyu.edu/login.aspx?direct=true&db=edsnba&AN=12B5CE7895167BB8 & site=eds-live

Kelman, I., & Stough, L. M. (2014). (Dis)ability and (Dis)aster. In I. Kelman & L. M. Stough (Eds.), *Disability and disaster: Explorations and exchanges* (pp. 3–14). Palgrave Macmillan.

Kent, M., & Ellis, K. (2015). People with disability and new disaster communications: Access and the social media mash-up. *Disability & Society, 30*(3), 319–431. https://doi.org/10.1080/09687599.2015.1021756

Knabb, R. D., Rhome, J. R., & Brown, D. P. (2005, December 20). *Tropical cyclone report: Hurricane Katrina, 23–30 August 2005.* National Hurricane Center. Retrieved January 10, 2022, from http://www.disastersrus.org/katrina/TCR-AL122005_Katrina.pdf

Livadas, G. (2005, September 11). Communication lines frayed for displaced deaf. *USA Today.* Retrieved December 5, 2019, from https://search-ebscohost-com.proxy.library.nyu.edu/login.aspx?direct=true&db=edsnba&AN=127C309259D098C8&site=eds-live

Magee, S. K. (2018, November 6). Mayor of tsunami-hit city stresses resilience and inclusivity at U.N. *The Japan Times.* Retrieved November 30, 2019, from https://www.japantimes.co.jp/news/2018/11/06/national/mayor-tsunami-hit-city-stresses-resilience-inclusivity-u-n/

Markwell, P., & Ratard, R. (2014). Deaths directly caused by Hurricane Katrina. *Louisiana Department of Health.* Retrieved December 5, 2019, from http://ldh.la.gov/assets/oph/Center-PHCH/Center-CH/stepi/specialstudies/2014Popwell Ratard_KatrinaDeath_PostedOnline.pdf

Misawa, S. (2011, April 20). Petition for countermeasures against East Japan Great Earthquake and Tsunami disasters. *DPI-Japan.*, Retrieved December 5, 2019, from http://dpi.cocolog-nifty.com

More barrier-free steps urged in disaster zone. (2012, June 27). *The Japan Times.* Retrieved November 30, 2019, from https://www.japantimes.co.jp/news/2012/06/27/national/more-barrier-free-steps-urged-in-disaster-zone/

Nakamura, K. (2009). Disability, destitution, and disaster: Surviving the 1995 Great Hanshin Earthquake in Japan. *Human Organization, 68*(1), 82–88. https://doi.org/10.17730/humo.68.1.bp20n61l0341l68x

National Council on Disability. (2006). *The Impact of Hurricanes Katrina and Rita on people with disabilities: A look back and remaining challenges.* Retrieved December 5, 2019, from http://www.ncd.gov/publications/2006/Aug072006

National Organization on Disability. (2005, October 5). *Report on Special Needs Assessment for Katrina Evacuees (SNAKE) Project.* Retrieved October 25, 2022, from https://tap.gallaudet.edu/Emergency/Nov05Conference/EmergencyReports/katrina_snake_report.pdf

Njelesani, J., Cleaver, S., & Tataryn, M. (2014). Practical strategies to meet the rights of persons with disabilities in disaster management initiatives. In D. Mitchell & V. Karr (Eds.), *Crises, conflict and disability: Ensuring equality* (pp. 84–89). Routledge. https://doi.org/10.4324/9780203069943

Ono, H. (2013, January). Impact of the Great East Japan Earthquake on persons with disabilities and support activities - through efforts by the JDF Miyagi Support Center. *Disability Information Resources.* Retrieved October 25, 2022, from https://www.dinf.ne.jp/doc/english/resource/JDF_201503/1-1-3.html

Osamu, N. (2014). The paradox of community-living and disaster. In D. Mitchell & V. Karr (Eds.), *Crises, conflict and disability: Ensuring equality* (pp. 142–146). Routledge. https://doi.org/10.4324/9780203069943

Otake, T. (2013, March 10). Filmmaker captures the 3/11 stress of Tohoku's deaf. *The Japan Times.* Retrieved November 30, 2019, from https://www.japantimes.co.jp/culture/2013/03/10/films/.filmmaker-captures-the-311-stress-of-tohokus-deaf/

Rouhban, B. (2014). Natural hazards: Enhancing disaster preparedness and resilience of people with disabilities. In D. Mitchell & V. Karr (Eds.), *Crises, conflict and disability: Ensuring equality* (pp. 75–83). Routledge. https://doi.org/10.4324/9780203069943

Singer, P. W. (2006, June 2). DHS seeks to better serve disaster victims with disabilities. *Government Executive: Web Edition.* Retrieved March 2, 2022, from https://www.govexec.com/defense/2006/06/dhs-seeks-to-better-serve-disaster-victims-with-disabilities/21956/

Stough, L. M., & Kelman, I. (2017). People with disabilities and disasters. Retrieved January 3, 2022, from https://oaktrust.library.tamu.edu/bitstream/handle/1969.1/165520/Stough%20%26%20Kelman-FINAL%20CLEAN%20COPY%206-19.pdf?sequence=1&isAllowed=y

Takahashi, R. (2019, October 14). Japan criticized for lack of foreign-language information during Typhoon Hagibis. Retrieved November 30, 2019, from https://www.japantimes.co.jp/news/2019/10/14/national/japan-criticized-lack-foreign-language-information-typhoon-hagibis/#.XdtnEuj7TIU

Takayama, K. (2017). Disaster relief and crisis intervention with deaf communities: Lessons learned from the Japanese deaf community. *Journal of Social Work in Disability & Rehabilitation, 16*(3-4), 247–260. https://doi.org/10.1080/1536710X.2017.1372241

Tokyo's Sumida ward spearheads project to assist disabled residents in times of disaster. (2016, February 21). *The Mainichi.* Retrieved November 30, 2019, from https://mainichi.jp/english/articles/20160221/p2a/00m/0na/004000c

Twigg, J., Kett, M., & Lovell, E. (2018, July). Disability inclusion and disaster risk reduction: Overcoming barriers to progress. Briefing note. *ODI.* Retrieved January 5, 2022, from https://www.odi.org/sites/odi.org.uk/files/resource-documents/12324.pdf

United Nations Digital Library. (2015, April 1). *Addressing the vulnerability and exclusion of persons with disabilities: The situation of women and girls, children's right to education, disasters and humanitarian crises: Note by the Secretariat.* Retrieved October 25, 2022, from https://digitallibrary.un.org/record/844726?ln=en

United Nations Office for Disaster Risk Reduction. (2013, October 10). *UN global survey explains why so many people living with disabilities die in disasters.* Retrieved October 25, 2022, from https://www.undrr.org/news/un-global-survey-explains-why-so-many-people-living-disabilities-die-disasters

U.S. Census Bureau. (2015, July 29). *Facts for features: Hurricane Katrina 10th anniversary: Aug. 29, 2015.* Retrieved December 5, 2019, from https://www.census.gov/newsroom/facts-for-features/2015/cb15-ff16.html

Upgrading anti-disaster measures. (2016, March 11). *The Japan Times.* Retrieved November 30, 2019, from https://www.japantimes.co.jp/opinion/2016/03/11/editorials/upgrading-anti-disaster-measures-2/

Walsh-Warder, M. (2016). The disproportionate impact of Hurricane Katrina on people with disabilities. *Verge, 13,* 2–20. Retrieved January 4, 2022, from https://mdsoar.org/bitstream/handle/11603/3744/Verge13_Walsh-WarderMolly.pdf?sequence=1&isAllowed=y

White, B. (2006). Disaster relief for Deaf persons: Lessons for Hurricanes Katrina and Rita. *Review of Disability Studies: An International Journal, 2*(3). Retrieved December 10, 2019, from https://www.rdsjournal.org/index.php/journal/article/view/336

White, G., Fox, M. H., Rooney, C., & Cahill, A. (2006, April 20). *Assessing the impact of Hurricane Katrina on Persons with Disabilities: Interim Report.* Law, Health Policy and Disability Center. Retrieved January 20, 2022, from https://disability.law.uiowa.edu/dpn_hi/345.pdf

Wisner, B. (2002). Disability and disaster: Victimhood and agency in earthquake risk reduction. *Radix—Radical Interpretations of Disaster.* Retrieved December 5, 2019, from http://www.radixonline.org/ disability2.html

Yamaguchi, M. (2020, March 5). Japan opens part of last town off-limits since nuclear leaks. *ABC News.* Retrieved January 10, 2022, from https://abcnews.go.com/International/wireStory/japan-opens-part-town-off-limits-nuclear-leaks-69377729

Zoraster, R. M. (2012). Vulnerable populations: Hurricane Katrina as a case study. *Prehospital and Disaster Medicine, 25*(1), 74–78. https://doi.org/10.1017/S1049023X00007718

CHAPTER 19

"Kept in a Padded Black Cell in Case He Accidently Said 'Piccaninny'": Disability as Humor in Brexit Rhetoric

Emmeline Burdett

After the divisive 2016 vote in favor of Brexit (Britain's vote to leave the European Union (EU)) a Facebook site called The Very Brexit Problems Club came into being. Its *raison d'être* was (and still is) that it should oppose Brexit in a humorous way—its tagline being "Laughing at Brexit Since 2016." The tagline is accompanied by a cartoon of a man wearing a Union Jack T-shirt running away from another man wearing a T-shirt with the European Union flag on it. The former is holding a saw and celebrating having extricated himself from the latter. The latter is looking down in puzzlement at the former's arm, which he has sawn off in his eagerness to get away. The cartoon demonstrates the Club members' view that Brexit is counterproductive; their commitment to using humor to express their opposition to it; and, arguably, their view that disability is something that can be laughed at. Though the cartoon's humor comes from the fact that the man in the Union Jack T-shirt has done something which harms only himself, but which he believes is a cause for celebration, he still has only one arm.

This ambiguity does rather set the stage for the Very Brexit Problems Club's attitude to disability. The members' anger at being forced out of the European Union against their will has been given striking expression in their willingness to diminish both prominent Brexit-supporting politicians and ordinary Brexiters in the eyes of others by claiming that these people have disabilities or

E. Burdett (✉)
University College London, London, UK

© The Author(s), under exclusive license to Springer Nature Switzerland AG 2023
M. S. Jeffress et al. (eds.), *The Palgrave Handbook of Disability and Communication*, https://doi.org/10.1007/978-3-031-14447-9_19

mental illnesses which "explain" their political views and their behavior. It is particularly remarkable that members should have chosen this method of attack, given that they openly deplore other forms of identity-based prejudice and stereotyping—most notably racism. That the humor that Club members have demonstrated is rather savage and angry in nature does not prevent it from *being* humor. Weaver (2022) has observed that.

> There has been an outpouring of humor, comedy, and satire on the EU Referendum and decision to leave the EU, or Brexit. Some of that humor is tendentious, forming mockery or ridicule of political opponents or the other side. Some of it is more obviously innocent humor, and not an attack on political opponents. (Weaver, 2022, p. 1)

The Very Brexit Problems Club's members' use of "humorous" claims that their opponents are disabled constitutes a form of latent violence, Shakespeare (1999) argued:

> There is an ambiguity about cultural responses to impairment, which both revels in the shared joke about the outsider, but also feels embarrassed about the violence which it perpetrates. (p. 48)

This being so, my methodology has been to apply disability studies theories to those posts which have criticized Brexit supporters by making unfounded claims that their views are the result of disability and/or mental illness.

Shakespeare claimed that those who use this type of humor feel embarrassed about doing so, but little or no such "embarrassment" appears to have made its way into the Brexit debate. This is probably due in part to the fact that the debate was (and in some respects still is) bitter and polarized. This means that no weapon is considered unfit to be used to criticize one's opponents. This polarization can be seen as partly rooted in Britain's adversarial political system, under which there is one governing party and one opposition party. As coalitions are seen as irremediably alien, there is little idea that compromising for the greater good could ever be advisable. It was perhaps inevitable that this tendency would translate into both Remainers and Leavers taking extremely unnuanced views of each other, and this was not helped by the behavior of the British government.

PORTRAYALS OF REMAINERS DURING THE BREXIT DEBATE

Both the current and previous Conservative administrations have portrayed Brexit as a national project and those opposed to it as elitist traitors. The former Prime Minister Theresa May made a speech to the 2016 Conservative Party Conference in which she claimed, "If you believe that you are a citizen of the world, you are a citizen of nowhere" (May, 2016). This remark was a criticism of cosmopolitanism, which May portrayed as being entirely negative—expressed in such things as being an employer who would rather employ cheap labor from abroad than show loyalty to the young people of the local area by employing them.

Prime Minister, Boris Johnson, continued this theme, by adopting "Get Brexit Done" as the official Conservative Party slogan for the 2019 General Election. This slogan reflected two things. Firstly, Brexit had still not fully happened, and was not scheduled to do so until January 2020. Secondly, Boris Johnson's government portrayed Brexit as a David versus Goliath battle, in which brave little Britain could not fulfill its true potential while it remained unable to make a clean break from the unbending, unwieldy, and overly bureaucratic European Union.

Thus, there are two main stereotypes of Remainers in general (and thus not only of members of the Very Brexit Problems Club). Firstly, that they are an out-of-touch elite with no loyalty to their place of birth. Secondly, that they lack understanding of the problems of ordinary people. It was quite likely that such polarizing stereotypes would have arisen anyway, but the views that Leavers had developed of them, and the extent to which these views were endorsed by the British government, meant that Remainers lost no time in developing a stereotype of Leavers. Their chosen method of attack was to draw attention to the educational shortcomings of Leavers. They insisted that these shortcomings were testament to Leavers' innately feeble mental attributes. This led Remainers to conclude that Leavers were unfit to make decisions.

"Leavers" Had Not Received a University Education

Ostensibly at least, the starting point for Remainers' uncharitable views of Leavers was a study carried out by the University of Leicester and published in the journal *World Development*. The study concluded that Leave won the 2016 referendum overwhelmingly because those who voted Leave had not received a university education (Stone, 2017). It is probably not very surprising that Leavers took exception to these findings. They perceived that they insulted both Leavers' intellectual caliber and their ability to make a decision. From this starting-point, Remainers could have gone on to have a serious discussion about the state of British education. Regrettably, however, they preferred to leap on every grammatical error and spelling mistake made by members of Leave groups on social media. This quickly escalated to claims that Leavers were generally incompetent. Remainers asserted that Leavers needed "carers" in their daily lives, that the right to vote should be dependent on successfully passing an IQ test, and, perhaps inevitably, a member of the Very Brexit Problems Club remarked that he was beginning to think that eugenics "was actually a pretty good idea" (Bowling, 2019).

Condemnation by Spelling Mistake

A Brexiter calling himself "Benny" is an example of this. Remainers seized upon a spelling mistake that he had made, seeing it as an opportunity to make all sorts of assumptions about his unsuitability to express an opinion on any topic, particularly one of import. "Benny" was the pseudonym of a Brexiter who, on Twitter, had had the temerity to tweet about his support for Brexit. In his tweet, "Benny" had mis-spelled the phrase "get-out clause" as "get out claws." A member of The Very Brexit Problems Club wrote that he regarded "Benny's" spelling as being less problematic than his stated reasons for wanting Britain to leave the European Union (Wilson, 2019). However, both the spelling mistake and the reasons given for wanting to leave the EU apparently condemned "Benny" as someone who, in the eyes of the Very Brexit Problems Club's members, was far too stupid to express an opinion. The Facebook responses to his reported tweet included: "Don't you just hate it when the semi-literate try and use big words?!"; "Utter gibberish from a confused mind"; "And Benny has the right to vote!"; and "Benny is happy in his world—no education, no job, no future."

Tyler (2008, p. 23) argues, "Laughter is always shared with a real or imagined community. Laughter is often at the expense of another, and when we laugh, we effectively 'fix' the other as the object of comedy."

This is what has happened with "Benny" and his tweet. This attitude to Brexiters already existed, but "Benny" is one of the instances of it becoming "fixed," as Tyler described. "Benny" was no longer seen as a moral equal with legitimate reasons for opposing Britain's membership of the European Union. Instead, he had become, in the minds of many in the Very Brexit Problems Club, a stereotype. They defined him by his bigoted stupidity, which was, they insisted, not only evident because of his spelling mistake, but was also his only relevant characteristic. This image of "Benny" only became more ingrained because it was shared with a community which (again going back to Tyler) was, in a sense, both real and imaginary. In imagining that support for Brexit could only be explained by low intelligence, Very Brexit Problems Club members were tacitly imagining themselves as intellectual giants, regardless of whether this was true.

Remainers extended the idea that Brexiters were inherently stupid (essentially that they had intellectual disabilities) when they used this claim to attack a speech made in the European Parliament by the newly elected MEP (Member of the European Parliament) Ann Widdecombe, in early July 2019. Widdecombe claimed in her speech that Brexit was akin to liberation from slavery. It is not surprising that these remarks caused fury among Remainers, but the chosen form of attack was to conclude that Widdecombe's remarks were the result of "dementia." One of the most vicious of these attacks occurred on The Very Brexit Problems Club, and ran as follows (Lawson, 2019):

This is Ann. Her friends call her Widders. She has been missing from her care in the community sheltered accommodation in Lowestoft since Sunday night. Ann suffers from advanced dementia which means she has no control over what she says and is prone to high-pitched rants against foreigners, ethnic minorities, and homosexuals. She also thinks she is an MEP.

We are getting very concerned as Ann hasn't had her special pants or her compression stockings changed since Sunday, which means she may be smelling of shit as well as talking it.

This raises three questions. Firstly, what happened to—in Tyler's words— "fix" in Remainers' minds the idea that support for Brexit (and, by extension, for any non-liberal philosophy) could be explained by either a lack of innate intelligence, or intelligence that had disappeared, in Widdecombe's case, supposedly as a result of "dementia." Secondly, how does the chosen method of attack on Widdecombe relate to Tom Shakespeare's concept of "violence"? Thirdly, is dementia a disability—and if it is, what difference does that make?

Low Intelligence as "Fixed" Explanation for Brexit

I earlier gave the example of Brexiter Benny's spelling mistake and showed that all the ideas that members of the Very Brexit Problems Club had about him stemmed not so much from the fact that he had made a spelling mistake, as from the idea that Brexiters were uneducated and, in all probability, inherently stupid. This, I argued, came from the University of Leicester's findings that the majority of Brexiters had not received a university education. But now we have moved far beyond the mere idea that Brexiters are not intelligent. We have moved to the idea that a Brexit-supporting politician could be attacked by making a completely unfounded claim that she had an illness which was in the process of destroying her mental powers. The crucial point is that such an attack would both "explain" the politician's extreme views and seek to portray her in a humiliating way.

Cameron (2014, p. xv) argues that disability is often seen as a regrettable attribute. Because it is seen as regrettable, it has the potential to reduce its bearer in the eyes of others. Seen from this point of view, there is little difference between noticing that someone has made a spelling mistake and claiming that someone is displaying aberrant behavior. This would be the case even if that behavior is supposedly caused by an illness which destroys the brain. Though different, these things are part of the same continuum. Thus, from this perspective they do not constitute an attack upon a person's identity. It is the possession of these "regrettable attributes" which is alone responsible for the bearer's "reduction" in the eyes of others. Making these attributes grounds for criticism is therefore seen as morally unproblematic. This was certainly the light in which Goffman (1963) viewed the matter in his book *Stigma: On the Management of Spoiled Identity.*

322   E. BURDETT

Cameron's comment above makes it clear that, as far as the disability movement is concerned, the kind of behavior that members of the Very Brexit Problems Club demonstrated in relation to both "Benny" and Ann Widdecombe is morally problematic. This is not simply because it is unpleasant.

DISABILITY HUMOR AS VIOLENCE

At the beginning of this chapter, I quoted Tom Shakespeare describing humor that has disabled people as its target as "perpetrating violence," but what does this mean? The "Widders" sketch quoted above was intended to provoke shared laughter among members of the Very Brexit Problems Club by portraying a relatively powerful political opponent as weak, powerless, and uncontrolled in every way (not only was Widdecombe supposedly unable to control what she said, but she was also incontinent). It was also savage and upsetting. This takes us back to Weaver's comment that one purpose of Brexit humor is the mockery or ridicule of political opponents. The "Widders' sketch falls into this category, but it also "perpetuates violence"—perhaps not physical violence, but certainly emotional and psychological violence.

Though McCann et al. (2010) were investigating homophobic humor in Australian masculine culture, some of their findings are relevant to this question. They argue, "Through language, ideas about acceptable social norms in a given society are transmitted using commonly understood symbols" (p. 506). They further say that

> Humour utilises the concept of "the other" to allow people to develop their own … identity by creating social, emotional and physical distances between themselves and those who are considered "failed" males … For hegemonic males, homophobic humour had a functional capacity to create their sense of heterosexuality … Thus, homosexuality becomes fodder for derision. Humour in general reaches beyond its immediate impact, allowing the ideas contained therein to permeate the social environment and influence non-verbal interaction. (p. 506)

As McCann et al. (2010) observe, humor disseminates ideas, and, in the case of the "Widders" sketch above, the idea disseminated is that dementia and its symptoms may be laughed at.

IS DEMENTIA A DISABILITY?

One thought that does occur when reading the "Widders" sketch is that symptoms such as losing control of one's utterances and bodily functions are quite difficult enough to cope with without having complete strangers decide that they are ripe for mockery. This is why it is important to view dementia as a disability. Doing this does not merely advance some idea that would result in the "Widders" sketch going from merely being unpleasant to being wrong. It changes the whole way in which dementia is viewed. The idea that dementia is a disability has profound social consequences.

The British Social Model of Disability distinguishes between *impairment* (a person's medical condition—in this case dementia), and *disability*, which describes the often-avoidable social consequences of having an impairment. The organization Lifted Care is not part of the disability movement as such, but it suggested that it was important that people with dementia should see their condition as a disability. It argued that doing so would bring to light the amount of discrimination that people with dementia suffer—the article mentioned lack of post-diagnostic support, with the implied message that they should go home and prepare to die. In addition, it found that information was given in inaccessible formats. People newly diagnosed with dementia have often been put under pressure to leave work. It has often been assumed that they lack capacity when no-one has assessed them, and so on (Lifted Team, 2018). In the United Kingdom, dementia is classed as a disability under the 2010 Equality Act, but the article makes the point that many people with dementia are reluctant to describe themselves as "disabled" (Lifted Team, 2018).

The reimagining of dementia as an impairment would make a great deal of difference to the way the "Widders" sketch was seen. One might say that, as one of nine "protected characteristics" under the Equality Act 2010, it should not be mocked in any way. The concept of "protected characteristics" was introduced to protect minority groups from being subjected to behavior which would disadvantage them much more than it would a member of the population at large. People with dementia would be disadvantaged by the idea that their symptoms were an appropriate subject for mockery. However, it is not necessary to view the matter through the "protected characteristic" prism. Seeing dementia as a disability does a great deal to repair the harm done by the "Widders" sketch. Instead of an isolated, struggling individual, whose deficiencies can be mocked, seeing dementia as a disability recreates a society, in which we all have responsibilities toward one another. Unlike homosexuality, which is just an aspect of human nature, dementia is an illness, but the point is that both homosexuals and people with dementia are just there. As they have done nothing wrong, they do not deserve to be made into means to somebody else's end.

In a similar vein to the "Widders" sketch is one about Dominic Raab. Raab was the UK Foreign Secretary at the time of the Brexit negotiations. A Sky News article reported that Raab had reacted to a fall in the value of the pound by saying that the European Union would have to adopt a more flexible approach to Brexit negotiations if it wanted to avoid Britain leaving with no deal. A link to the article was published on the Facebook page of the Very Brexit Problems Club. The member who posted the link accompanied it with his own comment on the situation (Milford, 2019): "As the pound hits parity with the Euro Cent, Mr Raab Esq can be seen dribbling in a corner, with two carers trying to tighten up his straitjacket."

324   E. BURDETT

Like the "Widders" sketch, this illustrates Weaver's (2022) comment that Brexit humor has been used as a tool to criticize political opponents. The comment is not really suggesting that Raab is mentally ill, but that portraying him as such is an acceptable way of attacking him. The same goes for a sketch about Boris Johnson which appeared in *The Guardian* in July 2019. The newspaper is left-wing, and thus its writers would be appalled at the idea of using racist, sexist, or homophobic stereotypes to get their message across. Thus, the fact that this writer saw fit to use unfounded allegations of mental illness as an appropriate way of criticizing Boris Johnson speaks volumes.

"Held Captive by His Carers for Four Weeks"

At the time the article was published, Johnson was the favored candidate in the contest to become leader of the Conservative Party, and, consequently, the next Prime Minister of the United Kingdom (Hyde, 2019). The article's jocular tone belies the fact that it does inform the reader about Boris Johnson's history, character, and ambitions. The problem comes with how this is done. The article tells us that Johnson had to be kept in a padded cell unless he used racist language or transgressed social norms (Hyde, 2019, unpaged).

Like the comment about Dominic Raab above, the tone of the article makes it clear that the writer is not really suggesting that Johnson requires "carers" or has actually been shut in a padded cell. Nevertheless, portraying him in this way is an acceptable method of attack. Like the "Widders" and Dominic Raab sketches discussed above, the article draws a connection between Johnson's supposed mental illness on the one hand, and his views (using outdated racist and homophobic language) and behavior (his sexual appetite). In this way, the article clearly implies that such things as bigotry and questionable morality can only be the result of mental imperfection.

Stereotyping

McCann et al. (2010) showed that humor was a particularly powerful way of fixing in minds the idea that a particular thing was deserving of mockery. The "Widders," Raab and Johnson sketches discussed above demonstrate the use of humor to denigrate political opponents. However, they also reveal a deep-seated contempt for anyone with the medical conditions satirized, or indeed with any of the symptoms satirized (such as incontinence). In other words, the sketches enforce stereotypes. Cameron (2014, p. 144) uses various definitions to explain what a stereotype is, including one from Baker (2005): "Stereotypes are vivid but simple representations which reduce people to a set of exaggerated, usually negative characteristics."

Firstly, the vote to leave the European Union can be "explained" by Leavers not having received a university education. It must therefore follow that Leavers are closed-minded and inherently stupid. There are an enormous number of reasons why people do not attend university, from financial concerns (even when university was less expensive than it now is), to perceptions that it is "elitist," and the idea that university merely teaches students how to think in a certain way (Hutchings & Archer, 2001). It would also be unrealistic to imagine that university was a good idea for someone who was already on a successful career path and who, by breaking off from this to do a university course, would only incur debt and delay.

Secondly, "Benny" had made a spelling mistake, which meant that he was a hopeless social outcast; he had no future; he had an uninquiring mind; his irremediable stupidity meant that he was unfit to have an opinion on any important topic. (In reality, Remainers cannot know whether any of these assumptions are at all true.)

Thirdly, Ann Widdecombe's bigoted views are the result of "dementia." Conditions which attack the brain might well lead to personality changes, but these would be complex, rather than merely being an opportunity for a glib assumption that they "explain" bigotry. Similarly, the claims that Widdecombe is "incontinent" and needs compression stockings are intended to make her look ridiculous. In reality, they would neither affect her ability to have an idea, nor influence what that idea might be.

Fourthly, Dominic Raab is portrayed as "dribbling in a corner," because obviously all mentally ill people do that. Like incontinence, it is ridiculous and contemptible, and fully deserves to be mocked.

Finally, like Ann Widdecombe's "dementia," Boris Johnson's "mental illnesses" explain his bigoted views and use of racist and homophobic language.

All these stereotypes that Remainers used against Leavers were ones which, in Cameron's words, "reduce them in the eyes of others." Remainers in general (and members of The Very Brexit Problems Club in particular) were using such stereotypes specifically against "the other side," and often as an expression of anger. "Benny," for example, had to be portrayed as being utterly ridiculous regardless of what he was actually like. If this did not happen, the points he made might have to be treated as though they were valid.

As Widdecombe, Raab, and Johnson occupied positions of power, Remainers saw no problem in portraying them in ways which made them look ridiculous. But this is only half of the story. As shown, many of the ways in which these prominent Leave-supporting politicians were portrayed involved "giving" them wildly exaggerated "characteristics" supposedly possessed by people with disabilities and mental illnesses (such as Dominic Raab "dribbling in a corner"), or which would have no effect on their ability to develop an opinion, or on that opinion's validity (such as being incontinent or needing compression stockings). This reveals Very Brexit Problems Club members' contempt for people who *are* mentally ill, or who have physical problems such as incontinence.

However, it also shows an assumption that due to shame or lack of capacity, no one with these problems will object to such depictions. Affected people will certainly not even consider rallying in their own defence. It is difficult to imagine that members of the Very Brexit Problems Club would be so keen to use such claims against their political opponents if they believed deeply that people who actually have the conditions specified really mattered. "Rallying in our own defence" is the fundamental concept behind any movement which seeks to advance the cause of a societal group but given the hegemonic view of disability as a tragic individual limitation (Cameron, 2014, p. xv), it has been hard for the disability movement to gain a place in the public consciousness. It has certainly been much harder than it has for movements based on race, gender, and so on. Additionally, stereotypes about disabled people are so ingrained that they are widely mistaken for reality (Cameron, 2014, p. 144). As well as being largely unable to gain a place in the public consciousness because the challenge which it represents to an established idea is too great, the disability movement is also yet to penetrate the consciousness of many Remainers.

REMAINERS AND *LITTLE BRITAIN*

Little Britain was a comedy show that ran on the British Broadcasting Corporation [BBC] from 2003–2007. It starred David Walliams and Matt Lucas, and its characters included Andy, a wheelchair-user played by Matt Lucas, and his support worker Lou, played by David Walliams. The "joke" of the Lou and Andy sketch was that Andy was in fact perfectly able to get out of his wheelchair. When Lou was not looking, he would get up and run about. On the surface, these characters recycled many insulting stereotypes of both disabled people and support workers. Such stereotypes included being dirty, ugly, badly dressed, and so on.

The way in which members of The Very Brexit Problems Club referenced Lou and Andy in the Brexit debate shows their lack of familiarity with disability theory. It also shows their fixed belief that disability can only ever be a subject for mockery and a depiction of individual incapacity and humiliation. It is not surprising that those outside a particular academic field would be unaware of developments within it, but one does not have to be an academic to see that a sketch may be read in more than one way.

The image that Very Brexit Problems Club members referenced involved a famous photograph of Lou and Andy. The photograph showed Andy sitting in his wheelchair wearing his habitual vacant expression. Lou is kneeling beside him, dressed in a distinctive red top. In 2019, in relation to the Brexit debate, this photograph appeared many times on social media, alongside a similar photograph of the Prime Minister of the United Kingdom, Boris Johnson, sitting on a bench alongside the BBC's Political Editor, Laura Kuenssberg.

Like Lou, Kuenssberg sported a bright red top. This underlined the intention that the viewer should see a similarity between the two photographs. In some of these photographic comparisons, Johnson was merely wearing a vacant expression like Andy's. In others, a speech-bubble showed Kuenssberg asking Johnson a question casting doubt on his mental capacity. An example of one of these questions is: "OK, you say you're the Prime Minister, and you live at 10 Downing Street. Is there a relative or a carer that I can phone to come and collect you?"

Montgomerie (2010) has provided an alternative reading of the Lou and Andy characters in *Little Britain*. In the context of this chapter, its significance is potentially profound. This is because, as Montgomerie argues, helper Lou believes unshakeably (and despite endless evidence to the contrary which he totally ignores) that he is in charge of Andy. His imagined position of power means that he needs to make decisions for Andy. Andy has no preferences of any importance, but Lou knows better anyway (Montgomerie, 2010, p. 98). On a slightly different note, Montgomorie also mentions another *Little Britain* character, Mrs. Emery, who has bladder incontinence, but she does not discuss what implications this might have for why the audience is supposed to find Mrs. Emery's incontinence funny.

Montgomerie's reading of the Lou and Andy sketch might have substantially changed the ideas of Remainers. Rather than having Kuenssberg saying "OK, you *say* you're the Prime Minister," Remainers would have had to recognize that Boris Johnson *was* the Prime Minister. Consequently, while ridiculing him might be satisfying, it did not affect him, and it also did not really address the matter in hand. This is a similar problem to the one which also arises with the examples we saw of Raab and Widdecombe—making them appear ridiculous was a powerful way of diminishing them, but it did nothing to address what they said or did. In other words, it showed opposition to them, but had no practical effect.

The same criticism could be made in relation to political satire, exemplified most strongly in the United Kingdom by the magazine *Private Eye* and the television sketch show *Spitting Image*. Political satire is supposed to ridicule political acts—but is implying that a political opponent is disabled or mentally ill commensurate with caricaturing a physical feature such as ears or noses?

Political Satire and Disability Prejudice

LeBoeuf (2007, p. 1) argues that satire implies criticism rather than stating it overtly, and that this helps to protect its creator from legal consequences. The obvious response to this is that by portraying a public figure in ways which are designed to make that figure appear to be ridiculous, one is not criticizing, but merely making the figure appear to be irrelevant. When this happens, the politician is being satirized, but the mode of satire being used is caricature. The problem is that, as shown in the "stereotypes" section of this chapter, a stereotype also relies on the exaggeration of certain characteristics, especially those which are negative. Caricature thus encompasses characteristics which the satire's intended audience is supposed to regard as relevant. They offer no direct comment on the politician's behavior, but make it easy to despise them.

Cameron (2014, p. 145) gives the example of the "dreadful, eyeless" Blind Pew in Robert Louis Stevenson's novel *Treasure Island*. Blind Pew is a villain, and the fact that he is eyeless is intended to increase the reader's fear of him. His blindness is, however, completely irrelevant to whether he is evil. Characteristics such as incontinence have a similar function and are also stereotypes. They denote helplessness and diminish the powerful in the eyes of others, Pritchard (2017) has argued that the cultural representation of people of restricted growth has a profoundly negative effect on the ways in which they are perceived. Not surprisingly, this can lead to people of restricted growth being badly treated by some members of mainstream society. The difficulty is that the examples which Pritchard uses clearly have particular motivations. For example, one interviewee of Pritchard's was a woman who was recalling her experience of visiting a friend who was appearing in a production of Snow White and the Seven Dwarves. When the interviewee and her friend went out for a meal, some strangers saw them and began singing "Hi-Ho!". This is the song from the production that the dwarves sing as they go off to work (Pritchard, 2017, p. 16).

These strangers may have recognized the friend from the production. Alternatively, they may have just seen two small people and assumed that singing a song referencing little people was witty rather than rude. Either way, they had a specific motivation for their actions. By contrast, those who portrayed Ann Widdecombe's behavior as being the result of "dementia" rather than bigotry had no such specific motivation. And this is, in my view, the crux of the problem.

Conclusion

The portrayal of unpopular political figures as having impairments or mental illnesses brings together several issues. It accuses political opponents of possessing characteristics which are supposed to be humiliating, and so render them less powerful by diminishing them in the eyes of others. They do not, however, possess these characteristics. Therefore, it cannot be political caricature. Those who make these accusations do not believe that disability can ever be a socio-political identity. They see it only as a source of individual shame. Partly because of this, they assume that anyone who does have these problems will be unable or unwilling to object.

This means that the use of such stereotypes is safe. The disability movement has shown that these stereotypes are not even thought to be stereotypes. This means that using them is even safer. But where does this leave "Benny"? He is not powerful, and thus does not "need" to be portrayed in a way which makes him look ridiculous. The characteristics imputed to "Benny" are not ones which it is perceived that he will feel entitled to complain about. Even if he does, regarding him as a stupid bigot makes it easier to dismiss him. This is particularly the case, because social media often takes away any real necessity for regarding one's opponents as real human beings. In short, the combination of disability prejudice, the perception that disability prejudice is not prejudice but a reflection of reality, the impersonality of social media, the binary nature of debate in Britain, and the bitterness of the Brexit debate, have all contributed to this issue.

In addition, the questions raised by all this are much wider than simply the humor that members of one Facebook group find acceptable. Greater public acceptance that dementia constitutes a disability would, potentially, make a very positive impact on the experiences of people with dementia and their families and friends. Greater public awareness is also needed that bigotry constitutes making sweeping statements about any categories of innocent people. It does not apply only to obvious categories such as race and gender. This awareness also needs to take root among the press. Perhaps most importantly, both the press and the public need to be aware that prejudices about disabled and mentally ill people are not reflections of reality.

References

Baker, C. (2005, August 31). Caption writers push for training. *The Washington Times*, p. C10. Retrieved December 5, 2019, from https://infoweb-newsbank-com.proxy.library.nyu.edu/apps/news/document-view?p=WORLDNEWS&docref=news/10C579939EAF54D8

Bowling, I (2019, February 1). Facebook. Retrieved December 10, 2019, from https://www.facebook.com/groups/theverybrexitproblemsclub/permalink/241068563484412/

Cameron, C. (2014). *Disability studies: A student's guide*. Sage.

Goffman, E. (1963). *Stigma: Notes on the management of spoiled identity*. Prentice-Hall.

Hutchings, L., & Archer, M. (2001). "Higher than Einstein": Constructions of going to university among working-class non-participants. *Research Papers in Education, 16*(1), 69–91. https://doi.org/10.1080/02671520010011879

Hyde, M. (2019, July 19). Held captive by his carers for four weeks, let's take a look at Boris Johnson's best bits. *The Guardian*. Retrieved December 10, 2019, from https://www.theguardian.com/commentisfree/2019/jul/19/held-captive-by-his-carers-for-four-weeks-lets-look-at-boris-johnsons-best-bits

Lawson, R. (2019, July 4). Facebook. Retrieved December 10, 2019, from https://m.facebook.com/groups/theverybrexitproblemsclub/permalink/333412987583302/

LeBoeuf, M. (2007). The power of ridicule: An analysis of satire [Unpublished doctoral dissertation]. University of Rhode Island. Retrieved December 27, 2021, from https://digitalcommons.uri.edu/srhonorsprog/63/

Lifted Team. (2018, September 19). Retrieved December 27, 2021, from https://www.liftedcare.com/dementia-disability-and-discrimination/

May, T. (2016, October 5). Full text: Theresa May's conference speech. *The Spectator*. Retrieved December 15, 2021, from https://www.spectator.co.uk/article/full-text-theresa-may-s-conservative-conference-speech/amp

McCann, D., Plummer, D., & Minichiello, V. (2010). Being the butt of the joke: Homophobic humor, male identity and its connection to emotional and physical violence for men. *Health Sociology Review 19*(4), 505–521). https://doi.org/10.5172/hesr.2010.1.9.4.505

Milford, P. (2019, July 29), Facebook. Retrieved December 10, 2019, from https://m.facebook.com/groups/theverybrexitproblemsclub/permalink/348750549382879/

Montgomerie, M. A. (2010). Visibility, empathy and derision. *Popular television representations of disability. Alter,* 4(2), 94–102. https://doi.org/10.1016/j.alter.2010.02.009

Pritchard, E. (2017). Cultural representations of dwarfs and their disabling effects on dwarfs in society. *Considering Disability, 1,* 1–31. '0_1985-cultural-representations-of-dwarfs-and-their-disabling-affects-on-dwarfs-in-society'(1).pdf

Shakespeare, T. (1999). Joking a part. *Body and Society,* 5(4), 47–52. https://doi.org/10.1177/1357034x99005004004

Stone, J., (2017, August 7). Brexit caused by low levels of education, study finds. *The Independent.* Retrieved December 10, 2019, from https://www.independent.co.uk/news/uk/politics/brexit-education-higher-university-study-university-leave-eu-remain-voters-educated-a7881441.html?amp

Tyler, I. (2008). Chav mum chav scum. *Feminist Media Studies,* 8(1), 17–34. https://doi.org/10.1080/14680770701824779

Weaver, S. (2022). *The rhetoric of Brexit humour: comedy, populism and the EU referendum.* Routledge.

Wilson, Z. (2019, August 10). Facebook. Retrieved December 10, 2019, from https://www.facebook.com/groups/theverybrexitproblemsclub/search/?query=BENNY&epa=SEARCH_BOX

CHAPTER 20

"Oh, We Are Going to Have a Problem!": Service Dog Access Microaggressions, Hyper-Invisibility, and Advocacy Fatigue

Robert L. Ballard, Sarah J. Ballard, and Lauren E. Chu

Though the language of the 1990 Americans with Disabilities Act (ADA) protects persons with disabilities (PWDs) who have service animals from being excluded from public access, societal acceptance of service dogs is far from guaranteed. As ambiguities in the law are misunderstood and public access inconsistently implemented (Glenn et al., 2017), it is critical to analyze the effects of the language used toward and by service dog handlers, especially by those negatively impacted by the encounter. Many handlers, especially those with invisible disabilities, report experiencing invasive inquiries, questions of legitimacy, unwanted attention, and discrimination (Mills, 2017 p. 646). Yet "the research on the social experiences of service dog handlers is in its infancy" (Mills, 2017, p. 640).

During casual, everyday interactions, at least one of the authors has overheard each of the following comments:

- Waiting for a table in a restaurant with our service dog, another person in line said, "What's next? Are they going to start allowing horses in here?"

R. L. Ballard (✉) • S. J. Ballard
Dog Training Elite Denver, Denver, CO, USA

L. E. Chu
The Penn State University, University Park, PA, USA

© The Author(s), under exclusive license to Springer Nature
Switzerland AG 2023
M. S. Jeffress et al. (eds.), *The Palgrave Handbook of Disability and Communication*, https://doi.org/10.1007/978-3-031-14447-9_20

331

- While shopping in a department store with our service dog, a woman remarked, "Jesus Christ. Why do people think they can just bring their dogs with them whenever they want."
- While in a grocery store with our service dog, another shopper commented, "It is disgusting they allowed that dog in here."

This chapter seeks to partly redress this gap and highlight the struggles faced by a growing population of service dog handlers by outlining three themes related to barely legal microaggressions (Keller & Galgay, 2010), handler hyper-invisibility, and advocacy fatigue (Basas, 2015) through the voices of handlers themselves. We employ a critical, qualitative framework through collaborative autoethnography and invite future research into this phenomenon.

Background on Service Dogs and the ADA

Determining the number of service dog handlers, let alone those impacted by discrimination, is difficult. An online source estimates there are at least 500,000 service dogs in the United States (Emma, 2022), and the American Kennel Club (AKC) estimates that a possible 80 million owners have service dogs or dogs in a working capacity (Karetnick, 2019). Assistance Dogs International, a worldwide coalition of not-for-profit programs that train and place assistance (guide, hearing, and service) dogs placed 16,766 assistance dogs in 2018 (Assistance Dogs International, 2019; see also Walther et al., 2017, for additional background). These variations indicate both the lack of consistent tracking and the difficulty in estimating how many service dogs work in the United States at any given time.

The lack of centralized regulation and certification of service dogs causes multiple problems. One is that estimates are inconsistent and potentially unreliable. Another is that, unlike handicap placards, which are regulated by state governments and are internationally recognized, service dogs are obtained at the discretion of individuals and no certifying agency legitimizes their status. This leads to confusion, ambiguity, and the possibility of fraud. In response to fraud, many states have enacted stringent penalties for those who pass off pets as service dogs (see Edelman, 2018). Because of this confusion and ambiguity, additional social pressure is placed on handlers to legitimize their use of a service dog and the validity of their disability.

Under the ADA, service animals are specifically defined as a dog "that has been individually trained to do work or perform tasks for an individual with a disability. The task(s) performed by the dog must be directly related to the person's disability" (U.S. Department of Justice, 2011, "Overview"). Service dogs, thus, are viewed as valuable and necessary medical assistive technology and equipment (Mills, 2017, p. 636; see also Partlow, 2019; Pierce, 2018), akin to eyeglasses, hearing devices, crutches, or wheelchairs, and "entities must permit service animals (an animal that is individually trained to do work or perform tasks for a person with a disability) to accompany people with disabilities in all areas where members of the public are allowed to go" (U.S. Department of Justice, 2011, "Overview"). Emotional support or therapy animals, which provide comfort to handlers or others are not classified in the same category as service dogs because they are not trained for specific tasks to assist those with documentable disabilities. Thus, emotional support and therapy dogs do not rise to the protected class of service dogs and therefore are not granted public access. At the same time, the confusion between these three classes of dogs is part of the reason there exists ambiguity about public access (Schoenfeld-Tacher et al., 2017). The ADA also does not require service dogs to wear a vest, ID tag, or harness that identifies them as service animals (although it is good practice), but the ADA does require that they be current on vaccinations. The ADA also excuses service dogs from some regulations that prohibit general animals from access, like self-service food lines, hotel rooms that prohibit pets, medical facilities, and housing regulation limits on the number of pets.

Regardless of access rights, the ADA is clear that a service dog must remain under handler control at all times and, if disruptive, loses its right to access, unless disruption is part of its trained task (i.e., alert qualified personnel through barking during a medical emergency). Service dogs do not have to be professionally trained or certified and can be self-trained. To determine if a dog is a service dog, businesses may ask only two questions:

(1) is the dog a service animal required because of a disability? and (2) what work or task has the dog been trained to perform? Staff are not allowed to request any documentation for the dog, require that the dog demonstrate its task(s), or inquire about the nature of the person's disability. (U.S. Department of Justice, 2011, "Inquiries")

The ADA provisions related to service dogs are aspirational and clear in concept, but ambiguous and contradictory in implementation. There are also exceptions. Service dogs are not allowed any places where public health may be compromised, such as sanitized areas in hospitals or in swimming pools. Religious institutions have the right to deny access to service dogs and their handlers (U.S. Department of Justice, 2015, "Q34"). Service dogs can also be denied access if the presence of the animal requires a change in the fundamental function of an organization (U.S. Department of Justice, 2015, "Q25"), which is vague at best and commonly controversial (Phillips, 2016). Additionally, the ADA has no protections for service dogs in training, and it is up to the individual states, local legislation, and facilities to decide such policies, which vary considerably. Indeed, some states and localities even allow public access for emotional support and therapy animals, marking inconsistency between jurisdictions and creating further ambiguity and confusion.

Because of confusion, ambiguity, and inconsistency, the process of simply bringing a service dog into a public space can lead to varying qualities of interactions. Business owners, for instance, may believe they have the legal right to deny access in more scenarios than they do. For example, allergies and phobias to dogs, unless they reach the point of being a disability themselves, are not valid reasons to deny access under the current law (Miles, 2010), yet business owners and employees may reasonably believe they are. The lack of coherence between federal, state, and local laws can also lead to states promulgating misinformation, such as suggesting that business entities require service dogs to show certification to gain access (all three authors have personally observed and encountered this), which is not legal. This also positions businesses to believe it is their responsibility to determine if the individual is disabled or not in order to minimize fraud. Huss (2010) states, "ADA regulations continue to leave the proprietors of public accommodations with little guidance on how to deal with situations where an individual without an apparent disability purports to be accompanied by a service animal" (p. 1212). The ample confusion around the law (Elliott & Hogle, 2013; Huss, 2017b; Huss & Fine, 2017; Lee, 2017) leads service dog handlers to face the unique challenge of having to both understand the law and effectively communicate their rights to others in order to thwart any unwanted interactions and gain public access. For service dog handlers, especially those with an invisible disability, interactions to justify the validity of their disability, and thus service dog, are often challenging, fraught with difficulty, and shrouded in a veil of suspicion.

Service Dogs: Positive Benefits, the ADA, and Invisible Disabilities

Much research has been conducted related to service dogs highlighting the positive outcomes and benefits of a service dog's presence in its handler's life, mostly related to hearing and mobility impairments. For instance, Guest et al.'s (2006) longitudinal study revealed that service dogs helped reduce handlers' hearing-related problems, anxiety, tension, and depression over time, and Rintala et al. (2008) showed how service dogs reduced both mobility and hearing impaired handlers' dependence on others and reduced their need to pay for additional assistance because of the effectiveness of their service dogs. Rodriguez, Bibbo, et al. (2020) found that service dogs led to significantly better psychosocial health including higher social, emotional, and work/school functioning for handlers as compared to those who had not yet received their service dog for assistance with physical disabilities. Yamamoto and Hart (2019) surveyed partners of service dog handlers and revealed an increase in independence, relationships, self-esteem, and life satisfaction alongside a decrease in anxiety, stress, and loneliness for the couples because of the service dog. However, professionally trained dogs decreased burdens and daily tasks more than self-trained dogs; the researchers recommend personalized service dog training that involves both handlers and their partners.

Interestingly, a systematic literature review by Rodriguez, Greer, et al. (2020) which examined research on mobility, hearing, guide, and medical assistant dogs, found that while "positive outcomes were noted in psychological, social, quality of life, and vitality domains," their results also indicated that "for most of the outcomes, having an assistance dog had no effect on [the domains of] psychosocial health and wellbeing" (p. 24). They caution, however, that high variation in rigor and methods could account for these inconsistencies and they encouraged more research. Another review by Lindsay and Thiyagarajah (2021) concluded similarly: service dogs provided positively reported benefits in terms of physical health, quality of life, self-esteem and self-confidence, lowered anxiety, improved stress management, enhanced social interactions at school and work, and improved relationship with one's dog. They also call for improved rigor and consistency.

In other research, the presence of a service dog dramatically increases social approaches and greetings toward a handler (Hart et al., 1987) as well as social acknowledgments (e.g., friendly glances, smiles, conversations), especially for children in generally overlooked settings (e.g., shopping malls) (Mader et al., 1989). Case studies involving individuals with physical disabilities revealed positive benefits for handlers including an increased sense of social integration and self-perceived health along with high levels of satisfaction with the dog's work and tasks and the handler-dog relationship (Lane et al., 1998).

A wide range of studies relate to the application and ambiguity of the ADA. Houghtalen and Doody (1995) point out how the vague language of the ADA creates unclear guidelines for the presence of a service dog in inpatient psychiatric hospitalizations and challenges are, therefore, created. Both Huss (2017a) and Muramatsu, et al. (2015) outline the issues and topics that should be addressed when considering service dogs for psychiatric care in institutions as related to need, intake, safety, policies, and guidelines. Others seek to define and clarify access in terms of context and setting and explore where the ADA could be both more expansive and restrictive in relation to the Fair Housing Act and the Air Carrier Access Act (Huss, 2010; see also Huss, 2017b).

Educational institutions are also affected by service dog access and the ADA: Hill et al. (2014) reviewed all state laws related to children with autism spectrum disorder and service dogs and show how the ADA has failed to provide sufficient guidance for local school districts and parents; Phillips (2016) delineates the difference between emotional support dogs and service dogs and the controversial issues raised on postsecondary institution campuses; and Sidhu (2008) shows how the ADA fails to provide clear guidelines for postsecondary institutions and individuals (students, faculty, and staff) with disabilities. Collectively, the research on service dogs and the ADA reveals what we've already stated: the ambiguity of the language in the ADA leads to confusion, uncertainty, and lack of clarity that makes application problematic in terms of both policy and practice.

Handbooks and resource guides exist for those focused on practitioners. Ensminger (2010) offers a comprehensive work addressing topics including the history of service dogs, the range of appropriate contexts and settings for their specialized work, the evolution of laws and regulations, and guidelines for handlers or others conducting trainings or starting animal assistance programs. Arkow (2021) and Fine (2019) both offer guidelines for those interested in the use of working dogs in service and animal-assisted therapy in activities including college courses, clinical and institutional settings, and a wide range of populations such as those with physical disabilities, anxiety, and depression, as well as with inmates, children, and the elderly.

Mills (2017), though, is the only scholarly work examining invisible disability and service dog interactions we could locate. Indeed, as Mills states, "No research to date has examined how these social experiences [service dog handling and related social interactions] may vary by disability type" (p. 640) as most research has "focused on people who use wheelchairs, a very visible disability" rather than invisible disabilities (p. 641). Drawing from an online survey of 482 service dog handlers, Mills found that 67.8% of service dog handlers, with either visible or invisible disabilities, self-reported everyday experiences of discrimination when accompanied by their service dog. Comparing those with visible disabilities versus those with invisible disabilities, 61.1% of invisibly disabled handlers reported everyday discrimination versus only 39.7% of those with visible disabilities. Mills uncovered three themes: that those with invisible disabilities consistently reported a higher percentage of 1) instances of invasive questioning (76.7% v. 56.5%), 2) unwanted attention (52.9% v. 29.41%), and 3) questioned legitimacy (82.0% v. 50.0%) than those with visible disabilities (p. 646).

Additionally, several variables predicted increased discrimination, including age, length of time as a handler, and frequency of use in public. The younger a handler, the longer she has used her dog, and the more she uses her dog in public, the more discrimination she can expect to face. Further, 49.5% of the full sample, both invisible and visible, agreed or strongly agreed that they sometimes choose not to bring their service dog into public due to unwanted attention, putting their health at risk in order to avoid discriminatory and uncomfortable social exchanges. Mills calls for both more research and education regarding access rights and the important role of service dogs.

Method: Collaborative Autoethnography and a Critical Framework

In this chapter, we enact a collaborative autoethnography, "a qualitative research method in which researchers work in community to collect their autobiographical materials and to analyze and interpret their data collectively in order to gain a meaningful understanding of sociocultural phenomena reflected in their autobiographical data" (Chang et al., 2013). We combined collaborative autoethnography with a critical viewpoint by building on personal experiences to critique cultural practices, employ reflexivity, reveal ourselves figuring out what to do amid challenging social interactions, and strive for social justice (Adams et al., 2015, pp. 1–2).

Following Chang et al. (2013), we engaged in an iterative, overlapping, multi-focal, collaborative data gathering, analysis, interpretation, and writing process. We drew upon personal memory as the source of data combined with self-seeking to interrogate our recalled experiences (pp. 73–94). We broadly followed an approach that allowed us to consider that "seeking social justice is not only about seeking social justice, but about critiquing and interrupting the minute moments of social injustice that permeate our everyday identity performances" (Toyosaki & Pensoneau-Conway, 2013, p. 561). We first began by freewriting at least three recalled memories each of difficult interactions that left us frustrated, challenged, struggling, or traumatized due to perceived social injustices. Some authors only had three, others had five; some authors included observations of close others, like a child or partner.

After initial drafts, we reviewed the collected memories together and chose the most rich and compelling eight stories. Working together, we narrowed it down to five, with one from Author 1, one from Author 2, and three from Author 3. Each author formalized their narratives, then the authors edited each other's narratives so that the writing reflected collaboration and consistent style.

Although we initially hoped to write a more evocative form of collaborative autoethnography (Chang et al., 2013, p. 22), during discussions it became apparent that we a) had too much data with five narratives and b) our work was foraying into new ground. We thus positioned ourselves as critical complements to Mills (2017), providing lived experience narratives that go beyond the quantitative results of Mills' three main themes of more invasive questioning, unwanted attention, and questioned legitimacy experienced more by people with invisible disabilities than those with visible disabilities.

Based on all the stories we generated and worked to write and rewrite, we developed our own three themes of (1) barely legal microaggressions (Keller & Galgay, 2010), (2) handler hyper-invisibility, and (3) advocacy fatigue (Basas, 2015). We believe these themes capture the lived experience and struggle while evoking the injustice that arose during invasive and challenging social interactions with service dogs. Due to space, we decided that we would provide one exemplar vignette that best captured that theme, with Author 3's experience for the barely legal and advocacy fatigue themes and Author 2's experience for the handler hyper-invisibility theme.

THREE THEMES AND SUPPORTING VIGNETTES

To present the three themes, we first introduce each theme followed by an extended vignette that encapsulates and exemplifies the theme. Then we map the vignette theme with analysis and interpretation.

Barely Legal

Microaggressions are "the everyday verbal, nonverbal, and environmental slights, snubs, or insults, whether intentional or unintentional, that communicate hostile, derogatory or negative messages to target persons based solely upon their marginalized group membership" (Sue, 2010, p. 3). Research by Keller and Galgay (2010) reveals that microaggressions against people with disabilities exhibit second-class citizenship, which "occurs when the rights of PWDs for equal access are construed by perpetrators as unreasonable, unjustified, and bothersome" (p. 256). These microaggressions can signal "that PWDs are likely to be a drain on people without disabilities on an individual, group, and societal basis" (p. 256). We label this experience as *Barely Legal*, meaning that legal rights are granted *reluctantly* and even remain under doubt while access is granted. In other words, PWDs with service dogs feel "barely legal." In the following vignette, Author 3 recounts difficulties with her college in order to gain access for her service dog. Author 3 uses Decker, a 60 lb. Goldendoodle, to provide critical mobility and balance support because her invisible disabilities make it difficult to safely walk unassisted.

Vignette #1
I was the first service dog handler to attend my university. Walking into my second class with Decker, I entered the room at the same time as my professor. She stopped me in the doorway and said "Oh, we're going to have a problem." (Notice it wasn't, "Hi. How are you? I'm professor so and so. Who is this? Will he be joining us in class this semester?") It turns out that she has an allergy to dogs. She asked me to sit in the back corner in order to protect her body and not distract other students. Often and at unpredictable times during the term, the professor would pause class to directly ask me, "Are you keeping up with us?" assuming I had a mental disability and unnecessarily spotlighting me to other students. I felt targeted by this professor and unsafe in this classroom because I had a service dog. Without Decker, I don't think I would've had a problem with this class. After a few weeks, I thought everything was going okay, but I was called into the campus disability services office only to be told that a "professor," who would not reveal her or his identity, said my dog was distracting others and requested something be done about it. The professor claimed that students were taking pictures of Decker during class and his presence was detracting from the value of their education. As a result, the director of student accessibility asked, "Is it possible for you to not bring the dog to class anymore?"

I was stunned. Decker was there for my safety, and it was suddenly my responsibility to keep other students from being distracted by my dog. At the time the requests seemed well-intentioned. I didn't want to be responsible for any allergies or distraction, but looking back, it was incredibly hurtful. The message was clear: my safety was less valuable than the education of other students. Hearing from the disability services staff, who are supposed to advocate for my rights, implying my service dog was an option and insinuating that the dog was a frivolous accessory and not a necessary medical device, left me feeling like no one was on my side. I was new to advocating for myself and Decker, and if it were not for some well-informed trainers and friends, I would have given up. I would have stayed at home with Decker when I was not feeling well so that I would not be a detriment to others.

The school made me feel like an inconvenience. They did not realize their legal liability as well as the medical liability I was without him. Before I got Decker, I was passing out daily, sometimes several times a day, in my dorm room and at work, alone. It was imperative he be there to ensure my safety. My perception is that they did not care to be in compliance with ADA, but rather wanted to avoid the "hassle" even if it was my legal right to have Decker accompany me. Further, the school overlooked not only that it was my legal right, but also the social and medical benefits to me, the student (and all future service dog handling students). I was even asked to withhold information on how I received accommodations so as not to burden the DSO with more requests for service dogs.

I continued to attend class with Decker, but the comments did not end. I was still asked to sit in the back, class was still paused when the professor would ask if I was keeping up, and the campus disability office never supported me. After that semester, I took medical leave for two years. While this experience was not the reason for my medical leave, it certainly didn't help nor did it offer me a sense of support or certainty upon my return. When I did return from medical leave, however, I was better prepared with legal and medical justification.

Mapping Themes in Vignette #1

In this case, second-class citizenship through microaggressions is apparent. From the opening greeting (*"Oh, we're going to have a problem"*), to pausing class (*"Are you keeping up with us?"*), to claiming the service dog and Author 3 were detrimental to the education process (*detracting from the value of other students' education*), to being asked by disability services if the service dog was optional (*"Is it possible for you to not bring the dog to class anymore?"*), each interaction reaffirmed this status. These microaggressions accord with Mills' (2017) three themes, especially when the professor paused class or when the disability director asked if the service dog was optional.

When the professor paused class, it was an invasive question that generated unwanted attention and questioned Author 3's mental fitness when her disability had nothing to do with her academic abilities. The director's question about whether or not Decker's presence was optional was invasive, capitalizing on unwanted attention when the professor exaggerated the impact of Decker's presence, and questioned the legitimacy of Author 3 needing a service dog (of course it is not optional). Piling microaggression upon microaggression, the request to withhold information situates Author 3 as a second-class citizen, asking her to be silent and marginalized.

Here, access does not mean equality or inclusivity. The situation was "barely legal." While Decker was allowed to continue in the classroom, his presence was barely tolerated and put under doubt. Author 3 continued to experience the same kinds of microaggressions and initially lacked support from the disabilities service office at her school (she received more support after returning from medical leave). Social interactions continued to situate Author 3 as marginalized, second class, uninvited, and even optional. ADA regulates public access; unfortunately, it does not regulate for social access. How Author 3 was treated is not illegal, but perhaps immoral, all because others are uncomfortable with the presence of a service dog, a medically assistive device necessary for Author 3 to function and be safe.

Handler Hyper-Invisibility

As noted by Hart et al. (1987) and Mader et al. (1989), the presence of a service dog increases social approaches, greetings, and acknowledgments, making one more visible (see also Kuzma, 2018, para. 23). Thus, if you have an invisible disability such as epilepsy, chronic fatigue syndrome, chronic pain, cystic fibrosis, severe hearing impairments, post-traumatic stress disorder, diabetes, or Ehlers-Danlos Syndrome, a service dog draws attention to this disability. However, an interesting phenomenon occurs in this drawing of attention: the person with the disability may actually become even less visible. If the person is acknowledged outside of the dog, then the interactions usually center on the disability of the individual, especially if the disability is an invisible one. We call this second theme *Handler Hyper-Invisibility*. Following the vignette, we explain handler hyper-invisibility within the context of other constructs such as invisibility, hypervisibility, and hyper-invisibility.

In Vignette #2, Author 2, a professor, explains how this handler hyper-invisibility has affected work interactions when she brings Oso, her 25 lb. Bordoodle service dog to work. Author 2 has Ehler Danlos Syndrome (EDS), "a group of inherited disorders that affect your connective tissues—primarily your skin, joints and blood vessel walls" (Mayo Clinic, 2020, para. 1). The effects of the disorders vary but often result in hypermobility and flexibility as well as chronic pain and fatigue. Oso helps Author 2 with mobility as well as retrieving items. EDS is considered an invisible disability.

Vignette #2
"Hi! Oso, right?!?" interjects my colleague in that baby talk voice that comes out around infants and puppies. "He's so cute! He's so sweet! How is he doing in the classroom?" I smile politely. She doesn't wait for my response, "Can I pet him? I know I'm not supposed to pet him, but can I?" I'm torn, I want to be nice. She's my friend, my colleague, and a good person. I want Oso to be accepted in his new position as my service dog. Having Oso has enabled me to continue my profession, especially on days where I teach three back-to-back classes.

But I'm exhausted. Just standing in the hallway is taking effort. I softly nod. Her smile wavers a bit, but the one-sided conversation continues. "The students must adore him! He must be so distracting!" I muster a polite chuckle and half-hearted smile. I'm so tired. "Well, I've got to go! Later, Oso! You be good!" As she walks away, I think about how this conversation would have gone a week earlier without Oso. She knows my daughter is also struggling with her health, that my husband has taken medical leave to care for her; she would have asked about that. She would have asked how school was going for my other two kids and what I had taught in my classes that day. She would have asked about my health and my pain. She would have shared an anecdote about her own child and plans for the holiday break. We would have grumbled together about the toils of grading. But those conversations don't happen anymore.

In general when I have Oso with me, people address the dog first and don't see me or say hello. At my place of work, students no longer give me eye contact in the hallway, regardless if they are students I know or not. "It's Oso!" "Is Oso coming to class?" "How is Oso?" "What's Oso doing today?" "Hi, Oso!" "You know, professor, people are going to be fighting to get into your classes next semester when they find out Oso is going to be there!" "So, now, what does this cutie do for you?" "OMG, he is soooooo cute, how can you even get any work done?" "Your dog is soooo adorable!" Thank you's, socially obligated smiles, and head nods flow from me in response to these well-meaning but marginalizing greetings. I constantly marvel at how invisible I feel even with all eyes on me.

With Oso accompanying me to work, people—students and faculty—now only see and speak to the dog. Even people who are "kind" enough to talk with me versus Oso always address the dog first. For those who do address me, my disability is the primary topic. Most of these conversations are shallow and cursory, but occasionally they are pointed and uncomfortably personal. "I had no idea you were so bad you needed a dog! What does he do?" "Why do you need him? What is your disability? How has that impacted you?" "I thought you had surgery on your back, isn't it better?" "So you have the same disease as your daughter, right? Is she getting better? Oh, you mean this never goes away? I'm so, so sorry to hear that…" These inquiries are immediately followed by uncomfortable silences and awkward looks of pity. In considering to get a service dog, I was not fully prepared for how much attention he would generate. But when he is with me, my invisible disability becomes visible, and I, the multifaceted person, become all but invisible.

Mapping Themes in Vignette #2

The idea of invisibility brings attention to the power dynamic whereby members of marginalized groups are denied recognition, legitimacy, authority, voice, and credibility in society (see Settles et al., 2019). If visibility, then, is where individuals of a group are fully regarded and recognized, granted power, voice, and credibility, hyper-visibility is where members of a marginalized group are subjected to heightened scrutiny and surveillance awaiting failures so that dominant groups can attribute their failures to all members of the marginalized group (see Settles et al., 2019). These three constructs (invisibility, visibility, and hyper-visibility) have often been applied to analyzing racial identity and racism (Richards, 2018; Settles et al., 2019), the intersection of race and gender (Mowatt et al., 2013), and workplace and gender (Buchanan & Settles, 2019). A related construct, hyper-invisibility, though, is now emerging (see Truong-Vu, 2022). A good definition of hyper-invisibility is "that, like the elephant in the room, someone can stand out easily in a crowd and yet be treated almost as if they don't exist—as if their presence, opinions, contributions, or experiences don't matter" (Bowden interview with Thomas, 2021). We think hyper-invisibility applies in the situation with Author 2 and her service dog. If invisibility and visibility tend to draw attention to structural levels of power, hyper-visibility and hyper-invisibility draw attention to interpersonal levels of interaction.

In vignette #2, the presence of the service dog creates a paradox. The service dog draws attention to the individual who needs one and also engenders the stigma of "widespread assumptions that people with disabilities are inferior to those without disabilities, and that people with disabilities are broadly incapable and a burden on their families and society" (Ostiguy et al., 2016, p. 311). Yet, the service dog simultaneously provides a "valuable type of assistive technology that can be used to mitigate numerous types of disabilities" (Mills, 2017, p. 636; see also Fairman & Huebner, 2001; Winkle et al., 2012), providing a small way to overcome these institutional barriers and inequities. The dog mitigates obstacles yet engenders stigmatization. The person is present, but in this kind of interaction, the dog becomes the focus. In other words, the individual has attention drawn to them because of the service dog but is ignored because of function of the service dog. Hyper-invisibility of the handler emerges.

Author 2's experience is one where colleagues and students have all rendered her hyper-invisible by addressing her service dog first (*"It's Oso!" "What's Oso doing today?"*). One comment implies that the professor is only valuable because of the service dog (*"You know, professor, people are going to be fighting to get into your classes next semester when they find out Oso is going to be there!"*), clearly favoring the dog over the human. It is interesting that the service dog is, at least in a technical sense, akin to a medically assistive device like a wheelchair, crutches, hearing aids, or eyeglasses, yet those are not addressed. (Imagine: "Hi, glasses! You're so cute!") Obviously, this is because a service dog is a living being and the prevailing perspective on dogs is that they are companions and pets. Yet, even when indicated that the dog is a service animal, both through visible markings on a vest and when disclosed, the dog maintains primary attention during the interaction.

Even when Author 2 is addressed subsequent to the service dog, she is stigmatized and addressed as a stereotype. Mills' (2017) three themes remain relevant. Invasive questioning (*"What is your disability?"*), unwanted attention (*"So you have the same disease as your daughter, right? Is she getting better? Oh, you mean this never goes away?"*), and questioned legitimacy (*"Why do you need him?"; "I thought you had surgery on your back, isn't it better?"*) all occur.

In Author 2's interactions, the conversations fizzle out after a variety of expressions—curiosity, surprise, pity, faux concern—are all centered on Author 2's dog. What is notable is less about what is spoken, but rather what is *not* spoken. No longer does Author 2 engage in conversations about her personhood and identity. The dog and the disability take up all of the conversation, and nothing about the rest of Author 2 is brought up, even though she longs for that kind of connection. She is rendered hyper-invisible—present, noticed, but not allowed to add nothing of significance. She is objectified and backgrounded. She is experiencing Handler Hyper-Invisibility.

We have no doubt that the students and faculty are good people, well-meaning, and trying to be polite. And we have no doubt that the students and faculty are uncomfortable discussing disability. They fall victim, though, to structurally perpetuated stigmas, uncertain and unclear about how to navigate a service dog and an invisible disability, but only able to view their coterminous presence outside of "normal" functioning. Yet, the solution is simple: address the handler as a whole person first, just like you would any other human being you encountered. The dog, while cute, is a medically assistive device and not the primary agent in the interaction.

Advocacy Fatigue and Vignette #3

For the third and final theme of *Advocacy Fatigue*, we start with the vignette where Author 3 describes a confrontation that violated her access rights in a nail salon:

In 2015, I left New York City to return home after a week of medical evaluations. After enduring days of being poked and prodded, I decided to reward myself with a manicure at the airport with my mother and Decker before flying out. As we entered the nail salon, I did not expect a conflict, but as soon as I saw a tall, white woman marching over to us with a sense of righteous indignation, I could not help but think, *Here we go again.* The woman blocked our entrance to the salon. While gesticulating with waved hands, she said loudly, "That dog needs to leave the salon." I replied with a firm, but matter-of-fact, "He's a service dog, ma'am." The woman, who was the manager, looked me up and down quickly and responded with an impertinent, "But you don't look disabled." My mother quickly interjected, "What does someone with a disability *look* like exactly? What would she need to look disabled in your eyes, a wheelchair or a cane?" The manager backed off a little, "The, um, exclusion, is, uh, unrelated to her disability. Um, it, uh, is that, um, local law prohibits any, um, animal from entering a salon. They say it's because, um, his [pointing to Decker, not even sure if it is a male or female dog], uh, hair could get into the nail polish." My mother interjected: "There's a difference between hair and fur," to which the woman responded, "Look, uh, fish are, um, not even allowed in, uh, here."

Despite her assertion this was based on New York state law, I challenged the manager and explained the Supremacy Clause: "Actually, federal law supersedes state law. That's in the Constitution." I couldn't believe I had to muster all of this knowledge and emotion just to prove that I was legally allowed to get my nails done with Decker. The manager said, "I'm going to call our corporate lawyers," which scared me. But after about ten minutes of waiting uncomfortably among other patrons who had observed the confrontation, the manager hung up the phone and said, "Well, they said we can allow it *just this once*" emphatically, as though she was doing us a favor. My mother interjected: "You aren't *allowing* us to do anything. You're just following *the law*."

By now, I was more exhausted than earlier. Since I was already dealing with the aches and pains of travel and testing, the emotional intensity of the interaction wore me down quickly. Internally, I was debating whether or not to even get the manicure. *Was it worth it? Did I need a manicure that badly? Do I want to give money to an establishment that would discriminate against me? If I leave to prove my point, don't they get what they wanted?*

I engaged in a lot of self-talk and self-motivation. *Don't let this derail you. The law is on your side. You "won" in the end. You still got what you wanted. The manager is just ignorant; don't hold it against her. You're doing the right thing. They are in the wrong.* But negative self-talk was also present. *What happens to the next handler that enters this establishment? Was I too pushy, and now the next person will face more discrimination? Am I truly disabled? Maybe I can go without Decker. Maybe that woman knows my condition better than I do. Maybe I should just pretend to be normal so I won't be so much of a bother. Am I acting entitled? Was she just doing her job, and I got her in trouble? This would all be so much easier if I weren't sick.*

In the end, I got the manicure. The manager basically avoided us. But I never really relaxed until we left. Despite having positive experiences elsewhere, I'm hesitant to return to salons with Decker because a public access denial can be embarrassing, traumatic, and emotionally draining. My service dog was supposed to open up my world and help me go more places with independence, but the negative encounters have shrunk my life to a few places I know I will be accepted without confrontation.

Mapping Themes in Vignette #3

Law professor Carrie Griffin Basas (2015) defines advocacy fatigue as:

> ...the increased strain on emotional, physical, material, social, and wellness resources that comes from continued exposure to system inequities and inequalities and the need to advocate for the preservation and advancement of one's rights and autonomy. Advocacy fatigue can diminish emotional and physical health, career prospects, and financial security because of the ongoing exposure to stress and discrimination. (p. 53)

While Basas employs a disability studies perspective that looked at families of two marginalized groups in the education system, students with special needs and students in an English Language Learner program, we think the concept applies well here.

Clearly, Author 3's encounter in the salon involved each of Mills' (2017) three themes—invasive questioning (*"But you don't look disabled"*), unwanted attention (*other patrons observed the tense interaction*), and questioned legitimacy (*"I'm going to call our corporate lawyers"*). In response, Author 3's language and expressions are matter-of-fact (*"He's a service dog, ma'am."*; *"Actually, federal law supersedes state law. That's in the Constitution"*) and Author 3's mother is adversarial and indignant (*"What does someone with a disability look like exactly?"*; *"You aren't allowing us to do anything. You're just following the law"*). Both are unbending and inflexible, articulating and asserting that the law supports access rather than denies it.

Notably, this encounter resulted in emotional strain (*the emotional intensity of this interaction wore me down quickly*), physical strain (*I was more exhausted than earlier*), social strain (*waiting uncomfortably*), mental strain (*I was debating whether or not to even get the manicure; I engaged in a lot of self-talk and self-motivation*), and even wellness and financial strain (*I'm hesitant to return to salons with Decker; the negative encounters have shrunk my life to a few places I know I will be accepted without confrontation*). Clearly, continually defending one's legal right to public access fulfills Basas' concept of Advocacy Fatigue.

In addition to being draining, Advocacy Fatigue has an impact on Author 3's sense of self. The "ongoing exposure to stress and discrimination" (Basas, 2015, p. 53) led Author 3 to question her worth (*Was it worth it? Did I need a manicure that badly?*) and doubt her own efforts, efficacy, and identity (*Was I too pushy, and now the next person will face more discrimination? Am I truly disabled?*). In other words, the more invasive, skeptical, and demeaning the language that is used toward PWDs, the more their own language changes to become adversarial. Prolonged use of such assertive language results in Advocacy Fatigue, questioning of self-worth, and self-doubt. Even though Author 3 "won," the negative interaction tainted the victory with lasting feelings of marginalization and exclusion. This is not merely about how the burden to enforce the law is shifted to those PWDs who have service dogs, but how the internal and external language impacts their sense of self and value.

Conclusion

This chapter is a complement and invitation. It explores the intersection of invisible illness, service dog handlers, and social discrimination. Our stories draw from and build upon Mills' (2017) study on the topic. Our collaborative autoethnography reveals lived experience, giving voice to service dog handlers and highlighting the language present in these discriminatory interactions. Background on the prevalence of service dogs, their legal access rights in the ADA, and the ambiguity and confusion created by the vague language and exceptions therein are presented.

Three autoethnographic vignettes reveal three emergent themes. Barely Legal microaggressions position PWDs as Second-Class Citizens (Keller & Galgay, 2010) reminding those who have service dogs that they may have legal access, but are still socially excluded and marginalized, and that their legal access always remains tenuous. Handler Hyper-Invisibility backgrounds PWDs with invisible disabilities but foregrounds the service dog, causing engagement but often an unwitting hyper-invisibility of the handler. Advocacy Fatigue, or a sustained strain on emotional, physical, material, social, and wellness resources emerging from a constant need to advocate for legal rights (Basas, 2015) leads PWDs to question their own identity and worth.

Through our lived experience as PWDs with service dogs and invisible disabilities as well as scholars, we have presented situations and interactions we hope illustrate these themes. Our hope is to build from and complement Mills (2017) by broadening beyond post-positivist approaches and into critical, qualitative frameworks. In doing so, we seek to follow Sheldon's (2017) call and encouragement "that disabled researchers need to use their subjectivity, their view of looking at the world, as a catalyst for transforming the experiences of other people with disabilities" (p. 995). Thus, this chapter is an invitation for others to pursue research into the ambiguous, negative, uncomfortable, and marginalizing interactions experienced by those whose disabilities are not visible but need the accompaniment of a service dog in order to work and live, especially for those for whom this represents lived, everyday occurrence.

We invite others, able-bodied and disabled, visible and invisible, service dog or no service dog, to explore how the three themes presented here point toward not just an interpersonal interaction that can be examined from a critical, qualitative, standpoint framework that gives voice to those who may not always have it. In this case, to give voice to PWDs who want their service dogs to accompany them without fear of feeling like a second-class citizen, invisible, and/or fatigue at having to constantly advocate for their rights.

At the outset of this chapter we presented three comments each of the authors has heard when bringing their service dog into the public. "*What's next? Are they going to start allowing horses in here?*"; "*Jesus Christ. Why do people think they can just bring their dogs with them wherever they want.*"; and "*It is disgusting they allowed that dog in here.*" These are everyday reminders that equality, inclusivity, and justice for PWDs with invisible disabilities and service dogs remain ambiguous, confusing, and fraught with social tension and discrimination. To the first comment about horses, we respond with, "We hope so!" because miniature horses can qualify as service animals under the ADA. To the second comment about bringing dogs wherever we want, we say, "No, we don't. We just want to be able to shop like you and we can't without their assistance." And to the third comment, we respond, "No, *you* are disgusting, because you have no compassion." We only want what you already have—access without barriers: legal, social, or otherwise.

REFERENCES

Adams, T. E., Jones, S. H., & Ellis, C. (2015). *Autoethnography*. Oxford University Press.

Arkow, P. (2021). *Animal-assisted therapy and activities: A study, resource guide and bibliography for the use of companion animals in selected therapies* (12th ed.). Animal Assisted Therapy.

Assistance Dogs International. (2019, August 30). *Member program statistics*. Retrieved January 11, 2022, from https://assistancedogsinternational.org/members/member-program-statistics/

Basas, C. G. (2015). Advocacy fatigue: Self-care, protest, and educational equity. *Windsor Yearbook of Access to Justice, 32*(2), 37–64. https://doi.org/10.22329/wyaj.v32i2.4681

Buchanan, N. T., & Settles, I. H. (2019). Managing (in)visibility and hypervisibility in the workplace. *Journal of Vocational Behavior, 113*, 1–5. https://doi.org/10.1016/j.jvb.2018.11.001

Chang, H., Ngunjiri, F. W., & Hernandez, K-A. C. (2013). *Collaborative ethnography*. Left Coast Press, Inc.

Edelman, A. (2018, May 5). *Collared: New laws crack down on fake service dogs*. NBCnews.com. Retrieved January 11, 2022, from https://www.nbcnews.com/politics/politics-news/collared-new-laws-crack-down-fake-service-dogs-n871541

Elliott, D., & Hogle, P. S. (2013). Access rights and access wrongs: Ethical issues and ethical solutions for service dog use. *International Journal of Applied Philosophy, 27*(1), 1–14. https://doi.org/10.5840/ijap20132716

Emma. (2022, January 9). *Most remarkable service dog statistics in 2022*. Pawsome advice. Retrieved October 28, 2022, from https://pawsomeadvice.com/dog/service-dog-statistics/

Ensminger, J. J. (2010). *Service and therapy dogs in American society: Science, law and the evolution of canine caregivers*. Charles C. Thomas Publisher Ltd.

Fairman, S. K., & Huebner, R. H. (2001). Service dogs: A compensatory resource to improve function. *Occupational Therapy in Health Care, 13*(2), 41–52. https://doi.org/10.1080/J003v13n02_03

Fine, A. H. (Ed.). (2019). *Handbook on animal-assisted therapy: Foundations and guidelines for animal-assisted interventions* (5th ed.). Elsevier.

Glenn, M. K., Foreman, A. M., Wirth, O., Shahan, K. M., Meade, B. J., & Thorne, K. L. (2017). Legislation and other legal issues relevant in choosing to partner with a service dog in the workplace. *Journal of Rehabilitation, 83*(2), 17–26. Retrieved January 11, 2022, from https://link.gale.com/apps/doc/A503309637/AONE?u=ucl_ttda&sid=bookmark-AONE&xid=613e0502

Guest, C. M., Collis, G. M., & McNicholas, J. (2006). Hearing dogs: A longitudinal study of social and psychological effects of deaf and hard-of-hearing recipients. *Journal of Deaf Studies and Deaf Education, 11*(2), 252–261. https://doi.org/10.1093/deafed/enj028

Hart, L. A., Hart, B. L., & Bergin, B. (1987). Socializing effects of service dogs for people with disabilities. *Anthrozoos, 1*(1), 41–44. https://doi.org/10.2752/089279388787058696

Hill, D. R., King, S. A., & Mrachko, A. A. (2014). Students with autism, service dogs, and public schools: A review of state laws. *Journal of Disability Policy Studies, 25*(2), 106–116. https://doi.org/10.1177/1044207313477204

Houghtalen, R. P., & Doody, J. (1995). After the ADA: Service dogs on inpatient psychiatric units. *The Bulletin of the American Academy of Psychiatry and the Law, 23*(2), 211–217. http://jaapl.org/content/jaapl/23/2/211.full.pdf

Huss, R. J. (2010). Why context matters: Defining service animals under federal law. *Pepperdine Law Review, 37*(4), 1163–1216. Retrieved June 17, 2022, from https://digitalcommons.pepperdine.edu/cgi/viewcontent.cgi?article=1054&context=plr

Huss, R. J. (2017a). Hounds at the hospital, cats at the clinic: Challenges associated with service animals and animal-assisted Interventions in healthcare facilities. *University of Hawaii Law Review, 40*(53), 53–113. Retrieved June 17, 2022, from https://papers.ssrn.com/sol3/papers.cfm?abstract_id=3249680

Huss, R. J. (2017b). Legal and policy issues for animal assisted interventions with special populations. *Applied Developmental Science, 21*(3), 217–222. https://doi.org/10.1080/10888691.2016.1231063

Huss, R. J., & Fine, A. H. (2017). Legal and policy issues for classrooms with animals. In N. R. Gee, A. H. Fine, & P. McCardle (Eds.), *How animals help students learn: Research and practice for educators and mental-health professionals* (pp. 27–38). Routledge.

Karetnick, J. (2019, September 24). *Service dogs 101—Everything you need to know.* American Kennel Club. Retrieved January 11, 2022, from https://www.akc.org/expert-advice/training/service-dog-training-101/

Keller, R. M., & Galgay, C. E. (2010). Microaggressive experiences of people with disabilities. In D. W. Sue (Ed.), *Microaggressions and marginality: Manifestation, dynamics, and impact* (pp. 241–267). Wiley.

Kuzma, C. (2018, November 16). *Everything you need to know before getting a service dog.* Vice.com. Retrieved January 11, 2022, from https://www.vice.com/en_us/article/j5zmak/everything-you-need-to-know-before-getting-a-service-dog

Lane, D. R., McNicholas, J., & Collis, G. M. (1998). Dogs for the disabled: Benefits to recipients and welfare of the dog. *Applied Animal Behaviour Science, 59*(1–3), 49–60. https://doi.org/10.1016/S0168-1591(98)00120-8

Lee, T. (2017). Criminalizing fake service dogs: Helping or hurting legitimate handlers? *Animal Law, 23*(325), 326–354.

Lindsay, S., & Thiyagarajah, K. (2021). The impact of service dogs on children, youth and their families: A systematic review. *Disability and Health Journal, 14*(3), 101012. https://doi.org/10.1016/j.dhjo.2020.101012

Mader, B., Hart, L. A., & Bergin, B. (1989). Social acknowledgments for children with disabilities: Effects of service dogs. *Child Development, 60*(6), 1529–1534. https://doi.org/10.2307/1130941

Mayo Clinic. (2020, October 16). *Ehlers-Danlos syndrome.* Retrieved January 11, 2022, from https://www.mayoclinic.org/diseases-conditions/ehlers-danlos-syndrome/symptoms-causes/syc-20362125

Miles, P. (2010, May 13). *Service dog v. allergies—ADA accommodation conflict* [Web log post]. Law Office Space. Retrieved January 11, 2022, from https://www.lawfficespace.com/2010/05/service-dog-v-allergies-ada.html

Mills, M. L. (2017). Invisible disabilities, visible service dogs: The discrimination of service dog handlers. *Disability & Society, 32*(5), 635–656. https://doi.org/10.1080/09687599.2017.1307718

Mowatt, R. A., French, B. H., & Malebranche, D. A. (2013). Black/female/body *hypervisibility* and *invisibility. Journal of Leisure Research, 45*(5), 644–660. https://doi.org/10.18666/jlr-2013-v45-i5-4367

Muramatsu, R. S., Thomas, K. J., Leong, S. L., & Ragukonis, F. (2015). Service dogs, psychiatric hospitalization, and the ADA. *Psychiatric Services, 66*(1). Online publication. https://doi.org/10.1176/appi.ps.201400208

Ostiguy, B. J., Peters, M. L., & Shlasko, D. (2016). Ableism. In M. Adams, L. A. Bell, D. J. Goodman, & K. Y. Joshi (Eds.), *Teaching for diversity and social justice* (3rd ed., pp. 299–337). Routledge.

Partlow, K. (2019, August). *12 misconceptions about service dogs and those who use them.* Animal Health Foundation. Retrieved January 11, 2022, from https://www.animalhealthfoundation.org/blog/2019/08/12-misconceptions-about-service-dogs-and-those-who-use-them/?sfw=pass1640721218

Phillips, M. (2016). Service and emotional support animals on campus: The relevance and controversy. *Research and Teaching in Developmental Education, 33*(1), 96–99. Retrieved January 11, 2022, from http://www.jstor.org/stable/44290251

Pierce, K. L. (2018, October 8). *Understanding and working with service dog handlers.* Counseling Today. Retrieved January 11, 2022, from https://ct.counseling.org/2018/10/understanding-and-working-with-service-dog-handlers/

Richards, M.-L. (2018). Hyper-visible invisibility: Tracing the politics, poetics and affects of the unseen. *Field Journal, 7*(1), 39–52. Retrieved January 11, 2022, from http://field-journal.org/wp-content/uploads/2018/01/3-Hyper-visible-Invisibility.pdf

Rintala, D. H., Matamoros, R., & Seitz, L. L. (2008). Effects of assistance dogs on persons with mobility or hearing impairments: A pilot study. *Journal of Rehabilitation Research and Development, 45*(4), 489–504. https://doi.org/10.1682/JRRD.2007.06.0094

Rodriguez, K. E., Bibbo, J., & O'Haire, M. E. (2020). The effects of service dogs on psychosocial health and wellbeing for individuals with physical disabilities or chronic conditions. *Disability and Rehabilitation, 42*(10), 1350–1358. https://doi.org/10.1080/09638288.2018.1524520

Rodriguez, K. E., Greer, J., Yatcilla, J. K., Beck, A. M., & O'Haire, M. E. (2020). The effects of assistance dogs on psychosocial health and wellbeing: A systematic literature review. *PloS ONE, 15*(12), e0243302. https://doi.org/10.1371/journal.pone.0243302

Schoenfeld-Tacher, R., Hellyer, P., Cheung, L., & Kogan, L. (2017). Public perceptions of service dogs, emotional support dogs, and therapy dogs. *International Journal of Environmental Research and Public Health, 14*(6), 642. https://doi.org/10.3390/ijerph14060642

Settles, I. H., Buchanan, N. T., & Dotson, K. (2019). Scrutinized but not recognized: (In)visibility and hypervisibility experiences of faculty of color. *Journal of Vocational Behavior, 113*, 62–74. https://doi.org/10.1016/j.jvb.2018.06.003

Sheldon, J. (2017). Problematizing reflexivity, validity, and disclosure: Research by people with disabilities about disability. *The Qualitative Report, 22*(4), 984–1000. https://doi.org/10.46743/2160-3715/2017.2713

Sidhu, D. (2008). Cujo goes to college: On the use of animals by individuals with disabilities in postsecondary institutions. *University of Baltimore Law Review, 38*(2), 276–303. https://scholarworks.law.ubalt.edu/ublr/vol38/iss2/3

Sue, D. W. (2010). Microaggressions, marginality, and oppression. In D. W. Sue (Ed.), *Microaggressions and marginality: Manifestation, dynamics, and impact* (pp. 3–24). Wiley & Sons.

Thomas, K. (2021, July 19). *Hyper-invisibility: What it's like to be Black in engineering: Biomedical-optics researcher Audrey Bowden discusses systemic racism, implicit bias, and five guiding principles for implement change*. SPIE: The International Society for Optics and Photonics. Retrieved January 11, 2022, from https://spie.org/news/hyper-invisibility-what-its-like-to-be-black-in-engineering-

Toyosaki, S., & Pensoneau-Conway, S. L. (2013). Autoethnography as a praxis of social justice: Three ontological contexts. In S. H. Jones, T. E. Adams, & C. Ellis (Eds.), *Handbook of autoethnography* (pp. 557–575). Left Coast Press.

Truong-Vu, K.-P. (2022). On the margins of hyperinvisibility and hypervisibility: The paradox of being an Asian-American during the COVID-19 pandemic. In M. Heath, A. K. Darkwah, J. Beoku-Betts, & B. Purkayastha (Eds.), *Global feminist autoethnographies during COVID-19: Displacements and disruptions* (pp. 199–210). Routledge.

U.S. Department of Justice. (2011). *Service animals*. Retrieved January 11, 2022, from https://www.ada.gov/service_animals_2010.htm

U.S. Department of Justice. (2015) *Frequently asked questions about service animals and the ADA*. Retrieved January 11, 2022, from https://www.ada.gov/regs2010/service_animal_qa.html

Walther, S., Yamamoto, M., Thigpen, A. P., Garcia, A., Willits, N. H., & Hart, L. A. (2017). Assistance dogs: Historic patterns and roles of dogs placed by ADI or IGDF accredited facilities and by non-accredited U.S. facilities. *Frontiers in Veterinary Science, 4*, 1–14. https://doi.org/10.3389/fvets.2017.00001

Winkle, M., Crowe, T. K., & Hendrix, I. (2012). Service dogs and people with physical disabilities partnerships: A systematic review. *Occupational Therapy International, 19*(2012), 54–66. https://doi.org/10.1002/oti.323

Yamamoto, M., & Hart, L. A. (2019). Professionally- and self-trained service dogs: Benefits and challenges for partners with disabilities. *Frontiers in Veterinary Science, 6*, 1–15. https://doi.org/10.3389/fvets.2019.00179

CHAPTER 21

"The Fuzzy Mouse": Unresolved Reflections on Podcasting, Public Pedagogy, and Intellectual Disability

Chelsea T. Jones, Jennifer Chatsick, Kimberlee Collins, and Anne Zbitnew

Dominate Language: Blending plain language and academic writing, this chapter describes the behind-the-scenes work of "The CICE Team" podcast—a public-pedagogy project rooted in disability justice and led by college students labelled with intellectual disabilities at Humber College in Toronto, Canada. Using podcast clips, focus group data, and students' writing, this co-authored reflection uncovers the tensions of non-disabled teachers and researchers doing disability justice-oriented broadcast and communication work with a group of disabled podcasters. These tensions include an ethical desire for disabled students to lead the podcasting, and non-disabled facilitators' conscious attempts to share power amid student-led media production and ableist digital divides (Shew, 2018). This chapter offers a mixed-methods account of podcasting through testimony from student podcasters and researchers working on a disability media studies project in a non-traditional classroom. Our reflections,

C. T. Jones (✉)
Brock University, St. Catharines, ON, Canada
e-mail: cjones@brocku.ca

J. Chatsick • A. Zbitnew
Humber College, Toronto, ON, Canada

K. Collins
University of Toronto, Toronto, ON, Canada

© The Author(s), under exclusive license to Springer Nature
Switzerland AG 2023
M. S. Jeffress et al. (eds.), *The Palgrave Handbook of Disability and Communication*, https://doi.org/10.1007/978-3-031-14447-9_21

351

including our thinking about how classroom accessibility must consider intersectional "knowing-making" (Hamraie & Fritsch, 2019), serve both as a methodological and pedagogical resource for those embracing the tensions around labelled people's vibrant contributions to knowledge production about themselves amid institutional inclusionism.

Plain language: An eight-episode podcast named "The CICE Team" was created in 2020 by nine intellectually disabled students in Toronto, Canada. All podcasters were part of a Humber College program called Community Integration through Co-operative Education (CICE). Their podcast production was part of a larger project called *Accessibility as Aesthetic: Three Films and a Podcast*. This project tasked students to make three films and a podcast (Jones et al., 2021). This reflexive account focuses exclusively on the podcast production. The four writers of this chapter supported the podcasters with the creation of each episode. We are white, non-intellectually disabled researchers and educators. The chapter includes our reflections on the experience, focusing on our thoughts about how we supported the creation of the podcast while trying to ensure we did not interfere with the decisions of the podcasters. Our hope is that this chapter can be used as a resource for others who want to collaborate with labelled people in a way that honors their stories.

It is important to us that we do our research and write in a way that is possible for labelled people, such as the CICE podcasters, to understand. We want to honor their knowledge because they made this project possible. For this reason, we have written this chapter in two ways: plain language and dominant language. As you read, you will move back and forth between plain and dominant language, experiencing the chapter in two ways. While this is not a solution for the ableism in academic writing, we hope that writing that includes plain language will invite more readers into this chapter, including "The CICE Team" podcasters and others who wish to make media with intellectual disability in mind.

Dominant language: The question driving this writing is: how do we "do" and represent critical intellectual disability-based communication scholarship and pedagogy without alienating the people whose creative work makes this inquiry possible? To face this question, we follow Laurel Richardson's (2003) directive to take writing as both methodology and method. To approach the question of how we "do" critical intellectual disability-based communication scholarship more equitably, we have included plain language sections to destabilize the usage of subsequent dominant language sections. Plain language translation is a method of writing, advocacy, and accessibility that is meant to be clear and understandable to a broad audience. By contrast, dominant language connects to linguistic imperialism that is at work when non-disabled people prioritize and conceptualize their communication style over others—as happens commonly in academic contexts that privilege high-level English writing over non-English, nonverbal, pictural, expressive, or signed modes of communication (Reagan, 2011; Rose & Conama, 2018). Our chimeric approach, which relies on both plain language and dominant language, is not meant to be repetitive or to split the narrative; rather, we orient our writing toward both the pluralities of intellectual disability-based inquiry and the labelled people who made this inquiry possible.

Intellectual disability is a slippery concept. Language around this concept changes over time and, like Licia Carlson (2016), we do not view "intellectual disability" as a binding, essential category. To reflect multiple, nuanced understandings of intellectual disability in this writing, we use various phrases, including commonly used person-first vernacular ("people with intellectual disability"), more political phrasing that challenges person-first vernacular ("intellectually disabled people"), and wording that acknowledges that this label is applied to people both with and without their consent ("labelled people").

AUTHOR'S POSITIONING

Plain language: The four writers of this essay have personal and professional connections with intellectual disability. Chelsea Temple Jones enjoys podcasting and grew up with a labelled brother. For almost 20 years, Jennifer Chatsick has worked with labelled adult students at a college and in the community. Kimberlee Collins is a researcher who has close connections with labelled people who have experienced institutionalization. Anne Zbitnew is a teacher and artist who has worked with labelled artists for over ten years.

Dominant language: Given our privileged positions, we write this chapter in an effort to confront, and be upfront about, the complex tensions involved in intellectual disability research and pedagogy, grounded as they are in our own entanglements with critical access and disability justice. We share the perspective that intellectual disability can be described and understood as an intersectional cultural phenomenon, rather than as a series of individual diagnoses. Too often, rhetoric of diagnoses dominates discourses around intellectual disability, as some researchers and readers alike long for a label and wonder what types of intellectual disability are at play. Because we do not subscribe to this longing, and because diagnostic labels have relevance neither in this project nor in knowledge creation around intellectual disability as a lived-out cultural phenomenon, we do not reveal participants' diagnostic label (Jones, 2016).

METHOD AND METHODOLOGY

Plain language: The goal of this project was to show that labelled people can be leaders in media production. Using the many creative methods described below, the podcasters used arts-based methods to produce "The CICE Team" podcast with support from media-makers and researchers between September 2019 and October 2020.

Podcasting

Plain language: Podcasting was our main method of research (Kinkaid et al., 2020). Podcasting allows people with internet access to listen to sound recordings online. Podcasting was chosen because the students could tell their stories in a way that could be widely shared with others. "The CICE Team" podcast involved labelled students, non-labelled students, and facilitators learning from each other. The non-labelled students shared information about how to use the equipment; the facilitators shared information about what a podcast is and what the different parts of a podcast are; and the labelled students shared their ideas and stories and decided what should be included in their podcast. This kind of work is sometimes called "knowing-making." The phrase "knowing-making" comes from Aimi Hamraie and Kelly Fritsch (2019). For these authors, "knowing-making" is a political way of world-building and world-dismantling "*by* and *with* disabled people and communities" that responds to the things going on around them (pp. 4–5).

Dominant language: Podcasting is embraced by critical disciplines because, unlike traditional forms of broadcast media production that privilege dominant voices and languages, podcasting can be made publicly available and "can foreground the voices and perspectives of nearly all individuals in the story" (Doane et al., 2017). Sonically influenced by radio—including the ways in which disability impacted early-twentieth-century radio production and vice versa—podcasting has gained tremendous public traction in the last 15 years (Kirkpatrick, 2017). Given its high potentiality for non-traditional narrativities and public knowledge sharing (Llinares, 2018), podcasting is an appealing method for social-justice-based projects such as our project, *Accessibility as Aesthetic*. Ultimately, this process resulted in a multifaceted podcast uniquely informed by labelled people's knowledge and process, or "knowing-making," described above.

Mixed Methods

Plain language: The podcast was made in three in-person sessions in a recording studio and three online sessions using Zoom. Each recording session was three hours long. The sessions included us (the researchers), and students Cody Bennett and Jacob Berc who taught the podcasters how to use the equipment and shared their reflections as part of this research. We used a variety of ways to communicate in-person and online: conversations, co-learning sessions, drawing, expressive writing, sound-making with objects and voices, and an online focus group. Sometimes podcasters used paper and markers to write or draw their thoughts and ideas. Some podcasters spoke and others were silent. During an online podcast session facilitated by a professional musician, the podcasters created a theme song by saying words, singing, and making sounds with household objects.

Dominant language: Our methodological approach began with the desire to re-orient our inquiry away from a focus on non-disabled communication practices toward new orientations of communication led by intellectual disability and embodied difference (Chandler et al., 2018; Rice et al., 2018). To this end, we embraced communication challenges and recognized the need to communicate in a wide variety of ways—even amid moments of misunderstanding and ambiguity (davis halifax et al., 2018; Jones & Cheuk, 2020). Our iterative methods were adapted to meet the communication needs of the podcasters: we supplied markers and paper for participants to draw and write out their thoughts and ideas, adding drawing and expressive writing to our methods (Jones, 2016). Some participants spoke while others participated quietly. We chose to embrace this silence as a way of contributing to the project (Jones & Cheuk, 2020). Ultimately, we relied on a flexible, mixed-methods approach that attended to Margaret Price and Stephanie Kerschbaum's (2016) instruction that critical disability studies (CDS) research in classrooms can be made accessible by allowing for flexibility and improvisation around method and methodology.

Outsider Participant Observation

Plain language: We also used a method called participant observation. Researchers took notes about what people were doing and saying as they produced "The CICE Team" podcast. These notes are important because later, when it was more difficult to connect due to COVID-19, we were unable to include intellectually disabled people in the writing of this chapter. This means that "insider" knowledge is missing. People with intellectual disabilities, such as the podcasters, can be considered insiders because they have lived experience of intellectual disability. People who do not have lived experiences of intellectual disability are "outsiders." We—the authors—are outsiders. Although we try to be careful to represent podcasters fairly, we consider this chapter to be incomplete without their input.

Dominant language: We bring to this piece collective uncertainty about how representation of "The CICE Team" and their podcast exists in tension with the justice-based approach this project is meant to espouse. While the podcasters' perspectives are freely, accessibly, and publicly available through "The CICE Team" podcast, our communication with many of the podcasters was limited during the coronavirus's global spread as the College closed and not all podcasters could access the internet. In other words, there were times when it was impossible for us to communicate with podcasters. Their perspectives are noticeably absent in this writing; this incompleteness as a result of contemporary digital divides characterizes our writing.

Literature Review

Intellectual Disability and Inclusion/ism in Pedagogical Research

Plain language: The CICE program believes in inclusion. This means that the people who run this program, and the students in it, want intellectually disabled people to be able to participate in college. Inclusion is an important part of disability history in Canada. However, inclusion does not work for everyone. In the past, institutions such as colleges have not supported disabled people. Today, some disability advocates argue that these places still do not support people even when they say that they are inclusive (Shanouda, 2019). This is called inclusionism (Mitchell et al., 2014). Because "inclusion" and "inclusionism" are ideas that overlap, we combine the words to describe this project as "inclusion/ist."

Dominant language: Though postsecondary education is increasingly becoming an option for intellectually disabled adults in Ontario, there is little written about critical, intersectional research conducted with labelled students in higher education. Labelled people who participate in research related to higher education often do so through programming designed with the rights-based principle of inclusion (Corby et al., 2020; Tucker et al., 2020). Inclusion is upheld as an important, long-fought-for goal for disabled communities hoping to access education (Porter & Richler, 1991; Jackson & Lyons, 2016). CICE programs have different legacies and philosophies across colleges. Humber's program describes itself as a "leader in building collaborative, inclusive communities" (CICE, 2020). CICE students report benefits from experiencing the "adult" side of college, wherein they are recognized as autonomous decision-makers (personal communication, Chatsick, J., July 21, 2020).

While it is clear to us that podcasters and other labelled people value their higher-education experiences of inclusion, a critical tension lingering throughout any pedagogical project linked to inclusion is the risk of inclusionism. Inclusionism refers to the ways in which educational institutions undermine social justice by merely tolerating disability without demanding change to their own disabling conditions or considering its intersectional facets (Mitchell et al., 2014). These disabling conditions have deep roots in Canadian higher education. Intellectual disability has long been present in higher education as a phenomenon deemed worthy of study, particularly when it is understood as a medical problem to be fixed or eradicated. As Jay Dolmage (2017) and other critical researchers explain, eugenics gained legitimacy in academia and is therefore included in higher education classrooms as a topic of study (Hazlewood, 2019; Kelly & Rice, 2020; Kelly et al., 2021; Zbitnew, 2015). Notably, the eugenic history of Humber College is not far out of reach for those involved in this project as it is the site of a former psychiatric hospital (Zbitnew, 2015). Consequently, research ethics boards often drastically overestimate the risks of labelled people participating in research, making it difficult to include intellectually disabled people in knowledge production about themselves (Jones et al., 2021; Santinele Martino & Fudge Schormans, 2018). Concurrently, intellectually disabled people's ongoing struggles to access higher education make it clear that inclusion-based agendas have not solved the problem of their chronic absence, and that their presence is still informed by a medicalized understanding of disability that would prefer labelled people be objects of knowledge production rather than knowledge producers (Siegal, 2011).

Intellectually disabled people's place in higher education remains precarious; it is possible for labelled people to experience real benefits of inclusion while also being folded into the assimilative agendas of institutional inclusionism, which blatantly aim to disempower and disavow intersectional, justice-based advocacy work. The substantial academic ableism intellectually disabled people face as inclusion and inclusion/ist agendas collides and continues to grow as higher education is forced toward emergency remote learning in pandemic times, which further exacerbates digital divides. The only time it ever seems to be overcome is when inclusionism achieves its primary purpose of "molding crip/queer bodies into tolerated neoliberal normativities" (Mitchell et al., 2014, p. 299; Shanouda, 2019). For this reason, we openly name *Accessibility as Aesthetic* as a project problematically positioned at the crux of inclusion/ism.

Disability Justice and Critical Access in Higher Education

Plain language: Disability justice is a type of activism founded by Indigenous people, Black people, and other people of color who identify as mad, disabled, d/Deaf activists and artists (Berne, 2015; Piepzna-Samarasinha, 2018). Disability justice is led by people like the CICE podcasters, some of whom are young people of color—people who may experience complex forms of oppression. Oppression is when one group of people is treated unfairly because of who they are (Making Space for Intimate Citizenship, 2016). Disability justice reminds us that disabled people are experts who have the skills and wisdom to resist oppression, including through "knowing-making" (Hamraie & Fritsch, 2019).

Dominant language: Our decision to critically consider access in the early stages of our project arose from the work of other CDS researchers who urged us to think beyond the promise of universal design (Dolmage, 2017; Hamraie, 2017; Shanouda, 2019). In an arts-based project like this one, we are aware that curative approaches to art therapy may risk reinforcing oppressive social structures in their delivery and design (Zappa, 2017). In her writing on disability justice, Mia Mingus (2011) urges us to "question a culture that makes inaccessibility even possible" (para. 6), while Hamraie (2017) stresses the importance of designing with disability in mind (instead of focusing on accommodation after the fact).

Designing with disability justice meant thinking about access to digital media as it is linked to civic engagement and as a necessary precursor to participation in learning (Ellcessor, 2016, p. 7). "The CICE Team" podcast consisted of creative people already engaged in their own arts-based work and world-making. Their process should be enveloped by their own iterative, "knowing-making" that allows them to create in ways that can be publicly available and therefore influential (p. 6). Following Elizabeth Ellcessor (2016), we conceptualized critical access through disability justice not only as necessary, but also as the justice-based process of labelled people's non-therapeutic cultural production and public knowledge creation from within the inclusion/ist boundaries of higher education.

Discussion

Beginning a College-Based Podcast

Plain language: In November 2019, Chatsick and Zbitnew invited a class of CICE students to make a podcast as part of this research. None of the students identified themselves as podcasters or podcast listeners, but many wished to participate. These students were interested in choosing a topic for the podcast. Chatsick and Zbitnew suggested making a podcast about disability and representation. CICE students wanted to choose a different topic on another day. The class ended with nine CICE students signing up to participate in podcasting.

Dominant language: Chatsick and Zbitnew made space for CICE participants to choose a different topic of their podcast, although this would mean explaining a change in plans to funders and the Humber Research Ethics Board. This points to the first lesson that emerges in intellectual disability research: if we believe in flexible methodologies directed by labelled people, we must be prepared to revise our plans and defend these revisions. Recalling this initial first step toward podcasting in her field notes, Zbitnew wrote, "had we persevered and forced the topic of representation of disability in the media, the project would not have been truly disability-led, as is often the case with intellectual disability [projects]" (Zbitnew, field note, July 14, 2020).

Early Podcast Recording Sessions

Plain language: Between February and April 2020, CICE students participated in three podcast recording sessions. Bennett and Berc guided CICE students through using the equipment. There were two goals for the first session: first, for everyone to draw a self-portrait and to write a short description of themselves, and second, for the group to collectively brainstorm a potential theme for the podcast. This way, audio descriptions of each podcaster would be recorded as well as a self-portrait image to include on the future podcast website. Using markers and paper, CICE students began to draw and write. They described themselves in many creative ways. For example, one podcaster said he "looked like a mountain." These two exercises introduced us to the many

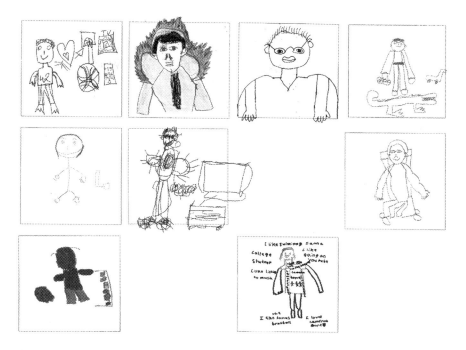

Fig. 21.1 A collection of ten different self-portraits, hand-drawn by members of "The CICE Team" in pen, pencil, marker, and pencil crayon. Some portraits are black and white, while others are very colorful. Each portrait is in a square box. Some show smiling figures with background objects such as a heart, a basketball, and an alligator. Other illustrations have text, including "I like Jonas Brothers." In each drawing, a figure of a podcaster is looking at the viewer

ways podcasters communicated. Below is a collection of self-portraits illustrated by podcasters (Fig. 21.1).

One podcaster offered a written visual description of themselves alongside the black-and-white portrait, below. The visual description reads: "I am wearing a black hoodie. I am wearing grey track pants. I [am] wearing running shoes. I [am] wearing glasses" (Fig. 21.2).

Dominant language: As the drawings above demonstrate, accessible podcasting took on different forms for each participant: some people dictated what they wanted written while Chatsick scribed for them, and one participant asked another student to draw his self-portrait while he verbally described himself. The audio recording picked up this conversation, as the students navigated this task together. In the transcription below, one student is asking another to draw

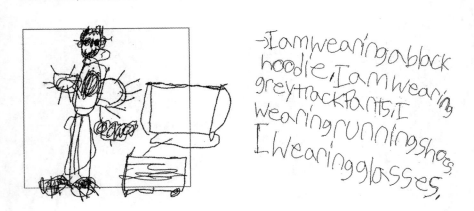

Fig. 21.2 A black and white hand-drawn self-portrait. In the portrait, the artist is facing the viewer and smiling, and appears to be standing beside a series of squares. The artist's image description is written on the right side: "I am wearing a black hoodie. I am wearing grey track pants. I wearing running shoes. I am wearing glasses"

him and his wheelchair. The conversation begins with drawing instructions, and veers off-topic:

Michael:	This is why I like college, because everybody wants to assist everybody....
Ermel:	Are you sure you want [the wheelchair] this size?
Michael:	Yeah.
Michael:	...here, in college, here I told you, you can do whatever you want.
Ermel:	Well, not really.
Michael:	Everybody treats you like an adult so it's only ... as long as you finish your classes and get good grades, they don't really bother you. And now they'll help you, and that's another thing. In college, people want to help people....
Ermel:	How many wheels?
Michael:	Two in the front, two in the back.

During their conversation described above, Ermel drew the following portrait of Michael (Fig. 21.3).

Plain language: The above conversation is an example of how some podcasters experienced inclusion/ism. When Michael explains that in college, "you can do whatever you want," Ermel immediately disagrees: "Well, not really." By disagreeing with Michael, we wonder if Ermel may be pointing out that there are barriers to justice in institutions, even if they claim to be inclusive.

Dominant language: This conversation also demonstrates a crucial moment of collaborative "knowing-making" (Hamraie & Fritsch, 2019). Bennett, who

Fig. 21.3 A black and white hand-drawn portrait. In the portrait, a figure is seated in a wheelchair and facing forward. The person is smiling and has their arms outstretched

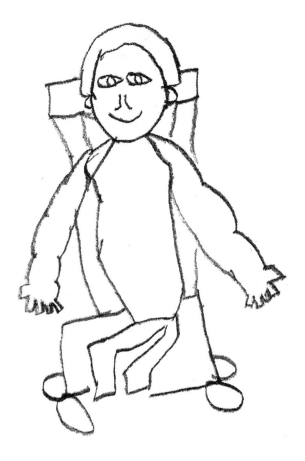

was pacing around the room with a microphone and video camera to capture the process, later wrote an entry in his field notes that reflected his witnessing of this conversational drawing process between two podcasters:

> The artist [Ermel] never once offered his opinion and asked for every single detail, from size of head, the inclusion of the mobility chair, whether he was standing or sitting, and if he had muscles. It provided a student with access that felt pure among peers. Capturing this moment illustrates the fundamentals of media accessibility. Do not create without those you are creating for. (Bennett, field notes, February 21, 2020)

The student's observation drives home the argument that barriers to co-creation and media production must be addressed in the early stages of production so that media representation does not occur without the input, or go

362   C. T. JONES ET AL.

against the interest, of marginalized people (Ellcessor, 2016, p. 6). This observation, combined with our learnings from early sessions that suggest intellectual disability-led podcasting takes a myriad of forms, teaches us that such
disability-led media-making must encourage an evolving set of practices.

Mutual Learning Through Podcast Production

Plain language: Throughout these podcast recording sessions, Bennett and
Berc recorded video and audio, introducing CICE students to the recording
tools. CICE students took turns holding up a large "boom" microphone and
introducing themselves. Berc explained that in the broadcasting industry, this
type of microphone is sometimes referred to as a "dead cat." The CICE students laughed at first, but they did not like picturing a dead cat. They decided
to rename this microphone. Renaming the microphone was an example of
intellectually disabled people making the podcast their own. Bennett recalled
this moment:

> The students' reaction is wild. They all laugh and start suggesting better names.
> One suggests dead rat, one suggests fuzzy, another suggests fuzzy mouse. I've
> never seen such a strong reaction to the term 'dead cat.' Being around the jargon
> all the time you don't take in the violence that comes with the name. Together
> the group decided it will now be called, 'the fuzzy mouse.' (Bennett, field notes,
> February 21, 2020)

Dominant language: The ability to participate in learning through media
production involves choices around technology—including the choice to
reclaim, rename, and hack technology to fit one's needs (Hamraie & Fritsch,
2019). Here, we witness an interchange of learning: CICE students are learning industry terms, and actively renaming and reclaiming their own equipment,
while a Broadcast Television/Videography student is challenged to rethink the
universality, and, as Bennett points out, the violence of dominant language.
What's more, by resistively renaming "the fuzzy mouse," podcasters expanded
the communication possibilities in the room. Bennett goes on:

> From there we had students take over the questioning completely as they took
> charge of the boom pole and point it at their friends to ask about their hobbies
> and interests outside of school time. Now there was room for silence as every
> student had something to say and revealed more and more information about
> themselves. (Bennett, field notes, February 21, 2020)

As podcasters interviewed each other, the podcast emerged not as a traditional, unified, easily explainable podcast, but as a public pedagogy production
with several logos, themes, and hosts who renamed and reclaimed elements of
the production including its gear—most notably the "fuzzy mouse"—and

whose creative work reflects the multifaceted nature of broadcast media production driven by intellectual disability.

Interviews About "Knowing-Making"

Plain language: Podcasters often interviewed one another for "The CICE Team" podcast. During the interviews they talked about their interests and college life. We also knew that two podcasters did their own "knowing-making" by writing stories with pen and paper. We asked if they might be interested in reading their stories for a podcast. When they agreed, another episode was planned around storytelling. In this episode, podcasters Jayson and Ermel explained when and how they prefer to write and offered advice for other writers. One podcaster described the importance of finding a quiet place to focus the mind on writing. In response, the interviewer, Jones, asked a follow-up question:

Jones: What kind of place is that for you?

Jayson: Well, … most of the stories I wrote was back when I was still in the Philippines. And back home in the Philippines, I used to go upstairs to a separate room because when we were at the Philippines before, me, my brother's room and my room were upstairs. So that's usually where I wrote stories before. Just to help me focus on what I'm writing.

Jones: Okay. And Ermel? How about you? Do you have any advice for people who may be interested in writing?

Ermel: If you feel like writing, if you feel like something is coming to you, towards you, and you feel like writing it on paper or in a book, you should go for it! If you've got, like, something that you imagined. Yeah.

Dominant language: These podcasters' engagement with expressive writing demonstrated the field of relations, knowledge, and practices that inform intellectually disabled people's artistic practices. In contrast to dominant forms of production *for* disability that too often inform disabled people's participation in arts-based media making, our choice was to lean into the "knowing-making" of these storytellers as they navigated intersectional systems of power. In the process, the authors designed their own stories (Hamraie & Fritsch, 2019). In addition to offering advice about writing, these authors also shared their writing. Below is an excerpt from Ermel's thriller, "The Mystery of the Missing Goldfish."

> The day started off just like any other. The sun rose in the sky. The school buses ran on time. The sweater Franke wanted to wear was once again stolen by Ermel. The breakfast Dylan ate before leaving for school was two eggs and two pieces of toast as he had every day. That is of course, unless he had human flesh instead.

The experience of blending "knowing-making" methods—writing and podcasting—revealed that project-based pedagogy that involves intellectual disability works well when it begins by honoring intellectually disabled people's already-existing knowledges and artistry, instead of positioning learners as technology "users" to be trained in podcasting.

Silent Podcasts

Plain language: Podcasters were sometimes completely silent during this project. This made our podcast unique because podcasts generally make extensive use of sound and spoken words. At first, we didn't know what to do about this. During the first podcast recording session, Zbitnew wrote in her field notes: "[We]are making a podcast and there is no sound! How is that going to work?" (Zbitnew, field notes, February 20, 2020). But we knew that even when they were silent, podcasters were still contributing to the project. For example, in one session, podcasters used markers and paper to draw a logo for "The CICE Team" podcast. One student sat apart from the group and silently drew. We remembered that silence is political. Disability justice is also political. This meant that being silent became another way of "knowing-making" through podcasting (Hamraie & Fritsch, 2019). Silence became a key characteristic of our podcast.

Dominant language: A silent podcast certainly poses a challenge to those of us accustomed to dominant modes of communication. We wondered: Is the recording still a podcast if parts of it are silent? Should the silent bits be cut in editing? We recognized, however, experiences of silence felt familiar to us. Our backgrounds working with intellectually disabled people made us familiar with silent moments, and we decided that these moments should not only be included in our research but also should characterize the podcast and contribute to its aesthetic.

Initially, we considered the politics of silence. Researchers elsewhere have shown concern that people who communicate silently, or in ways that cannot be recorded by traditional modes of data collection such as audio recordings, might be dismissed in qualitative research (Jones & Cheuk, 2020), although a field of qualitative research inquiry does argue for silence as a critical and meaningful part of research (Freund, 2013; Mazzei, 2007). Silence can also indicate an ethics of refusal, whereby researchers and research participants together decide not to make particular information available for use within the academy (Zahara, 2016). Refusal is a constructive characteristic of communication research; it is through the politics of refusal that disabled and other marginalized groups have forged space in the western cultural imagination (San Pedro, 2015; Wemigwans, 2018).

Moments of silence exist in this research and contribute to the sensorial experience of listening to "The CICE Team" podcast as sound comes and goes. Silence characterizes the production. Following Carlson's (2016) music-based work with labelled people, the podcasting experience is one that can be "valuable and valued for its own sake" without having to be therapeutic, inclusion/ist, or contained by dominant language and expected broadcast forms (p. 5). The integration of silence into the "The CICE Team" podcast asserts a new form of communication that we recognize as embodied, creative, and expressive, coming, as it does, from intellectual disability "knowing-making" that has yet to be fully described.

Conclusion

Plain language: In this chapter we describe important learning moments in the *Accessibility as Aesthetic* project, including the discovery of the "fuzzy mouse." These moments taught us some important lessons. Some of the lessons we learned from this process are listed below.

1. Thinking about accessibility as an ongoing process led by people who are already "knowing-making" pushes back against inclusionism and helps support a disability justice approach to media production.
2. Research around intellectual disability-led media making must be prepared to change in response to what labelled people want to make and do (such as drawing portraits).
3. There is value in creating something like a podcast for its own sake, at its own pace, and at its own volume—even if this means silently.
4. While podcasting is a vibrant method, intellectual disability-informed podcasting holds opportunities for new ways of podcasting, such as a flexible show filled with many logos, themes, hosts, stories, and new names for the technologies (such as "the fuzzy mouse").

Dominant language: In the *Accessibility as Aesthetic* project, we produced a critical access-based podcast that centered labelled people's cultural production from within the inclusion/ist boundaries of higher education. Our findings, listed above, demonstrate some possibilities of considering podcasters' intersectional "knowing-making," (Hamraie & Fritsch, 2019) both as a methodological resource for those embedded in institutional research and pedagogy with labelled people. Yet, in writing about our experience, we still think this chapter is incomplete because not all podcasters could be present in this writing as a result of the digital divides mentioned earlier and the difficulty navigating these divides during a global pandemic. We have tried to make the chapter more accessible by writing in plain language and in dominant language. The challenge of writing both in plain language and in dominant language was significant. The incongruities between these communication styles are stifling, sometimes causing the narrative to skid and falter. For these reasons, we consider our reflections unresolved. Moving forward, it is our challenge as educators and researchers to involve intellectually disabled people in the analysis of their "knowledge-making" so that writing like this can more fully prioritize insider perspectives.

References

Berne, P. (2015). Disability justice—A working draft by Patty Berne. Retrieved February 21, 2022, from http://sinsinvalid.org/blog/disability-justice-a-working-draft-by-patty-berne

Carlson, L. (2016). Music, intellectual disability, and human flourishing. In N. Lerner, J. N. Straus, S. Jensen-Moulton, & B. Howe (Eds.), *The Oxford handbook of music and disability studies* (pp. 37–53). Oxford University Press.

Chandler, E., Changfoot, N., Rice, C., LaMarre, A., & Mykitiuk, R. (2018). Cultivating disability arts in Ontario. *Review of Education, Pedagogy, and Cultural Studies, 40*(3), 249–264. https://doi.org/10.1080/10714413.2018.1472482

CICE (2020). Community Integration through Co-operative Education (CICE). Faculty of Health Sciences & Wellness. Humber College. Retrieved February 22, 2022, from https://healthsciences.humber.ca/programs/cice-ontario-college-certificate.html

Corby, D., Taggart, L., & Cousins, W. (2020). The lived experience of people with intellectual disabilities in post-secondary or higher education. *Journal of Intellectual Disabilities, 24*(3), 339–357. https://doi.org/10.1177/1744629518805603

davis halifax, n.v, Fancy, D., Rinaldi, J., Rossiter, K., & Tigchelaar, A. (2018). Recounting Huronia faithfully: Attenuating our methodology to the "fabulation" of truths-telling. *Cultural Studies, Critical Methodologies, 18*(3), 216–227. https://doi.org/10.1177/1532708617746421

Doane, B., McCormick, K., & Sorce, G. (2017). Changing methods for feminist public scholarship: Lessons from Sarah Koenig's podcast serial. *Feminist Media Studies: Feminist Reception Studies in a Post-Audience Age: Returning to Audiences and Everyday Life, 17*(1), 119–121. https://doi.org/10.1080/14680777.2017.1261465

Dolmage, J. T. (2017). *Academic ableism: Disability and higher education.* University of Michigan Press.

Ellcessor, E. (2016). *Restricted access: Media, disability, and the politics of participation.* New York University Press.

Freund, A. (2013). Toward an ethics of silence? Negotiating off-the-record events and identity in oral history. In A. Sheftel & S. Zembrzycki (Eds.), *Oral History off the record: Toward an ethnography of practice* (pp. 221–238). Palgrave Macmillan.

Hamraie, A. (2017). *Building access: Universal design and the politics of disability.* University of Minnesota Press.

Hamraie, A., & Fritsch, K. (2019). Crip technoscience manifesto. *Catalyst, 5*(1), 1–33. https://doi.org/10.28968/cftt.v5i1.29607

Hazlewood, J. (2019, September 25). New Guelph exhibit reveals history of eugenics education in Ontario. *CBC.* Retrieved February 22, 2022, from https://www.cbc.ca/news/canada/kitchener-waterloo/eugenics-ontario-guelph-museum-exhibit-1.5293653

Jackson, R., & Lyons, M. (2016). *Community care and inclusion for people with an intellectual disability.* Floris Books.

Jones, C. T. (2016). *Writing intellectual disability: Glimpses into precarious processes of re/making a cultural phenomenon* (Unpublished doctoral dissertation). York University.

Jones, C. T., Collins, K., & Zbitnew, A. (2021). Accessibility as aesthetic in broadcast media: Critical access theory and disability justice as project-based learning.

Journalism & Mass Communication Educator, 77(1), 24–42. https://doi.org/10.1177/10776958211000198

Jones, C. T., & Cheuk, F. (2020). Something is happening: Encountering silence in disability research. *Qualitative Research Journal, 21*(1), 1–14. https://doi.org/10.1108/QRJ-10-2019-0078

Kelly, E. & Rice, C. (2020, January 16). Universities must open their archives and share their oppressive pasts. *The Conversation.* Retrieved February 11, 2022, from https://theconversation.com/universities-must-open-their-archives-and-share-their-oppressive-pasts-125539

Kelly, E., Manning, D. T., Boye, S., Rice, C., Owen, D., Stonefish, S., & Stonefish, M. (2021). Elements of a counter-exhibition: Excavating and countering a Canadian history and legacy of eugenics. *Journal of the History of the Behavioral Sciences, 57*(1), 12–33. https://doi.org/10.1002/jhbs.22081

Kinkaid, E., Emard, K., & Senanayake, N. (2020). The Podcast-as-method? Critical reflections on using podcasts to produce geographic knowledge. *Geographical Review, 110*(1–2), 78–91. https://doi.org/10.1111/gere.12354

Kirkpatrick, B. (2017). "A blessed boon": Radio, disability, governmentality and discourse of the "shut-in," 1920–1930. In E. Ellcessor & B. Kirkpatrick (Eds.), *Disability media studies.* New York University Press.

Llinares, D. (2018). *Podcasting: New aural cultures and digital media.* Palgrave Macmillan. https://doi.org/10.1007/978-3-319-90056-8

Making Space for Intimate Citizenship, (2016). "Let us show you"—Shona Casola. Retrieved February 21, 2022, from https://makingspaceforintimatecitizenship.wordpress.com/

Mazzei, L. A. (2007). *Inhabited silence in qualitative research: Putting poststructural theory to work* (Vol. 318). Peter Lang.

Mingus, M. (2011, August 22). *Moving toward the ugly: A politic beyond desirability.* Femmes of Color Symposium keynote speech, Oakland, CA. Retrieved February 21, 2022, from http://leavingevidence.wordpress.com/2011/08/22/moving-toward-the-ugly-a-politic-beyond-desirability/

Mitchell, D. T., Snyder, S. L., & Ware, L. (2014). "[Every] child left behind": Curricular cripistemologies and the crip/queer art of failure. *Journal of Literary & Cultural Disability Studies, 8*(3), 295–314. https://doi.org/10.3828/jlcds.2014.24

Piepzna-Samarasinha, L. L. (2018). *Care work: Dreaming disability justice.* Arsenal Pulp Press.

Porter, G. L., & Richler, D. (1991). *Changing Canadian schools: Perspectives on disability and inclusion.* The Roeher Institute.

Price, M., & Kerschbaum, S. L. (2016). Stories of methodology: Interviewing sideways, crooked and crip. *Canadian Journal of Disability Studies, 5*(3), 18–56. https://doi.org/10.15353/cjds.v5i3.295

Reagan, T. (2011). Ideological barriers to American Sign Language: Unpacking linguistic resistance. *Sign Language Studies, 11*(4), 606–636. https://doi.org/10.1353/sls.2011.0006

Rice, C., Chandler, E., Liddiard, K., Rinaldi, J., & Harrison, E. (2018). Pedagogical possibilities for unruly bodies. *Gender and Education, 30*(5), 663–682. https://doi.org/10.1080/09540253.2016.1247947

Richardson, L. (2003). Writing: A method of inquiry. In Y. S. Lincoln & N. K. Denzin (Eds.), *Turning points in qualitative research: Tying knots in a handkerchief* (pp. 379–396). AltaMira Press.

Rose, H., & Conama, J. B. (2018). Linguistic imperialism: Still a valid construct in relation to language policy for Irish Sign Language. *Language Policy, 17*(3), 385–404. https://doi.org/10.1007/s10993-017-9446-2

San Pedro, T. J. (2015). Silence as shields: Agency and resistances among Native American students in the urban Southwest. *Research in the Teaching of English, 50*(2), 132–153. https://www.jstor.org/stable/24890030

Santinele Martino, A., & Fudge Schormans, A. (2018). When good intentions backfire: University research ethics review and the intimate lives of people labeled with intellectual disabilities. *Forum: Qualitative Social Research, 19*(3). https://doi.org/10.17169/fqs-19.3.3090

Shanouda, F. (2019). *The Politics of passing: Disabled and mad students' experiences of disclosure in higher education.* (Unpublished doctoral dissertation). University of Toronto.

Shew, A. (2018). Different ways of moving through the world. *Logic, 5.* Retrieved February 21, 2022, from https://logicmag.io/failure/different-ways-of-moving-through-the-world/

Siegal, A. (2011, August 13). The education of Ashif Jaffer. *BBC* [The Documentary Podcast BBC World Service]. Retrieved February 21, 2022, from https://www.bbc.co.uk/programmes/p02rth23

Tucker, E. C., Jones, J. L., Gallus, K. L., Emerson, S. R., & Manning-Ouellette, A. L. (2020). Let's take a walk: Exploring intellectual disability as diversity in higher education. *Journal of College and Character, 21*(3), 157–170. https://doi.org/10.1080/2194587X.2020.1781659

Wemigwans, J. (2018). *A digital bundle: Protecting and promoting Indigenous knowledge online.* University of Regina Press.

Zahara, A. (2016, March 21). Refusal as research method in discard studies. Retrieved February 21, 2022, from https://discardstudies.com/2016/03/21/refusal-as-research-method-in-discard-studies/

Zappa, A. (2017). Beyond erasure: The ethics of art therapy research with trans and gender-independent people. *Art Therapy, 34*(3), 129–134. https://doi.org/10.1080/07421656.2017.1343074

Zbitnew, A. (2015). Visualizing absence: Memorializing the histories of the former Lakeshore Psychiatric Hospital. Retrieved February 21, 2022, from https://visualizingabsence.wixsite.com/visualizing-absencel-space-gallery

CHAPTER 22

Organizational Communication and Disability: Improvising Sense-Sharing

Amin Makkawy and Shane T. Moreman

We offer a disability-centered approach to organizational communication to underscore the practicality and the creativity that disability catalyzes within organizations and therefor within the study of organizational communication. As scholars of organizational communication have well established, the creation, sharing, and understanding of meaning are wonderfully complex processes within organizations. Most recently, Ashcraft (2020) has argued for an ontological turn within organizational communication studies that focuses on relationality and communicative practice. In this chapter, we take up Ashcraft's call by examining disability as a powerful catalyst for organizational communication. Specifically, we argue that a cripistemological approach to disability can activate new ways of organizing and establishing meaning within groups. If epistemology is the nature of knowledge, then cripistemology is a focus on the denaturing of knowledge so as to know the range of realities experienced by disabled persons and their communities. In this chapter we are attentive to how a cripistemological approach generates improvisational acts of meaning within the contexts of organizations.

We write from our respective backgrounds as an organizational communication scholar and an intercultural communication scholar as well as our intersectional positionalities. We are particularly interested in the forms of knowledge and communication practiced by marginalized groups that have only recently been recognized as valuable within the communication discipline. Our

A. Makkawy (✉) • S. T. Moreman
California State University, Fresno, CA, USA
e-mail: amakkawy@mail.fresnostate.edu

© The Author(s), under exclusive license to Springer Nature
Switzerland AG 2023
M. S. Jeffress et al. (eds.), *The Palgrave Handbook of Disability and Communication*, https://doi.org/10.1007/978-3-031-14447-9_22

369

combined positionalities represent both sides of the following dialectics, provided here in random order: border-state-raised/Midwest-raised, disabled/nondisabled, married/single, middle-aged/young, Muslim/Latinx, sighted/blind, straight/gay, tenure-track/tenured. To be intersectionally aware requires being cognizant of one's advantages (Yep, 2016), so we also acknowledge our shared privileges as cisgendered males, who use the pronouns he/him/his, enjoy birthright U.S. citizenship, have doctorates in communication, and are gainfully employed at the same U.S. public university. These identities guide our research interests and our research findings (Lindlof & Taylor, 2019; Madison, 2020; Tracy, 2020).

Our positionalities also make this research particularly timely. The U.S.'s continual involvement in Middle Eastern and Latin American conflicts have resulted in Latinxs and Muslims being discursively rediscovered each time they are subject to public attention. Despite a longstanding U.S. presence, Muslims and Latinxs tend to become national concerns only when debate intensifies over who belongs in the U.S. and what space should be allotted to these "new" Brown subjectivities. Similarly, the Americans with Disabilities Act has only been ratified since 1990, making its requirements appear sudden and oppressive to some, while effectively obscuring a long history of disabled persons being integral contributing members of U.S. society. We embrace our own dynamic positionalities as assets for understanding modern organizational cultures with their own continually changing dynamics and demographics. To more fully explain our approach to organizational communication, in the next section we elucidate our understanding of organizational culture as well as the foundational disciplinary literature that informs us.

THE PERFORMANCE OF ORGANIZATIONAL CULTURES

Pacanowsky and O'Donnell-Trujillo (1982, 1983, 1990) maintain that organizations have cultures and, more specifically, organizations are cultures constituted through communication. "From our point of view, organizations are places where people work and do a whole lot of other things, and all of these work things and other things constitute life in that organization" (Pacanowsky & O'Donnell-Trujillo, 1982, p. 117). The tasks of the job are only a part of the overall culture of an organization. "So for now, it seems appropriate to construe organizations as places where people do things together, to the extent that what they do together involves communication" (Pacanowsky & O'Donnell-Trujillo, 1982, p. 122). The organizational culture, a composite of varying types of communication performances, is the whole of the organization's meaning and value. An organizational culture lens on organizations provides a way to recognize the organizational uniqueness that is, somewhat ironically, both derived from and in resistance to structures that are common across all organizations (e.g., meetings, human resources departments, labor laws). As Pacanowsky and O'Donnell-Trujillo (1983) put it, "If... we pay attention to the variability in the patterns of performances, we can expect that we will develop a more subtle appreciation both of particular organizational cultures and the more general processes that bring them into being" (pp. 146–147). Paying attention to organizational culture means paying attention to what makes an organization both typical and unique.

We adhere to the performance studies paradigm that acknowledges the agency of organizational members (i.e., they act) and the embodied materiality of the organizational reality (i.e., they present actions). Trujillo (1985) encourages attending to an organization's symbolic and rhetorical functioning through communicative performances. From the researcher's perspective, performance helps define organizations in three different ways: (1) "it encourages researchers to look closely at communicative action as it occurs in organizational contexts"; (2) it "encourages researchers to consider the senses of identity and culture the organizational communication creates"; and (3) it "may motivate organizational researchers to begin making more 'rhetorical' judgments about organizational communication phenomena" (Trujillo, 1985, pp. 220–221). Today, organizational culture is well recognized as a phenomenon in both academic and non-academic settings. Eisenberg and Riley (2001) note that by the turn of the twenty-first century, multiple studies had adopted this performance approach to studying organizational cultures: "As these studies indicate, culture as performance moved far beyond early notions of significant 'symbols' and artifacts and began to embrace a multivocal, eclectic, contradictory, and celebratory sense of organizational culture" (p. 299). What remains to be seen, however, is to what extent these studies have also considered the significance of disability within organizational culture.

A performance-focused approach to organizational communication yields research that is described through the embodied and symbolic acts of its organizational members. "Using the symbolic-performance lens allows the researcher to examine how culture is brought into being" (Keyton, 2014, p. 556). Because exploring organizations through this lens sheds light on how organizations are constituted through their members, it also provides insight into strategies for organizational inclusivity. Harter et al. (2006), for example, conduct a narrative ethnography of a non-profit organization that offers a way for disabled people to perform counter-narratives against delimited views of who they are. Sass (2000) explores how nursing home caregivers perform emotional labor within their task and relational roles. Scott (2012) does not examine organizational culture per se, but does explore the struggles and successes of 26 physically disabled professionals to capture how they performatively embody resilience within their often-challenging work environments. Also, Scott (2018) extends a discussion of embodiment that is performed within varying contexts including health and educational institutions. We find the above studies valuable, but argue that performance approaches to embodiment could still improve with greater attention to intersectionality—by which we mean, the discursive interconnections of socio-political positionalities within and across one another. In the following section, we review crip theory with a specific focus on communication and connect it to a more intersectionally inclusive conceptualization of disability.

CRIP THEORY IN COMMUNICATION

Organizational culture studies in communication lean toward an interactional methodology of data collection techniques such as ethnography, participant observation, and unstructured interviews. From these methods, the performances of the organizational members are categorized. As Keyton explains (2011), "the symbolic performance perspective examines the way in which organizational performances reveal cultural meaning, as well as how the performance itself is developed, maintained, and changed" (p. 83). To assemble those embodied and symbolic performances in a way that intensifies an intersectional organizational representation, we coordinate those meanings through crip theory. Broadly, "crip theory is an interdisciplinary sourced lens for understanding the interplay between space, minds, bodies, and meaning out of the positionalities of disabled persons and their communities" (Makkawy & Moreman, 2019, p. 402). Developed by Sandahl (2003, 2006, 2008, 2018) through a performance studies framework, crip theory attends to the generative meanings of disabled people's expressed experiences.

Crip theory often places binaries in tension with one another—for example, the tragic with the ludic—so as to account for the complexity and humanity of disabled persons. The theory has also evolved from primarily being applied in artistic settings to offering a broader societal analysis (Kafer, 2013; McRuer, 2006, 2018; Puar, 2017). For scholars like McRuer (2018), the praxis of crip theory is a praxis of common sense social justice: "attend to those who are not you, to those who are different from you (different embodiments, different minds, different behaviors), and attempt in that interdependent attending to apprehend the web of social relations in which we are currently located—social relations can (of course) be figured, and that can (of course) be changed" (p. 217). Crip, as both theory and method, offers a framework for theorizing and researching the human experience that interrupts and then rescripts nondisableist discourses. Yet crip studies are still not robustly researched within the communication discipline. To the extent that crip is included in communication research, it ranges from expressive synonym to productive metaphor to transformative concept. For example, crip has sometimes been directly equated with disability as a way to present resistance to nondisableist communication theory and practice (Scott, 2012; St. Pierre, 2015). Addressing compulsory ablebodiedness more directly, Mann (2018, 2019) looks at how crip rhetorically congeals progressive solidarity and revamps nondisableist-privileging concepts of time. Makkawy and Moreman (2019) explore how crip, as methodology, potentially changes the theorization of communication. Fletcher and Primack (2017) present a crip media analysis that ultimately betters narrative coherence. For Yep (2013), crip is an additional entrée into intersectional perspectives of positionality. And for Ferris (2008), crip addresses how to reconceptualize the presentation of knowledge and ultimately change what is respected *as* knowledge. Taken together, these crip studies demonstrate not only the diversity of crip theory and method, but also the ways that communication is forming crip from our co-created, shared understanding perspective. Nonetheless, there is still more work to be done.

Organizational communication scholarship has sought to attune itself to contemporary identities of difference found within organizations (Allen, 2011; Ashcraft, 2017). An identity framework in organizational studies offers opportunities for "novel and nuanced theoretical accounts, to produce rich empirical analyses that capture the inter-subjectivity of organizational life in a thoughtful and empathetic fashion, and to demonstrate how individual and collective self-constructions become powerful players in organizing processes and outcomes" (Alvesson et al., 2008, p. 7). By paying attention to changing demographics, organizational communication scholars are also highlighting the changing ways how meaning is created, shared, and understood within organizations. Valuing difference but rejecting a narrow focus on language as sense-making, Ashcraft (2020) moves the communication discipline toward affect as a way to explain sense-sharing. Encouraging us to look beyond words and the individual, Ashcraft theorizes an ontological turn that understands sense-sharing as an accomplishment of the full body and mind in collaboration with other bodies and minds and with the surrounding contexts. "To be affected is to be an absorbent body [and mind] emerging as a self with the surround, through energetic flow between bodies [and minds]" (Ashcraft, 2020, p. 574). Crip theory, too, is experientially based and is relationally manifested, all from subjectivities at the margins of the normative. A coalition of non-normatives (e.g., physically diverse altered, gender nonconforming, neurodiverse, or racially disenfranchised), crip is both intersectional and inclusive in its transformative possibilities. In the following section, we explain how making a crip ontological turn requires attending to the affect of non-normative energy flows of bodies and minds whose presences are often uncertainly performed and co-performed.

CRIPISTEMOLOGY OF ORGANIZATIONAL COMMUNICATION

For people of difference, our affective sense-sharing may consistently offer a troubled affect. While disability is a personal experience, it is also a social experience that is created beyond the individual. Using the term "affect trouble," Forrest (2020) describes how crip persons experience their disability subjectivity beyond the normative. To develop the term, he overlaps crip theory (McRuer, 2006), gender trouble (Butler, 2006), and Brown sense-making (Muñoz, 2006). As Puar (2009) puts it, "If affect is impersonal, emotion is the expression or capture of affect, the subjective content and sociolinguistic fixing of the quality of experience which is from that point onward defined as personal" (p. 161). Affect trouble is the voluntary or involuntary misalignment of social expectations with compulsory affective norms that becomes a personal experience. For example, the personal challenge for some is access to the organizational space so that their bodies can participate in sense-sharing. For others, it is the personal awkwardness of, once having accessed the space, being able to engage physically, emotionally, or cognitively within these spaces. It all depends and it is not at all dependable. Even an embrace of crip theory is troubling insofar as crip is an ever-shifting perspective that fails compulsory ideals of predictability and often exceeds or evades definition. Very often, crip "has the fabulous potential to be simultaneously flamboyantly identarian (as in, we are crip and you will acknowledge that!) and flamboyantly anti-identarian (as in, we reject your categories or the capacity of languages saturated in ableism to describe us!)" (McRuer, 2018, p. 20). We take up crip's deviations and divergences in order to shed light on how organizational communication is constituted through performative acts of meaning. Following Ashcraft's (2020) ontological turn, we understand these performative acts to be about sense-sharing, especially a crip sense-sharing that may be troubling for some, but for others may be a sharing that finally, if fleetingly, makes common sense.

Cripistemology is the practice of knowing disability through a crip theoretical lens. More directly, cripistemology is an approach to knowledge that accounts for "rejected and extraordinary [bodies/minds] and at the same time... [explores] disability at the places where [bodily/mental] edges and categorical distinctions blur or dissolve (where the disabled [body/mind] as literal referent is, if not dematerialized, then differently materialized)" (Johnson & McRuer, 2014, p. 134). Put another way, the cripistemological troubles the ontological, and it does so in a productive way. Johnson and McRuer (2014) point in particular to the women of color/queer of color thinkers who have founded critical work in bodily experience. This legacy "attended to what was happening, differentially, to bodies and minds caught up in the transformations taking place, rejected processes of pathologization and making-deviant, and gestured outward to new ways of being-in-common together" (Johnson & McRuer, 2014, p. 138). Cripistemology purposefully refocuses on the ways and forms of knowing of non-ideal bodies and frames the minds as an agent of data collection and interpretation. With its intentional exploration of crip spaces, times, and consciousness, cripistemology honors the totality of the human experience via the exploration of crip life, while it also seeks to share such experiences in ways that could bring people together.

Cripistemology grants expression of the experiences of crip persons and their communities beyond the nondisableist subject and toward a solidarity with one another and with others. It seeks to reimagine beyond what is normal. Our adopted definition of organizational communication is simple: "the interaction required to direct a group toward a shared goal" (Eisenberg et al., 2017, p. 4). By integrating cripistemology, our adapted definition of organizational communication gets more complicated. We are interested in understanding the ways in which organizational culture manifests in the performed, embodied and symbolic acts of its members. We appreciate how the ontological turn within communication studies can "(a) inform transmission as a constitutive activity, (b) expand what counts as communication to include overlooked forms of message exchange, and (c) recover disappeared ways that power operates communicatively" (Ashcraft, 2020, p. 2). With a cripistemological approach to organizational communication, we offer ways that crip's troubling affects are opportunities to rescript the sense-sharing performances of organizations. These rescriptings produce potentialities for constituting flows of signification that allow for wider understandings of the what and the who of sense-sharing. To further explain, we offer three cripistemological themes for organizational communication that are borne from crip troubling affects that provoke a sense-sharing toward a goal of valuing disability.

CRIPISTEMOLOGICAL THEMES FOR ORGANIZATIONAL COMMUNICATION

Drawing on a performance of organizational culture framework, we suggest three cripistemological themes for organizational communication: (1) improving interactions, (2) improvising group members, and (3) improvising shared goals. These are crip improvisations that both materialize disabled subjectivity but also seek to transform disability from a static identarian construct toward a recognition of humanity. Disability has often been used as a staged storytelling device to signify character struggle (e.g., visual impairment in *Oedipus* or neurodiversity in *Richard III*) (Kuppers, 2017). U.S. disability history exposes the many ways in which organizations have sought to manage the disabled through "diagnostic regimes" ranging from the curative (i.e., fix the disabled) to the custodial (i.e., oversee the disabled) (Snyder & Mitchell, 2006, p. 71). Historically, the interactions between disabled persons and nondisabled persons within organizations are fraught with challenge. As such, we approach the communicative encounter as one that "informs the material contact and movement involved in language and representation (step one) and expands the bodies and modes of communication eligible to partake in the transmission of sense (step two)" (Ashcraft, 2020, p. 20).

Our focus on organizational communication cultural encounters foregrounds disability via an ontological turn as a transmission and a constitution but also an expanded sense to avoid the curative and the custodial. And we are not the first to do so. The artist and activist, Terry Galloway, has developed an Ethic of Accommodation that is drawn from her personal and professional history of seeking and adapting organizational fit (Galloway, 2009, 2016; Galloway et al., 2007; Moreman, 2019). We summarize the four components of the Ethic of Accommodation as: (1) gratefully pursue difficult changes proposed by the few; (2) listen; (3) prioritize complex negotiations; and (4) be receptive to creative inspiration. We find Galloway's positive emotional approach to accommodation to be particularly refreshing in the way it fully recognizes the arduousness of the tasks, but also underscores the improvisational joy of it all. Similarly, Puar (2009) emphasizes the conviviality of the encounter or, put another way, the intentional positive affect of reframing disability as the stimulant for transformative sense-sharing.

Rather than understanding the encounter as trouble between the disabled person and nondisabled person, Puar (2017) reconfigures the encounter in terms of the capacities and debilities within the transmission and constitution of the exchange. While disability is often defined through its debilities or weaknesses, Puar encourages to also understand it through its capacities or strengths. However, by couching the disabled/nondisabled encounter as concerning capacity and debility, we should not lose grasp on how disability is more likely to be a statistical likelihood for disenfranchised communities. While disability may be the primary signifier within the encounter, that signifier often overlaps with the capacities and debilities of race, gender, sexuality, socio-economic status, and employment status. The encounter is one of multiple differences. Indeed, all of our differences can be understood because of and beyond their identarian categorizations as attributes that intersectionally shape the capacities and debilities of the transmission, constitution, and affect of the encounter. What are the relational, collaborative, envisioned capacities or debilities exposed by the tension between disability and nondisability? Using a framework of capacity and debility lends a more generous understanding of the interaction, the group, and the shared goals. Bringing this all back to a performance framework, the encounter between disability and nondisability is an improvisational synergy between cultural norms and innovations. As a crip praxis, these improvisations are not necessarily "how to" but we hope they are inspirations for "why not?" Next, we improvise three cripistemological themes for organizational communication: improvising interactions, improvising group members, and improvising shared goals.

Improvising Interactions in Crip Organizational Communication

As manifested through the interactions of its organizational members, organizations are structured by organizational rules in the form of policies, laws, and rituals. Organizational actors, in turn, either follow the reified organizational scripts or they agentically improvise. Operating from a positionality of affect trouble, crip members improvise interaction in the organizational context and, in doing so, perform potentially new structural norms. Michalko (2010) explains how his blindness combined with others' sight "marks the beginning for sight to see itself" (para. 20). As the blind and the sighted coordinate with one another, disability is recast as crip capacity (i.e., sense-sharing that generates a self-reflexivity about what is normative) and nondisabled debility (i.e., an obliviousness to a limited world view). By reframing how interactions transmit and constitute organizational culture, cripistemology provides the tools to transform agency from an optional pursuit to an ongoing pursuit for more agile and innovative organizational interactions. It also reorganizes interactions in a way that increases synchronicity and potentially rescripts organizational futures.

Improvising Group Members in Crip Organizational Communication

While the structural elements of an organization may determine the organizational roles, the people of the organization determine the outcomes derived from those roles. To fulfill an organization's mission and vision, organizational members must interdependently coordinate as teams, departments, or units. To be an ensemble, group members must act collectively and collaboratively, while also playing off their own idiosyncrasies. Crip's troubling affect productively disrupts the rhythm of organizational flows. As organizations strive toward inclusivity, crip workers require an improvisational rescripting of inclusion that demands neither assimilation (e.g., be like the nondisabled) nor segregation (e.g., be separate from the nondisabled). Focusing on the failures of crip group membership, Mitchell et al. (2014) promote attention to the crip person's idiosyncrasies. The ironies, tensions, and individual incongruities revealed by crip experience have the potential to "create more flexibility within majoritarian norms and within crip/queer subcultures themselves" (Mitchell et al., 2014, p. 308). All group members benefit from the failures because all group members learn how the shared-meanings of non-normativity can transform the organizational scripts.

Improvising Shared Goals in Crip Organizational Communication

An organization is also manifested through the shared goals of its organizational members. These shared goals become the larger purpose that drives organizational members to do their work, and, over time, organizational members perform the culture of organization. While the goals may be shared, the collective sharing happens between members with individual perspectives, therefore offering an organization of unified, even if fragmented, intentions. Crip's troubling affect introduces improvisation that can cause discontinuity within an organization but also reveals the perpetual interpretive unrest of the organization's shared goals. Chen (2012) focuses upon the non-neutral energy or flows among and between the animate and inanimate, including the crip disabled. These energies are shaped by the context, by institutions, by people, and by flora and fauna—and Chen refuses to erase the role of race and sexuality in these flows. A crip perspective on the organizing process challenges organizations to reconsider the fragmented flows of shared goals as productively unifying forces. Crip invites those on and off the stage to improvise both their interpretations and their enactments. As a result of crip's energies, the stage is transformed into a self-aware space in which shared goals are recoded in ways that can give organizational culture new life.

Conclusion

Organizational communication continues to develop ways to understand how humans communicate and make and share meaning with one another. We offer a cripistemological approach that is informed by Ashcraft's (2020) ontological turn, and that seeks to combine communication theory with organizational communication studies. Johnson and McRuer point out that "[c]ripistemology is everywhere in theory, once you start looking for it" (Johnson & McRuer, 2014, p. 130), and we find it within organizational communication as organizational sense-sharing. By understanding the organization as a culturally performed phenomenon, we consider how the affect trouble of crip exposes the absent or erased experiences of disability. But beyond revealing such absences and erasures, we want to highlight and build commonalities between disability and nondisability by reframing their encounter in terms of capacity and debility. Moreover, we seek to move beyond the limitations of language because "language is not *the* mode of communication that helps human bodies translate one kind of energetic mattering into another" (Ashcraft, 2020, p. 17). A crip perspective thus seeks to broaden sensory reception by exploring both organizational capacities and organizational debilities. In this way, organizational culture is a form of sense-sharing that goes beyond the mere symbolic and linguistic to operate through other corporeal and perceptual means.

The bodies and minds of organizational members engage the debilities of an organization through their own given capacities; these capacities are both individual and collective. Puar (2009) acknowledges that the goal is to move past the individual isolations and conflicts of identitarian politics. "[T]he challenge before us is how to craft convivial political praxis that does not demand a continual reinvestment in its form and content, its genesis or its outcomes, the literalism of its object nor the direction of its drive" (p. 169). Offering forth crip improvisations does not dismantle difference but it does demonstrate how differences are opportunities to relearn debilities as capacities and vice versa. Unfinished and uncertain, these crip improvisations help to reconfigure the "prepersonal (i.e., precedes, or exceeds, the self) and transpersonal (i.e., traverses bodies, forming interdependent selves)" (Ashcraft, 2020, p. 4) so that the world-making effect is as inspiring as it is innovating. Importantly, we do not want to promote crip as being in service to the neoliberal profit project. Also, as St. Pierre and Peers (2016) note, the crip theoretical project is not one of self-definition: "De-composing ourselves through crooked and crip tellings is to cultivate the types of interruptions and disorientations through which we find ourselves given over and responsive to each other" (para. 15). When organizations enact crip improvisations, innovation drives the sense-sharing flows of the encounter. And with innovation as the shared goal, an improvised, inclusive praxis is sure to follow and then lead.

References

Allen, B. J. (2011). *Difference matters: Communicating social identity* (2nd ed.). Waveland Press.

Alvesson, M., Ashcraft, K. L., & Thomas, R. (2008). Identity matters: Reflections on the construction of identity scholarship in organization studies. *Organization, 15*(1), 5–28. https://doi.org/10.1177/1350508407084426

Ashcraft, K. L. (2017). "Submission" to the rule of excellence: Ordinary affect and precarious resistance in the labor of organization and management studies. *Organization, 24*(1), 36–58. https://doi.org/10.1177/1350508416668188

Ashcraft, K. L. (2020). Communication as constitutive transmission? An encounter with affect. *Communication Theory, 31*(4), 571-592. https://doi.org/10.1093/ct/qtz027

Butler, J. (2006). *Gender trouble: Feminism and the subversion of identity* (2nd ed.). Routledge.

Chen, M. Y. (2012). *Animacies: Biopolitics, racial mattering, and queer affect.* Duke University Press.

Eisenberg, E. M., & Riley, P. (2001). Organizational culture. In F. M. Jablin & L. L. Putnam (Eds.), *The new handbook of organizational communication* (pp. 291–322). Sage. https://doi.org/10.4135/9781412986243

Eisenberg, E. M., Trethewey, A., LeGreco, M., & Goodall, H. L., Jr. (2017). *Organizational communication: Balancing creativity and constraint* (8th ed.). Bedford/St. Martin's.

Ferris, J. (2008). Thirteen ways of looking at crip poetry. *Text and Performance Quarterly, 28*(1–2), 6–7. https://doi.org/10.1080/10462930701754275

Fletcher, B., & Primack, A. J. (2017). Driving toward disability rhetorics: Narrative, crip theory, and eco-ability in *Mad Max: Fury Road. Critical Studies in Media Communication, 34*(4), 344–357. https://doi.org/10.1080/15295036.2017.1329540

Forrest, B. J. (2020). Crip feelings/feeling crip. *Journal of Literary & Cultural Disability Studies, 14*(1), 75–90. https://doi.org/10.3828/jlcds.2019.14

Galloway, T. (2009). *Mean little deaf queer: A memoir.* Beacon Press.

Galloway, T. (2016). On being told "no": Keynote for *Celebrating disability through performance,* Georgia Southern's Patti Pace Performance Festival 2016. *Text and Performance Quarterly, 36*(2–3), 149–155. https://doi.org/10.1080/10462937.2016.1195507

Galloway, T., Nudd, D. M., & Sandahl, C. (2007). "Actual lives" and the Ethic of Accommodation. In P. Kuppers & G. Robertson (Eds.), *The community performance reader* (pp. 227–234). Routledge.

Harter, L. M., Scott, J. A., Novak, D. R., Leeman, M., & Morris, J. F. (2006). Freedom through flight: Performing a counter-narrative of disability. *Journal of Applied Communication Research, 34*(1), 3–29. https://doi.org/10.1080/00909880500420192

Johnson, M. L., & McRuer, R. (2014). Cripistemologies: Introduction. *Journal of Literary & Cultural Disability Studies, 8*(2), 127–147. https://doi.org/10.3828/jlcds.2014.12

Kafer, A. (2013). *Feminist, crip, queer.* Indiana University Press.

Keyton, J. (2011). *Communication & organizational culture: A key to understanding work experiences* (2nd ed.). Sage.

Keyton, J. (2014). Organizational culture: Creating meaning and influence. In L. L. Putman & D. K. Mumby (Eds.), *The Sage handbook of organizational communication: Advances in theory, research, and methods* (3rd ed., pp. 549–568). Sage.

Kuppers, P. (2017). *Theatre & disability.* Palgrave.

Lindlof, T. R., & Taylor, B. C. (2019). *Qualitative communication research methods* (4th ed.). Sage.

Madison, D. S. (2020). *Critical ethnography: Methods, ethics, and performance* (3rd ed.). Sage.

Makkawy, A., & Moreman, S. T. (2019). Putting crip in the script: A critical communication pedagogical study of communication theory textbooks. *Communication Education, 68*(4), 401–416. https://doi.org/10.1080/03634523.2019.1643898

Mann, B. W. (2018). Rhetoric of online disability activism: #CripTheVote and civic participation. *Communication, Culture and Critique, 11*(4), 604–621. https://doi.org/10.1093/ccc/tcy030

Mann, B. W. (2019). Autism narratives in media coverage of the MMR vaccine-Autism controversy under a crip futurism framework. *Health Communication, 34*(9), 984–990. https://doi.org/10.1080/10410236.2018.1449071

McRuer, R. (2006). *Crip theory: Cultural signs of queerness and disability.* New York University Press.

McRuer, R. (2018). *Crip times: Disability, globalization, and resistance.* New York University Press.

Michalko, R. (2010). What's cool about blindness? *Disability Studies Quarterly, 30*(3/4). https://doi.org/10.18061/dsq.v30i3/4.1296

Mitchell, D. T., Snyder, S. L., & Ware, L. (2014). "[Every] child left behind": Curricular cripistemologies and the crip/queer art of failure. *Journal of Literary & Cultural Disability Studies, 8*(3), 295–314. https://doi.org/10.3828/jlcds.2014.24

Moreman, S. T. (2019). Accommodating desires of disability: A multi-modal approach to Terry Galloway and the Mickee Faust Club. *QED: A Journal of GLBTQ Worldmaking, 6*(3), 149–162. https://doi.org/10.14321/qed.6.3.0149

Muñoz, J. E. (2006). Feeling brown, feeling down: Latina affect, the performativity of race, and the depressive position. *Signs: Journal of Women in Culture and Society, 31*(3), 675–688. https://doi.org/10.1086/499080

Pacanowsky, M. E., & O'Donnell-Trujillo, N. (1982). Communication and organizational cultures. *Western Journal of Speech Communication, 46*(2), 115–130. https://doi.org/10.1080/10570318209374072

Pacanowsky, M. E., & O'Donnell-Trujillo, N. (1983). Organizational communication as cultural performance. *Communication Monographs, 50*(2), 126–147. https://doi.org/10.1080/03637758309390158

Pacanowsky, M. E., & O'Donnell-Trujillo, N. (1990). Communication and organizational cultures. In S. R. Corman, S. P. Banks, C. R. Bantz, & M. E. Mayer (Eds.), *Foundations of organizational communication* (pp. 142–153). Longman.

Puar, J. K. (2009). Prognosis time: Towards a geopolitics of affect, debility and capacity. *Women & Performance: A Journal of Feminist Theory, 19*(2), 161–172. https://doi.org/10.1080/07407700903034147

Puar, J. K. (2017). *The right to maim: Debility, capacity, disability.* Duke University Press.

Sandahl, C. (2003). Queering the crip or cripping the queer? Intersections of queer and crip identities in solo autobiographical performance. *GLQ: A Journal of Lesbian and Gay Studies, 9*(1-2), 25–56. https://muse.jhu.edu/article/40804

Sandahl, C. (2006). More than just funny: Reading Galloway from a disability perspective. *Liminalities: A Journal of Performance Studies*, *2*(3), 1–7. http://liminalities. net/2-3/san.htm

Sandahl, C. (2008). Why disability identity matters: From dramaturgy to casting in John Belluso's *Pyretown*. *Text and Performance Quarterly*, *28*(1–2), 225–241. https://doi.org/10.1080/10462930701754481

Sandahl, C. (2018). Using our words: Exploring representational conundrums in disability drama and performance. *Journal of Literary & Cultural Disability Studies*, *12*(2), 129–144. https://doi.org/10.3828/jlcds.2018.11

Sass, J. S. (2000). Emotional labor as cultural performance: The communication of caregiving in a nonprofit nursing home. *Western Journal of Communication*, *64*(3), 330–358. https://doi.org/10.1080/10570310009374679

Scott, J.-A. (2012). "Cripped" heroes: An analysis of physically disabled professionals' narratives of performance of identity. *Southern Communication Journal*, *77*(4), 307–328. https://doi.org/10.1080/1041794X.2012.673852

Scott, J.-A. (2018). *Embodied performance as applied research, art and pedagogy*. Palgrave Macmillan.

Snyder, S. L., & Mitchell, D. T. (2006). *Cultural locations of disability*. University of Chicago Press.

St. Pierre, J. (2015). Cripping communication: Speech, disability, and exclusion in liberal humanist and posthumanist discourse. *Communication Theory*, *25*(3), 330–348. https://doi.org/10.1111/comt.12054

St. Pierre, J., & Peers, D. (2016). Telling ourselves sideways, crooked and crip: An introduction. *Canadian Journal of Disability Studies*, *5*(3), 1–11. https://doi. org/10.15353/cjds.v5i3.293

Tracy, S. J. (2020). *Qualitative research methods: Collecting evidence, crafting analysis, communicating impact* (2nd ed.). Wiley Blackwell.

Trujillo, N. (1985). Organizational communication as cultural performance: Some managerial considerations. *Southern Speech Communication Journal*, *50*(3), 201–224. https://doi.org/10.1080/10417948509372632

Yep, G. A. (2013). Queering/quaring/kauering/crippin'/transing "other bodies" in intercultural communication. *Journal of International and Intercultural Communication*, *6*(2), 118–126. https://doi.org/10.1080/17513057.2013.777087

Yep, G. A. (2016). Toward thick(er) intersectionalities: Theorizing, researching, and activating the complexities of communication and identities. In K. Sorrells & S. Sekimoto (Eds.), *Globalizing intercultural communication: A reader* (pp. 85–93). Sage.

PART V

Advocacy, Policy, and Action

CHAPTER 23

Overlooked and Undercounted: Communication and Police Brutality Against People with Disabilities

Deion S. Hawkins

In September 2019, 24-year-old Brady Mistic was driving through the streets of Colorado, planning to stop by a laundromat. What was intended to be a peaceful day filled with mundane errands quickly turned chaotic. Brady, who is deaf in both ears, was shocked to find out he was being approached by law enforcement. Unaware of his infraction, Brady was startled and confused. A mere moments after exiting his vehicle, Brady's vision was blurred by police lights; police lights *should* be a sign of comfort, but for Brady, it was the polar opposite. Officers shouted at Brady, but Brady could not hear the audible warnings (Hernandez, 2021b; Low, 2021). Next, chaos and violence ensued. Officers wrongfully assumed Mistic was being purposely defiant, but in reality, Brady *did* attempt to communicate using American Sign Language (ASL) (Hernandez, 2021b). However, officers misinterpreted his hand gestures as aggressive and claimed he resisting arrest; in turn, officers used force to get him to "comply," (Hernandez, 2021b; Low, 2021). Not only was Brady thrown to the ground by one officer and tased by the other, but he spent four months in jail because of the ordeal (Pelisek, 2021). Unfortunately, Brady's case is not unique.

In October 2021, individuals were outraged when the story of Clifford Owensby hit the news and went viral. Owensby, of Dayton, Ohio, is a

---

D. S. Hawkins (✉)
Emerson College, Boston, MA, USA
e-mail: deion_hawkins@emerson.edu

© The Author(s), under exclusive license to Springer Nature
Switzerland AG 2023
M. S. Jeffress et al. (eds.), *The Palgrave Handbook of Disability and Communication*, https://doi.org/10.1007/978-3-031-14447-9_23

385

paraplegic, and officers repeatedly asked him to get out of the vehicle (Hernandez, 2021a; Li & Ciechalski, 2021). Owensby first asked for probable cause, but then informed officers he could not physically exit the vehicle in the requested manner because of limited mobility in his legs. Despite being documented on body cameras, this did not curb the officers' violence. Officers forcefully dragged Clifford out of his car by his shoulders and dreadlocks; next, they threw him to the ground with one officer placing a knee on his back (Li & Ciechalski, 2021).

While horrifically tragic, both Brady and Clifford survived, but brutality against people with disabilities often ends on a much more somber note. Several cases illustrate this unfortunate truth. Charleena Lyles, a pregnant woman diagnosed with bipolar disorder, called law enforcement to report a burglary (Green, 2021). Police arrived at her home and described her as "delusional," "hysterical," and "unruly"; all of these are a direct result of her mental health condition that is supposed to be covered by the Americans with Disabilities Act (ADA). Police fired over 13 times and killed Charleena even though *she called* asking for assistance (Levin, 2017). Robert Ethan Saylor, a 26-year-old quadriplegic man with Down syndrome, was forcefully dragged out of his wheelchair and removed from a movie theater in handcuffs and restraints. Police forced him out of the theater after he accidentally presented the wrong ticket, and when approached, officers claimed Saylor "freaked out." Saylor's outbursts prompted officers to use force, fracturing his larynx, making it difficult for him to breathe. Saylor was pronounced dead at a local hospital. His death was ruled a homicide as a result of asphyxia (Vargas, 2018).

Although jarring, the stories above are not outliers; instead, they serve as evidence of a pattern and highlight an often unspoken fact: people with disabilities repeatedly face intense violence from law enforcement (Thompson, 2021). Despite the ADA's intent to protect Americans with disabilities from violence at the hands of law enforcement, people with disabilities experience brutality at an elevated rate (Jones, 2020; Perry & Carter-Long, 2016). Often, these fatal encounters are the result of law enforcement failing to use de-escalation tactics, a flaw frequently rooted in the lack of adequate communication training and/or understanding of people with disabilities. The communication tactics of people with disabilities are often misinterpreted as violent, and in turn, police use excessive force.

STATEMENT OF PROBLEM

As our country rightfully grapples with the harsh reality of police brutality against racial minorities, we cannot forget other systematically marginalized groups. This is especially true considering disability heavily intersects with and influences racial perceptions. In fact, for many more "notable" cases of brutality against Black bodies (including Sandra Bland, Eric Garner, Tamir Rice, and Laquan MacDonald), the victim's disability has been ignored if not blatantly erased from the narrative (Abrams, 2020; Thompson, 2021). Perry and

Carter-Long (2016) note, "when disabled Americans get killed and their stories are lost or segregated from each other in the media, we miss an opportunity to learn from tragedies, identify patterns, and push for necessary reforms" (p. 2).

We do not know the full toll of police brutality against people with disabilities because no federal database exists (Srikanth, 2021). While the Federal Bureau of Investigation (FBI) does collect *some* information about people killed by police officers, the agency has yet to establish mandatory reporting requirements. Thus, only 3% of police precincts provide information regarding the number of civilians harmed or killed by law enforcement (Davis & Lowery, 2015). While the number of U.S. law enforcement agents killed while on duty is documented, official, reliable, and verifiable data related to individuals killed *by* law enforcement are virtually nonexistent (Krieger et al., 2015). At best, we have rough estimates. According to a 2016 report released by the Ruderman Family Foundation, a disability rights organization, at least a third, if not half of the people who die at the hands of law enforcement have some form of a disability (Perry & Carter-Long, 2016). Kim (2020) notes, "Historically, in the U.S, people who were labeled as deviant, unproductive, dangerous, unworthy and unfit were disabled and killed by the police force or arrested and incarcerated in large, segregated institutions" (p. 1). The labels of "dangerous," "deviant," and "unproductive" are often applied heavily to BIPOC communities. Disability often intersects with other factors such as race, class, and gender, exacerbating bias and violence from law enforcement. Understanding the role of communication and how intersecting identities interact with law enforcement is critical to curbing police violence against people with disabilities.

CHAPTER PREVIEW

The vow to protect and serve should not be bound by a civilian's physical or mental capabilities; therefore, further analysis of brutality against people with disabilities is needed. People with disabilities ought to have the right to adequate protection, regardless of any physical or mental classification. Communication plays a vital role in saving lives and bolstering police-community relations (Bain, 2016; Giles et al., 2012; Italiano et al., 2021).

Thus, this chapter will:

(1) first, define police brutality and unpack various uses of force
(2) then, briefly explore key tenets of the Americans with Disabilities Act by outlining protected conditions, both mental and physical
(3) isolate the role communication plays in exacerbating police violence against people with disabilities by analyzing the (a) lack of adequate tailored communication-oriented trainings and (b) stigmatized media framing and erasure
(4) propose practical solutions.

Before continuing, it is important to note that language in the context of disabilities is of the utmost importance. A frequent debate emerges when individuals are asked if people-first (for example: a person who is hard of hearing, a person with Autism) compared to identify-first language, for example: deaf person, an Autistic person, a disabled person) is preferred. As a scholar who identifies as a member of the disabled community, I will be using people-first language; however, I wholeheartedly acknowledge and respect the individuals who prefer identity-first language. I am aware of the difference, but because there is not a consensus, I would like to acknowledge and respect both viewpoints. However, for the sake of clarity, consistency, and readability, I will use people-first language throughout this chapter.

Police Brutality and Use of Force Continuum

There is no single, universally agreed-upon definition of police brutality. At best, the current literature uses two concepts loosely related to police brutality: excessive force and death by legal intervention. Fatalities resulting from the use of force by law enforcement agents on duty are known as "legal interventions" (DeGue et al., 2016). It is important to note that "death by legal intervention" classifications carry significant implications (Arseniev-Koehler et al., 2021). Because these deaths are often legally upheld but highly contested, research surrounding brutality is stunted as public officials become more interested in saving face/reputation than holding officers accountable.

As a means of personal and public safety, officers have the right to use force to curb potential threats (Alpert & Dunham, 2009). The National Institute of Justice (2020) explains, "use of force is an officer's last option—a necessary course of action to restore safety in a community when other practices are ineffective" (p. 1). However, this chapter argues people with disabilities are often met with *excessive force*. The institute elaborates: "the level of force an officer uses varies based on the situation. Because of this variation, guidelines for the use of force are based on many factors, including the officer's level of training or experience" (p. 1).

Again, the frequency and impact of excessive police force are difficult to estimate as no national database exists. Guided by the Department of Justice's Office of Justice Programs, all precincts that receive federal funding are expected to adhere to a "Use-Of-Force" continuum (National Institute of Justice, 2020). The continuum outlines what force is appropriate for certain situations; in virtually every circumstance involving an individual with a disability, the situation could have been de-escalated or thwarted by using less intense force and more effective communication. The National Institute of Justice's continuum (2020) can be seen in Table 23.1.

Alpert and Dunham (2009) write, "excessive force refers to situations where government officials legally entitled to use force exceed the minimum amount necessary to diffuse an incident" (p. 21). Both excessive force and death by

23 OVERLOOKED AND UNDERCOUNTED: COMMUNICATION AND POLICE... 389

Table 23.1 Use of force continuum table

Type of force	Definition	Example
Officer presence	No force is used. Presence alone deters crime or diffuses a situation	– Officer shows up to 911 call and individuals cease activity.
Verbalization	Force is not physical	(1) Officer issues calm, nonthreatening commands – "ID, please" (2) Officers may increase volume and intensity. "stop," and/or "don't move."
Empty hand control	Officers use bodily force to gain control	(1) *Soft technique*: Officers use grabs, holds, and joint locks to restrain individuals. (2) *Hard technique*: Officers use punches and kicks to restrain individuals.
Less lethal methods	Officers use less-lethal technologies to control situation	(1) *Blunt impact*: Officers will use baton or projectiles to immobilize. (2) *Chemical*: Officers may use chemical sprays to restraint individuals (ex: pepper spray) (3) *Conducted Energy Devices(CEDs)*: Officers may use CEDS to immobilize an individual. CEDs discharge a high-voltage, low-amperage jolt electricity at a distance (ex: Tasers).
Lethal force	Officers use lethal weapons to gain control of situation	– Officers use firearms to stop an individual

legal intervention encompass *some* aspects of brutality, but a comprehensive definition is still needed.

Thus, for this chapter, police brutality can be defined as a police action that harms, dehumanizes, or degrades its target. Excessive use of physical violence constitutes brutality, but not all brutality stems from excessive force. Police brutality also includes: false arrests, verbal abuse, intimidation, and corruption (Alpert & Dunham, 2009). Some scholars support this notion that brutality extends past physical violence and includes emotional violence, verbal assault, and psychological intimidation (Alang et al., 2017). It is also important to note that brutality *does not require intent*; dehumanization and degradation can occur in the absence of intent.

AMERICAN WITH DISABILITIES ACT: AN OVERVIEW

Under the ADA, people who have disabilities are entitled to the same services law enforcement provides to anyone else. Legislation prevents individuals with disabilities from being: excluded or segregated from services, denied services, or treated differently than other people. Usually, in other settings, a reasonable accommodation is proffered or recommended. For example, if one is employed but has limited mobility, they may receive a reserved parking spot or an office located closest to the door. However, similar accommodations are virtually non-existent in law enforcement, even when the communicative accommodations are relatively simple. For example, when interacting with people with deafness, the ADA's official website (2020) recommends officers accommodate by using: (1) visual aids/cue cards with simple commands, (2) a pad and pencil for written notes, and/or (3) an assistive listening system.

Psychiatric Disabilities

Analysis and narratives clearly indicate people with disabilities are not receiving adequate accommodations and are treated differently by law enforcement. This is true even in situations when their disability is well known and documented. For example, Morgan (2021) notes that individuals with psychiatric disabilities are especially vulnerable in medical facilities, the very place they are seeking care. When an individual is in the midst of a mental health crisis, police officers are frequently called, often resulting in violence. Additionally, when discussing certain mental health conditions covered under the ADA, such as schizophrenia or Tourette's syndrome, individuals are often arrested or brutalized as a direct result of being labeled "disruptive" or "disorderly" (Morgan, 2021). This is all true *despite* the ADA's supposed protections.

Like other cases of police shootings, much of the violence inflicted against people with disabilities is the result of law enforcement failing to communicate effectively and utilize de-escalation tactics. The level of force used by law enforcement often far exceeds what is necessary to ensure public safety (Mizner, 2018; Lewis, 2015; Kim, 2020) In 2015, the U.S. Supreme Court heard *San Francisco v. Sheehan*. Police were called to take Sheehan, who was in the midst of a mental health crisis, to the hospital, but instead of helping secure treatment, they shot her five times. Sheehan survived the encounter and sued the city's police department (Hurley, 2015). The court ruled in favor of the officers, finding that their use of force did not violate the constitution or the ADA. Sheenan's case highlights a troubling reality: police officers frequently injure individuals with mental health or behavioral issues and are exonerated for these violent offenses.

Individuals with psychiatric disorders are automatically presumed to be a threat to themselves and others. To law enforcement, a Black male experiencing a mental crisis is inherently unstable and dangerous. LaQuan McDonald, a Black teenager suffering from post-traumatic stress disorder (PTSD) and other mental health issues, was killed by police outside a Burger King in Chicago. Jason Harrison, Anthony Hill, and Kajieme Powell had similar violent confrontations with police; they were all Black teens with psychiatric disabilities.

Perry and Carter-Long (2016) note police officers have become de facto first responders when dealing with individuals with mental disabilities, but an unfortunate pattern exists where an individual experiences a mental health crisis, and the police are called in to calm that person down or escort the person to a facility. The communication quickly breaks down. When the person in crisis fails to adhere to commands, officers escalate and frequently draw their weapons, aggravating the crisis. After seeing guns, the civilian may feel threatened and may yield a weapon, prompting the officers to fire. It is important to remember the individual is not a criminal; instead, they are in the midst of a health-related event related to their disability. In these events, the person with a disability rarely survives the encounter; yet, police officers often face little to no consequences for their actions.

Physical Disabilities

In addition to mental disabilities, police officers have a history of misunderstanding and harassing individuals with physical disabilities (Perry, 2017). For instance, even when police officers know a person is deaf or hard of hearing, they often treat them as uncooperative. Because sign language inherently requires one to use their hands *and* officer commands also usually involve hands being shown, a miscommunication with deadly consequences often emerges.

In the case of McCray v. City of Dothan, officers knew the plaintiff, a Black man in Alabama, was deaf and could not read lips; however, this did not stop them from slamming McCray's head on a table, putting him in a chokehold, and forcefully removing him from the premises. McCray's story is not an isolated incident. Lewis (2015) sheds light on similar cases. After being pulled over, Pearl Pearson, a 64-year-old deaf man, was attempting to show an officer a place card that read "I am deaf." The officer assumed Pearson, who is Black, was reaching for a weapon, yanked him from his car, and beat him. Immediately after the incident, the officer ran Pearson's license plate and learned he was deaf; this finding did not matter. Local courts ruled that the officer had not violated any rules and Pearson was charged with resisting arrest. In February 2013, Jonathan Meister was leaving his friend's home with a bag of items and officers mistook him for a burglar. Meister attempted to use sign language, but officers perceived his "frantic" movements as a sign of aggression; they tased and choked him until he was unconscious.

Persons with disabilities like epilepsy, autism, diabetes, and cerebral palsy have symptoms that are often misinterpreted to be signs of intoxication or drug use. In 2010, Garry Palmer was driving and accidentally hit a dog. He rightfully reported the accident, but when officers arrived, they arrested him for drunk driving because he was slurring his words—this was a result of his cerebral palsy, not alcohol intoxication (Perry & Carter-Long, 2014). Next, take the case of Schreiner vs. City of Gresham in 2010 where the plaintiff was experiencing severe hypoglycemic shock and was unresponsive to officer orders. Even though she was wearing a medical alert necklace, Schreiner was handcuffed and thrown to the ground, resulting in a broken hip and bruised lung.

The Role of Communication in Brutality Against People with Disabilities

The narratives highlighted above outline a problem that is often overlooked and under discussed. Violence should not be the default response to anyone's disability, and disabling conditions should not be criminalized. As previously articulated, in most instances, more effective communication could be used to neutralize the situation. In this section, I isolate two areas of communication that play a role in exacerbating this issue: (1) media framing and erasure and (2) inadequate communication training.

Media Framing and Erasure

Through the process of framing, purveyors of news often select elements of a story and combine those elements to tell a narrative that promotes a particular interpretation (Entman, 2007). Because of the frames presented, and the promotion of certain ideas within those frames as salient or important, audiences are primed to perceive, evaluate, and internalize issues in a particular way (Kim et al., 2002).

In one of the few studies connecting the dots between media framing and brutality against people with disabilities, Perry and Carter-Long (2016) outlined two noteworthy patterns. First, disability goes unmentioned or is listed as an attribute without context, and second, a medical condition or "mental illness" is used to blame victims for their deaths. Simply put, media coverage rarely discusses one's disability, and when it is mentioned, it is embedded in stigma as a means to blame the victim for the violence.

To illustrate how these ideas manifest in the real world, we can assume a case study approach. First, let's unpack the erasure of disability. Generally speaking, coverage of police violence against people with disabilities only included the date of altercation and where the incident took place (Perry & Carter-Long, 2016). For example, let us take the high-profile case of Freddie Gray. Media coverage of Gray's case rightfully centered on his race, but neglected to mention his disability; from childhood, Gray was a known victim of lead poisoning. He even received small financial compensation as a result of his condition (McCoy, 2015). Lead poisoning can lead to intellectual disabilities, developmental delays, and altered attention span (Perry & Carter-Long, 2016). All of these symptoms could impact interactions with law enforcement, but despite this, not a single article centered Gray's disability until an exposé by the *Washington Post* (McCoy, 2015).

The most common type of interaction between law enforcement and people with disabilities usually involves a psychiatric disability, notably bipolar disorder and schizophrenia. Perry and Carter-Long (2016) found that (1) coverage may mention "mental illness" without contextualizing/framing it as a disability recognized by the ADA and (2) individuals with psychiatric disabilities were repeatedly blamed for their actions. One of the most troubling phrases that repeatedly appeared in coverage was that individuals died by "suicide by cop" (Voorhees, 2014).

Media generally depicts disability through a medical model/lens of impairment, making the condition of the disabled person the reason for violence. This framing allows stigma about mental illness (psychiatric disabilities) to flourish and to inform reporting. The framing also suggests that people with psychiatric disabilities are likely to be violent and that police and the public have reason to fear them. Such framing creates a situation where a police officer no longer perceives themselves as a public servant aiding a civilian with a disability; instead, they are there to neutralize an unruly threat. This framing reinforces the systemic dehumanization of people with disabilities.

Inadequate Communication Training

In addition to media framing and stigmatization, the lack of adequate communication training also plays a vital role. When one analyzes these interactions, a paradox emerges. While people with disabilities are much more likely to have encounters with law enforcement, they are also more likely to have communication difficulties that can lead to misunderstandings. Research shows a police officer's perceptions about individuals with disabilities can be changed over time, and are heavily influenced by personal life experience, job training, and field experience (Diamond & Hogue, 2021; Henshaw & Thomas, 2011). However, even though officers self-report a higher level of understanding of individuals with disabilities, their actions reveal a disconnect as they often fail to identify and understand who is disabled (Perry & Carter-Long, 2016). Without more robust training, officers literally do not have the ability to identify who is disabled, and thus, fail to adjust their behavior. Additionally, police officers frequently conflate various learning disabilities, behavioral issues, and autism spectrum disorders as mental illness (Henshaw & Thomas, 2011; Perry & Carter-Long, 2016; Diamond & Hogue, 2021). Research also shows the lack of formal disability training heightens officer anxiety on the job as they are unprepared and uneducated on issues of disability (Gardner et al., 2018).

Currently, because exchanges between law enforcement and people with disabilities often escalate and require force, trainings on how to handle these situations typically fall under sessions related to Use of Force protocol. According to the Department of Justice (DOJ), on average, police officers receive around 843 hours of basic training, and of those 843 hours, 168 are specifically dedicated to teaching use of force continuum and appropriate tactics (Anderson, 2019; Diamond & Hogue, 2021). However, according to the National Center on Criminal Justice and Disability (ARC), the number of hours or percentage of training dedicated to interacting with people with disabilities greatly varies and typically focuses on intellectual disabilities exclusively (Whelan et al., 2020). In turn, this leaves other types of disabilities in the shadows, leading officers to act on problematic assumptions. Moreover, these trainings are inherently reactive, asking officers to identify the force needed to neutralize the "threat," but the best trainings would prevent escalation and use of force entirely.

This lack of training clearly translates into problematic policing practices, especially when communication is centered. Take the example of a civilian with a severe speech impediment. To an officer, a long pause can be perceived as abnormal nervousness or anxiety driven by guilt; but in reality, it may be the result of a medical condition. Someone with Tourette's syndrome may make uncontrollable movements or blurt out offensive words, also open to misinterpretation. Without understanding these are symptoms of a medical condition, officers could easily escalate the situation and use violence when patience and verbal commands would suffice. Let us take a situation where an officer is called to aid a person with an autism spectrum disorder, a condition often marked by chronic fleeing and/or sensory perceptions issues (Burke, 2021). In this circumstance, the lights may cause an intense reaction, and render one unable to adequately communicate their concerns.

SOLUTIONS: A CALL FOR CRITICAL MEDIA FRAMING AND COMMUNITY PARTICIPATORY TRAININGS

The analysis above illuminates a law enforcement problem within the United States. Luckily, there are multiple solutions that could and should be developed and implemented; it is imperative that communication, not brute force, is at the center. It is impossible to change the legacy and practices of policing overnight, but we can move the needle of equity forward and save lives in the process.

There are several ways the media can better advocate for people with disabilities. First, it is imperative that reporters and journalists be more aware of mentioning disabilities when reporting. Perry and Carter-Long (2016), write, "we ask reporters to be cognizant of the potential for anyone to be disabled and to consider it a key aspect in linking causes, concerns and a contributing element in police use of force" (p. 39). One tangible way for the media to help is by avoiding stigmatizing language when reporting. In 2021, the National Center on Disability and Journalism, released its most updated style guide (Loeppky, 2021). In it, they advise communication professionals to avoid stigmatized language such as: "stricken with," "suffers from," and "victim of" as it assumes suffering is a prerequisite of disability. People living with disabilities can and do live whole, fulfilling lives.

In addition to this, Perry and Carter-Long (2016) give more concrete steps on avoiding stigmatized language when discussing disability and policing. Many outlets would publish a piece that calls a victim "crazy" "delusional," and erratic" but journalists should make sure quotations do not center ableist language. Journalists should manage ableist language in the same way they would handle language ripe with sexism, racism, or any other form of discrimination: by not publishing it. Finally, when reporting, the media usually accepts the narrative that blames the victim, depicting it as an unavoidable tragedy influenced by someone's disability, but a different framing exists. Media ought to provide the full context of the situation by: (1) mentioning one's disability, (2) discussing the use of force continuum, and (3) mentioning the behavior/demeanor of the law enforcement official.

Media framing can help alleviate the issue, but more must be done on the ground via trainings to ensure police officers can more effectively communicate with people with disabilities. It is important to note many advocates argue that a larger cultural and systemic shift away from law enforcement being *de facto* first responders is the key to curbing this issue. Mental health professionals and social work-oriented Crisis Intervention Teams should be the default when discussing people with disabilities, especially those with psychiatric needs (Lewis, 2015; Abrams, 2020; Loeppky, 2021; Kim, 2020). Some states, like Maryland, have passed legislation to ensure more tailored training exists. After the high-profile death of Ethan Saylor, Maryland passed legislation entitled "The Law Enforcement Training Bill," mandating community-oriented police trainings that center individuals with intellectual and developmental disabilities (Anderson, 2019). This legislation could serve as a model for other states.

However, until we reach a large shift, we must advocate for better trainings. Funneling more resources to police budgets is not the solution, especially considering police budgets often trade off with forms of social services. Instead, we must alter how we train police officers and how they perceive and respond to disabilities. Mizner (2018) notes, "officers need different training—not additional training. It shouldn't be a one-week training to learn how to work with people with disabilities. We need different police training altogether from the ground up, starting at the police academy" (p. 1). The traditional "command and control" framework should only be utilized when there is evidence of an actual crime taking place.

Right now, police trainings are geared toward a basic awareness of the ADA, but a better model exists. Diamond and Hogue (2021) advocate for a shift in content as well as who delivers the trainings. First, they recommend police officers receive training that allows officers to gain knowledge and awareness on how to recognize disabilities, not just what they are. After one has the ability to recognize, one must be taught how to adjust. Communication Accommodation Theory would argue for access to multiple communication strategies, visual and verbal. For example, an officer could be trained to ask "Are you deaf?" in ASL or carry a laminated card asking "do you have any of these conditions?"

Equally as important, we must pay attention to who is conducting the trainings. Police officers prefer a collaborative approach to training with a trainer (e.g., disability specialist, special educator, and a police officer (e.g., Peace Officer) because collaboration increases buy-in among officers (Diamond & Hogue, 2021). However, this dyadic approach ignores a key demographic: people with disabilities. Diamond and Hogue (2021) argue that trainings related to people with disabilities must feature the voices and lived experiences of the community. Simply put, if one is being trained on how to deal with a person with Down syndrome, the training should be led by someone with Down syndrome. Lastly, all trainings should: (1) assess an officer's current ability to accurately identify (or ask about) one's disability; (2) discuss traditional verbal and nonverbal cues that may not work for people with disabilities; (3) provide best communication practices; (4) provide realistic role plays via case studies; (5) analyze previous body camera footage as applicable; and (5) conduct a post-assessment to ensure growth. After this initial training, it is recommended that disability awareness training be weaved into mandatory, annual trainings.

CONCLUSION

Despite its prevalence, police brutality against people with disabilities remains largely under discussed. These heinous and usually preventable acts of state-inflicted violence are often rooted in communicative misunderstandings. To mitigate this violence against a systemically silenced population, paradigm shifts of police trainings as well as media framing are needed. The rights of the disabled ought to be defended with the same rigor and passion as other social justice issues. Disability rights are human rights that must be protected. We must work to ensure that law enforcement officials truly adhere to their creed—to protect and serve. Calling for help should not ever be a death sentence.

REFERENCES

Abrams, A. (2020, June 25). Black, disabled people at higher risk in police encounters. *Time*. Retrieved October 31, 2021, from https://time.com/5857438/police-violence-black-disabled/

ADA National Network. (2020, January). *I heard that miniature horses are considered to be service animals by the ADA. Is this true?* Retrieved January 11, 2022, from https://adata.org/faq/i-heard-miniature-horses-are-considered-be-service-animals-ada-true

Alang, S., McAlpine, D., McCreedy, E., & Hardeman, R. (2017). Police brutality and Black health: Setting the agenda for public health scholars. *American Journal of Public Health, 107*(5), 662–665. https://doi.org/10.2105/ajph.2017.303691

Alpert, G., & Dunham, R. (2009). *Understanding police use of force*. Cambridge University Press.

Anderson, M. (2019, April 13). How one mother's battle is changing police training on disabilities. *NPR*. Retrieved November 2, 2021, from https://www.npr.org/2019/04/13/705887493/how-one-mothers-battle-is-changing-police-training-on-disabilities

Arseniev-Koehler, A., Foster, J. G., Mays, V. M., Chang, K.-W., & Cochran, S. D. (2021). Aggression, escalation, and other latent themes in legal intervention deaths of Non-Hispanic Black and white men: Results from the 2003–2017 National Violent Death Reporting System. *American Journal of Public Health, 111*(S2), S107–S115. https://doi.org/10.2105/ajph.2021.306312

Bain, A. (2016). Positive policing: Communication and the public. In A. Bain (Ed.), *Law enforcement and technology* (pp. 47–61). Palgrave. https://doi.org/10.1057/978-1-137-57915-7_4

Burke, M. (2021, April 23). Father says son with autism was slammed to ground, punched by officer. *NBCNews.com*. Retrieved November 2, 2021, from https://www.nbcnews.com/news/us-news/father-says-son-autism-was-slammed-ground-punched-officer-n1265142

Davis, A. C., & Lowery, W. (2015, October 7). FBI director calls lack of data on police shootings 'ridiculous,' 'embarrassing'. *The Washington Post*. Retrieved November 2, 2021, from https://www.washingtonpost.com/national/fbi-director-calls-lack-of-data-on-police-shootings-ridiculous-embarrassing/2015/10/07/c0ebaf7a-6d16-11e5-b31c-d80d62b53e28_story.html?utm_term=.30dae2e6b3a0

DeGue, S., Fowler, K. A., & Calkins, C. (2016). Deaths due to use of lethal force by law enforcement. *American Journal of Preventive Medicine, 51*(5/S3), S173–S187. https://doi.org/10.1016/j.amepre.2016.08.027

Diamond, L. L., & Hogue, L. B. (2021). Preparing students with disabilities and police for successful interactions. *Intervention in School and Clinic, 57*(1), 3–14. https://doi.org/10.1177/1053451221994804

Entman, R. M. (2007). Framing bias: Media in the distribution of power. *Journal of Communication, 57*(1), 163–173. https://doi.org/10.1111/j.1460-2466.2006.00336.x

Gardner, L., Campbell, J. M., & Westdal, J. (2018). Brief report: Descriptive analysis of law enforcement officers' experiences with and knowledge of autism. *Journal of Autism and Developmental Disorders, 49*(3), 1278–1283. https://doi.org/10.1007/s10803-018-3794-4

Giles, H., Linz, D., Bonilla, D., & Gomez, M. L. (2012). Police stops of and interactions with Latino and white (non-Latino) drivers: Extensive policing and communication accommodation. *Communication Monographs, 79*(4), 407–427. https://doi.org/10.1080/03637751.2012.723815

Green, S. J. (2021, February 16). Appeals Court rules Charleena Lyles wrongful-death suit against Seattle police can proceed. *The Seattle Times*. Retrieved October 31, 2021, from https://www.seattletimes.com/seattle-news/crime/appeals-court-rules-charleena-lyles-wrongful-death-suit-against-seattle-police-can-proceed/

Henshaw, M., & Thomas, S. (2011). Police encounters with people with intellectual disability: Prevalence, characteristics and challenges. *Journal of Intellectual Disability Research, 56*(6), 620–631. https://doi.org/10.1111/j.1365-2788.2011.01502.x

Hernandez, J. (2021a, October 10). Police dragged a paraplegic man from his car after he told them he couldn't get out. *NPR*. Retrieved October 31, 2021, from https://www.npr.org/2021/10/10/1044884579/police-dragged-a-paraplegic-man-from-his-car-after-he-told-them-he-couldnt-get-o

Hernandez, J. (2021b, September 29). A deaf man who couldn't hear police commands was tased and spent 4 months in jail. *NPR*. Retrieved October 31, 2021, from https://www.npr.org/2021/09/29/1041562502/deaf-man-tased-police-colorado-lawsuit

Hurley, L. (2015, May 18). The Supreme Court just sided with 2 San Francisco cops who shot a mentally ill woman wielding a knife. *Business Insider*. Retrieved November 1, 2021, from http://www.businessinsider.com/r-us-top-court-backs-police-over-arrest-of-mentally-ill-woman-2015-5

Italiano, R., Ramirez, F., & Chattopadhyay, S. (2021). Perceptions of police use of force among U.S. adults and the role of communication accommodation in improving police–civilian interactions. *Journal of Applied Communication Research, 49*(6), 669–686. https://doi.org/10.1080/00909882.2021.1930103

Jones, S. (2020, June 19). 33–50 percent of police use-of-force incidents involve a person who is disabled. *WTHR.com*. Retrieved October 31, 2021, from https://www.wthr.com/article/news/33-50-percent-of-police-use-of-force-incidents-involve-a-person-who-is-disabled-has-disability/531-011bddff-a5f0-4d2a-9ad2-6964623bc32d

Kim, E. (2020, April). More trainings are not the answer to police violence against disabled people. Retrieved November 2, 2021, from https://www.criminallegalnews.org/news/2020/mar/18/more-trainings-are-not-answer-police-violence-against-disabled-people/

Kim, S.-H., Scheufele, D. A., & Shanahan, J. (2002). Think about it this way: Attribute agenda-setting function of the press and the public's evaluation of a local issue. *Journalism & Mass Communication Quarterly, 79*(1), 7–25. https://doi.org/10.1177/107769900207900102

Krieger, N., Chen, J. T., Waterman, P. D., Kiang, M. V., & Feldman, J. (2015). Police killings and police deaths are public health data and can be counted. *PLOS Medicine, 12*(12). https://doi.org/10.1371/journal.pmed.1001915

Levin, S. (2017, June 19). Seattle woman killed by police while children were home after reporting theft. *The Guardian*. Retrieved October 31, 2021, from https://www.theguardian.com/us-news/2017/jun/19/seattle-police-shooting-charleena-lyles-mother

Lewis, T. A. (2015, April 26). Police brutality and deaf people. *American Civil Liberties Union*. Retrieved November 1, 2021, from https://www.aclu.org/blog/national-security/police-brutality-and-deaf-people

Li, D., & Ciechalski, S. (2021, October 9). Paraplegic man pulled from car, thrown to ground by police in Ohio. *NBCNews.com*. Retrieved October 21, 2021, from https://www.nbcnews.com/news/us-news/paraplegic-man-pulled-car-thrown-ground-police-ohio-n1281148

Loeppky, J. (2021, October 26). When reporting on disability, advice about language is simple: Just ask. *Poynter*. Retrieved November 2, 2021, from https://www.poynter.org/reporting-editing/2021/when-reporting-on-disability-advice-about-language-is-simple-just-ask/

Low, R. (2021, October 9). Idaho Springs cops face another Taser lawsuit after using weapon on deaf man. *FOX3* Retrieved October 31, 2021, from https://kdvr.com/news/local/idaho-springs-cops-face-another-taser-lawsuit-after-using-weapon-on-deaf-man/

McCoy, T. (2015, April 29). Freddie Gray's life a study on the effects of lead paint on poor Blacks. *The Washington Post*. Retrieved November 2, 2021, from https://www.washingtonpost.com/local/freddie-grays-life-a-study-in-the-sad-effects-of-lead-paint-on-poor-blacks/2015/04/29/0be898e6-eea8-11e4-8abc-d6aa3bad79dd_story.html.

Mizner, S. (2018, May 11). Police "command and control" culture is often lethal—especially for people with disabilities. *American Civil Liberties Union*. Retrieved November 3, from https://www.aclu.org/blog/criminal-law-reform/reforming-police/police-command-and-control-culture-often-lethal-especially

Morgan, J. M. (2021). Policing under disability law. *Stanford Law Review*, *73*(6), 1401–1405. Retrieved November 1, 2021, from https://www.stanfordlawreview.org/print/article/policing-under-disability-law/

National Institute of Justice. (2020, March). *Overview of police use of Force*. Retrieved November 1, 2021, from https://nij.ojp.gov/topics/articles/overview-police-use-force

Pelisek, C. (2021, September 30). Deaf Colorado man says he was arrested after not obeying police commands he couldn't hear: Lawsuit. *People.com*. Retrieved October 30, 2021, from. https://people.com/crime/deaf-colorado-man-arrested-not-obeying-police-commands-could-not-hear-lawsuit/

Perry, D. M. (2017, September 25). 4 disabled people dead in another week of police brutality. *The Nation*. Retrieved November 1, 2021, from https://www.thenation.com/article/four-disabled-dead-in-another-week-of-police-brutality/

Perry, D. M., & Carter-Long, L. (2014, May 6). How misunderstanding disability leads to police violence. *The Atlantic*. Retrieved November 21, 2021, from https://www.theatlantic.com/health/archive/2014/05/misunderstanding-disability-leads-to-police-violence/361786/

Perry, D. M., & Carter-Long, L. (2016). *The Ruderman White paper on media coverage of law enforcement use of force and disability*. Retrieved October 31, 2021, from https://rudermanfoundation.org/wp-content/uploads/2017/08/MediaStudy-PoliceDisability_final-final.pdf

Srikanth, A. (2021, March 17). National Database on police killings tracked 1,127 deaths last year. *The Hill*. Retrieved November 1, 2021, from https://thehill.com/changing-america/respect/equality/543712-national-database-on-police-killings-tracked-1127-police

Thompson, V. (2021, February 10). Understanding the policing of Black, disabled bodies. *Center for American Progress*. Retrieved October 31, 2021, from https://www.americanprogress.org/issues/disability/news/2021/02/10/495668/understanding-policing-black-disabled-bodies/

Vargas, T. (2018, April 24). Settlement reached in police-custody death of man with Down Syndrome. *The Washington Post*. Retrieved October 31, 2021, from https://www.washingtonpost.com/local/settlement-reached-in-police-custody-death-of-man-with-down-syndrome/2018/04/24/7d53c0ca-47fe-11e8-827e-190efaf1f1ee_story.html

Voorhees, J. (2014, August 27). "Suicide by cop" is a horrible, misleading phrase. We need to stop saying it. *Slate Magazine*. Retrieved November 3, 2021, from https://slate.com/news-and-politics/2014/08/suicide-by-cop-the-dangerous-term-that-stops-us-from-asking-hard-questions-about-police-shootings.html

Whelan, D., Askey, C. J., & Mann, C. P. (2020). Disability awareness training: A train the trainer program for first responders. *The National Center on Criminal Justice & Disability*. Retrieved February 1, 2022, from https://thearc.org/policy-advocacy/legal-advocacy/#what_arc_doing

CHAPTER 24

Critical Disability Studies in Technical Communication: A 25-Year History and the Future of Accessibility

Leah Heilig

For more than two decades, technical communicators have used critical disability studies in our field to improve multimodal design (Walters, 2010), teach accessibility to novice web developers (Youngblood, 2013), use accessibility in service-learning (Browning & Cagle, 2017), evaluate the accessibility of online writing instruction (Oswal & Melonçon, 2014; Oswal & Melonçon, 2017), study usability, and explore other material and social discourses. This entry to the *Handbook* offers an abbreviated history of the approximately 25-year relationship between technical communication and critical disability studies, mapping its impact on accessible communication design. Following this history, I introduce contemporary demands for accessibility practices that go beyond conformance standards like the Web Content Accessibility Guidelines (WCAG 2.1) to promote inclusivity and to position access as a "collective responsibility" (Zdenek, 2018, p. 6) in technical communication's social justice turn. This entry then moves toward the future, presenting three ways in which technical communication as a discipline might further expand the margins of accessible communication design: (1) broadening accessibility to include sociospatial factors for interactive environments, (2) considering "hierarchies of impairment" and the historical exclusion of the neurodivergent and those with non-physical disabilities from accessibility best practices, and (3) promoting accessibility as

L. Heilig (✉)
University of Rhode Island, Kingston, RI, USA
e-mail: leah_heilig@uri.edu

© The Author(s), under exclusive license to Springer Nature
Switzerland AG 2023
M. S. Jeffress et al. (eds.), *The Palgrave Handbook of Disability and Communication*, https://doi.org/10.1007/978-3-031-14447-9_24

401

402   L. HEILIG

an act of human dignity to "re-center" accessibility through a technical communication lens.

Before beginning this history, I would like to offer an acknowledgment of its limitations, constraints, and politics. This history is derived solely from prominent scholarly sources; as such, it is grounded in systems of power that privilege white, male, able-bodied/minded narratives, among others, and is therefore not excused from its own critiques. I also acknowledge the limitations of my own knowledge. This history is meant not to be a comprehensive representation of every article on disability and technical communication but rather to identify important movements and turns within technical communication that have shaped discourses on accessibility. I invite additions, amendments, and further conversations that build upon, enrich, and contest this history.

AN ABBREVIATED HISTORY OF TECHNICAL COMMUNICATION AND DISABILITY

Disability studies as a field "seeks to advance the cause of the disabled and promote social change" (Wilson & Lewiecki-Wilson, 2001, p. 9) and is "a location and a means to think critically about disability" (Linton, 1998, p. 1). Scholarship that emerged from disability advocacy groups solidified under the umbrella of disability studies in the 1980s and 1990s (Wilson & Lewiecki-Wilson, 2001) and has since been in interdisciplinary conversation with a variety of fields, including but not limited to cultural/American studies (Garland-Thomson, 1997), feminist/gender studies (Hall, 2011), queer theory (McRuer, 2006), rhetoric (Wilson & Lewiecki-Wilson, 2001), composition/writing studies (Dolmage, 2008), and, of course, design and technical communication.

Although "disability" has been discussed in its sister field of rhetoric since the Classical era (such as Plato's *Phaedrus* comparing love to madness), disability studies' relationship to technical communication is more nascent. Undeniably, the focal point of said relationship is accessibility. Accessibility can briefly be defined as the removal of barriers between people and environments and information. In the realm of technical communication, this often takes shape in material discourses and/or the design of communication—such as the improvement of online writing instruction for students with disabilities (Oswal and Melonçon, 2014) or the accessibility and rhetoricity of closed captioning (Zdenek, 2015). While technical communicators have and continue to do work in critical theory of disability, this piece traces *how* such work has influenced accessibility in particular.

Usability and Accessibility

In the 1980s and 1990s, amid the rapid global increase in personal computing technologies, technical communication researchers and practitioners were among those designing and developing new web content. The host of accessibility barriers that accompanied these new modalities of communication was inevitably brought to the discipline's attention. Early responses in technical communication to web accessibility errors were centered on making content work with other technologies (Ray & Ray, 1998). Attention was particularly placed on adaptive technologies, or "special versions of already existing technologies or tools that provide enhancements or different ways of interacting with the technology" (Adaptive Computing Technology Center, 2021), to promote accessible communication in web content. Such adaptive technologies are often situated in single-context, or one-to-one, scenarios "depend[ing] on the specific technology as well as the individual" (Ray & Ray, 1998, p. 573). By themselves, they do not enable more universal accessibility.

For wider approaches, technical communicators studied accessibility in its relationship to usability, or "how well a specific user in a specific context can use a product/design to achieve a defined goal effectively, efficiently, and satisfactorily" (Interaction Design Foundation, 2021) along with adaptive technology. Initial studies focused on how to make web content better for specific populations, such as blind and low-vision users (Bayer & Pappas, 2006; Theofanos & Redish, 2003; Theofanos & Redish, 2005) and aging populations (Lippincott, 2004; O'Hara, 2004). Through this work emerged exploratory research that attempted to "understand the relationship" between accessibility and usability as well as "develop research-based guidelines" for creating best practices in content development—particularly for the web (Theofanos & Redish, 2003, p. 36). Goals for early technical communication research therefore appeared to be twofold: (1) accommodate designs or content to adaptive technologies and (2) create best practices for accessibility that account for as many users as possible, improving overall usability of communication design.

In 2005, Theofanos and Redish stated a need for a paradigm shift in how technical communicators approached the relationship between accessibility and usability. Rather than an accessibility that accounted for as many users as possible, or an accessibility that relied on websites being accommodating to adaptive technologies, they argued for a model that holds "a wide range of flexibility" and "portability" (Theofanos & Redish, 2005, p. 19) and acknowledges the diversity of users with disabilities—moving against a one-site-fits-all model of web design. This new paradigm emphasized the importance of varied experiences in navigating web content and called for web developers to acknowledge diversity in their designs. Said call reflected earlier insights from researchers to be mindful of disabilities from the beginning of the design process (Ray & Ray, 1998) and to conduct accessibility evaluation with actual users with disabilities (Bayer & Pappas, 2006). While the call is over 15 years old, this shift is where technical communicators currently reside in accessibility praxis, as critiques against universal design's reification (see: Dolmage, 2017) continue to rise and content developers further recognize the complexity and fluidity of disability's relationship to technology. By the early 2000s, technical communication

404 L. HEILIG

scholarship broadened to other issues of social and material discourses, further integrating critical disability theory into its work on accessibility.

Accessibility and Material and Social Discourses

Among the first technical communication studies to make explicit use of disability studies as a theoretical frame was Wilson's (2000) work, which used the lens of disability to analyze medical and scientific discourse. Wilson's (2000) research provided the initial connection between technical communication and disability studies that was then expanded in Jason Palmeri's (2006) landmark article. Drawing on foundational disability studies literature (primarily Davis, 1995; Garland-Thomson, 1997; Linton, 1998) and connecting it to technical communication's previous work in cultural studies (primarily Longo, 1998, 2000; Scott, 2003), Palmeri argued for technical communication scholars and practitioners to interrogate the roles of social constructivism in the creation of "disability and normalcy" (p. 50). Workplace research, he claimed in particular, served as "a vital area for exploring the material consequences of the social construction of disability" (p. 51) through how the accessibility of the workplace is manufactured by policies such as the Americans with Disabilities Act (ADA). The importance of such workplace research is evidenced in Donna Kain's (2005) study which discusses the sociopolitical and metacommunicative importance of genre in the development of a reference guide to the ADA. In sum, Palmeri's (2006) work served as a call for expanding disability studies research into technical communication. It established that it was no longer suitable to approach accessibility from a utilitarian perspective: rhetorical work and cultural critique in technical communication practices were undeniably needed.

By the end of the first decade of the 2000s, several technical communication scholars were integrating rhetorical practices, disability, and cultural theory into their research on accessibility (see: Spinuzzi, 2007; Walters, 2010; Zdenek, 2009; Zdenek, 2011). Notable was Lisa Melonçon's (2013) edited collection, which furthered the discipline as being well suited to contribute to disability studies. In her introduction, Melonçon positioned technical communicators as being uniquely situated for reciprocity toward disability studies scholars as "one of the primary arenas for social change and for moving toward universal access is through changing the discourse and through changing the material conditions" (p. 4). Technical communicators, "As self-identified rhetoricians" (p. 3), can further disability scholarship through skills such as technological expertise, the rhetorical addressing of audiences, rhetorical analysis of documents and policy, usability of interfaces and materials, and teaching and training (pp. 10–11).

Of special consideration is the teaching and training of accessibility in technical communication, as addressed in the literature (Pass, 2013; Youngblood, 2013), marking a steady and increasing interest in the field toward accessible design. However, Oswal and Melonçon (2014) later asked the field at large whether technical and professional communication (TPC) programs and instructors were adequately (1) addressing disability and accessibility, (2) engaging in best practices for creating accessible online educational spaces, and (3) taking the lead within institutions to advocate for improved access to online education for students with disabilities (p. 272). Citing a shortage in the field of discussions of online accessibility, technical communication, and pedagogy (see: Pass, 2013; Oswal & Hewett, 2013; Youngblood, 2013), Oswal and Melonçon stressed the need for technical communication instructors to "pay attention" to the technologies used in the classroom and how they affect accessibility. The article emphasizes accountability for technical communication instructors and advocates for ethical praxis in the design of online educational spaces, arguing that technical communicators have not been "paying attention to the politics of the interface" (p. 285).

This ethical call to pay attention—to be accountable—became more present in conversations surrounding accessibility following the social justice turn in technical communication.

The Social Justice Turn and Expanding the Margins

Technical communication's social justice turn (see Agboka, 2013; Jones et al., 2016) has brought an increased consideration on highlighting the disparities in material and social discourses, as well as re-centering the narratives of marginalized storytellers. In considerations of communication design, scholarship has addressed the importance of retaining human dignity in design research (Walton, 2016), designing for vulnerable populations (Rose, 2016), and incorporating narrative into the design process as a means of social justice (Jones, 2016). With the Association of Teachers of Technical Writing (ATTW), a major conference in the field, calling for work in social justice (Jones & Scott, 2017) and accountability (Yu & Moeller, 2018), disability studies is clearly an important area to continue work in technical communication and design.

And more work is undeniably still needed. Literature has shown that issues of accessibility identified in the late 1990s/early 2000s persist. The central issue of accessible communication design is that accessibility is still treated as a problem of retrofitting rather than an exercise in inclusivity. This treatment takes different forms but can include reducing accessibility practices to checklist-driven approaches for legal compliance, focusing on accommodation, or relying on adaptive technologies instead of integrating accessibility from the ground up in content development. The problem with a retrofitted accessibility, as eloquently stated by Sushil Oswal (2014), is that "In a great many situations, the screen reader's job becomes that of a virtual hotel maid who cleans up after the software designers and web developers have left after finishing their exclusionary projects" (p. 15). Expecting adaptive technologies to do the work of accessibility is, simply put, *not* accessibility.

Calls have since been made to expand accessibility practices—to push beyond the boundaries of sole reliance on web standards or retrofitted technologies or actions (Oswal & Melonçon, 2017; Zdenek, 2017). In a special issue of *Communication Design Quarterly*, Zdenek's (2018) introduction asks, "How can we disable technical and professional communication" to challenge access as it is defined by the default user and motivate those in privilege to "notice barriers and do something about them?" (p. 5). Returning to the principle of accountability (Oswal & Melonçon, 2014; Oswal, 2014; Yu & Moeller, 2018), Zdenek states, "Access is our collective responsibility" (p. 6).

Accessibility as collective responsibility has progressed in conversations within technical communication. Early suggestions were to include those with disabilities in the usability testing process (Bayer & Pappas, 2006; Theofanos & Redish, 2003; Theofanos & Redish, 2005). Participatory design was later advocated, moving from inclusion to active partnerships as those with disabilities are involved from the very outset of content development and are active contributors of the design process (Oswal, 2014). Some current approaches to collective accessibility include practicing accessibility assessment through the lens of virtue ethics across university partnerships (Huntsman et al., 2018); considering the importance of language access in crafting and sharing digital research (Gonzales, 2018); and making crowdsourced, activist syllabi accessible as part of social justice coalitions (Bivens et al., 2020). It is increasingly clear that collaboration is a necessary part of accessibility.

From the beginning of the literature of our field, it has been established that we need to partner with people with disabilities to make successful designs. Additionally, the field should make better efforts to recognize that some technical communicators are disabled themselves; to do otherwise risks falling into the trap of what Palmeri (2006) called "rehab science" (p. 55), assuming that technical communicators are all outsiders working to solve problems for the disability community. We need to work as collectives to, as Zdenek calls for, "Expand the margins" (2017) of accessible design.

FUTURE DIRECTIONS FOR ACCESSIBILITY IN TECHNICAL COMMUNICATION

In this last section of this contribution, I'd like to present three ways in which technical communicators might consider new, future directions for accessibility. First, I suggest an applied version of accessibility in broadening its design to include sociospatial factors for wider networks of interactivity. In this section, I argue that accessibility should combat the naturalization of spaces and relationships in technology, incorporating critical disability frameworks into our accessibility practices that account for disabling built environments. Such practices would help move accessible design beyond single-task scenarios into more complex systems.

Second, I consider what Lewthwaite and Swan (2013) call a "hierarchy of impairment" (p.161) in how we approach practices of accessibility. Traditionally, accessibility praxis focuses on physical disabilities, and as a result those with learning, cognitive, mental, or psychiatric disabilities are historically under-served in technical communication. In this contribution, I call attention to the gaps in accessible communication design for mental or psychiatric disabilities, also conditions known as belonging to neurodivergence.

Finally, addressing Rebecca Walton's (2016) call to adopt principles of human rights in human-centered design, I close this contribution by reflecting upon what accessibility means in the realm of human dignity. This reflection ties together arguments from the past, such as the importance of individuating accessibility and treating users as valued partners, and moves toward contemporary issues, such as the field's current interest in accessibility as a collective. The chapter concludes with how said collective action might take shape in the future, and what that might look like through a technical communication lens, specifically.

Environmental and Sociospatial Factors in Communication Design

Historically, the body of technical communication scholarship on accessibility draws on the World Wide Web Consortium's (W3C) Web Content Accessibility Guidelines (WCAG 2.1) for quality assurance. As affirmed by the W3C itself, these guidelines are meant to serve as baseline recommendations for assessing accessibility and inclusive design. Other means of evaluation are necessary to account for context of use, general user experience, and other framing issues (Web Access Initiative, 2016). Scholarship within the last 20 years supports this affirmation, with conclusions from studies indicating that WCAG 2.1 has clear limitations when used as an isolated tool for quality assurance in web interface accessibility (Alonso et al., 2010; Kelly et al., 2009).

Initially, technical communication research set a precedent of positioning accessibility as a one-to-one problem. Now, the majority of technical communication scholars acknowledge that the interaction between user and technology no longer operates in isolation. Technical communication scholars in Experience Architecture (XA), for example, posit that users and technologies are part of "ecosystems of activity" (Potts & Salvo, 2017, p. 4). Designing for ecosystems, or rather having an active consideration of user scenarios, user profiles, and the networked contexts and technologies between them, goes beyond the practice of accounting for "single task scenarios" (Potts & Salvo, 2017, p. 4). In this vein, the technical communicator's approach to accessibility and inclusive communication design needs to be similarly expanded by accounting for the interactivity between users and technologies in activity ecosystems. While current scholarship in technical communication has identified the need for more comprehensive approaches to accessible design, more work still needs to be done on how this approach might be implemented in our design practices. Multiple technologies, multiple users, multiple environments, and multiple tasks all intersect in communication design, and these intersections need to be reflected in technical communication accessibility practices.

A common goal of designers is to build intuitive, natural experiences and environments with their interfaces. To contend with the "increasing complexity and volume of information" that exists in environments, built or physical, technical communicators have turned toward practices of information design as "information overload has become a major problem" (Albers & Mazur, 2014, p. 1). Contemporary designers of mobile technologies attempt to tap into "cognitive unconsciousness" (Farman, 2012, p. 28) by assuming the cognitive behaviors, information needs, and sensory experiences of their users in physical space. The built environments assembled by human designers therefore necessitate certain user performances in routing, orientating, and spatial problem solving. If effective, these constrained digital environments are "naturalized" (Barton & Barton, 1993) by their users—a process where visualizations are taken-for-granted as being natural, real, or objectively true and definitive, often at the expense of ignoring the socio-ideological motives behind their designs.

Disability scholars have challenged this process of naturalization, of neutral space, in a variety of ways, such as the sociospatial model of disability and the political/relational model that state disability is built into social environments (Hamraie, 2013; Kafer, 2013). These models are similar in their approach to disability being in "inaccessible buildings, discriminatory attitudes, and ideological systems that attribute normalcy and deviance to particular minds and bodies" (Kafer, 2013, p. 6). Locating disability in the body and mind, under these models, is inseparable with how we build, depict, interact with, and navigate environments. It is important then, in disability studies and spatial humanities, that space is not a neutral terrain but something designed. And when designed for normative users, or with accessibility as a single-task need, social space alienates or oppresses those who do not fit the preconstructed models or interactions of embodiment.

As technical communicators begin to progressively develop content ubiquitous within built, interactive environments, it becomes important to consider how naturalization might influence communication design practices—and account for accessibility practices thereof. While technical communicators are skilled in accessibility for web development, one area of consideration is how to improve accessible design practice that accounts for sociospatial factors (Heilig, 2018) in interactive, communication designs. Future technical communication praxis must consider critical theories of disability and accessibility that account for complexity with the same level of exigence that the field considers when designing for user experience.

A "Hierarchy of Impairment"

In accessibility praxis, driving heuristics like WCAG 2.1 focus nearly entirely on *physical* disability. Technical communication scholars have critiqued this emphasis in the past, stating that standards like WCAG 2.1 support "hierarchies of impairment" that ignore the experiences and needs of those with cognitive, affective, learning, or mental disabilities (Lewthwaite & Swan, 2013, p. 161). The blanketing of the term "disability" in WCAG 2.1 language omits important, diverse needs and experiences that exist among the broad population of users with disabilities. WCAG 2.1 guidelines, when not supplemented by responsible design practices and accommodations, discursively construct who a disabled person is, what obstacles they will encounter, and how they will interact with the interface. The disabled body, as it is imagined by the WCAG 2.1 guidelines, is thus a body with only physical barriers, excluding neurodivergent users or those with non-physical disabilities. Most broadly defined, neurodiversity can mean the divergence of thinking from what society deems as "normal," which is typically defined as autism, ADHD, and dyslexia but can/has included mental, psychiatric, and affective disabilities. To be blunt, technical communication scholarship does little service for this population.

As technical communication "increasingly constructs itself as a profession that assists users with disabilities" (Palmeri, 2006, p. 50), we need to listen to and partner with those who are traditionally de-centered. Studies advocating for disability and neurodiversity and/or mental disability, autism, and mental illness have been better served in our sister fields of rhetoric (see Price, 2011; Uthappa, 2017; Yergeau, 2018) and engineering (the *IEEE* journal alone hosts 179 entries on "mental illness"), so why not technical communication? Even when there are calls to expand research in our field regarding disability (Zdenek, 2017)? When it comes to approaches from disability studies that center on neurodiversity, our field has used very little—particularly from neurodivergent scholars, practitioners, and designers (for an example of technical communication research that *does* include neurodivergent users, see Elmore, 2013). We might account for neurodiversity in accessible communication design by returning to participatory design (Oswal, 2014) and coalitional accessibility (Bivens et al., 2020) efforts. Simple matters such as recruitment go a long way in identifying accessibility barriers (Bayer & Pappas, 2006) and the wide spectrum of neurodiversity necessitates involving actual users in the process of design—one-size-fits-all communication is not possible (Theofanos & Redish, 2005), nor should it be. It's important to recognize the neurodivergent as experts, who can contribute valuable understandings to the accessible design process.

To that end, technical communicators ought to critically reflect upon the design process that endorses only neurotypical thinking. Returning to Theofanos and Redish's (2005) more than 15-year call to support a flexible and portable accessibility, it is important not to become mired in an accessible design process that follows a linear and hegemonic design thinking.

Actionable Items for Human Dignity in Accessibility

Rebecca Walton (2016) argues that "TPC [technical and professional communication] struggles with the complexities of determining which humans are at the center of our work" (p. 402). She posits that it is "embracing human dignity and human rights as the first principle of communication and the foundational value of the TPC field" (p. 402) which should unify our work as we move toward the social justice turn—going from critical theory to critical action. While Walton's work is not explicitly about accessibility, the topic of centering—of who deserves attention in the field of technical communication, of dignity and rights—is a predominant one in its conversations. Because "centers" inherently imply margins, and as this contribution has addressed, it's time to go beyond them, to *re-center,* as they relate to disability and technical communication. Human dignity and human rights, the "notion that every person has intrinsic worth" (Walton, 2016, p. 402), is important groundwork to establish when it comes to communication design practice.

Because as addressed nearly a decade later (Oswal, 2014), issues identified by early technical communication scholars regarding accessibility continue. Recruitment of users with disabilities for design projects (Bayer & Pappas, 2006) could still be improved, *especially* for non-adaptive technology projects. Accessibility is still viewed as an act of legal compliance instead of "more than a checklist" (Oswal & Melonçon, 2017) or something that acknowledges the complexity and diversity of users with disabilities (Theofanos & Redish, 2005). Technical communicators still run the risk of lacking acknowledgment that technical communicators with disabilities exist, and that they can and do serve as accessibility and usability experts in the fields of design. In short, these historical problems are still current. There is still work to be done.

As we, as a discipline, look to the future of accessibility, accountability is going to be the driving force of re-centering. As experts in material and social discourses (Palmeri, 2006; Melonçon, 2013), technical communicators should *all* see accessibility as part of their calling toward social and critical action. If we claim usability, user experience, and communication design as areas of expertise, it goes without saying that accessibility needs to be a central part of technical communicators' curriculum (Pass, 2013; Youngblood, 2013) and pedagogical responsibility (Oswal & Melonçon, 2014). It's no longer enough to have accessibility be a niche skill of interested designers; this needs to be, as Zdenek (2018) said, *collective responsibility.* To reiterate Walton (2016), we need to rethink who's at the center of our work. We need to think of who we're depriving of human rights and dignity by exclusionary praxis.

SUGGESTIONS FOR FUTURE ACCESSIBILITY WORK IN TECHNICAL COMMUNICATION

I'd like to close this contribution with some actionable items that technical communicators can take, in this moment, to better our accessibility practices. These items are not definitive, nor are they perfect, but they are starting points in which to have conversations and continue practices of accountability as we move forward as a discipline.

The first is to make active efforts to recruit users with disabilities in our design work. This is far from a new suggestion (Bayer & Pappas, 2006). Recruitment will always be an ongoing effort for technical communicators, but it is important to make active efforts to engage users with disabilities as valued partners in design with usability expertise.

The second is to integrate accessibility into coalitional social justice work. Technical communicators are well-situated to provide feedback and service in making materials accessible for social justice efforts, to include archiving, translation, usability, plain language, and other inclusionary practices. The skillsets of technical communicators enable us to have resources that are well-suited toward enacting social change regarding matters of accessibility (Melonçon, 2013).

The third is to recognize hierarchies of impairment in current accessible design praxis. We need to identify when and advocate for users who are excluded from "best practices" of accessibility. These populations include but do not limit users with learning, cognitive, mental, psychiatric, or mood disabilities. Future accessibility research should make more concentrated efforts to specifically recruit users from these populations and elicit their expert feedback.

And, finally, contemporary work in accessible communication design must continue to respond to calls beyond the margins. As technical communication increasingly concerns itself with matters of social justice and coalition building (see: Walton et al., 2019), it is no longer appropriate for technical communicators to shed responsibility for accessible design. As specialists in material discourses (Melonçon, 2013), rhetoricians (Palmeri, 2006; Melonçon, 2013, among others), and members of disabled communities ourselves, we have an ethical obligation to enact best practices informed by and partnered with users with disabilities. We must keep moving accessible design forward and hold ourselves and members of our discipline accountable.

Conclusion

Over a period of approximately 25 years, technical communicators have been using critical disability studies to enhance knowledge and practice of accessibility. Since the late 1990s, technical communicators have moved from approaching accessibility as only an issue of adapting technology to broader considerations of cultural critique, social justice, and accountability in communication design. Turning to the future, technical communicators can continue to develop accessibility praxis in three areas: 1) broaden communication design to account for sociospatial factors and de-naturalize built environments, 2) make more concentrated efforts to include neurodiversity in accessibility, and ultimately 3) re-center human dignity in the communication design process. Practical suggestions for technical communicators are to actively recruit users with disabilities for design work, integrate accessibility into social justice initiatives, recognize hierarchies of impairment in current practices, and, most

412 L. HEILIG

importantly, continue to hold themselves and others in the field accountable for inclusive communication design.

REFERENCES

Adaptive Computing Technology Center. (2021). *What is adaptive technology?* Retrieved May 14, 2021, from https://actcenter.missouri.edu/about-the-act-center/what-is-adaptive-technology/

Agboka, G. Y. (2013). Participatory localization: A social justice approach to navigating unenfranchised/disenfranchised cultural sites. *Technical Communication Quarterly, 22*(1), 28–49. https://doi.org/10.1080/10572252.2013.730966

Albers, M. J., & Mazur, M. B. (Eds.). (2014). *Content and complexity: Information design in technical communication.* Routledge.

Alonso, F., Fuertes, J. L., González, Á. L., & Martínez, L. (2010). On the testability of WCAG 2.0 for beginners. *Proceedings of the 2010 International Cross Disciplinary Conference on Web Accessibility (W4A), 9.* https://doi.org/10.1145/1805986.1806000

Barton, B. F., & Barton, M. S. (1993). Ideology and the map: Toward a postmodern visual design practice. In N. Roundy Blyler & C. Thralls (Eds.), *Professional communication: The social perspective* (pp. 49–78). Sage.

Bayer, N. L., & Pappas, L. (2006). Accessibility testing: Case history of blind testers of enterprise software. *Technical Communication, 53*(1), 32–38. https://www.ingentaconnect.com/content/stc/tc/2006/00000053/00000001/art00005

Bivens, K. M., Cole, K., & Heilig, L. (2020). The activist syllabus as technical communication and the technical communicator as curator of public intellectualism. *Technical Communication Quarterly, 29*(1), 70–89. https://doi.org/10.1080/10572252.2019.1635211

Browning, E. R., & Cagle, L. E. (2017). Teaching a "critical accessibility case study": Developing disability studies curricula for the technical communication classroom. *Journal of Technical Writing and Communication, 47*(4), 440–463. https://doi.org/10.1177/2F0047281616646750

Davis, L. J. (1995). *Enforcing normalcy: Disability, deafness and the body.* Verso.

Dolmage, J. T. (2008). Mapping composition: Inviting disability in the front door. In C. Lewiecki-Wilson & B. J. Brueggemann (Eds.), *Disability and the teaching of writing: A critical sourcebook* (pp. 14–27). Bedford/St. Martin's.

Dolmage, J. T. (2017). *Academic ableism: Disability and higher education.* University of Michigan Press.

Elmore, K. (2013). Embracing interdependence: Technology developers, autistic users, and technical communicators. In L. Melonçon (Ed.), *Rhetorical accessability: At the intersection of technical communication and disability studies* (pp. 15–38). Routledge.

Farman, J. (2012). *Mobile interface theory: Embodied space and locative media.* Routledge.

Garland-Thomson, R. (1997). *Extraordinary bodies: Figuring physical disability in American culture and literature.* Columbia University Press.

Gonzales, L. (2018). Designing for intersectional, interdependent accessibility: A case study of multilingual technical content creation. *Communication Design Quarterly, 6*(4), 35–45. https://doi.org/10.1145/3309589.3309593

Hall, K. Q. (2011). *Feminist disability studies*. Indiana University Press.

Hamraie, A. (2013). Designing collective access: A feminist disability theory of universal design. *Disability Studies Quarterly*, *33*(4). https://doi.org/10.18061/dsq.v33i4.3871

Heilig, L. (2018). Silent maps as professional communication: Intersections of sociospatial considerations and information accessibility. *Business and Professional Communication Quarterly*, *81*(4), 421–439. https://doi.org/10.1177/2F2329490618802446

Huntsman, S., Colton, J. S., & Phillips, C. (2018). Cultivating virtuous course designers: Using technical communication to reimagine accessibility in higher education. *Communication Design Quarterly*, *6*(4), 12–23. https://doi.org/10.1145/3309589.3309591

Interaction Design Foundation. (2021). *What is usability?*. Retrieved May 14, 2021, from https://www.interaction-design.org/literature/topics/usability

Jones, N. N. & Scott, J. B. (2017). *Call for proposals: Precarity and possibility: Engaging technical communication's politics*. Association of Teachers of Technical Writing.. Retrieved May 14, 2021, from http://attw.org/attw-2018-conference-2/

Jones, N. N., Moore, K. R., & Walton, R. (2016). Disrupting the past to disrupt the future: An antenarrative of technical communication. *Technical Communication Quarterly*, *25*(4), 211–229. https://doi.org/10.1080/10572252.2016.1224655

Kafer, A. (2013). *Feminist, crip, queer*. Indiana University Press.

Kain, D. J. (2005). Constructing genre: A threefold typology. *Technical Communication Quarterly*, *14*(4), 375–409. https://doi.org/10.1207/s15427625tcq1404_2

Kelly, B., Nevile, L., Sloan, D., Fanou, S., Eliison, R., & Herrod, L. (2009). From web accessibility to web adaptability. *Disability and Rehability: Assistive Technology.*, *4*(4), 212–226. https://doi.org/10.1080/17483100902903408

Lewthwaite, S., & Swan, H. (2013). Disability, web standards and the majority world. In L. Melançon (Ed.), *Rhetorical accessability: At the intersection of technical communications and disability studies* (pp. 157–174). Routledge.

Linton, S. (1998). *Claiming disability: Knowledge and identity*. New York University Press.

Lippincott, G. (2004). Gray matters: Where are the technical communicators in research and design for aging audiences? *IEEE Transactions on Professional Communication*, *47*(3), 157–170. https://doi.org/10.1109/TPC.2004.833687

Longo, B. (1998). An approach for applying cultural study theory to technical writing research. *Technical Communication Quarterly*, *7*(1), 53–73.

Longo, B. (2000). *Spurious coin: A history of science, management, and technical writing*. State University of New York Press.

McRuer, R. (2006). *Crip theory: Cultural signs of queerness and disability*. New York University Press.

Melançon, L. (2013). Introduction. In L. Melançon (Ed.), *Rhetorical accessability: At the intersection of technical communication and disability studies* (pp. 1–14). Routledge.

O'Hara, K. (2004). "Curb cuts" on the information highway: Older adults and the internet. *Technical Communication Quarterly*, *13*(4), 426–445. https://doi.org/10.1207/s15427625tcq1304_4

Oswal, S. K. (2014). Participatory design: Barriers and possibilities. *Communication Design Quarterly, 2*(3), 14–19. https://doi.org/10.1145/2644448.2644452

Oswal, S. K., & Hewett, B. L. (2013). Accessibility challenges for visually impaired students and their online writing instructors. In L. Melonçon (Ed.), *Rhetorical accessability: At the intersection of technical communication and disability studies* (pp. 135–156). Routledge.

Oswal, S. K., & Melonçon, L. (2014). Paying attention to accessibility when designing online courses in technical and professional communication. *Journal of Business and Technical Communication, 28*(3), 271–300. https://doi.org/10.1177/2F105065 1914524780

Oswal, S. K., & Melonçon, L. (2017). *Saying no to the checklist: Shifting from an ideology of normalcy to an ideology of inclusion in online writing instruction. WPA: Writing Program Administration-Journal of the Council of Writing Program Administrators, 40*(3) https://wpacouncil.org/aws/CWPA/asset_manager/get_file/400647?ver=526

Palmeri, J. (2006). Disability studies, cultural analysis, and the critical practice of technical communication pedagogy. *Technical Communication Quarterly, 15*(1), 49–65. https://doi.org/10.1207/s15427625tcq1501_5

Pass, E. (2013). Accessibility and the web design student. In L. Melonçon (Ed.), *Rhetorical accessability: At the intersection of technical communication and disability studies* (pp. 115–134). Routledge.

Potts, L., & Salvo, M. (Eds.). (2017). *Rhetoric and experience architecture*. Parlor Press.

Price, M. (2011). *Mad at school: Rhetorics of mental disability and academic life*. University of Michigan Press.

Ray, D. S., & Ray, E. J. (1998). Adaptive technologies for the visually impaired: The role of technical communicators. *Technical Communication, 45*(4), 573–579. https://www.jstor.org/stable/43088583

Rose, E. J. (2016). Design as advocacy: Using a human-centered approach to investigate the needs of vulnerable populations. *Journal of Technical Writing and Communication, 46*(4), 427–445. https://doi.org/10.1177/2F0047281 616653494

Scott, J. B. (2003). *Risky rhetoric: AIDS and the cultural practices of HIV testing*. Southern Illinois University Press.

Spinuzzi, C. (2007). Accessibility scans and institutional activity: An activity theory analysis. *College English, 70*(2), 189–201. https://doi.org/10.2307/25472260

Theofanos, M. F., & Redish, J. (2003). Bridging the gap: Between accessibility and usability. *Interactions, 10*(6), 36–51. https://doi.org/10.1145/947226.947227

Theofanos, M. F., & Redish, J. G. (2005). Helping low-vision and other users with web sites that meet their needs: Is one site for all feasible? *Technical Communication, 52*(1), 9–20. https://www.ingentaconnect.com/content/stc/tc/2005/00000052/00000001/art00002

Uthappa, N. R. (2017). Moving closer: Speakers with mental disabilities, deep disclosure, and agency through vulnerability. *Rhetoric Review, 36*(2), 164–175. https://doi.org/10.1080/07350198.2017.1282225

Walters, S. (2010). Toward an accessible pedagogy: Dis/ability, multimodality, and universal design in the technical communication classroom. *Technical Communication Quarterly, 19*(4), 427–454. https://doi.org/10.1080/10572252.2010.502090

Walton, R. (2016). Supporting human dignity and human rights: A call to adopt the first principle of human-centered design. *Journal of Technical Writing and Communication, 46*(4), 402–426. https://doi.org/10.1177/2F0047281616653496

Walton, R., Moore, K. R., & Jones, N. N. (2019). *Technical communication after the social justice turn: Building coalitions for action*. Routledge.

Web Accessibility Initiative. (2016). Web Accessibility Initiative (WAI) Highlights. World Wide Web Consortium. Retrieved May 14, 2021, from http://www.w3.org/WAI/highlights/archive#x20131220a

Wilson, J. C. (2000). Making disability visible: How disability studies might transform the medical and science writing classroom. *Technical Communication Quarterly, 9*(2), 149–161. https://doi.org/10.1080/10572250009364691

Wilson, J. C., & Lewiecki-Wilson, C. (2001). *Embodied rhetorics: Disability in language and culture*. Southern Illinois University Press.

Yergeau, R. (2018). *Authoring autism: On rhetoric and neurological queerness*. Duke University Press.

Youngblood, S. A. (2013). Communicating web accessibility to the novice developer from user experience to application. *Journal of Business and Technical Communication, 27*(2), 209–232. https://doi.org/10.1177/2F1050651912458924

Yu, H., & Moeller, M. (2018). *Accountability in technical communication*. Association for Teachers of Technical Writing. Retrieved May 4, 2020, from http://attw.org/2019-conference-cfp/

Zdenek, S. (2009). Accessible podcasting: College students on the margins in the new media classroom. *Computers and Composition Online*, 1–21. http://www.cconline-journal.org/Zdenek_Word_version_CConline.pdf

Zdenek, S. (2011). Which sounds are significant? Towards a rhetoric of closed captioning. *Disability Studies Quarterly, 31*(3). https://doi.org/10.18061/dsq.v31i3.1667

Zdenek, S. (2015). *Reading sounds: Closed-captioned media and popular culture*. University of Chicago Press.

Zdenek, S. (2017). Call for proposals: Reimagining accessibility and disability in technical and professional communication. *Communication Design Quarterly*. Retrieved May 14, 2021, from http://readingsounds.net/wp-content/uploads/CFP-CDQ-2017/CFP-ReimaginingAccessibility-CDQSpecial-Issue.html

Zdenek, S. (2018). Guest editor's introduction: Reimagining disability and accessibility in technical and professional communication. *Communication Design Quarterly, 6*(4), 4–11. https://doi.org/10.1145/3309589.3309590

CHAPTER 25

Communication Infrastructures: Examining How Community Storytelling Facilitates or Constrains Communication Related to Medicaid Waivers for Children

Whittney H. Darnell

Access to affordable and adequate health care is important to all Americans. For persons with disabilities who often require complex and expensive care, adequate coverage is not always available in the private market. To address this disparity, Medicaid was established in 1965 to ensure that persons with limited income from specific vulnerable groups, such as persons with disabilities, had access to basic medical insurance. Medicaid, as a public insurance program option, is jointly funded by the federal government and the states (Center on Budget Policy and Priorities, 2000). Although conceptualized as a way to meet long-term care needs through institutionalized facilities, disability advocates' efforts have resulted in Medicaid now allowing some individuals to apply for funds to support home care programs (U.S. Department of Health and Human Services [USHHS], 2010), such as home- and community-based (HCBS) waivers. States have considerable flexibility in designing their programs, resulting in a great degree of variance in the offerings and eligibility requirements for Medicaid and Medicaid waivers from state to state. In recent years, the number of persons eligible for Medicaid programs has grown substantially, leading to serious questions about how such programs should operate moving forward.

W. H. Darnell (✉)
Northern Kentucky University, Highland Heights, KY, USA
e-mail: darnellw1@nku.edu

© The Author(s), under exclusive license to Springer Nature Switzerland AG 2023
M. S. Jeffress et al. (eds.), *The Palgrave Handbook of Disability and Communication*, https://doi.org/10.1007/978-3-031-14447-9_25

417

Medicaid's Balancing Incentive Program (BIP) encourages states to lower their percentage of HCBS spending, while also allowing more individuals to be served within their own homes and communities (Medicaid.gov, 2020). In this chapter, a brief history of disability health care is provided as a backdrop to the current study, which explores the unique role that custodial caregivers occupy in accessing and facilitating the use of home and community-based waivers for their children with disabilities. For this chapter, custodial caregivers refer to individuals with whom a child resides and who are legally and directly responsible for their day-to-day care, for example, parents, relatives, and legal guardians who are responsible for the health and well-being of children with a disability. Included in the work of custodial caregivers is the skill and communication required to learn about and navigate Medicaid waiver offerings in their communities as a means of health care for the children relying upon them. Access to Medicaid programs is often critical to affordable health care for children with disabilities. Williams and Musumeci (2021) found that "families of Medicaid/CHIP-only children with special health care needs are more likely to face financial difficulty, they find their health care more affordable than those with private insurance only due to Medicaid's cost-sharing protections" (para 4). This chapter utilizes communication theory to shed light on the physical and psychosocial conditions that can constrain or facilitate custodial caregivers' ability to access and share stories and information related to Medicaid waivers.

Disability Health Care: A Complex History

Prior to the 1970s, the primary health care option for persons with disabilities who required complex medical care was institutionalization. Over time, suspicion grew about the quality of care provided by institutions (Lakin et al., 1985; The Minnesota Governor's Council on Developmental Disabilities, 2022). A series of notable court battles, largely brought about through family- and community-level advocacy, successfully exposed a pattern of abuse and neglect occurring within many institutional facilities across the United States (Lakin et al., 1985; The Minnesota Governor's Council on Developmental Disabilities, 2022), which led to revolutionary changes in the health care system for persons with disabilities, including waiver-based care. Since then, several laws and protections have been established to offer those with disabilities and their family caregivers additional choices and access to care within the community rather than having them rely on care facilities (American Bar Association, 2017).

In 1981, HCBS waivers funded through Medicaid were instituted in many states to help support individuals and caregivers in their efforts to access quality health care in their own communities. The term "waiver" is significant because when recipients of the HCBS waivers become eligible for Medicaid funding, they are also given permission to "waive" currently existing Medicaid rules that require individuals with complex needs to receive health care services exclusively in an institutional setting. Essentially, by law, individuals must apply for and be given permission to waive a condition requiring that they leave their communities and families to access advanced health care. In doing so, the beneficiaries (i.e., persons with a disability), or legal caregivers on behalf of the persons with a disability, agree to coordinate their own specialized care within their own homes and communities.

Medicaid waivers are utilized by more than 10 million individuals with disabilities in the United States (Medicaid and CHIP Payment and Access Commission [MACPAC], 2017). As the number of individuals choosing to access Medicaid waivers has grown, so too have the costs of managed care programs, including those for people on HCBS waiver. In 2002, waiver programs costs were an estimated $93 billion; by 2015 costs had swelled to nearly $158 billion (MACPAC, 2017). Faced with a growing national debt, lawmakers at the state and federal levels have expressed an interest in exploring opportunities that reduce the cost of care for long-term supports such as HCBS waiver programs (Gibson et al., 2003). As recently as January 2018, the Centers for Medicare and Medicaid Services (CMS) released new guidelines for states pursuing waivers (e.g., imposing work requirements in Medicaid as a condition of eligibility). It remains to be seen whether or not these new requirements will be enforced, what other provisions CMS might approve, and how these changes to the waiver system will affect the costs, access, enrollment, and burden experienced by waiver recipients and their families (KFF, 2018).

Kentucky's Michelle P. Waiver

The Michelle P. Waiver (MPW) is one of six HCBS waivers offered in the state of Kentucky and covers more than 10,000 people in the state. Through the MPW waiver, individuals receive a medical card as well as additional coverage for medical expenses that fall beyond the scope of traditional health insurance. The MPW was created as a settlement in response to a lawsuit filed in 2002 against Kentucky's Protection and Advocacy Services Division by the Cabinet for Health and Human Services. At the time of the lawsuit, Kentucky's Supports for Community Living (SCL) waiver, another Medicaid waiver that provides community-based residential services, included over 3000 adults with disabilities on the waiting list, meaning thousands of families were left waiting for the health care their loved ones needed. The lawsuit was named after Michelle Phillips, a young woman living with a disability with the support and help of her parents. The suit contended that Kentucky was not sufficiently addressing the number of individuals like herself who were waiting for services. The six-year-long litigation resulted in a court-ordered expansion of Medicaid and the creation of the MPW.

The MPW is one of only two Medicaid waivers in Kentucky for which children with disabilities qualify. There are two features of the MPW that make it especially attractive to families of children (under the age of 18) with disabilities. First, and unlike other Medicaid waivers, the MPW does not offer residential care at a facility, but rather includes the option to hire qualified providers to administer in-home and community care in the caregiver's home, school, or community environments. Second, the MPW waiver is especially popular among families with young children with disabilities because it is robust in its benefit offerings and also one of the few Medicaid resources that does not include custodial caregivers' income as a qualifying factor in eligibility. As of 2021, the waiting list for the MPW has swelled to more than 8000 individuals, many of whom are children (Complex Child Magazine, 2021).

Custodial Caregivers

Custodial caregiving is a significant factor for families with disabled children. According to Young (2021), in a review of 2019 U.S. Census Bureau data, "an estimated 2.6 million households had at least one child in the home with a disability, representing 7.2 percent of the 36.7 million households in the United States that had children under the age of 18" (p. 1). Most custodial caregivers are not paid for advanced care that they provide, which is often clinical and/or therapeutic in nature. According to Fuith and Trombley (2020), "unpaid caregiving is a widely occurring part of family life in the United States" (p. 162). The emergence of COVID-19 has further exacerbated the U.S. health care system's reliance on custodial caregivers (Dhiman et al., 2020). Custodial caregivers have expressed concern about their ability to successfully navigate the new challenges that have stemmed from the pandemic, such as continuously fluctuating continuity of care and treatment, changing modes of educational instruction, food insecurity, digital inequity, and even greater job insecurity (Dhiman et al., 2020; Greer & Pierce, 2021).

Meanwhile, it remains true that children with disabilities often have the most to gain from community supports and early intervention access (CDCP, 2022). Studies show that a young child's level of exposure to early intervention is positively associated with improved health outcomes (Center on the Developing Child at Harvard University, 2007); increased language and communication ability (American Speech-Language-Hearing Association, 2008); and improved cognitive and social/emotional development (Hebbeler et al., 2008). Families of children with disabilities also benefit from such early intervention. Past studies have linked early intervention to decreased stress in the household and improved family relationships (Hebbeler et al., 2008). However, many custodial caregivers of children with complex care needs feel overwhelmed by the level of care their child requires, which may delay their decision-making and seeking of health care resources. Therefore, in studying health disparities among children with disabilities, research must expand its focus to those intimately involved in the caregiving and decision-making for children with disabilities; these caregivers are most likely to be the parents.

Communication Infrastructures

Few studies have explored how custodial caregivers go about seeking, processing, and sharing information about their child's disability (Baumbusch et al., 2018; Haw & Leustek, 2015). Given the aim of the MPW, which is to meet the needs of individuals with disabilities who prefer to receive specialized services and treatment in their home or community to institutional settings, it seems likely that individuals' connections to supportive networks in the community are critical to the achievement of desired health outcomes. Past studies have defined the powerful benefits and relationships that persons with disabilities have derived from direct participation in their communities as the procurement of "social capital" (Ellenkamp et al., 2016; Jeffress & Brown, 2017). Putnam (1993) describes social capital as "properties of social life" such as "trust, norms and networks" that promote "cooperation between participants and thereby enhance society's efficiency" (p. 167). Jeffress and Brown (2017) explored social capital as it related to the access of persons with disabilities to sport, power soccer specifically. In this study, we consider social capital as components of families' communication infrastructure, that is, those spaces and places available (or not) for custodial caregivers and parents of children eligible for the MPW to find out about and discuss the MPW.

Communication Infrastructure Theory

As both an ecological and a communication-focused theory, communication infrastructure theory (CIT) emphasizes the environmental conditions that contribute to community members' individual, interpersonal, organizational, and societal decision-making within a geographic region (Matsaganis & Golden, 2015). The CIT perspective positions researchers better to explain how interactions and the sharing of ideas and values among various levels of a social ecology contribute to individual-level health behavior. CIT provides a specific lens through which researchers can examine a communicatively constructed environment and to make sense of the communication actions that occur within it (Kim & Ball-Rokeach, 2006). Specifically, through CIT, researchers define a communication infrastructure as a socially constructed product of the community's storytelling network (STN) and the community's communication action context (CAC).

The Storytelling Network

Storytelling from a CIT perspective is defined as any type of communicative action that addresses residents, their local communities, or their lives in these communities (Ball-Rokeach et al., 2001). The STN operates at multiple levels and includes micro-, meso-, and macro-level social actors (Ball-Rokeach et al., 2001; Kim & Ball-Rokeach, 2006). Micro-level actors within a community include the physical residents and their close interpersonal networks (i.e., friends, family, neighbors). Meso-level storytellers, also known as community-level actors, include community organizations, community-oriented media, and grassroots or aggregated networks that focus on a particular area or population. Meso-level storytellers are focused on a particular section of the city or segment of a population (Kim & Ball-Rokeach, 2006). Local media are also considered members of the meso-level community. Finally, macro-level storytelling involves those messages received from mass-media organizations (e.g., national news media) and other larger governing institutions and organizations (e.g., state and national governments) that help shape the culture, stories, and experiences of a community. According to Kim and Ball-Rokeach (2006), "When residents talk about their community in neighborhood council meetings, at a neighborhood block party, at the dinner table, or over the fence with neighbors, they become local storytelling agents themselves—participating in an active imagining of their community" (p. 179). Importantly, past research shows that individuals' connectedness to an integrated STN can have a positive impact on their receptivity and access to critical health messages (Manos et al., 2001).

The Communication Action Context

The communication action context is the physical, psychological, sociocultural, economic, and technological properties that exist in a community and actively enable or constrain communication between members of an STN (Ball-Rokeach et al., 2001). When communities have physical spaces for their residents (including community organizations and media) to connect and talk to one another, stories can be told, and resources can be shared more easily (Wilkin & Ball-Rokeach, 2011). CIT assumes that communities are built through discourse, and that storytelling is a key channel for discourse to occur. According to Kim and Ball-Rokeach (2006), "Local communities are based on resources for storytelling about the community; without any resources for constructing stories about the local community and sharing them with others, it is impossible to build a community" (p. 177). Evaluating the CAC of a particular community, therefore, includes a consideration of the community's physical layout (e.g., the built environment), its psychological environment (e.g., the community members' perception of safeness or stigma), its "communication hotspots" (e.g., places and spaces where residents gather to talk), and its comfort zones (e.g., community institutions that help residents feel connected) (Wilkin et al., 2011).

CIT also posits that the degree of connectedness between individuals and all three levels of the STN can influence their goal attainment. In previous work, Kim and Ball-Rokeach (2006) found that a greater degree of connection to the STN is oftentimes positively associated with increased civic engagement, levels of belonging, collective efficacy, and civic participation. Further, when social actors are more connected to local resources at each level, they are more likely to be knowledgeable about diseases, outcomes, and resources (Kim et al., 2011), and they will also show more interest in actively seeking health information (Kim & Kang, 2010). CIT allows researchers to analyze the relationships among the different communication infrastructure levels and health outcomes for populations facing health disparities.

RESEARCH QUESTION

The objective of this research was to identify the discursive elements of custodial caregivers' CAC. This included identifying the psychosocial conditions of the community that constrained the sharing of stories and information related to the MPW, and also to locate the physical places and spaces (i.e., communication hotspots) that were available for discussing the MPW at the meso level (Villanueva et al., 2016; Wilkin & Ball-Rokeach, 2006). In order to better understand the environmental context of meso-level (i.e., community-level) storytelling related to the MPW and its influence on custodial caregivers' management experiences, the following research question was proposed: What environmental barriers or facilitators within the communication action context constrain or enable custodial caregivers' ability to manage the MPW?

METHOD

Participants

Eligible participants for this study were custodial caregivers who were at least 18 years old and currently providing care for a child (under 18) with an intellectual or developmental disability receiving benefits through the MPW. Following IRB approval, participants who agreed to take part in the study were also asked to provide informed consent and some basic demographic information (see Table 25.1) via a Qualtrics survey. Participation included the completion of the demographic survey and a semi-structured, narrative interview conducted by the author between October 2018 and January 2019. Interview length ranged between 52 and 119 minutes. Of the 31 total participants, one participant elected to meet face-to-face (3.23%), with all others choosing the phone interview ($n = 30$; 96.77%). All interviews were recorded using a university secured iPad and the Rev. recording app. Rev. transcription services were used to complete the transcripts within 24 hours of each interview. Completed transcriptions were then reviewed by the author. All participant names and identifying details were removed, and pseudonyms were given to each participant. Original and deidentified transcriptions were saved to a university secured drive, accessible only to the researcher. The final sample included all 31 custodial caregivers ($n = 27$ female caregivers, $n = 4$ male caregivers) who were interviewed for this study. All but one female caregiver were the biological mothers of the children. One female caregiver was the aunt of the child but had obtained legal custody. All male parental caregivers were the

Table 25.1 Parental caregiver demographic information

Characteristic	N	%
Gender		
Female	27	87.1
Male	4	12.9
Relationship to child		
Mother	26	83.87
Father	4	12.9
Other (i.e. aunt)	1	3.23
Racial/Ethnic Background		
White/Caucasian	30	96.77
Asian/Asian American	1	3.23
Relationship status		
Single/ Never married	1	3.23
Serious relationship	1	3.23
Married	27	87.1
Other (did not describe)	2	6.44
Education		
High school/GED	1	3.23
Some college	6	19.35
Two-year degree/Associate	1	3.23
Four-year degree/ Bachelor	12	38.71
Master's degree	5	16.13
Doctoral degree	4	12.9
Professional (MD, JD, etc....)	2	6.45
Current employment status		
Full-time	10	32.25
Part-time	3	9.68
Full-time at home caregiver	10	32.25
Student full-time	1	3.23
Other (i.e., irregular, self-employed)	4	12.9
Did not answer	3	9.68
Annual household income		
Below $20,000	2	6.45
$20,000–$39,999	3	9.68
$40,000–$60,000	2	6.45
$60,000–$79,999	4	12.9
$80,000–99,999	8	25.81
$100,000 and above	11	35.48
Prefer not to answer	1	3.23

biological fathers of the children. This final sample included participants from 26 different zip codes in the state of Kentucky. The participants ranged from 31 to 52 years of age.

Interview Protocol

The aim of the narrative interview was to gather data about custodial caregivers' particular experiences communicating about the MPW by asking them questions meant to prompt a storied response. A semi-structured method allows the researcher to conduct the interview in a way that is intimate and informative using open-ended questions to elicit detailed narratives and stories (DiCicco-Bloom & Crabtree, 2006). The interview questions for this study were theoretically guided by Ball-Rokeach et al.'s (2001) CIT and encouraged the sharing of stories specifically related to custodial caregivers' experience in learning about and accessing the MPW waiver (e.g., "Can you think of a time when you heard about the Michelle P. Waiver or waiver services in general discussed on the local news, Facebook, a newsletter, a flyer at the library, or some other public venue?" "How did this experience help you find information or support related to the MPW?" "What community resources were available or unavailable that made this decision more or less difficult?").

Recruitment

Convenience sampling (Etikan et al., 2016), which is a type of nonprobability or nonrandom sampling was utilized in order to broadly recruit participants across the state. Convenience sampling is useful when populations are not easily identified or hard-to-reach. Participants were members of the target population (i.e., custodial caregivers of children with disabilities in Kentucky utilizing the MPW) and were accessible either geographically or through a shared connection or organization known to the researcher. Prior to participation, potential participants were provided with an IRB-approved consent letter informing them of the purpose of the research and the activities involved in participation, which included a face-to-face or phone interview and the completion of a short Qualtrics survey. Participants were remunerated for their participation with a $20 Visa gift card. Participants were recruited through social media; this included a recruitment post on Facebook which resulted in 15 interviews, and also through a statewide disability network listserv. Recruitment through the listserv, which included disability-related agencies and support service providers across the state, resulted in 16 interviews.

Thematic Narrative Analysis

To make sense of the interview data, which resulted in over 600 pages of transcripts, three coders employed thematic narrative analysis, a method for interpreting texts in their storied form (Riessman, 2008). The goal of narrative analysis is not to evaluate the truthfulness of the narrator's story but rather to understand the human experience (Saldaña, 2009). While traditional thematic analysis emphasizes the content of the narrator or the narrative, a thematic narrative analysis is also attuned to the telling of stories, including the "how," "to whom," and "for what purposes" the story is told, or untold (Riessman, 2008). For this research project, a narrative thematic analysis allowed the researchers to preserve the participants' "whole stories," and ultimately provided robust insights regarding the discursive and physical conditions that custodial caregivers recounted in their narratives that they felt made discussions about the MPW more or less accessible.

The three coders (the author, one graduate student, and one undergraduate student), all with training in communication research, analyzed the transcripts that resulted from the 31 interviews. Guided by the principles of CIT (Ball-Rokeach et al., 2001), the coders read the narratives as a whole, looking to extract moments of the story that exemplified participants telling of barriers to and facilitators of MPW access and management within their own CAC. A barrier included any physical or psychosocial feature or condition of the community that constrained storytelling between individuals and meso-level entities about the MPW, thus hindering participants' ability to effectively access and manage the MPW. A facilitator, then, included those physical or psychosocial features or conditions that enabled storytelling about the MPW between the individual and meso-level entities and contributed to the adaptive access and management of the MPW.

During the initial round of coding, the first author created a Microsoft Excel spreadsheet that was provided to the coders, along with a copy of the transcripts. Pseudonyms were given to participants, and identifying information was removed before coding materials were shared. Each coder was instructed to individually copy and paste to their Microsoft Excel file all instances wherein participant stories described a psychosocial or physical barrier or facilitator to MPW information or storytelling. Transcript page numbers were also documented for reference. The coding team then met to discuss and organize their initial codes. Coders recorded many of the same instances during this first round. For those instances wherein coders had observed the same story and were in agreement that the coded exemplar was a barrier or facilitator, a discussion was held about how much of the story was needed to showcase and preserve as a whole unit (Riessman, 2008). The use of longer excerpts is common in narrative research (Polkinghorne, 1995) and allows the researcher to showcase "how and why a particular outcome came about" (p. 19). Discussion continued until consensus had been reached for each of the exemplars coded by the research team. The research team agreed to conduct a second round of coding to ensure that all relevant data had been captured.

In a second meeting, the coding team was able to quickly confer and come to agreement on all remaining codes. Next, the following thematic classification was determined: three barrier themes (lack of systematic entry, poor case management, and constraints due to social control), and two subfacilitator themes (online neighborhoods and disability networks). At the end of this second meeting, the team agreed to individually review the themes and exemplars a third time before conducting a member check and then finalizing the analysis.

Member Checking

A member check of synthesized data (Birt et al., 2016) was used to "explore whether results have resonance with the participants' experience" (p. 1805). Using an online random name draw, six participants (20%) from the sample were invited to participate in a member-checking activity that included a summarized version of the results. Participants were first contacted to confirm their willingness to participate and then provided a written summary of the findings to review before a follow-up interview. Interviews were conducted in the first two weeks of February 2018. Those participants interviewed as part of the member check universally supported the findings, with much of the interview dialogue resulting in expressions of gratitude from the participants for the opportunity to share their story and for giving them a sense of doing something to "make things easier for the next family." Harper and Cole (2012) found that participants often describe member-checking experiences as an opportunity to feel validated and to see they are not alone in their experiences. It became clear to the research team that our research facilitated participants' desire to share their MPW experiences. For many of our participants, this was the first time anyone asked about the MPW. This realization strengthened the resolve of the research team to want to share the following participant stories through publication.

FINDINGS

Ultimately, the analysis of this data revealed several physical and psychosocial barriers of the communication action context that constrained communication between custodial caregivers and their meso-level community—lack of systematic entry, poor case management, and constraints due to social control—and that these thus also challenged caregivers' ability to adaptively manage the MPW. In addition, several features of the CAC that enabled communication at the meso level were identified—in particular, online neighborhoods and disability networks—which seemed to connect caregivers to resources, support, or information that helped them effectively manage the MPW. These are illustrated in Fig. 25.1.

Barriers in the Communication Action Context

No Systematic Entry Point
Perhaps the most consistent theme in the data was the lack of systematic entry into the MPW. Each participant learned about the waiver from a different community source, often years after learning the diagnosis of their child. Next, several participant exemplars are shared to support these findings.

Taylor explained, "There is nowhere to find information in our little town, unless you are getting it from me or someone else that has it. Ninety-five percent of people have no idea what a waiver is." Becca felt that there is no easy

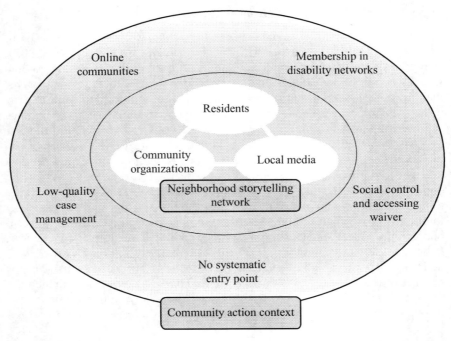

Fig. 25.1 Conceptually illustrates the current findings. (Modified for the current study based on *Metamorphosis, 2020* by Annenberg School for Communication, USC)

way for caregivers to learn about the MPW in the community. She was especially frustrated that medical providers—whom most people learn to rely on for health-related information—do not suggest the MPW, and she blamed this lack of a systematic process for introducing families to the MPW for her child's delayed access to the program. Becca stated,

> I do think, that it is something that needs to be put out there, even if it's just a suggestion; to say, "Listen, we offer this to all of our patients that have a child with a mental disability. There is a program called MPW." Maybe even have a brochure or a handout to say, "Here, this is what the program is, and if you're interested, you need to contact. That would have helped me. I ran around looking for an answer and had to find it the hard way years down the line."

Several other caregivers also expressed their surprise and frustration in learning that pediatricians and other health care providers do not have information related to the MPW to share with disability families. For instance, Nancy said,

> I think it starts with the pediatrician. I think that has to be the first point of contact for most individuals who will need a referral for a diagnostic battery. Every pediatrician should have information. I don't know why it doesn't happen. Maybe it's just not seen as a priority.

Mary also wished that the medical community were more knowledgeable about the MPW so that finding out about the waiver was a more straightforward process. She said,

> I wish there was a better way, that I don't know, the doctor, or hospital, social worker, somebody who says, "Okay, you got this diagnosis, here's things that we're going to do to help you. Here's the Michelle P. Waiver if you need it." Instead of just saying, "Here's the diagnosis, have fun with your autistic child."

In sum, caregivers expected information about the MPW to come from a medical source (e.g., pediatrician) and were surprised that there was no systematic process in place to alert potential candidates about it. This absence of a systematic entry was particularly problematic for caregivers who struggled to find information from the medical community.

Low-Quality Case Management

Poor or unavailable case management arose as a barrier to many families' ease in accessing waiver information or other related health services. Participants often discussed their lack of confidence in the validity of information provided by case management agencies because of past incidents wherein they received inaccurate information. Andrea shared how incorrect information provided by a past case manager led to their daughter losing access to a specialty doctor:

> Her case worker told us she couldn't have other insurance and stay eligible for the MPW. So, for a year and a half, I was told that, and it's not true, not the correct information. We lost her doctor in Baltimore because a case worker in Kentucky did not know what they were talking about.

In another example, Stacie discussed being discouraged by her case manager to apply for the MPW. "We asked our case manager about the MPW, they were like, 'No, no, there's no way.' They just shut us down … I mean, some of the case workers act like the services are coming out of their pocket sometimes." Some participants talked about case manager turnover as an issue that considerably reduces their trust in their management team. According to Andrea, when case managers moved on, she never knew what to expect regarding the quality of their replacements. "I've had a couple of case workers that have been really good and have given me suggestions about places to take [child's name] for physical therapy. But then I've had some, and they don't know anything."

Taylor is currently working with her fifth case manager since her child became waiver-eligible seven years ago. Taylor said that in her experience, she is usually better off finding answers to her questions about the MPW from her own sources because the case managers' knowledge is usually limited. "It wasn't that we had anyone that was particularly bad, but we definitely had case managers that only knew the basics…Like I said, I feel like they try; but I will get better information if I poke around myself."

By and large, several of the participants in this study expressed a common skepticism about case managers' knowledge and ability to provide accurate and useful information about the MPW. In many cases, the lack of quality case management ultimately delayed their child's application and access to the MPW.

Social Control in Accessing the Waiver

Many participants discussed the stringent processes and rules imposed by various meso-level authorities that made it difficult to effectively manage the MPW. Participants felt that inconsistent instructions from Medicaid created an obstacle to their child's access to health care by inhibiting open communication. For example, Nancy spoke about the indirect paper trail and the redundancy of work required by Medicaid as factors that delayed her child's access to care. She said,

> I had to provide all the documentation and sign releases of information for every doctor we'd ever seen, write down every medication, every procedure that had been done. It was ridiculous; I literally carried my entire tub of paperwork from the first two years of her life to the Medicaid office, never knowing what they might need. And then, even though I had just jumped through the hoops of Michelle P., I had to jump through the hoops again with Medicaid.

Madeline also discussed feeling that the complexity of Medicaid was a barrier to access care for her child. It took Madeline almost three years of persistence to apply for the waiver successfully. She explained,

> I got bounced around a lot. I would go to the Social Security office and they would say, "Oh, no, you're at the wrong office, you've gotta go to Cabinet for Families and Children." I remember this one day in particular. I drove to Lexington, had an appointment with Social Security because that's where I thought I was supposed to go. Sat there and waited—an hour or plus. Then, I finally got my appointment, sat down for literally 30 seconds, [and] she said, "You don't need to be here. You need to be at Cabinet for Families and Children." And I was like, "What the heck? And where is that?" Probably took us two and a half to three years to go from starting the process to being accepted.

June wondered if the process of applying for the waiver was purposely complex to discourage people from accessing it, acknowledging that she knew several families that had given up on trying to access the waiver for their children. "I know tons of families that started the process that gave up, knowing that their child was going to benefit greatly from the program." They were like, "I have a job. I cannot do another job; this is a job."

In sum, findings revealed three elements of the CAC (i.e., lack of systematic entry, poor case management, and social control through Medicaid) that created major barriers for custodial caregivers when seeking information about the MPW. Participants shared several instances in which they felt that the information flow regarding the MPW was overly complex or unreliable.

25 COMMUNICATION INFRASTRUCTURES: EXAMINING HOW COMMUNITY... 431

Facilitators in the Communication Action Context

The CAC can enhance communication within a community by creating communication hotspots—places where community members tend to engage with one another in dialogue. In the present study, participant narratives revealed two communication hotspots within the CAC of custodial caregivers that facilitated communication about the MPW: online neighborhoods and disability networks/nonprofits.

Online Communities

Several caregivers discussed the importance of connecting with other waiver families through social media outlets. In some cases, it was through their engagement with online communities that caregivers first learned about the MPW. For example, Nancy recalled, "I didn't know about the waiver, other than through the community, the Facebook community of the Down Syndrome Association of Central Kentucky (DSACK), where I heard rumors of waivers."

Taylor also discussed the impact of joining online communities, which she considers her most trusted source of MPW-related information:

> Everything that we've ever been able to get for our daughter—the reimbursement of insurance, the waiver programs, figuring out how to do timesheets, all the things that we do, everything I've learned that actually helped us—we have learned from parents through Facebook support groups, or just by polling parents.

Reece discussed how social media has made it easier to connect with other families and share resources at a pace that she feels is best for her and her family, thereby facilitating her use of information-seeking.

> When [child's name] is having a particular issue, I go look online for information. There is Autism Speaks, there are all kinds of support groups on Facebook. I mean, there's just anything you want support on in Facebook...Even for the waiver itself, I pretty much get all my information from other people that are in those communities that are on the program.

In summary, online communities enable the sharing of resources among custodial caregivers by providing a space where caregivers could talk openly about their experiences. These forums also served as a form of informational and social support that aided the management of the MPW.

Membership in Disability Networks

Membership in disability networks (e.g., Human Development Institute, Down Syndrome Association, Autism Speaks) also facilitated MPW-related communication among caregivers. These nonprofit entities were instrumental in creating opportunities, whether by hosting a meeting, a website, or a Facebook page for families to communicate with each other and with knowledgeable advocates. For example, Rachel described how her membership in state and international disability networks had recently led to an opportunity to be an ambassador for one of the networks. Her task will be to help disseminate diagnosis and resource information, such as a list of programs—like the MPW—for which families might be eligible:

> Once we did the [disability-specific] page, then we found there's a central Kentucky special-needs parent page, and then we found there's a [treatment type] support page. We met one other kid that has [child's name's] diagnosis, and the rest of them are spread all over the world. The [disability-specific] foundation is working on an ambassador program, so they're seeking out people like me in each state that can collect all the resources, like stuff about the waivers in each state, and to put it in one place so that as people are diagnosed, we can literally hand them a sheet and say, "Here are the things in Kentucky your kid will automatically qualify for." Or, "Here's the way these are processed, do this."

For Jenny, it was through her membership with a disability network that she finally learned how to successfully apply for the MPW:

> I started going to [disability network]. I e-mailed them. I was Googling something, and I found them, and I was like, "Hey, this is what my kid has. Can you guys serve him?" They said yes…They have a parent organization, which I'm just starting to become a part of, where we go out there and talk to parents and say, "Hey, you need any support?" They will ask you, "Do you have this? Have you tried this?" They will go through the entire list. They pushed me to apply for Michelle P. again. He goes, "You've asked the wrong questions when you've gone in there. You have to apply, and you will get it." And we did get it, which was huge for us.

When asked "Can you think of a time where you learned something that helped you navigate the MPW better or differently?" Madeline shared an example of an important connection she was able to make through her association with a disability network. As a result of the association, she gained access to both social and informational support:

> I think probably the biggest thing is that connecting to [disability network] makes you feel like you've got support. So that if you do feel like you're in a spot where things are not completely known, or you don't know where to go or where to turn, at least you have resources to reach out to. And some of those resources are nationally known people that do this every day.

These participant narratives illustrate several ways the CAC either connected custodial caregivers to resources that positively impacted the health of their children or constrained communication between custodial caregivers and their meso-level community, thus challenging caregivers' ability to adaptively manage the MPW. Next, the implications of these findings are discussed.

Discussion

Over half a century after Medicaid was signed into law, there remains a dearth of rigorous and intentional research to guide policy makers when making decisions about Medicaid funding. In this study, communication theory was used to explore the barriers to and facilitators of community-level (meso-level) communication surrounding the MPW, a HCBS waiver in the state of Kentucky that is especially attractive to custodial with children who have a disability. This focus allowed the research team to identify common challenges and roadblocks within custodial caregivers' available communication infrastructure that delayed caregivers' education and involvement with the MPW. We also identified community storytelling infrastructures that facilitated custodial caregivers' introduction to the MPW and provided spaces and places to talk about their experience and the experiences of others. A number of potential implications are offered as considerations for disability studies researchers and policy makers working to rethink how home- and community-based waivers offered through Medicaid are structured and communicated.

Implications

The findings of this study offer important insights for addressing barriers to home- and community-based waiver storytelling in the community, and suggestions for building on current community infrastructures that have shown success in creating spaces and places where Medicaid waiver stories can be shared.

Barriers to Medicaid Waiver Storytelling in the Community

Given that states have substantial flexibility in the design of their Medicaid programs, one priority might be the development of a systematic entry point to knowledgeable MPW storytellers in the community. Ensuring custodial caregivers' access to knowledgeable sources in the community is likely to improve the rate at which families apply for waivers like the MPW for children who are eligible. Healthy People 2020 states that states and local communities should improve health for people with disabilities by educating individuals, institutions, and systems about existing laws that protect people with disabilities (HealthyPeople.gov, 2021). The current study exposes a lack of consistent storytelling at the local level. Custodial caregivers in the current study often expressed a desire for their pediatricians to become credible authorities regarding the MPW. Additional research is needed to understand if and how pediatricians should become informants about waiver-based care.

Second, case management concerns were echoed by many of the custodial caregivers interviewed for this study. This finding is consistent with recent studies exploring the role of case management as a key resource for persons with disabilities and their families (Bogenschutz et al., 2015). Such issues included inadequate training, turnover, and excessive workload. Unfortunately, there has been very little research that has explored the interactions between persons with disabilities and their families and the case manager. Further, case management roles vary widely from state to state (Amado, 2008; Lightfoot & LaLiberte, 2006). Examining the current availability of resources and continuing education specific to home- and community-based waivers for case managers may be a useful next step to removing this barrier.

Finally, several participants discussed their desire to have the application process and maintenance work for persons with disabilities and their family caregivers examined. Participants felt that the required processes are purposely complex and confusing, and thought that the processes were designed to discourage access. As states work to specifically redesign their Medicaid waivers in order to qualify for incentives offered by Medicaid's Balancing Incentive Program, a close examination of the application process from a usability and health literacy perspective seems to be warranted.

Facilitators of Medicaid Waiver Storytelling in the Community

Community-level communication remains an important source of waiver education for custodial caregivers of children with disabilities. Specialized or informal community storytellers were essential to many participants' progress in learning about the waiver, accessing the waiver, and utilizing the waiver more fully. From a CIT perspective, this study shows that conceptualizations of *community*, specifically in terms of belongingness, residency, and connectedness, should be expanded to account for custodial caregivers' influential memberships with specialized community groups (e.g., disability networks, diagnosis-specific entities, online communities). Most research in CIT has explored health behaviors and communication storytelling among ethnic communities that lived together in identifiable and proximal parts of a city or neighborhood (Ball-Rokeach et al., 2001). Members of disability communities are less likely to share the same level of geographical proximity. Current findings suggest that the criteria for "community" are likely context-specific, especially in cases related to the disability health care experience. To access community knowledge about the MPW, building community with other persons who were experienced with public health care in the state (i.e., the MPW in Kentucky)—rather than building community within a neighborhood's geography—was the more important criterion for establishing locality.

The growing number of applications for HCBS waivers across the country suggests that family and custodial caregivers prefer to care for their loved ones in their homes and in their own communities. In the current study, we found that community networks, such as disability networks, online communities, churches, social media pages, and other disability-specific groups, contributed to custodial caregivers' sense of belongingness and connectedness to the communities they lived in and opened up opportunities for storytelling about the

MPW that were unavailable within their more immediate interpersonal networks (e.g., family and friends).

LIMITATIONS

Like any study, this study is not without its limitations. First, a sample of 31 custodial caregivers in the state of Kentucky is too small a sample size to draw conclusions about waiver-based care more generally, and thus this constrains the transferability of these findings. In addition to the limited number of participants, this sample also lacked ethnic diversity. Given that cultural characteristics are known to play a role in how individuals view their health, and how they experience structural barriers and institutional discourse, it is essential that in future recruitment efforts, researchers find effective channels through which to access a more diverse sample. A disturbing fact about this sample was that custodial caregivers with higher levels of income were overrepresented. This raises important questions about who is accessing the waiver, and how the experiences of custodial caregivers of different incomes and education levels may impact available STNs and CACs. The length of time that custodial caregivers had been managing the MPW for their children also may have affected the narratives they told. Some participants were among the first to access the waiver and had experienced little wait time, whereas others waited up to five years before their child was finally approved. The fact that the study was not designed to examine these temporal differences is a limitation to consider. The possibility of recall bias is a factor to consider when interpreting participants' stories. Finally, there are some demographic concerns about the final sample. For instance, only four participants (12.9% of the sample) were fathers to a child with disabilities receiving health care through the MPW. Additionally, all but one of the participants reported their ethnicity as White. Hence, the sample may not reflect the actual population of custodial caregivers of children with disabilities in Kentucky.

There are also several limitations in the scope of this exploratory study that could provide insight for future directions in disability policy research. For example, in this study, the perceived communication infrastructures of custodial caregivers related to the MPW were generally explored as a whole. This study did not critically examine the communication infrastructure of specific storytelling instances such as MPW application and interview procedures that may encourage or dissuade custodial caregivers to pursue access to the waiver. Careful examination of these individual processes could lend valuable practical guidance to custodial caregivers and the community providers working with them. In addition, this study prioritized only the experiences of custodial caregivers. Interviewing case managers, family resource providers, pediatricians, and other community-level sources of MPW-related information may uncover additional opportunities or gaps in the communication infrastructure.

Conclusion

By recognizing the community-level impact of communication on the everyday lives and decisions of custodial caregivers, community partners can begin to address the barriers to management created by ambiguous processes and nonexistent points of access to information. The present findings have important implications for improving health in the context of caregiving and home- and community waiver-based care, which is a primary means of access to health care for thousands of people with disabilities in the United States. Families have made clear that they prefer home- and community-based waivers over institutionalized care options for their children with disabilities. Kentucky's MPW, like similar waivers in other states, makes more affordable a wide range of medical and long-term care services, many of which are not covered or are only partially covered through private insurance, for custodial caregivers. Communities must continue to create and improve communication related to such waivers so that families and eligible providers can knowledgeably communicate about home- and community-based waivers and feel empowered to take the steps necessary to apply for and utilize the waivers to provide care for children with disabilities. Continued research and community discussion about the role of custodial caregiving and HCBS waivers in U.S. health care is critical, as several legislative proposals at the state and federal levels are currently exploring ways in which to reduce or eliminate the funding of Medicaid, including waiver programs.

References

Amado, A. N. (2008). *Innovative models and best practices in case management and support coordination*. Institute on Community Integration, University of Minnesota.

American Bar Association. (2017). *Introduction: Disability rights under siege*. Retrieved March 1, 2020, from https://www.americanbar.org/publications/crsj-human-rights-magazine/vol%2D%2D42/vol-42-no-4/introduction%2D%2Ddisability-rights-under-siege.html

American Speech-Language-Hearing Association. (2008). *Roles and responsibilities of speech-language pathologists in early intervention: Position statement*. Retrieved March 1, 2020, from https://www.asha.org/policy/PS2008-00291/

Ball-Rokeach, S. J., Kim, Y. C., & Matei, S. (2001). Storytelling neighborhood: Paths to belonging in diverse urban environments. *Communication Research, 28*(4), 392–428. https://doi.org/10.1177/009365001028004003

Baumbusch, J., Mayer, S., & Sloan-Yip, I. (2018). Alone in a crowd? Parents of children with rare diseases' experiences of navigating the healthcare system. *Journal of Genetic Counseling, 28*(2), 1–12. https://doi.org/10.1007/s10897-018-0294-9

Birt, L., Scott, S., Cavers, D., Campbell, C., & Walter, F. (2016). Member checking: A tool to enhance trustworthiness or merely a nod to validation? *Qualitative Health Research, 26*(13), 1802–1811. https://doi.org/10.1177/2F1049732316654870

Bogenschutz, M., Nord, D., & Hewitt, A. (2015). Competency-based training and worker turnover in community supports for people with IDD: Results from a group randomized controlled study. *Intellectual and Developmental Disabilities, 53*(3), 182–195. https://doi.org/10.1352/1934-9556-53.3.182

Brown, L. X. Z., Ashkenazy, E., & Giwa Onaiwu, M. (Eds.). (2017). *All the weight of our dreams: On living racialized autism*. DragonBee Press.

Center on Budget Policy and Priorities. (2000). *Policy basics: Introduction to Medicaid*. Retrieved December 21, 2021, from https://www.cbpp.org/research/health/policy-basics-introduction-to-medicaid

Center on the Developing Child at Harvard University. (2007). *A science-based framework for early childhood policy: Using evidence to improve outcomes for learning, behavior, and health for vulnerable children*. http://developingchild.harvard.edu/index.php/download_le/-/view/63

Centers for Disease Control and Prevention. (2022). *What is early intervention*. Retrieved December 1, 2019, from https://www.cdc.gov/ncbddd/actearly/parents/states.html

Complex Child Magazine. (2021). *Kentucky*. Retrieved January 17, 2022, from http://www.kidswaivers.org/ky

Dhiman, S., Sahu, P. K., Reed, W. R., Ganesh, G. S., Goyal, R. K., & Jain, S. (2020). Impact of COVID-19 outbreak on mental health and perceived strain among caregivers tending children with special needs. *Research in Developmental Disabilities, 107*, 103790. https://doi.org/10.1016/j.ridd.2020.103790

DiCicco-Bloom, B., & Crabtree, B. F. (2006). Making sense of qualitative research. *Medical Education, 40*(4), 314–321. https://doi.org/10.1111/j.1365-2929.2006.02418.x

Ellenkamp, J. J., Brouwers, E. P., Embregts, P. J., Joosen, M. C., & van Weeghel, J. (2016). Work environment-related factors in obtaining and maintaining work in a competitive employment setting for employees with intellectual disabilities: A systematic review. *Journal of Occupational Rehabilitation, 26*(1), 56–69. https://doi.org/10.1007/s10926-015-9586-1

Etikan, I., Musa, S. A., & Alkassim, R. S. (2016). Comparison of convenience sampling and purposive sampling. *American Journal of Theoretical and Applied Statistics, 5*(1), 1–4. https://doi.org/10.11648/j.ajtas.20160501.11

Fuith, L., & Trombley, S. (2020). COVID-19 and the caregiving crisis: The rights of our nation's social safety net and a doorway to reform. *University of Miami Race & Social Justice Law Review, 11*(2), 159–184. Retrieved January 17, 2022, from https://repository.law.miami.edu/cgi/viewcontent.cgi?article=1132&context=umrsjlr

Gibson, M. J., Gregory, S. R., & Pandya, S. M. (2003). *Long-term care in developed nations: A brief overview*. Retrieved December 1, 2021, from http://research.aarp.org/health/2003

Greer, M., & Pierce, C. (2021). Examining the impact of the COVID-19 pandemic on caregivers of children with complex and chronic conditions. *Research, Advocacy, and Practice for Complex and Chronic Conditions, 40*(1), 1–26. https://doi.org/10.14434/rapcc.v40i1.33294

Harper, M., & Cole, P. (2012). Member checking: Can benefits be gained similar to group therapy. *The Qualitative Report, 17*(2), 510–517. https://doi.org/10.46743/2160-3715/2012.2139

Haw, M. H., & Leustek, J. (2015). Sharing the load: An exploratory analysis of the challenges experienced by parent caregivers of children with disabilities. *Southern Communication Journal, 80*(5), 404–415. https://doi.org/10.1080/1041794X.2015.108197

HealthyPeople.gov. (2021). Disability health. Retrieved December 1, 2019, from https://www.healthypeople.gov/2020/law-and-health-policy/topic/disability-and-health

Hebbeler, K., Barton, L. R., & Mallik, S. (2008). Assessment and accountability for programs serving young children with disabilities. *Exceptionality, 16*(1), 48–63. https://doi.org/10.1080/09362830701796792

Jeffress, M. S., & Brown, W. J. (2017). Opportunities and benefits for powerchair users through power soccer. *Adapted Physical Activity Quarterly, 34*(3), 235–255. https://doi.org/10.1123/apaq.2016-0022

Kasier Family Foundation (KFF). (2018). Medicaid waivers: Sharing state experiences. Retrieved https://www.ncsl.org/Portals/1/Documents/fiscal/Robin_Rudowitz_Presentation.pdf

Kim, Y. C., & Ball-Rokeach, S. J. (2006). Civic engagement from a communication infrastructure perspective. *Communication Theory, 16*(2), 173–197. https://doi.org/10.1111/j.1468-2885.2006.00267.x

Kim, Y. C., & Kang, J. (2010). Communication, neighborhood belonging and household hurricane preparedness. *Disasters, 34*(2), 470–488. https://doi.org/10.1111/j.1467-7717.2009.01138.x

Kim, Y. C., Moran, M. B., William, H. A., & Ball-Rokeach, S. J. (2011). Integrated connection to neighborhood storytelling network, education, and chronic disease knowledge among African Americans and Latinos in Los Angeles. *Journal of Health Communication, 16*(4), 393–415. https://doi.org/10.1080/10810730.2010.546483

Lakin, K. C., Hill, B., & Bruininks, R. H. (1985). *An analysis of Medicaid's intermediate care facility for the mentally retarded (ICF-MR) program.* Retrieved December 1, 2019, from https://mn.gov/mnddc/parallels2/pdf/80s/85/85-AMI-UMN.pdf

Lightfoot, E. B., & LaLiberte, T. L. (2006). Approaches to child protection case management for cases involving people with disabilities. *Child Abuse & Neglect, 30*(4), 381–391. https://doi.org/10.1016/j.chiabu.2005.10.013

MACPAC. Medicaid and CHIP Payment and Access Commission. (2017). *People with disabilities.* Retrieved December 12, 2019, from https://www.macpac.gov/subtopic/people-with-disabilities

Manos, M. M., Leyden, W. A., Resendez, C. I., Klein, E. G., Wilson, T. L., & Bauer, H. M. (2001). A community-based collaboration to assess and improve medical insurance status and access to health care of Latino children. *Public Health Reports, 116*(6), 575–584. https://doi.org/10.1093/phr/116.6.575

Matsaganis, M. D., & Golden, A. G. (2015). Interventions to address reproductive health disparities among African-American women in a small urban community: The communicative construction of a "field of health action." *Journal of Applied Communication Research, 43*(2), 163–184. https://doi.org/10.1080/00909882.2015.1019546

Medicaid.gov (2020). *Quality of care: Home and community based services (HCBS) waivers.* Retrieved January 5, 2022, from https://www.medicaid.gov/medicaid/quality-of-care/improvement-initiatives/hcbs/index.html

Polkinghorne, D. E. (1995). Narrative configuration in qualitative analysis. *International Journal of Qualitative Studies in Education, 8*(1), 5–23. https://doi.org/10.1080/0951839950080103

Putnam, R. (1993). The prosperous community: Social capital and public life. *The American Prospect, 13*(4), 249–263. Retrieved January 5, 2022, from http://www.prospect.org/print/vol/13

Riessman, C. K. (2008). *Narrative methods for the human sciences.* Sage.

Saldaña, J. (2009). *The coding manual for qualitative researchers.* Sage.

The Minnesota Governor's Council on Developmental Disabilities. (2022). *Parallels in time. A history of developmental disabilities.* Retrieved June 15, 2023 from https://mn.gov/mnddc/parallels/five/5a/6.html

U.S. Department of Health and Human Services. (2010). *Understanding Medicaid home and community services.* Retrieved December 1, 2019, from https://aspe.hhs.gov/system/files/pdf/76201/primer10.pdf

Villanueva, G., Broad, G. M., Gonzalez, C., & Ball-Rokeach, S. (2016). Communication asset mapping: An ecological field application toward building healthy communities. *International Journal of Communication, 10,* 2704–2724. https://ijoc.org/index.php/ijoc/article/viewFile/5335/1674

Wilkin, H. A., & Ball-Rokeach, S. J. (2006). Reaching at risk groups: The importance of health storytelling in Los Angeles Latino media. *Journalism, 7*(3), 299–320. https://doi.org/10.1177/2F1464884906065513

Wilkin, H. A., & Ball-Rokeach, S. J. (2011). Hard-to-reach? Using health access status as a way to more effectively target segments of the Latino audience. *Health Education Research, 26*(2), 239–253. https://doi.org/10.1093/her/cyq090

Wilkin, H. A., Stringer, K. A., O'Quin, K., Montgomery, S. A., & Hunt, K. (2011). Using communication infrastructure theory to formulate a strategy to locate "hard-to-reach" research participants. *Journal of Applied Communication Research, 39*(2), 201–221. https://doi.org/10.1080/00909882.2011.556140

Williams, E. & Musumeci, M. (2021). *Children with special health care needs: Coverage, affordability, and HCBS access* (Issue Brief). Kaiser family Foundation. Retrieved June 15, 2022 from https://www.kff.org/medicaid/issue-brief/children-with-special-health-care-needs-coverage-affordability-and-hcbs-access/

Young, N. A. (2021). Childhood disability in the United States: 2019. (Issue Brief ACSBR-006), U.S. Department of Commerce, U.S. Census Bureau. Retrieved January 1, 2022, from https://www.census.gov/content/dam/Census/library/publications/2021/acs/acsbr-006.pdf

CHAPTER 26

Governing Deaf Children and Their Parents Through (and into) Language

Tracey Edelist

Informed choice and consent are central tenets of the Canadian health care system. While seemingly straightforward, meaning that people have the right to choose whether or not to consent to a specific health care treatment after being informed of such treatment and any alternatives, in practice, what it means to provide informed choice and obtain informed consent is rather murky, especially in the case of parents making health care decisions for their children. How society values and understands disability can direct how informed choice and consent are understood and presented by institutions and experienced by parents. In this chapter, through an interpretive disability studies approach, I examine how a specific health care institution, Ontario's Infant Hearing Program (IHP), has historically framed informed choice and consent to parents of young infants through the meanings of language and deafness presented to parents during their infants' hearing screening and diagnostic process. I discuss some of my findings from an interpretive analysis of IHP texts and interviews with parents whose children have received services from the IHP, expanding on findings discussed in my doctoral dissertation. IHP texts exemplify how certain types of information are presented and understood as unbiased or objective while conveying how language and deafness are organized and conceptualized in our society. Societal understandings of disability, deafness, language, and cultural difference have framed the IHP's discourse and practice within a medicalized understanding of deafness, making it

T. Edelist (✉)
Université du Québec à Trois-Rivières, Trois-Rivières, QC, Canada
e-mail: tracey.edelist@mail.utoronto.ca

© The Author(s), under exclusive license to Springer Nature Switzerland AG 2023
M. S. Jeffress et al. (eds.), *The Palgrave Handbook of Disability and Communication*, https://doi.org/10.1007/978-3-031-14447-9_26

441

acceptable for the IHP to not inform parents about sign language as a viable communication option, despite a policy of fully informed choice and consent.

The IHP's discourse, also reflective of the ideologies of speech-language pathology and audiology professions, perpetuates the idea that the ability to hear and to speak is necessary for communication and language development, hence discounting sign language as a viable option for communication and ignoring the importance and vibrancy of Deaf culture. These understandings of deafness as a problem that can and should be fixed with hearing technologies, and the assumed superiority of spoken language over sign language, govern parents toward a "right" choice of spoken language for their deaf children. This choice is also supported by hearing parents' own understandings of deafness and language and the inclination to want their child to hear and speak.

Recently, the IHP has modified their protocols and communications to parents, seemingly in an attempt to be more neutral in their discourse and to provide more information about the option of sign language. However, the new documents also make clear that the IHP will only provide services for sign language OR spoken language. Considering that most parents of deaf children are themselves hearing, it remains unlikely that parents would forego spoken language services to learn sign language. To end the chapter, I suggest a reconceptualization of informed choice and discuss how a fluid and flexible understanding of language, deafness, and parental choice could allow parents the opportunity to use multiple communication options to both strengthen parent-child interactions and increase language development opportunities for deaf infants.

THE ONTARIO INFANT HEARING PROGRAM

Ontario's Infant Hearing Program (IHP) is the official abbreviated title for The Infant Hearing Screening and Communication Development Program, which came into effect in 2002. There are three major components of the program: Universal newborn hearing screening (which usually occurs prior to discharge for babies born in hospital and in the community for babies born with midwifery care, or for those who did not get screened in hospital); assessment (audiology assessment and medical management); and follow-up support and services (family support, information access, hearing technologies, and communication development) (Ontario Ministry of Health and Long Term Care, 2002). The IHP also provides referrals to related services, such as one of the three Cochlear Implant (CI) programs in Ontario (most services move from the IHP to the hospital's CI Program if the child receives a CI), and the preschool Home Visiting Program, which offers a teacher of the deaf to work with the child and family in their home, provided by the Ontario Ministry of Education. The IHP has a goal to screen at least 95% of babies born in Ontario (Canadian Working Group of Childhood Hearing, 2005, p. 83), and between 2006 and 2016 (the last available dataset), over 130,000 babies were screened each year (Ministry of Children, Community and Social Services, 2016).

Universal Newborn Hearing Screening (UNHS) has therefore become a regular part of the birth experience for new parents in Ontario.

When an infant is identified as deaf or hard of hearing during audiology assessment, they then receive follow-up services, including services to support communication development. One of the principles of Ontario's IHP is "Every aspect of this program will be provided based on fully informed parent/guardian choice and consent" (Ontario Ministry of Health and Long Term Care, 2002, p. 2). The IHP previously provided three options for communication development: spoken language, sign language, or a dual approach (both spoken and sign). However, despite these three options, the vast majority of parents chose an exclusive spoken language approach for their child (MCYS Program Consultant, personal communication, January 2015; Small & Cripps, 2012). As I demonstrate in this chapter, this outcome is not simply based on a decision parents make after being "fully informed" of all communication options as stated in the IHP's policy; it instead reflects the governing of parents toward this spoken language decision. It is likely that choosing a spoken language approach has become easier for hearing parents, since as of April 2018, the IHP removed the dual approach as a service option, effectively promoting the idea that sign language and spoken language are incompatible (Ministry of Children and Youth Services, 2018).

Governing Through Language During Screening: Deafness as Unthinkable

Interpretive Analyses of IHP Screening Documents and Parent Experiences

In this chapter, I examine how children and their parents are governed through language, into particular forms of language, through interpretive discourse analysis of IHP texts and parental interviews, informed by the work of Foucault. Foucault's related concepts of governmentality, "a 'conduct of conducts' and a management of possibilities" (Foucault, 2003, p. 138), and bio-power, "the organization of power over life," (Foucault, 1978, p. 139), have been used by disability studies scholars to examine how disabled bodies are controlled with a goal to normalize (e.g., Sullivan, 2015; Hughes, 2015). As my focus is on the control of disabled bodies through and into language, my analysis is also informed by the idea of "language governmentality" proposed by critical linguistic theorists. Language governmentality seeks to examine the many different ways that language governs people, beyond formal state imposed language policies, and reiterates the importance of how language is conceptualized and expected to be used (Flores, 2014, p. 2).

I conducted in-depth textual analyses of IHP screening texts, including information pamphlets given to parents at the time of screening and information provided verbally by the screeners. This analysis was supplemented by other IHP policy and implementation documents, as well as national speech-language pathology and audiology association position papers related to childhood hearing. I also analyzed the text of parental interviews, obtained for my doctoral research. I interviewed 12 parents of deaf and hard of hearing children between June and November 2016. The children were aged one to ten years at the time of the interviews, and had recently used or were using Ontario's IHP services. I obtained University of Toronto Research Ethics Board approval for these interviews in December 2015. Interpretive analyses of both IHP texts and parent interviews provided rich sources of information, as I could examine parents' descriptions of their experiences with IHP text and the documents themselves. In my analysis, I paid particular attention to the socio-political history of the texts to question how the IHP made language and deafness meaningful to parents and how informed choice was produced through the texts via relations of power.

Whether or not their child becomes identified as deaf or hard of hearing, parents encounter certain meanings of deafness throughout the screening process. The IHP carefully scripts how information is presented to parents (information about the hearing screening procedure and the result of their baby's hearing screening) to ensure protocol is followed and to manage parental action, all the while presenting hearing loss as a problem. An IHP protocol document states, "...the screener's behaviour, style, and tone can have a major effect on the family's cooperation, giving of informed consent, satisfaction with the screening experience, and adherence to follow-up instructions" (Ministry of Children, Community, and Social Services, 2019, p. 15), an explicit reference to how parents are deliberately governed through language. In this and other ways to be discussed below, the IHP screening texts demonstrate how the IHP exercises power via a form of governmentality.

The screener must first obtain parental consent to perform the screening which happens within the first 24 hours of a hospital birth, or within days of a community birth. If parents consent to the hearing screening, explicit consent is also sought for a risk factor screen, which tests the newborn blood spot sample for genetic mutations and cytomegalovirus (Ministry of Children, Community, and Social Services, 2019). Screening is presented to parents as necessary to avoid undiagnosed hearing loss, and all the potential speech, language, behavior, educational and emotional problems their child may have by not getting early support and services if needed (e.g., Government of Ontario, 2022a). Legally, parents have a right to decline the screening, a fact included in newer protocols (Ministry of Children, Community, and Social Services, 2019) but previously largely ignored in past protocols that outline how to obtain consent for what the IHP deemed a necessary, unquestionable, routine test (Sinai Health System, 2012). These protocols suggested a moral judgment associated with screening that situated screening as the right thing to do, blurring the line between medical and moral (Conrad, 1992; Illich, 1977). I do not mean to suggest that hearing screening is not important; rather, I am pointing out a problem inherent in informed consent when the medical establishment has determined the value of a certain procedure: parents who do not agree to the procedure are considered difficult or non-compliant, rather than as autonomous people making an informed decision for their child (Young et al., 2006). I found this to be just the first of such judgments that parents encounter during the screening and assessment process.

After parental consent is obtained and the screening test completed, the screener gives parents information pamphlets related to their baby's screening result. The possible screening results are: pass, refer for more testing, no result, or bypass hearing screen to get a full assessment (Government of Ontario, 2022b). Both the verbal script of the screener and the information pamphlets comprise IHP texts that can influence the actions parents take, which are dependent on the meanings they attribute to their child's diagnosis of deafness, which are in turn shaped by meanings presented to them through text. The screening texts do more than simply provide information to parents about the screening procedure and outcomes, they present a particular way to think about and react to deafness, which governs parents toward a spoken language approach.

Governing Toward Spoken Language

Hearing Loss as Problem

There are a few ways the screening texts govern parents toward a spoken language approach. To begin, the screening texts make it clear hearing loss is a problem. Even for babies who "pass," or those whose parents decline the screening, parents are expected to monitor their baby's speech and language for signs of delayed development that may signify the problem of possible hearing loss (Ministry of Children, Community, and Social Services, 2019). For any screening result other than a pass, hearing loss has been presented as a problem expected to cause worry. To circumvent parental concern over hearing loss, the parents I interviewed were told of the unlikelihood that a refer result could mean a problem with hearing, consistent with the pamphlets provided at that time. Although this is reflective of test outcomes (around 5% of babies with normal hearing fail the screening) (Ontario Ministry of Health and Long Term Care, 2002), parents were also warned that an undetected hearing loss could lead to delayed language, which could lead to behavioral and emotional problems and difficulties with school (e.g., Government of Ontario, 2014a). The statistical unlikelihood of hearing loss was used to reassure parents after a refer result that their child's hearing was likely "fine," while the developmental issues that could result from undetected hearing loss were used to create enough concern for parents to follow-through with another screening and/or diagnostic audiology. This manipulation of parental worry situates hearing loss as both an unthinkable concept and a material problem requiring fast solutions.

The pamphlets given to parents describe speech and language problems as potential developmental concerns that may arise from hearing loss AND as indicators for potential hearing loss. Parents are told that the goal of screening is to prevent speech and language delays through early hearing loss identification and intervention: "Identifying hearing loss shortly after birth is important. It allows families to work with health care professionals to determine the best way to help their child learn language and avoid delays in communication and social development" (Government of Ontario, 2014a). However, parents are also told to "pay attention," because if hearing loss is not identified early, then speech and language delay may indicate a potential hearing loss: "It is important to pay close attention to your baby's speech and language development, because problems with speech and language development can be a sign of hearing loss" (Government of Ontario, 2014b).

Language delay can serve as an indicator for the main "problem" of hearing loss, but the potential for delayed language is also presented as the principal justification for identifying hearing loss early (to prevent language problems), creating a circular relationship between speech, language, and hearing. The IHP's focus on the relationship between speech, language, and hearing from the first stage of screening leaves little consideration (implicit or explicit) that language development could be anything other than spoken language development. What can be imagined as language and communication has therefore been precisely governed by how the IHP presents information to parents. In terms of informed choice and consent, this means parents are governed, from the beginning of screening, toward "choosing" spoken language services as a way to "fix" the problem of deafness as framed by the IHP, within wider societal understandings of deafness and disability.

The Duality of Chance as Risk and Chance as Opportunity

Another way parents are governed toward spoken language is through the rhetoric of chance. The pamphlets now given to parents are more streamlined and generic with tick boxes to indicate the screening outcome, rather than separate pamphlets for each outcome (see the "fact sheets" available on the Infant Hearing Program webpage of the Government of Ontario's website (Government of Ontario, 2022b)). At the time of my parent interviews, however, babies who passed but were deemed at risk for future hearing loss received a separate pamphlet. Although there is less information in the newer pamphlets and a notable attempt to be "factual" and "objective," the rhetoric of chance is still implied.

The pamphlet for the "pass at risk" result provided information about the benefits of early identification and early access to services, to ensure parental follow-through with subsequent testing for babies at risk of hearing loss,

> When hearing loss is found early there is more time to take advantage of all the services that are available. Most deaf and hard of hearing children whose hearing loss is identified early, and who receive the support they need, will have the same

chance to develop language skills as other children their age. (Government of Ontario, 2014c)

The pamphlet informs parents that the IHP provides many services to help deaf and hard of hearing children learn language, services that must be accessed as early as possible for their child to have a "chance" of developing language like "normal" children, and "most [other] deaf and hard of hearing children." If parents do not follow the IHP's recommendations to access services quickly, their child may be one of the few deaf and hard of hearing children who do not have the same chance to be like other children, since "most" participate in this chance. The risk of identifying hearing loss too late for the baby to have the same chance as hearing babies is used to persuade parents to continue with screenings; the IHP makes the small chance of hearing loss an urgent concern due to the risk of not accessing early language support.

This rhetoric of chance in the pamphlet presents parents with both negative and positive meanings of "chance": for babies at risk, there is "a small chance that a hearing loss may develop over time," but early identification will allow for access to services and "the same chance to develop language skills as other children." This duality of chance governs parents to access IHP screening services and any necessary follow-up audiology and speech and language services. The pamphlet tells parents to worry about the potential risk of hearing loss, but only just enough to go for testing. Parents are also told not to worry about the refer result because if their child does have hearing loss, early identification and accessing IHP support would mitigate the problem of delayed language development. This duality of chance as risk and opportunity establishes the potential of hearing loss as both something to be feared (based on the assumption parents will already fear hearing loss) and something that can/should be fixed. These conflicting meanings of chance manage parental action and hence the assessment and interventions they seek for their baby, all the while maintaining hearing loss as a significant risk parents should worry about. In this way, the IHP asserts bio-power to seek parental cooperation in the identification and circumscribed treatment of possible hearing loss (Foucault, 1978, p. 139). Within this duality of chance, hearing loss can only be conceptualized as a problem in need of fixing, establishing the necessity of services for hearing technologies and spoken language.

Hearing Loss as an Excludable Type
Parents have also been governed toward an exclusive spoken language approach through the IHP's presentation of hearing loss as an "excludable type" (Titchkosky, 2007). For example, when the baby obtains a "refer" result after screening, they are scheduled for another test in a couple of weeks. Despite not passing the screening, a training video for screeners indicates that parents should be reassured of the unlikeliness of hearing loss: "We didn't get a pass today...it doesn't mean that there's a hearing loss..." (Sinai Health System, 2012). Consistent with the recollections of the parents I interviewed, the

screener on the training video tells parents that waiting a couple of weeks can allow time for fluid or debris in the baby's ears to clear "so we can have a better chance of passing" (Sinai Health System, 2012). The act of passing is presented as the goal of the test, a goal that can be achieved through collaboration between the screener, the infant, and the parents. On the training video, the screener does not mention what would happen if the baby does not pass the second screening. This evasion of the possible need for diagnostic audiology combined with a pass result being the unquestioned desired outcome, constructs hearing loss as an unthinkable problem connected to a collaborative "we" who do not want or expect the problem to emerge. As the justification for screening is to identify hearing loss in infancy, yet hearing loss is presented as an unthinkable outcome of screening, hearing loss is therefore only included as an excludable type (Titchkosky, 2007).

The IHP's screening of most babies born in Ontario means deafness is included in the everyday lives of newborns and parents, yet at the same time, has excluded deafness as a possible outcome of screening. Titchkosky (2007) explains how disability can be both included and excluded in everyday life:

> A deep provocation lies in the fact that the very ways that disability is included in everyday life are, also, part of that which structures the continued manifestation of disabled people as a non-viable type. It is, for example, provocative to think about how disability is both excluded and included simultaneously in the interstices of our lives, or included as an excludable type. (p. 5)

The possibility of permanent childhood hearing loss and the need for early intervention is the justification for universal newborn hearing screening (UNHS), yet the very condition the screening was developed to identify has historically been presented to parents as an unimaginable outcome throughout the screening process. Making deafness unthinkable in this way reflects a desire for normalcy so prominent in society (Davis, 1995), while making habilitation (i.e., making a deaf child learn to hear and speak) the only acceptable parental action in response to a deaf diagnosis, to give normalcy a "chance" to be recovered. The newer screening scripts remove the emphasis of the unlikelihood of deafness, instead telling parents that "more testing is needed" to find out "how well your baby hears" (Ministry of Children, Community, and Social Services, 2019, pp. 51, 52). It would be important to interview parents to understand how these newer changes are reflected in practice.

Fully Informed? A Medical Lens of Objectivity

Rather than assuming that IHP texts are objective sources of information that only explain hearing screening procedures, audiological assessments, and communication services, an interpretive analysis shows how the texts enact their meaning of deafness. The IHP's principle of fully informed choice and consent suggests parents are informed of all communication options for their deaf child in an objective manner. At the time of my parent interviews, IHP documents indicated that a family support worker (FSW) would be available to discuss all possible options with parents as soon as possible after diagnosis:

> This individual must be completely unbiased in terms of choices for communication. The main purpose of this individual will be to support, counsel and assist the family; and to serve as a short term case coordinator to ensure that they receive all the information on communication options and meet with all the stakeholders that represent those options. (Ontario Ministry of Health and Long-Term Care, 2001, p. 17)

Although it may seem the IHP is fulfilling their obligation to fully inform parents in an unbiased manner with the provision of an FSW, the experiences of parents I interviewed indicate many parents came to make the decision of spoken language before even meeting with the FSW, and after having to do their own research to get information.

For example, one parent waited six months after diagnosis (when the audiologist responded to her questions by simply telling her to "accept it") before meeting with the FSW. Another parent stated that by the time she met with the FSW, "I knew more about hearing loss at that point than she did." In addition, although this support person is still made available when requested by parents, it seems that the task of discussing language development options is now placed on the audiologist at the time hearing loss is confirmed, although the "IHP Audiologist should offer the involvement of other service providers (e.g., SLPs, ASL/LSQ Consultants" (Ministry of Children and Youth Services, 2018, p. 21). As parents generally indicated to me that their audiologists were not forthcoming with information, let alone unbiased information, unless these service providers can be accessed quickly it remains unclear whether the IHP's principle of informed choice is upheld.

The IHP's presentation of deafness as an unthinkable problem to be fixed with hearing technologies and spoken language, along with societal understandings of deafness and disability and the thoughts parents themselves bring to this decision-making, governs parents toward choosing an exclusive spoken language approach for their children before being informed of other options. I found this to be at least in part a function of quick referrals to a Cochlear Implant Program for deaf infants considered good candidates for cochlear implantation, as parents often decided on cochlear implants and an exclusive spoken language approach before meeting with the FSW. In addition, when they did meet with the FSW, parents recalled being told of either sign language or spoken language, but not about the dual option of both sign and spoken language. Others didn't recall being told about sign language at all, only learning about sign language later when a teacher of the deaf came for a home visit. The lack of services for a dual approach has been confirmed with the IHP's removal of the option for both sign and speech services, and is also unsurprising since many of the parents chose cochlear implantation and were told to

450   T. EDELIST

focus on auditory-verbal language and not sign language for their child to be considered a candidate (see also Edelist, 2019; Snoddon, 2009).

Professional Standpoints: SLPs and Audiologists

Another factor governing parents toward spoken language is how audiologists, the first professionals to discuss the diagnosis with parents and tasked with presenting information about communication in an unbiased manner, and speech-language pathologists, who provide speech and language services, bring a professional imperative to promote listening and speaking into their relationships with parents. The ideologies and professional policies and practices of audiologists and speech-language pathologists (SLPs) and other professionals who provide services are reflected within IHP discourse. This discourse presents deafness as a problem and hearing technologies and spoken language as the solution. As such, the IHP frames "informed choice and consent" within a medical understanding of deafness.

The Health Care Consent Act, which became law in Ontario in 1996, stipulates that health care providers must obtain informed consent before beginning treatment. As regulated health professionals, SLPs and audiologists must obtain voluntary, informed consent from the parents/guardians of infants and young children before providing a health service (Health Care Consent Act, 1996). Speech-Language and Audiology Canada (SAC) (previously CASLPA) is a national association that promotes SLP and audiology and offers national clinical certification (SAC, 2018a). SAC also provides professional resources and guidelines, including position papers on universal newborn hearing screening (UNHS), and cochlear implants in children. A brief analysis of these position papers demonstrates how audiologists and SLPs are expected to promote cochlear implants (CI) for deaf children, while positioning spoken language as the only desirable language outcome.

Position Paper on Cochlear Implants in Children

SAC's 2006 CI position paper reiterates that cochlear implants improve "auditory-only speech understanding" (i.e., understanding speech without lip-reading, manual gestures or signs) and recommends rehabilitation to develop a child's listening skills within an oral communication context (CASLPA, 2006, Background, para 2). The text acknowledges that individual speech and language outcomes after CI vary significantly, but also claims that despite this variability in expressive communication outcomes, "all cochlear implants have been shown to be effective in improving auditory-only speech understanding" (CASLPA, 2006, Background, para 6). With this focus on auditory-only speech understanding, and no mention of sign language, SAC's support of cochlear implants makes sign language irrelevant for deaf children, and even counterproductive to the imperative to improve auditory-only speech understanding.

The one reference to Deaf culture is a cautionary statement that hearing professionals should be prepared to counsel parents and children around issues that Deaf culture members have with cochlear implants in young children (CASLPA, 2006). Knowledge of Deaf culture is presented as necessary to reactively counsel parents in their decision to choose CI, rather than for proactive educational purposes to assist parents in deciding whether to agree to a CI for their child in the first place. Cochlear implants are therefore positioned in opposition to Deaf culture (and sign language); knowledge of Deaf culture and sign language in and of themselves is not presented as valuable and important for deaf children.

SAC updated their position paper in support of cochlear implants in children in 2018 to acknowledge the auditory access available with bilateral cochlear implantation (cochlear implants in both ears rather than only one ear) in young children, and to support the use of CI, due to technological advances, in children with conditions and/or residual hearing that previously discounted implantation (SAC, 2018b). This revised text also acknowledges that communication "may also include augmentative communication systems or sign languages," followed by a list of factors that should be considered when helping a family choose a communication method (SAC, 2018b, p. 3). How these factors relate to SAC's support of early CI is unclear, but seem to be part of a "[thorough exploration] of parental expectations and commitment to implantation and (re)habilitation," (p. 3), which I interpret as a commitment to an exclusive spoken language approach to communication. Although SAC recognizes sign language as a means of communication, it is not one suited to cochlear implantation. The exception SAC makes to this stipulation, is for families who already use sign language. Although an important change, this is presented as a way to include deaf children of signing deaf adults as candidates for cochlear implantation, rather than acknowledgment and support of all implanted children learning and using sign language.

Position Paper on Universal Newborn Hearing Screening
SAC's position paper in support of universal newborn hearing screening (UNHS) in Canada (2010) further demonstrates the profession's focus on spoken language for deaf infants. The position paper explains the necessity of UNHS to detect permanent childhood hearing loss in infancy "and initiate intervention for auditory and communication development" (2010, p. 20). Furthermore, SAC states that "extended periods of auditory deprivation have a significant impact on the overall brain development and sensory integration of the child" (SAC, 2010, p. 2). The position paper presents the value of UNHS as the identification of hearing loss to prevent auditory deprivation through the use of hearing technologies, rather than to prevent language deprivation (spoken or signed) and providing the opportunity to begin teaching the child a visual-based sign language while they are young.

According to this position paper, for a deaf child to develop to their full potential and avoid deprivation, they must use hearing technologies to access sound and develop their brain through spoken language. Indeed, the position paper identifies the underlying premise of UNHS to be the importance of early identification and early auditory stimulation, and the development of "speech, language, cognitive and psychosocial abilities" (SAC, 2010, p. 3). Within this position paper, communication for deaf children is assumed to be spoken language supported by hearing technologies: "coupled with advances in hearing aids and cochlear implants, UNHS has improved the outcomes for communication development for children with all degrees of hearing loss" (SAC, 2010, p. 4). This link between hearing technologies and communication effectively eliminates sign language and other non-verbal modes of communication as viable and desirable ways for deaf children to communicate.

The Medical Construction of Objectivity

These position papers show how audiologists and SLPs have professional guidelines against teaching deaf children sign language, notions that are brought forward into their interactions with parents of newly identified deaf children. With the benefit of UNHS stated to be the early use of hearing technologies to improve communication, spoken language is prioritized and a medical perspective of deafness is upheld. This medicalization of deafness and the assumption that deaf children should be habilitated to hear and speak, brings into question how audiologists and SLPs can follow IHP policy and provide parents with "unbiased information" regarding the use of hearing technologies and communication modalities. The IHP's presumption that an audiologist can and will fully inform parents by presenting unbiased information about communication neglects the obvious fact that audiologists are professionally mandated to treat hearing loss through technology, not by teaching sign language.

Although audiologists may attempt to provide unbiased information with good intentions, whether these professionals, who have extensive knowledge about how to treat deafness from a medical perspective, can do so should be questioned. Rather than assuming professional neutrality is possible or necessary for parents to make a well-informed decision, I instead suggest parents should be made aware of the differing positions and tensions between Deaf culture and the medical establishment. Parents need information about hearing technologies and spoken language development, as well as information about sign language and Deaf culture, and other communication methods, from people who have the appropriate knowledge and experience, most importantly, those who live with deafness.

As SLPs and audiologists work toward habilitating deaf children to hear and speak within a normalizing medical system, it should not be expected they would (or should) provide parents with adequate information about all communication options. Recognizing how objectivity reflects normalcy and is influenced by professional and societal values explains how parents can be governed toward a particular choice amid discourse of fully informed choice. In MacKinnon's (1989) discussion on objectivity within the legal system in relation to men's point of view as the valued norm, she explains how female perspectives were not included as reasonable or objective:

It [objectivity] legitimates itself by reflecting its view of society, a society it helps make by so seeing it, and calling that view, and that relation, rationality. Since rationality is measured by point-of-viewlessness, what counts as reason is that which corresponds to the way things are. (p. 162)

In the case of the IHP's objective (or unbiased) information for parents of deaf children, objectivity reflects the norm of hearing and spoken language, while the perspectives of those who promote sign language are not considered reasonable or objective.

The objective solution of hearing technology and spoken language follows from the "objective" assumption that deafness is a problem. The IHP's assumption that their professionals provide parents with value-neutral objective information works to govern parents toward a spoken language approach. Such governing is problematic because it influences which services the IHP makes readily available to parents, how parents are told of the available services and by whom, how parents come to make decisions for their children, and how the IHP evaluates these decisions as rational or not. Understanding the medical construction of objectivity explains how the IHP can support spoken language over sign language in their communications with parents despite "IHP core principles of informed family/caregiver choice and consent" and "timely provision of unbiased information based on the best available scientific evidence" (Ministry of Children, Community and Social Services, 2019, p. 8). As audiologists and SLPs often provide information regarding communication options to parents, their professional bias toward a spoken language approach to communication suggests the IHP's principle of providing fully informed choice and consent must be problematized and reconceptualized.

The Danger of "Objectivity"

The IHP's objective presentation of options is a decidedly moral one that suits a medical/normalcy-based hearing society. My analysis has shown how rather than supporting parents in making informed choices, the IHP governs parents toward the goal of producing deaf children who will become culturally hearing, English-speaking citizens who can in turn be governed. Equating a medical perspective of deafness with an objective, unbiased presentation is dangerous in a couple of different ways. The first is that not all deaf children with hearing aids or CIs learn to listen and speak to the standards expected by hearing society (Humphries et al., 2012). The gap between deaf and hearing children in language development, reading skills, and educational achievement that the IHP is working to close through UNHS and language development services, is not made better for these children. Deaf children who do not develop speech and language as expected may be introduced to sign language later in life, but by then, years of opportunity using a visual language would have been missed.

A few parents in my study for example, after concern over their children falling behind in speech and language milestones as they grew older, and after discovering the IHP did offer sign language services, advocated for their children to access those services. However, parents described having to fight for this access because of limits to sign language services placed on children with CI, demonstrating again how informed choice and consent is narrowly defined within medical parameters. The IHP has recently placed further roadblocks in the way of families learning sign language by only providing services for spoken or signed languages and not both. This means that children with cochlear implants will only have the opportunity to receive government-funded spoken language services (Ministry of Children and Youth Services, 2018). The IHP's focus on audition and speech may result in the opposite of the desired outcome: no access to sign language may result in language and communication problems for those children who are not able to pass as hearing despite hearing technologies and speech-language therapy. A second danger in the IHP assuming the objectivity of a medical perspective is the message deaf children receive that their own unique perspective of the world is insignificant; they come to learn the only way to be accepted in a hearing society is to learn to listen and speak and pass as hearing.

Reconsidering Deafness and What It Means to "Fully Inform" Parents

My interpretive analysis has shown how the phrases "unbiased information" and "fully informed choice and consent" have complicated social meanings in relation to parents' experiences of their child's deafness. These phrases govern parents toward a particular choice, while being cloaked in legislation meant to ensure parental autonomy over the right to make decisions for their child and influenced by parents' preconceived ideas about what it means to be deaf. This finding points to the obscure meaning of "choice and consent" within medical discourse, particularly when influenced by the complexity of parents making decisions for children who stray from normative expectations of childhood (e.g., Mol, 2008; Showalter Salas, 2011). The way the IHP provides information exemplifies "a tension between the provision of information to promote informed choice and the provision of information to promote participation in a particular activity, the benefits of which may already have been accepted as health or social good" (Young et al., 2006, p. 327). Providing taken-for-granted objective information to govern parents into a specific choice fits a neoliberal system where individuals are assumed to be responsible for their own decisions, while the encompassing social forces that construct their choices remain hidden.

The IHP's narrow understanding of language and choice restricts deaf children's possibilities for learning language and coming to learn about themselves. The IHP must, at the very least, make parents aware of alternate modes of communication and their importance to deaf children, and provide the opportunity for parents to choose to communicate and learn language in ways best suited to their children, without pressure to conform to disciplinary control and normative expectations. It is therefore important that the IHP provide parents comprehensive information about communication for deaf children, and that parents have time to do further research and understand this information *before* they are referred to a CI Program. At the same time, the IHP should be aware there is no guarantee that providing comprehensive information will "fully inform" parents. On the contrary, it is unlikely parents could be fully informed about communication decisions and their potential consequences at any one point in time.

Rather than assuming parental decision making as a singular, static event, a reframing of "choice" as a fluid and flexible process and acknowledging the ongoing socio-political debate between signed and spoken language is necessary, as circumstances and child and family needs change over time. Many of the parents I interviewed, including those whose children had CIs and were following an exclusive spoken language approach, used multiple communication methods with their children. Mauldin (2012) also found that "parents of children with CIs do sometimes create their own 'gray areas' and reject the strict divide between the two approaches to deafness" (p. 229). This indicates parents intuitively foster flexible communication, even while working toward developing standard spoken language. In addition, some parents considered other modes of communication after their child did not develop spoken language as expected. One parent described frustration in discovering the numerous communication options available almost two years after diagnosis: "there are so many options out there...now I've been open to a world that it's not just spoken language or sign language... But those options aren't given until it's too late." In making parents choose between signed language and spoken language in infancy, and only providing services in line with one or the other, the IHP places harmful limits on deaf children's communication possibilities.

At an early point during the IHP's planning and implementation phase, there seemed to be an intent to include alternate knowledges:

> ...every effort should be made to provide access to parents of children who use sign language; parents of children who use oral language; parents of children who are bilingual/bicultural; deaf/hard of hearing adults who sign; deaf/hard of hearing oral adults; deaf/hard of hearing bilingual/bicultural adults; different programs or agencies that provide the various methods of communication. (Ontario Ministry of Health and Long-Term Care, 2001, p. 17)

However, unlike the heavily documented standardized screening and audiology procedures, there seem to be no procedures to ensure parents have access to deaf people who communicate in ways other than, and/or in addition to, spoken language. Many IHP documents detail screening and audiological protocols, but I found none that outline how the IHP should provide information from deaf people or parents of deaf children, and nothing prior to the 2018 guidelines that outline how to inform parents of their options. Perhaps if the

IHP were to revisit earlier documents in which the involvement of signing deaf people was intended, the IHP could establish a system for parents to meet people with different experiences of being deaf and having language. At minimum, a pamphlet providing information about deaf history, Deaf culture, sign language, and bilingual-bicultural education, developed by a deaf-run organization, should be included in an information package for parents.

At the time of screening, there is another way the IHP can include deaf knowledges and experiences as valuable sources of information for parents. Rather than presenting a deaf diagnosis as unwanted and unexpected during screening, the IHP should make parents aware of the slight possibility of deafness, which is after all, the reason for screening. It seems the IHP has changed the screening protocol to inform parents that a refer result could mean the baby does not hear. However, this information continues to be presented as deafness-as-problem. In addition to explaining how following through with further testing after a refer result could mean early identification and access to early language development services, I suggest the IHP assist parents in developing an awareness that deaf children experience the world differently than hearing people and that there may be benefits and joys experienced by knowing and embracing their deaf ways of being. Appreciating and embracing these deaf ways of knowing and being rather than trying to remove them with a sole focus on listening and speaking, would also entail that IHP allows parents to adjust communication methods whenever and however appropriate and support the development of sign language. This would entail changing the current policy that restricts services to either spoken language or sign language.

Conclusion

The IHP's normative assumptions, also reflective of assumptions held within society, govern deaf children and their parents by presenting deafness as an unthinkable, problematic outcome of screening, and spoken language services as the "right" way to handle this unexpected outcome. My analysis has shown how IHP discourse sets parents searching for normalizing solutions to the unexpected problem of hearing loss, governing them and their children through language and into (spoken) language. The IHP also presumes professionals will objectively fully inform parents about communication options. However, audiology and speech-language professionals are mandated to normalize hearing, speech and language, not inform parents about sign language and Deaf culture.

Rather than presenting deafness as an unthinkable problem and providing parents with limited communication options which restrict parent-child interactions and language development opportunities for deaf infants, I suggest that IHP develop a fluid and flexible understanding of language, deafness, and parental choice. As a medical institution in contact with most new parents in Ontario, the IHP has an opportunity to share conceptions of deafness that counter the hegemonic bio-medical and audist understanding of deafness as only a problem to be fixed. I propose that IHP change their discourse to appreciate deafness as a valued sensory experience, as opposed to a failure judged against the hearing and speaking norm. In this way, the IHP could help parents consider what deafness and language may mean to their child outside a medicalized framework.

REFERENCES

Canadian Working Group of Childhood Hearing. (2005). *Early hearing and communication development: Canadian working group of childhood hearing (CWGCH) Resource Document*. Minister of Public Works and Government Services Canada. Retrieved November 2015, from https://publications.gc.ca/collections/Collection/H124-10-2005E.pdf

CASLPA. (2006). *Position paper on cochlear implants in children*. SAC-OAC. Retrieved November 2016, from http://www.sac-oac.ca/sites/default/files/resources/Cochlear_implants_%20in_children_Oct_2006.pdf

Conrad, P. (1992). Medicalization and social control. *Annual Review of Sociology, 18*(1), 209–232. https://doi.org/10.1146/annurev.so.18.080192.001233

Davis, L. J. (1995). *Enforcing normalcy: Disability, deafness and the body*. Verso.

Edelist, T. (2019). *Constructing parental choice in deaf diagnostic and intervention practices in Ontario*. (Publication No. 13421479) [Doctoral Dissertation, University of Toronto]. ProQuest Dissertations Publishing.

Flores, N. (2014). Creating republican machines: Language governmentality in the United States. *Linguistics & Education, 25*, 1–11. https://doi.org/10.1016/j.linged.2013.11.001

Foucault, M. (1978). *The history of sexuality. Volume 1, An introduction*. Penguin.

Foucault, M. (2003). The subject and power. In P. Rabinow & N. Rose (Eds.), *The essential Foucault: Selections from essential works of Foucault, 1954–1984* (pp. 126–144). The New Press.

Government of Ontario. (2014a). *Newborn hearing screening: Parents are important partners* (Publication No. 018853) [Pamphlet]. Queen's Printer for Ontario. Retrieved February 2016, from http://www.children.gov.on.ca/htdocs/English/documents/earlychildhood/hearing/screening-parents/Screening-Parents-EN.pdf

Government of Ontario. (2014b). *Your baby needs a hearing assessment* (Publication No. 019573) [Pamphlet]. Queen's Printer for Ontario. Retrieved February 2016, from http://www.children.gov.on.ca/htdocs/English/documents/earlychildhood/hearing/assessment/Assessment-EN.pdf

Government of Ontario. (2014c). *Your baby has passed the screening but is at risk* (Publication #019609) [Pamphlet]. Queen's Printer for Ontario. Retrieved February 2016, from http://www.children.gov.on.ca/htdocs/English/documents/earlychildhood/hearing/at-risk/At-Risk-EN.pdf

Government of Ontario. (2022a). *Your baby's hearing screen* [Pamphlet]. Infant Hearing Program. Retrieved January 12, 2022, from http://www.children.gov.on.ca/htdocs/English/documents/earlychildhood/hearing/screening/HearingScreen-EN.pdf

Government of Ontario. (2022b). *Infant Hearing Program*. Queen's Printer for Ontario. Retrieved January 11, 2022, from https://www.ontario.ca/page/infant-hearing-program#results

Health Care Consent Act, Government of Ontario, S.O. 1996, c. 2, Sched. A (1996). https://www.ontario.ca/laws/statute/96h02

Hughes, B. (2015). What can a Foucauldian analysis contribute to disability theory? In S. Tremain (Ed.), *Foucault and the government of disability* (pp. 78–92). University of Michigan Press.

Humphries, T., Kushalnagar, P., Mathur, G., Napoli, D., Padden, C., Rathmann, C., & Smith, S. (2012). Language acquisition for deaf children: Reducing the harms of zero tolerance to the use of alternative approaches. *Harm Reduction Journal, 9*(16), 1–9. https://doi.org/10.1186/1477-7517-9-16

Illich, I. (1977). Disabling professions. In I. Illich, K. Zola, J. McKnight, J. Caplan, & H. Shaiken (Eds.), *Ideas in progress: Disabling professions* (pp. 11–39). Marion Boyars.

Mauldin, L. K. (2012). *Parents of deaf children with cochlear implants: Disability, medicalization and neuroculture* (Publication No. 3508706) [Doctoral dissertation, The City University of New York]. UMI Dissertation Publishing.

Ministry of Children and Youth Services. (2018). *Language development services guidelines: Ontario Infant Hearing Program* (Version 2018.02). Retrieved January 11, 2022, from https://www.uwo.ca/nca/pdfs/clinical_protocols/IHP%20Language%20Development%20Services%20Guidelines_2018.01.pdf

Ministry of Children, Community and Social Services. (2016). *Ontario Infant Hearing Program screening statistics* [Data set]. Government of Ontario. Retrieved February 2018, from https://data.ontario.ca/dataset/ontario-infant-hearing-program-ihp-screening-statisticsI

Ministry of Children, Community, and Social Services. (2019, July 15). *Protocol for universal newborn hearing screening in Ontario* (Version 2019.01). Retrieved January 11, 2022, from https://www.uwo.ca/nca/pdfs/clinical_protocols/IHP%20Screening%20Protocol%202019.01_Final_July_2019.pdf

Mol, A. (2008). *The logic of care: Health and the problem of patient choice.* Routledge.

Ontario Ministry of Health and Long-Term Care. (2001). Infant Hearing Program: Universal infant hearing screening assessment and communication development: Local implementation support document.

Ontario Ministry of Health and Long-Term Care. (2002). *Infant Hearing Program: Well-baby (DPOAE) screening protocol and training manual.* Retrieved June 2016, from www.mountsinai.on.ca/care/infant-hearing-program/documents/midwives-protocol.pdf

SAC. (2010). *SAC Position paper on universal newborn hearing screening in Canada.* Retrieved January 10, 2022, from https://www.sac-oac.ca/professional-resources/resource-library/sac-position-paper-universal-newborn-hearing-screening-2010?_ga=2.220293402.382556165.1641852772-1275366536.1641852772

SAC. (2018a). *About SAC.* Retrieved April 2018, from https://www.sac-oac.ca/about-sac/about-sac

SAC. (2018b). *SAC position paper on cochlear implants in children.* Retrieved January 11, 2022, from https://www.sac-oac.ca/sites/default/files/resources/SAC-OAC-Cochlear_Implants_PP_EN.pdf

Showalter Salas, H. (2011). Cochlear implants and deaf children. In D. Diekema, M. Mercurio, & M. Adam (Eds.), *Clinical ethics in pediatrics: A case-based textbook* (pp. 154–159). Cambridge University Press.

Sinai Health System. (2012). *Communicating with parents: Sample scripts for each pamphlet.* [Video File]. Retrieved October 2017, from https://vimeo.com/61719338

Small, A., & Cripps, J. (2012). On becoming: Developing an empowering cultural identity framework for deaf youth and adults. In A. Small, J. Cripps, & J. Côté (Eds.), *Cultural space and self/identity development among deaf youth* (pp. 29–41). Canadian Cultural Society of the Deaf.

Snoddon, K. (2009). *American sign language and early literacy: Research as praxis* (Publication No. NR61098) [Doctoral Dissertation, University of Toronto]. ProQuest Dissertations Publishing.

Sullivan, M. (2015). Subjected bodies: Paraplegia, rehabilitation, and the politics of movement. In S. Tremain (Ed.), *Foucault and the government of disability* (pp. 27–44). University of Michigan Press.

Titchkosky, T. (2007). *Reading & writing disability differently: The textured life of embodiment.* University of Toronto Press.

Young, A., Carr, G., Hunt, R., McCracken, W., Skipp, A., & Tattersall, H. (2006). Informed choice and deaf children: Underpinning concepts and enduring challenges. *Journal of Deaf Studies and Deaf Education, 11*(3), 322–336. https://doi.org/10.1093/deafed/enj041

CHAPTER 27

#ImMentallyIllAndIDontKill: A Case Study of Grassroots Health Advocacy Messages on Twitter Following the Dayton and El Paso Shootings

Sarah Smith-Frigerio

At the time of writing, in June 2022, mass shooting events in Buffalo, New York and Uvalde, Texas have garnered significant national attention and calls for gun control legislation, increased mental health services, better community policing, and means to address increases in hate and white nationalist inspired violent crime. Yet, these calls are not new. According to Mass Shooting Tracker (n.d.), there have been nearly 4700 mass shooting events in the United States since January 1, 2013. This chapter focuses on two mass shootings that occurred in the United States in August 2019, a month that experienced 49 mass shootings with 253 individuals injured and 93 individuals killed. There is no consensus between law enforcement officials, scholars, and journalists as to what constitutes a mass shooting event, but Mass Shooting Tracker (n.d.) defines a mass shooting as when four or more individuals are shot during one event.

The two mass shootings that garnered national attention in August 2019 occurred in a Wal-Mart in El Paso, Texas on August 3, 2019, and in the Oregon District of Dayton, Ohio on August 4, 2019. In addition to reporting on the timeline of events and the victims of the two shootings, media coverage

S. Smith-Frigerio (✉)
University of Tampa, Tampa, FL, USA
e-mail: ssmithfrigerio@ut.edu

© The Author(s), under exclusive license to Springer Nature Switzerland AG 2023
M. S. Jeffress et al. (eds.), *The Palgrave Handbook of Disability and Communication*, https://doi.org/10.1007/978-3-031-14447-9_27

461

described then President Trump's response to the shootings. President Trump's official statement was, initially, in support of background checks and denounced "racism, bigotry and white supremacy," (Rupar, 2019, para. 2), but quickly transitioned into proposing social media monitoring to "detect mass shooters before they strike," (Rupar, 2019, para. 3) reopening mental institutions, involuntary hospitalization of individuals with mental health diagnoses before they possibly commit a violent crime, and even the expansion of the death penalty—particularly reducing the amount of time those individuals sentenced to death have to appeal their cases through the judicial system (Rupar, 2019). This is similar to comments President Trump has made elsewhere about the alleged connection between mental health concerns and violence (Smith-Frigerio & Houston, 2018). What makes these comments so problematic is the alleged connection between mental health concerns and violent crime is not supported by research. As an aside, I use the term mental health concerns throughout this chapter to describe mental illness, as some individuals do not ascribe to the idea that they are ill, but that their physiology or brain chemistry is not "typical." This is similar to how individuals who have an autism spectrum diagnosis may not agree they are ill or disordered, but non-neurotypical.

Individuals experiencing mental health concerns only constitute 3 to 5% of all violent crimes (Appelbaum & Swanson, 2010). According to Knoll et al. (2016), less than 1% of all mass shootings can be attributed to individuals in a mental health crisis. This is well below the rate of violent crime perpetrators in the general population, which sits around 15% (Appelbaum & Swanson, 2010), and well below the incidence rate of diagnosable mental health concerns in the United States in any given year, which is approximately 20 to 25% (World Health Organization, 2017). Individuals experiencing a mental health crisis are approximately 11 times more likely to be the victim of violent crime than the perpetrator (Appelbaum & Swanson, 2010), largely due to the stigmatization of individuals with mental health concerns as dangerous criminals.

This helps explain the pushback by many Twitter users when President Trump's comments were reported. Several hashtags, including #ImMentallyIllAndIDontKill, #StopTheStigma, #EndTheStigma, #EndGunViolence, #MentalIllnessIsNotToBlame and #RacismIsNotAMentalIllness cropped up, starting on August 5, 2019. Using these hashtags, Twitter users expressed frustration for the further stigmatization of mental health concerns the President's comments could bring. Additionally, individuals (many of whom self-identified as experiencing mental health concerns) tweeted responses that sought to educate and persuade others on Twitter to not view mental health concerns as connected to mass shootings. There were also efforts to organize, through protests and support of policy change. Twitter users were, on a grassroots level, advocating against the idea that mental health concerns are directly linked to committing acts of mass violence.

This chapter, employing a case study approach, outlines the grassroots advocacy strategies and tactics that Twitter users posting with the aforementioned hashtags engaged in during the two weeks following President Trump's comments on the El Paso and Dayton shootings. I describe how individuals who tweeted sought to bring awareness through humanizing mental health concerns, how they relied on experts and research to educate their followers, how they organized—both online and offline—through protests, reaching out to their elected officials, and policy support, and how those tweeting sought to provide an inclusive environment by decentering the narrative that mental health concerns equate to violence. As will be described later in this study, the one advocacy strategy missing in the data was fundraising.

To situate these advocacy strategies, I briefly discuss the activities individuals with stigmatized health conditions engage in online, the ways individuals with mental health concerns can engage in advocacy/activism online, and how online health advocacy/activism can relate to disability advocacy/activism. Then, I discuss the importance of such research in expanding our understanding of how individuals can advocate for themselves and others online, the implications of such research, and recommend future directions for this line of academic inquiry. First, I describe the online activities of individuals with stigmatized health conditions.

Coping and Disability Advocacy Online

Scholars have explored the types of activities and the reasons why individuals with stigmatized health conditions engage with online content about their health conditions (Naslund et al., 2016; Rains, 2018; Smith-Frigerio, 2019; Thompson, 2012; White & Dorman, 2001; Zhu et al., 2017). These studies have described anonymous information seeking, developing a connected community with others who share experiences or health concerns, sensemaking, and even grassroots advocacy work. One concise description offered by Rains (2018), proposed a model of the different coping behaviors that individuals with health concerns engage in online. Rains' (2018) coping strategies model provides a starting point for understanding how individuals with health concerns interact with content and others online. That said, coping is not the best lens for exploring the tweets presented in this case study.

Twitter users who posted under these hashtags were focused on advocacy work. The interdisciplinary field of disability studies can provide some insight into grassroots advocacy and activism online; Ferguson and Nusbaum (2012) described disability studies, at its core, as "the academic side of the disability rights movement," (p. 71). Advocacy has been integral to the disability rights movement (and its successes) since its inception (Bower & Sheppard-Jones, 2020; Charlton, 1998). Yet, disability studies' contributions to health advocacy constructs can be expanded further (Petri et al., 2017, 2020), as can inclusion of mental health concerns as disability (Thomas, 2007). This study sought to contribute to our understanding of mental health advocacy/activism online in a manner that can also augment scholars' understanding of disability advocacy/activism.

464   S. SMITH-FRIGERIO

Servaes and Malikhao (2010) described how health communication professionals should craft campaigns to focus on advocacy and organizing work. The authors argue health advocacy work "be viewed in conjunction with social support and empowerment strategies," (p. 43) for communication professionals and their audiences and stakeholders. Servaes and Malikhao (2010) proposed that health advocacy work includes: awareness-raising and support of policy initiatives, addressing health inequalities and social determinants of health, as well as citizen and community engagement in participatory health communication. Their focus centered on communication professionals assisting those with lived experience and individuals working to resolve health issues. With mental health concerns, this privileges the voices and experiences of those diagnosed with a mental health concern, followed by organizations and agencies that serve the population.

Following Servaes and Malikhao's (2010) work, Smith-Frigerio (2020) found advocacy strategies are present in social media content for grassroots mental health advocacy groups with strong online presences, and 80% of audience members of such groups reported employing advocacy strategies in their posts, comments, and other content. The advocacy strategies Smith-Frigerio (2020) observed varied and were employed by both organizations and audience members. These strategies fell into the following types, awareness-raising, policy (and policy change) support, fundraising efforts, and work toward creating more inclusive audiences. Smith-Frigerio (2020) called for future work to explore if advocacy strategies around mental health are present in other types of content and with other organizations because online health advocacy work and advocacy work around mental health concerns are under explored and undertheorized. To answer this call for additional research, the following research question was posed:

RQ1: What, if any, advocacy strategies and tactics were employed using the Twitter hashtags responding to President Trump's statements linking mass shootings with mental health concerns?

METHOD

A qualitative case study was conducted to answer the research question. Case study is an excellent method for exploring events or phenomena bound either by time or location to develop a deeper understanding of events or phenomena (Small, 2009; Stake, 1995; Yin, 2013). Scholars have argued that it is possible to derive natural generalizations (Stake, 1995) and theoretical generalizations (Flyvbjerg, 2006) from a single case, provided there is abundant data to support data triangulation and theoretical transferability. This case study contributes understanding to other existing studies of health advocacy online—specifically as it relates to mental health—providing an opportunity to further theorize health advocacy strategies online.

From August 5, 2019 to August 20, 2019, tweets, replies, and retweets with comments using the hashtags #ImMentallyIllAndIDontKill (11 pages of collected tweets), #EndGunViolence along with #StopTheStigma (3 pages) and #EndTheStigma (15 pages), #MentalIllnessIsNotToBlame (195 pages), and finally #RacismIsNotAMentalIllness (246 pages) were collected. The hashtags #EndTheStigma and #StopTheStigma needed to be combined with the trending #EndGunViolence hashtag to ensure the collected tweets were relevant to the study. This is because several stigmatized health conditions now use stigma-related hashtags. Collected tweets included words and associated visuals, including photographs, infographics, and memes, resulting in 470 total pages of tweets collected for analysis. Although tweets collected for this study were publicly available and did not require IRB approval, I have chosen to not provide usernames, for the privacy of individuals disclosing what remains a highly stigmatized group of health concerns. For those who are elected officials, I redacted the username and instead inserted their title and name.

Analysis consisted of multiple readings of the collected tweets, similar to the constant comparative analysis first proposed by Glaser and Strauss (1967) and expounded upon by Fram (2013) and Charmaz (2014). After the first reading—focused on becoming familiar with the data—tweets were coded for the advocacy strategies of awareness-raising, education, inclusion, policy promotion, organizing, and fundraising. I was careful to remain open to any emergent codes, due to limited understanding of the nuances and scope of advocacy strategies that may be undertaken online surrounding mental health issues. Then, codes were collapsed further into themes, and themes were compared between hashtags, with only one difference in the advocacy strategies used found between the different hashtags, which is described in the findings. The final reading ensured themes provided rich detail for understanding the strategies employed by those tweeting with these hashtags but did not exclude important codes identified in prior readings.

Several themes emerged from the data. Themes include bringing awareness by humanizing mental health concerns, incorporating experts and research studies to educate followers, creating an inclusive area online by decentering the "mental illness equals violence" narrative, and organizing efforts and policy change support—including protest, contacting elected officials, and supporting specific policy changes—both online and offline, all of which will be described below. I will also touch upon why fundraising strategies were likely absent.

FINDINGS

The research question focused on what health advocacy strategies and tactics were used by individuals posting with hashtags associated with the backlash against President Trump's statement on the Dayton and El Paso shootings. The most prevalent strategy was raising awareness, particularly through efforts to humanize mental health concerns.

Raising Awareness by Humanizing Mental Health Concerns

Approximately 33% of tweets analyzed focused on raising awareness, and this was largely accomplished by individuals tweeting their diagnoses, their photographs, and their intention to never harm anyone. Many tweets describe providing a "personal account" or "sharing my story." These tweets were typically short, given the nature of Twitter's platform, but several tweets included threads and many tweets included photographs of those who were posting, showing smiling faces, and individuals enjoying common life moments (e.g., a cup of coffee, etc.). For instance, one tweet stated, "My name is {redacted}. I have anxiety, a panic disorder, and PTSD but have never once committed or been motivated to commit mass murder. Mental illness is not the problem," above a brightly smiling face. Another tweet stated, "Hi, I'm {redacted}. I have borderline personality disorder, major depressive disorder, and generalized anxiety disorder. Never once have I considered hurting others due to my mental illness," over the picture of a smiling young person, holding up a large cup of coffee. These tweets used humanizing tactics to show that individuals with mental health concerns were not violent and "not monsters." Including a photograph of a cheerful person appears to be very important to changing the narrative that mental health concerns equate to violence or mass shootings. As I will discuss in the conclusion, this is in line with what scholars, such as Hinshaw (2007), have said is required for reducing stigma, prejudice, and discrimination.

It is important to note the awareness strategy is the only strategy where there were differences between hashtags included in the study. In all other themes, the strategies were present across all hashtags at roughly the same rates. Most tweets using awareness strategies occurred with the hashtags #ImMentallyIllAndIDontKill and #MentalIllnessIsNotToBlame. This is likely due to attempts by two individuals to persuade others to share their stories under these hashtags. For instance, one of these included the following tweet, "I'm a victim of childhood sexual abuse. Seven years ago, I nearly died by suicide. I take prescriptions 2x/day. I live with anxiety, depression, & PTSD. I've never shot anyone. Share YOUR #mentalhealthstory. Let's get this trending." These two hashtags contained many of the tweets employing the awareness-raising strategy. They also contain other strategies. Additionally, the other hashtags contained awareness-raising tweets, just not at the same level as these two. Instead, many tweets were employing educational health advocacy strategies.

Educating with Expert Testimony and Research

Tweets employing educational strategies comprised approximately 30% of all tweets in the collected data. While, in many ways, educational strategies could also be considered raising awareness, there was a distinct difference between the personal narratives and disclosures of individuals tweeting under the hashtags, and those using experts and research studies to provide context to the issue of mental health and the potential for violence. After comparing both, I thought it prudent to present each as its own strategy and not two different tactics within the same strategy, given the distinct differences in aims and presentation.

While raising awareness sought to put a human face on mental health concerns to disrupt stigmatizing narratives, educating sought to bring evidence to light that would disrupt the connection between mental health concerns and mass shootings. This included quoting studies, linking to the studies themselves, or both. One tweet included a synopsis and then linked to a *Science Daily* article, "Counter to a lot of public opinion, having a mental illness does not necessarily make a person more likely to commit gun violence. According to a new study, a better indicator of gun violence was access to firearms." Another linked to a study published in the *Journal of Preventative Medicine*, "Our problem is more so: anger and access to guns. The study found that ONLY hostility was able to predict threatening others with a gun, and there was NO connection with mental health symptoms." In addition to media coverage of recent studies and direct links to medical and research journals, individuals tweeting under these hashtags included official statements from organizations such as the National Alliance for Mental Illness, the American Psychological Association, the National Association of School Psychologists, and others. All of these organizations reiterated that a predisposition to anger and prior violence, access to firearms, substance abuse, and even radicalization online were stronger indicators of the potential to commit a mass shooting than mental health concerns.

Beyond quoting or linking to research studies and official statements, educating strategies included bringing experts into the conversation. For the most part, these experts were doctors, researchers, and media professionals. One such example came from a medical doctor, who was copied on a thread with another individual tweeting with the hashtags, who then responded by stating, "Blaming mental illness does not paint a clear picture of what's going on... it's a scapegoat and is dangerous because it further stigmatizes a population that doesn't need further stigmatization." Another tweet came from a practicing psychologist, and they stated, "In my twenty years as a psychologist, at times working with young people with the most severe mental illnesses, none of them have ever shot anyone. Never." Oftentimes, the doctors, researchers, and experts who involved themselves in the conversation would link to their work, whether it was medical journals, academic journals, or news stories. This is important for several reasons; the first is to demonstrate mental health concerns are not predictive of or inextricably linked to mass shootings. The second reason is that expert "testimony" would be important to combat President Trump's official statement. As President of the United States, not only did Trump possess a significant amount of sway over his supporters, but any statement of his would command attention, both in traditional media and social media platforms. His stance on the connection between mental health concerns and mass shootings quickly spread; multiple experts speaking out online and offline would be needed to effectively contradict the inaccurate connection between mental health concerns and mass shootings.

As will be seen in the next theme, stigmatizing comments such as the President's statement are often linked to discriminatory behaviors (i.e., monitoring social media and phones, involuntary hospitalization, etc.). Destigmatizing mental health concerns and appealing to other active Twitter groups became important tactics within the promoting inclusivity advocacy strategy.

Inclusivity Through Decentering the Mental Health Concerns Equals Violence Narrative

Servaes and Malikhao (2010) described how health advocacy should focus on the empowerment of those within a health community, and they, in part, envisioned this as actively working to address health disparities and the social determinants of health. Together, these items can be described as health equity or health inclusivity. There is an argument to be made for the term health inclusivity over health equity. Health inclusivity allows for the recognition that expression or treatment of some health conditions cannot be made "equal," as their presentation, prevalence, or treatment will differ between gender groups, racial and ethnic groups, etc. There are several ways to address health inclusivity, but within this theme, there were two notable tactics, by decentering mental health concerns as responsible for mass shootings and centering firearms, racism and domestic violence, and by involving members of the disability community on Twitter, who then jumped into the conversation using the hashtags.

Inclusivity advocacy strategies composed approximately 7% of tweets using these hashtags, but the example tweets of such work were striking. Examples of destigmatizing mental health concerns and decentering them as the cause of mass shootings often looked like the following tweet, "Blaming gun violence on mental illness is only adding to the hundreds of years of fearing and stigmatizing mental illness. It's an oversimplified answer to a complex question." This directly addressed the fact that mental health concerns are highly stigmatized, and that tropes of dangerousness and violence have been around for a significant period (Klin & Lemish, 2008; Wahl, 1992). Additional tweets included, "Mental illness is not a prerequisite for hatred, violence, or white nationalism. Let's please stop affiliating these things." One might expect to see such tweets under the #RacismIsNotAMentalIllness hashtag, but in fact, tweets including racism, domestic violence, and access to firearms as precursors to mass violence were present across all hashtags.

The other tactic used by individuals posting with these hashtags was to appeal to and include the disability community on Twitter. This growing group of disability activists and supporters have been in the news in recent years for their trending hashtags, such as #ThingsDisabledPeopleKnow, #DisabledCompliments, #AbledsAreWeird, and #CripTheVote. The

#CripTheVote hashtag was prominent in tweets employing the organizing and supporting policy change advocacy strategy, which will be described in the next theme. Tweets focused on inclusion posted by disability advocates called for the voices of those individuals experiencing a mental health concern to be heard, such as in this tweet by a disability activist, "Please read the work by disabled people on why this rhetoric & conflation is harmful to the disability community {username redacted} & everyone else giving their hot takes on the #ElPasoShooting." Another tweet stated, "Please read this amazing piece by {redacted} and {redacted} to learn more about the criminalization and surveillance of people with mental health disabilities."

Decentering the narrative about mental health concerns and mass shootings, and instead centering other predictors, including racism, was a powerful step. Privileging and promoting the voices of those who have experienced a mental health concern, as the disability community on Twitter did, was also an important and powerful step. The next theme discusses how individuals tweeting with these hashtags called for more direct action, including offline action.

Organizing and Policy Change Support, Online and Offline

The organizing and policy change support health advocacy strategy comprised 30% of the tweets using the studied hashtags. In particular, tweets using this strategy focused on speaking directly to elected officials online, calls to contact elected officials by other means, calls to vote for elected officials that would support policy changes, directly discussing support of policy changes (e.g., gun control measures for domestic assault offenses), and organizing protests. Many of the tweets describing policy change included the #CripTheVote hashtag, as mentioned previously, and examples include:

> Mentally ill people are far more likely to be victims - not perpetrators - of gun violence. #StopTheStigma Removing guns from hateful people saves lives. Tell {then Senate Majority Leader Mitchell McConnell} #GiveUsAVote on bipartisan gun background checks bills #HR8 and #HR1112 that the House already passed!

Other tweets discussed the possibility items President Trump mentioned in his official statement, such as social media monitoring and involuntary hospitalization, might contradict existing health laws such as HIPPA and human rights laws, "This has huge consequences for the disability community & is a major civil liberties/human rights issue." Also, some tweets were directed to elected officials, even Democrats, such as this tweet which was not in support of mental health tracking databases:

> NO. This Democrat strongly rejects mental health databases. It is wacky ideas like this that further stigmatize access to mental health services. {New York Governor Andrew Cuomo} you are terrifying my community and owe us an explanation for your harmful and dangerous words.

Finally, it is important to mention the offline peaceful protest that was initiated by one individual on Twitter using these hashtags. Other individuals jumped in to organize the protest in Union Square in New York City, and then to record their participation in the protest on Twitter using these hashtags. For example, one individual posted pictures of themselves with a sign they made, which stated, "I have schizophrenia and I am NOT a MONSTER! Stop blaming mental health for a gun problem." Other individuals created and posted signs and t-shirts that had the slogan, "I'm mentally ill, and I don't kill" on them. It is unclear from Twitter posts how many attended this protest. Regardless, this organizing of an offline event on a social media platform supports scholarship that found social media use was important to organizers involved with the Arab Spring in Egypt (Lim, 2012; Tufekci & Wilson, 2012). While liking a tweet or posting with a trending hashtag is not as overt an action as contacting one's elected officials or participating in a peaceful protest, there is evidence that individuals posting on Twitter were doing more than what is typically termed "slacktivism."

The Lack of Fundraising Appeals

The data collected for this study presented a lack of fundraising appeals. Only two tweets possessed a fundraising appeal, and both were for someone's treatment/care, and not for larger advocacy work in the area of mental health concerns or disassociating mental health concerns from mass shootings. This was an unexpected result of the analysis, as other scholarship in health advocacy strategies, such as Smith-Frigerio's (2020) work, found that fundraising appeals were a small but important strategy employed by mental health advocacy organizations. While this was a grassroots movement involving individuals posting with particular hashtags, and not mental health organizations or agencies, the ability for individuals to fundraise through avenues such as GoFundMe and Kickstarter should not be dismissed. This has occurred around many other causes or issues on social media platforms. Perhaps individuals tweeting with these hashtags were unaware of other fundraising activities, such as the National Alliance for Mental Illness and their existing campaigns. Perhaps individuals considered the most pressing advocacy strategies were raising awareness and educating. It is important to understand why fundraising may be absent here, but the presented rationale is speculation at this point, and additional scholarship in this area should explore further when and why fundraising may be employed as an advocacy strategy in online contexts.

Nevertheless, the themes identified in this study present an interesting case, with varied strategies and nuanced tactics being employed on Twitter. The conclusions that can be drawn from this research are presented below.

Discussion

Individuals tweeting under these hashtags following President Trump's call to monitor and involuntarily hospitalize individuals with mental health concerns employed several health advocacy strategies. Raising awareness became an opportunity to humanize mental health concerns with personal diagnosis disclosures, photographs of everyday individuals enjoying their lives, and proclamations that they had never even considered harming other individuals. Education relied heavily on bringing expert voices into the discussion, and reliance on research disproving the connection between mental health concerns and violence. Efforts toward inclusion involved decentering the mental health concerns equates to mass shootings narrative and involved disability advocates on Twitter. Organizing and support for policy changes started online but moved into offline endeavors, such as the peaceful protest in New York City.

Additionally, the larger disability community on Twitter showed up in support of their use of the hashtags as well. Finally, there were no fundraising endeavors in the tweets collected in this study, and the lack of this health advocacy strategy may be explained by the perceived need for the present strategies. The tweets were not from mental health communication professionals working for specific organizations or agencies. The focus was on awareness, education, organizing, promoting policy change, and inclusivity. Furthermore, these strategies may have had an impact in 2022, when mass shootings again garnered significant national attention and calls for drastic change. The tone shifted among news media and policymakers. While there were calls for increased community mental health services from some lawmakers, the calls for universal background checks, red-flag laws, raising the age limit to purchase a modern sporting or assault rifle, and other approaches dominated the conversation. The immediate desire to blame individuals with mental health concerns for acts of mass violence appeared to lessen.

This study provides theoretical contributions, particularly at a time when health and disability advocacy/activism may be undertheorized (Zoller, 2005; Zoller & Kline, 2008). As Servaes and Malikhao (2010) described in their work, there is a lack of advocacy theorizing in health communication. Petri et al. (2017, 2020) also describe a need for more work in disability advocacy. Scholars should incorporate what we know of advocacy from multiple subdisciplines, expand upon it, and tailor it to the specific nature and requirements of different groups. This study contributes to this by building upon Servaes and Malikhao's (2010) and Smith-Frigerio's (2020) work, which involved mental health advocacy groups. Extending our understanding of health and disability advocacy strategies surrounding mental health lends credence to the types of strategies we should expect to see. Exploring tactics used within these strategies provides us with a nuanced understanding of what resonated with individuals posting with these hashtags, and what they believe resonated with their followers.

Health advocacy deserves a fuller explication so professionals can develop best practices around their goals. The themes identified here provide mental health communication professionals and grassroots advocates/activists with practical implications that can be employed in their mental health messaging campaigns. As scholars such as Hinshaw (2007) and Corrigan et al. (2003) have pointed out, there is a significant need for awareness-raising and educational endeavors when it comes to communicating about mental health concerns. Hinshaw (2007) advocated for the use of narratives of everyday persons who have experienced a mental health concern in destigmatization efforts involving other media channels. Corrigan et al. (2003) argue that it is not enough to simply remove stigmatizing content (i.e., for politicians to stop using the mental health concerns equates to mass shootings narrative), but that for stigmatization to stop, negative content must be removed and replaced with affirming content. Given that awareness-raising and educational strategies were prominent strategies found here, and the tactics used to achieve these strategies were very specific to those posting with the hashtags in this study, mental health communication professionals can take note and incorporate similar tactics into their health messaging campaigns.

There are limitations to this study. For instance, while approximately 470 pages of tweets containing the relevant hashtags were collected for analysis, there is ambiguity surrounding whether Twitter's API captures all tweets using those hashtags in the timeframe requested, regardless of the approach or software program used to interface with Twitter. For example, I had to "weed out" promoted and sponsored tweets that were embedded in the collected tweets, as well as repeated tweets posted under more than one hashtag. Another limitation to this study is that the analysis was conducted by a sole researcher. To overcome this limitation, theoretical triangulation, data triangulation (through the use of multiple hashtags), and thick description of the themes presented in the analysis were undertaken. Future research in this same vein by scholars can lend credence to or further refine the theoretical generalizations presented in this chapter.

There are several exciting avenues for future research. Servaes and Malikhao's (2010) call for specific health advocacy strategies should continue to be explored in other platforms and among other health communities. Audience reactions to such strategies need to be explored and compared to the intentions of content creators. With a better understanding of the possible health advocacy strategies and tactics used—particularly for highly stigmatized conditions—a model can be proposed, and the success of such health and disability advocacy strategies could be measured and further refined. Finally, tracking the strategies used and how narratives surrounding mental health concerns and acts of mass violence may have changed is certainly warranted. In sum, this study is one piece in a larger effort to both understand health and disability advocacy strategies and work toward destigmatizing mental health concerns in the hopes that more individuals will seek treatment and live successful and fulfilling lives.

REFERENCES

Appelbaum, P. S., & Swanson, J. W. (2010). Law & psychiatry: Gun laws and mental illness: How sensible are the current restrictions? *Psychiatric Services, 61*(7), 652–654. https://doi.org/10.1176/ps.2010.61.7.652

Bower, W., & Sheppard-Jones, K. (2020). Advocacy: History of the Disability Rights Movement in the United States. In D. A. Harley & C. Flaherty (Eds.), *Disability studies for human services: An interdisciplinary and intersectionality approach* (pp. 75–90). Springer.

Charlton, J. (1998). *Nothing about us without us: Disability oppression and empowerment.* University of California Press.

Charmaz, K. (2014). *Constructing grounded theory.* Sage.

Corrigan, P., Markowitz, F. E., Watson, A., Rowan, D., & Kubiak, M. A. (2003). An attribution model of public discrimination towards persons with mental illness. *Journal of Health and Social Behavior, 44*(2), 162–179. https://doi.org/10.2307/1519806

Ferguson, P. M., & Nusbaum, E. (2012). Disability studies: What is it and what difference does it make? *Research and Practice for Persons with Severe Disabilities, 37*(2), 70–80. https://doi.org/10.1177/154079691203700202

Flyvbjerg, B. (2006). Five misunderstandings about case-study research. *Qualitative Inquiry, 12*(2), 219–245. https://doi.org/10.1177/2F1077800405284363

Fram, S. M. (2013). The constant comparative analysis method outside of grounded theory. *The Qualitative Report, 18*(1), 1–25. http://www.nova.edu/ssss/QR/QR18/fram1.pdf

Hinshaw, S. P. (2007). *The mark of shame: Stigma of mental illness and an agenda for change.* Oxford University Press.

Klin, A., & Lemish, D. (2008). Mental disorders stigma in the media: Review of studies on production, content, and influences. *Journal of Health Communication, 13*(5), 434–449. https://doi.org/10.1080/10810730802198813

Knoll, I. V., James, L., & Annas, G. D. (2016). Mass shootings and mental illness. In L. H. Gold & R. I. Simon (Eds.), *Gun violence and mental illness* (pp. 81–104). American Psychiatric Association Publishing.

Lim, M. (2012). Clicks, cabs, and coffee houses: Social media and oppositional movements in Egypt, 2004–2011. *Journal of Communication, 62*(2), 231–248. https://doi.org/10.1111/j.1460-2466.2012.01628.x

Naslund, J. A., Aschbrenner, K. A., Marsch, L. A., & Bartels, S. J. (2016). The future of mental health care: Peer-to-peer support and social media. *Epidemiology and Psychiatric Sciences, 25*(2), 113–122. https://doi.org/10.1017/S2045796015001067

Petri, G., Beadle-Brown, J., & Bradshaw, J. (2017). "More Honoured in the Breach than in the Observance"—Self-advocacy and human rights. *Laws, 6*(4), 26. https://doi.org/10.3390/laws6040026

Petri, G., Beadle-Brown, J., & Bradshaw, J. (2020). Redefining self-advocacy: A practice theory-based approach. *Journal of Policy and Practice in Intellectual Disabilities, 17*(3), 207–218. https://doi.org/10.1111/jppi.12343

Rains, S. A. (2018). *Coping with illness digitally.* MIT Press.

Rupar, A. (2019, August 5). "Mental illness and hatred pulls (*sic.*) the trigger": Trump's speech about shootings ignored the real problem. *Vox.* http://www.vox.com/2019/8/5/20754770/trump-el-paso-dayton-speech-white-house-mental-illness-video-games-guns

Servaes, J., & Malikhao, P. (2010). Advocacy strategies for health communication. *Public Relations Review, 36*(1), 42–49. https://doi.org/10.1016/j.pubrev.2009.08.017

Small, M. L. (2009). 'How many cases do I need?' On science and the logic of case selection in field-based research. *Ethnography, 10*(1), 5–38. https://doi.org/10.1177/2F1466138108099586

Smith-Frigerio, S. (2019). Coping, community and fighting stereotypes: An exploration of multidimensional social capital in personal blogs discussing mental illness. *Health Communication, 35*(4), 410–418. https://doi.org/10.1080/10410236.2018.1564959

Smith-Frigerio, S. (2020). Grassroots mental health groups' use of advocacy strategies in social media messaging. *Qualitative Health Research, 30*(14), 2205–2216. https://doi.org/10.1177/1049732320951532

Smith-Frigerio, S., & Houston, J. B. (2018). Crazy, insane, nut job, wacko, basket case, and psycho: Donald Trump's tweets surrounding mental health issues and attacks on media personalities. In M. Lockhart (Ed.), *President Donald Trump and his political discourse* (pp. 114–130). Routledge.

Stake, R. E. (1995). *The art of case study research.* Sage.

Thomas, C. (2007). *Sociologies of disability and illness: Contested ideas in disability studies and medical sociology.* Macmillan International Higher Education.

Thompson, R. (2012). Screwed up, but working on it: (Dis)ordering the self through E-stories. *Narrative Inquiry, 22*(1), 86–104. https://doi.org/10.1075/ni.22.1.06tho

Tufekci, Z., & Wilson, C. (2012). Social media and the decision to participate in political protest: Observations from Tahrir Square. *Journal of Communication, 62*(2), 363–379. https://doi.org/10.1111/j.1460-2466.2012.01629.x

Wahl, O. F. (1992). Mass media images of mental illness: A review of the literature. *Journal of Community Psychology, 20*(4), 343–352. https://doi.org/10.1002/1520-6629(199210)20:4%3C343::AID-JCOP2290200408%3E3.0.CO;2-2

White, M., & Dorman, S. M. (2001). Receiving social support online: Implications for health education. *Health Education Research, 16*(6), 693–707. https://doi.org/10.1093/her/16.6.693

World Health Organization. (2017). 'Depression: let's talk' says WHO, as depression tops list of causes of ill health. http://www.who.int/en/news-room/detail/30-03-2017%2D%2Ddepression-let-s-talk-says-who-as-depression-tops-list-of-causes-of-ill-health

Yin, R. K. (2013). *Case study research: Design and methods* (5th ed.). Sage.

Zhu, X., Smith, R. A., & Parrott, R. L. (2017). Living with a rare health condition: The influence of a support community and public stigma on communication, stress, and available support. *Journal of Applied Communication Research, 45*(2), 179–198. https://doi.org/10.1080/00909882.2017.1288292

Zoller, H. M. (2005). Health activism: Communication theory and action for social change. *Communication Theory, 15*(4), 341–364. https://doi.org/10.1111/j.1468-2885.2005.tb00339.x

Zoller, H. M., & Kline, K. N. (2008). Theoretical contributions of interpretive and critical research in health communication. *Annals of the International Communication Association, 32*(1), 89–135. https://doi.org/10.1080/23808985.2008.11679076

References

"Disabled." (n.d.). Oxford Dictionary. Retrieved October 16, 2019, from https://www.lexico.com/en/definition/disabled

"Fit." (n.d.). Merriam Webster Dictionary. Retrieved May 20, 2020, from https://www.merriam-webster.com/dictionary/fit

5 years after Fukushima meltdowns, off-limits zone in Iitate languishes. (2016, March 9). *The Mainichi*. Retrieved November 30, 2019, from https://mainichi.jp/english/articles/20160309/p2a/00m/ 0na/021000c

Abbott, D., & Porter, S. (2013). Environmental hazard and disabled people: From vulnerable to expert to interconnected. *Disability & Society, 28*(6), 839–852. https://doi.org/10.1080/09687599.2013.802222

Abidin, C. (2020). Mapping internet celebrity on TikTok: Exploring attention economies and visibility labours. *Cultural Science Journal, 12*(1), 77–103. https://doi.org/10.5334/csci.140

Abrams, A. (2020, June 25). Black, disabled people at higher risk in police encounters. *Time*. Retrieved October 31, 2021, from https://time.com/5857438/police-violence-black-disabled/

ADA National Network. (2020, January). *I heard that miniature horses are considered to be service animals by the ADA. Is this true?* Retrieved January 11, 2022, from https://adata.org/faq/i-heard-miniature-horses-are-considered-be-service-animals-ada-true

ADA National Network. (2021, December 30). *What is the definition of disability under the ADA?* ADATA. https://adata.org/faq/what-definition-disability-under-ada

Adams, T. E., Jones, S. H., & Ellis, C. (2015). *Autoethnography.* Oxford University Press.

Adaptive Computing Technology Center. (2021). *What is adaptive technology?* Retrieved May 14, 2021, from https://actcenter.missouri.edu/about-the-act-center/what-is-adaptive-technology/

Afifi, T. D., Caughlin, J. P., & Afifi, W. A. (2007). The dark side (and light side) of avoidance and secrets. In B. H. Spitzberg & W. R. Cupach (Eds.), *The dark side of interpersonal communication* (2nd ed., pp. 61–92). Lawrence Erlbaum Associates. https://doi.org/10.4324/9780203936849

© The Author(s), under exclusive license to Springer Nature Switzerland AG 2023
M. S. Jeffress et al. (eds.), *The Palgrave Handbook of Disability and Communication*, https://doi.org/10.1007/978-3-031-14447-9

476 REFERENCES

Agboka, G. Y. (2013). Participatory localization: A social justice approach to navigating unenfranchised/disenfranchised cultural sites. *Technical Communication Quarterly, 22*(1), 28–49. https://doi.org/10.1080/10572252.2013.730966

Agne, R. R., Thompson, T. L., & Cusella, L. P. (2000). Stigma in the line of face: Self-disclosure of patients' HIV status to health care providers. *Journal of Applied Communication Research, 28*(3), 235–261. https://doi.org/10.1080/00909880009365573

Aguado-Delgado, J., Gutierrez-Martinez, J. M., Hilera, J. R., de Marcos, L., & Otón, S. (2020). Accessibility in video games: A systematic review. *Universal Access in the Information Society, 19*(1), 169–193. https://doi.org/10.1007/s10209-018-0628-2

Alang, S., McAlpine, D., McCreedy, E., & Hardeman, R. (2017). Police brutality and Black health: Setting the agenda for public health scholars. *American Journal of Public Health, 107*(5), 662–665. https://doi.org/10.2105/ajph.2017.303691

Albers, M. J., & Mazur, M. B. (Eds.). (2014). *Content and complexity: Information design in technical communication.* Routledge.

Albert, A. B., Jacobs, H. E., & Siperstein, G. N. (2016). Sticks, stones, and stigma: Student bystander behavior in response to hearing the word "retard." *Intellectual and Developmental Disabilities, 54*(6), 391–401. https://doi.org/10.1352/1934-9556-54.6.391

Alexander, D., Gaillard, J. C., & Wisner, B. (2012). Disability and disaster. In B. Wisner, J. C. Gaillard, & I. Kelman (Eds.), *The Routledge handbook of hazards and disaster risk reduction* (pp. 413–423). Routledge. https://doi.org/10.4324/9780203844236.ch34

Allen, B. J. (2011). *Difference matters: Communicating social identity* (2nd ed.). Waveland Press.

Alonso, F., Fuertes, J. L., González, Á. L., & Martínez, L. (2010). On the testability of WCAG 2.0 for beginners. *Proceedings of the 2010 International Cross Disciplinary Conference on Web Accessibility (W4A), 9.* https://doi.org/10.1145/1805986.1806000

Alper, M. (2015). Augmentative, alternative, and assistive: Reimagining the history of mobile computing and disability. *IEEE Annals of the History of Computing, 37*(1), 96. https://doi.org/10.1109/MAHC.2015.3

Alper, M. (2017). *Giving voice: Mobile communication, disability, and inequality.* MIT Press.

Alper, M. (2019). Future talk: Accounting for the technological and other future discourses in daily life. *International Journal of Communication, 13,* 715–735. https://ijoc.org/index.php/ijoc/article/view/9678

Alpert, G., & Dunham, R. (2009). *Understanding police use of force.* Cambridge University Press.

Alvesson, M., Ashcraft, K. L., & Thomas, R. (2008). Identity matters: Reflections on the construction of identity scholarship in organization studies. *Organization, 15*(1), 5–28. https://doi.org/10.1177/1350508407084426

Amado, A. N. (2008). *Innovative models and best practices in case management and support coordination.* Institute on Community Integration, University of Minnesota.

Amanda, B., & Shevyrolet. (2012, June 13). *Danth's law.* Know Your Meme. Retrieved April 4, 2021, from https://knowyourmeme.com/memes/danths-law

American Bar Association. (2017). *Introduction: Disability rights under siege.* Retrieved March 1, 2020, from https://www.americanbar.org/publications/crsj-human-rights-magazine/vol%2D%2D42/vol-42-   no-4/introduction%2D%2Ddisability-rights-under-siege.html

American Psychiatric Association. (2013). *Diagnostic and statistical manual of mental disorders* (5th ed.). American Psychiatric Association.

American Speech-Language-Hearing Association. (2008). *Roles and responsibilities of speech-language pathologists in early intervention: Position statement.* Retrieved March 1, 2020, from https://www.asha.org/policy/PS2008-00291/

Americans with Disabilities Act information for law enforcement. (2020, December 1). *Americans with Disabilities Act: Information for Law Enforcement.* https://www.ada.gov/lawenfcomm.htm

And I can count to potato. (n.d.). Meme Maker. Retrieved May 30, 2021, from https://www.mememaker.net/meme/and-i-can-count-to-potato/

Anderson, M. (2019, April 13). How one mother's battle is changing police training on disabilities. *NPR.* Retrieved November 2, 2021, from https://www.npr.org/2019/04/13/705887493/how-one-mothers-battle-is-changing-police-training-on-disabilities

Angel, J. (2020, August 5). A warning about fake face mask exemption cards. *New England ADA Center Blog.* https://www.newenglandada.org/blog/warning-about-fake-face-mask-exemption-cards

Annamma, S. A., Connor, D., & Ferri, B. (2013). Dis/ability critical race studies (DisCrit): Theorizing at the intersections of race and dis/ability. *Race Ethnicity and Ethnicity, 16*(1), 1–31. https://doi.org/10.1080/13613324.2012.730511

Annenberg School for Communication. (2020). *Theory.* Retrieved December 2021, from https://www.metamorph.org/research/theory/

Anonymax. (2012, April 13). *Heidi Crowter ("I can count to potato" girl)—Midlands Today 12/04/12 (Internet Trollers).* Retrieved April 4, 2021, from https://www.youtube.com/watch?v=BYowYqNOjUQ

Antonelli. (2012, November 29). *Video games: 14 in the collection, for starters.* Retrieved May 18, 2021, from https://www.moma.org/explore/inside_out/2012/11/29/video-games-14-in-the-collection-for-starters/

Appelbaum, P. S., & Swanson, J. W. (2010). Law & psychiatry: Gun laws and mental illness: How sensible are the current restrictions? *Psychiatric Services, 61*(7), 652–654. https://doi.org/10.1176/ps.2010.61.7.652

Arendt, H. (1958). *The human condition.* University of Chicago Press.

Aristotle. (1942). *Generation of animals* (A. L. Peck, Trans.). Harvard University Press. (Original work published ca. 4th century B.C.E).

Arkrow, P. (2021). *Animal-assisted therapy and activities: A study, resource guide and bibliography for the use of companion animals in selected therapies* (12th ed.). Animal Assisted Therapy.

Arseniev-Koehler, A., Foster, J. G., Mays, V. M., Chang, K.-W., & Cochran, S. D. (2021). Aggression, escalation, and other latent themes in legal intervention deaths of Non-Hispanic Black and white men: Results from the 2003–2017 National Violent Death Reporting System. *American Journal of Public Health, 111*(S2), S107–S115. https://doi.org/10.2105/ajph.2021.306312

Asasumasu, K. A. (2017a). Things about working with "emotionally disturbed" children that will break your heart. In L. X. Z. Brown, E. Ashkenazy, & M. Giwa Onaiwu (Eds.), *All the weight of our dreams: On living racialized autism* (pp. 76–84). DragonBee Press.

Asasumasu, K. A. (2017b). Plea from the scariest kid on the block. In L. X. Z. Brown, E. Ashkenazy, & M. Giwa Onaiwu (Eds.), *All the weight of our dreams: On living racialized autism* (pp. 106–111). DragonBee Press.

478 REFERENCES

Ashcraft, K. L. (2017). "Submission" to the rule of excellence: Ordinary affect and precarious resistance in the labor of organization and management studies. *Organization, 24*(1), 36–58. https://doi.org/10.1177/1350508416668188

Ashcraft, K. L. (2020). Communication as constitutive transmission? An encounter with affect. *Communication Theory, 31*(4), 571-592. https://doi.org/10.1093/ct/qtz027

Ashinoff, B. K., & Abu-Akel, A. (2021). Hyperfocus: The forgotten frontier of attention. *Psychological Research, 85*(1), 1–19. https://doi.org/10.1007/s00426-019-01245-8

Assistance Dogs International. (2019, August 30). *Member program statistics*. Retrieved January 11, 2022, from https://assistancedogsinternational.org/members/member-program-statistics/

Baggs, A. (2007, January 14). *In my language* [Video]. YouTube. https://www.youtube.com/watch?v=JnylM1hI2jc&list=PL70BB95AC2A07D6B2&index=3&t=0s

Baggs, M. (2020). Losing. In S. K. Kapp (Ed.), *Autistic community and the neurodiversity movement: Stories from the frontline* (pp. 77–86). Palgrave Macmillan. https://doi.org/10.1007/978-981-13-8437-0

Bailey, B., & Arciuli, J. (2020). Indigenous Australians with autism: A scoping review. *Autism, 24*(5), 1031–1046. https://doi.org/10.1177/1362361319894829

Bain, A. (2016). Positive policing: Communication and the public. In A. Bain (Ed.), *Law enforcement and technology* (pp. 47–61). Palgrave. https://doi.org/10.1057/978-1-137-57915-7_4

Baker, C. (2005, August 31). Caption writers push for training. *The Washington Times*, p. C10. Retrieved December 5, 2019, from https://infoweb-newsbank-com.proxy.library.nyu.edu/apps/news/document-view?p=WORLDNEWS&docref=news/10C579939EAF54D8

Baker, S. A., & Michael, J. M. (2018). 'Good morning Fitfam': Top posts, hashtags and gender display on Instagram. *New Media & Society, 20*(12), 4553–4570. https://doi.org/10.1177/1461444818777514

Baker, S., Gallois, C., Driedger, S. M., & Santesso, N. (2011). Communication accommodation and managing musculoskeletal disorders: Doctors' and patients' perspectives. *Health Communication, 26*(4), 379–388. https://doi.org/10.1080/10410236.2010.551583

Baker-Sperry, L., & Grauerholz, L. (2003). The pervasiveness and persistence of the feminine beauty ideal in children's fairy tales. *Gender & Society, 17*(5), 711–726. https://doi.org/10.1177/0891243203255605

Baliey, M., & Mobley, I. A. (2019). Work in the intersections: A black feminist disability framework. *Gender & Society, 33*(1), 19–40. https://doi.org/10.1177/0891243218801523

Ballard, R. L., Ballard, S. J., & Chue, L. E. (2022). Invisible marginalizations of service-dog handlers: The tensions of legal inclusion and social exclusion. In M. S. Jeffress, J. M. Cypher, J. Ferris, & J.-A. Scott (Eds.), *The Palgrave handbook of disability and communication*. Palgrave.

Ballard, R. L., Ballard, S. J., & Chue, L. E. (2023). Invisible marginalizations of service-dog handlers: The tensions of legal inclusion and social exclusion. In M. S. Jeffress, J. M. Cypher, J. Ferris, & J.-A. Scott (Eds.), *The Palgrave handbook of disability and communication*. Palgrave.

Ball-Rokeach, S. J., Kim, Y. C., & Matei, S. (2001). Storytelling neighborhood: Paths to belonging in diverse urban environments. *Communication Research, 28*(4), 392–428. https://doi.org/10.1177/009365001028004003

REFERENCES 479

Banet-Weiser, S. (2012). *Authentic™: The politics of ambivalence in a brand culture.* New York University Press.

Barker, C. (2002). *Making sense of cultural studies: Central problems and critical debates.* Sage. https://doi.org/10.4135/9781446220368

Barton, B. F., & Barton, M. S. (1993). Ideology and the map: Toward a postmodern visual design practice. In N. Roundy Blyler & C. Thralls (Eds.), *Professional communication: The social perspective* (pp. 49–78). Sage.

Barzilai-Nahon, K. (2009). Gatekeeping: A critical review. *Annual Review of Information Science and Technology, 43*(1), 1–79. https://doi.org/10.1002/aris.2009.1440430117

Basas, C. G. (2015). Advocacy fatigue: Self-care, protest, and educational equity. *Windsor Yearbook of Access to Justice, 32*(2), 37–64. https://doi.org/10.22329/wyaj.v32i2.4681

Bascom, J. (2011, November 23). On "quiet hands." *Just Stimming.* http://www.thinkingautismguide.com/2011/11/on-quiet-hands.html

Battle, D. E. (2015). Persons with communication disabilities in natural disasters, war, and/or conflicts. *Communication Disorders Quarterly, 36*(4), 231–240. https://doi.org/10.1177/2F1525740114545980

Baudrillard, J. (1994). *Simulacra and simulation* (S. F. Glaser, Trans.). University of Michigan Press.

Baumann, S. (2008). The moral underpinnings of beauty: A meaning-based explanation for light and dark complexions in advertising. *Poetics, 36*(1), 2–23. https://doi.org/10.1016/j.poetic.2007.11.002

Baumann, S., & de Laat, K. (2012). Socially defunct: A comparative analysis of the underrepresentation of older women in advertising. *Poetics, 40*(6), 514–541. https://doi.org/10.1016/j.poetic.2012.08.002

Baumbusch, J., Mayer, S., & Sloan-Yip, I. (2018). Alone in a crowd? Parents of children with rare diseases' experiences of navigating the healthcare system. *Journal of Genetic Counseling, 28*(2), 1–12. https://doi.org/10.1007/s10897-018-0294-9

Baxter, L. A., & Montgomery, B. M. (1996). *Relating: Dialogues and dialectics.*

Baxter, L. A. (2011). *Voicing relationships: A dialogic approach.* Sage.

Bayer, N. L., & Pappas, L. (2006). Accessibility testing: Case history of blind testers of enterprise software. *Technical Communication, 53*(1), 32–38. https://www.ingentaconnect.com/content/stc/tc/2006/00000053/00000001/art00005

BBC News. (2021, February 11). Covid: Disabled people account for six in 10 deaths in England last year—ONS. https://www.bbc.com/news/uk-56033813

Been a meme since 2010. (n.d.). Retrieved June 1, 2021, from http://memegenerator.net/instance/19515463/i-can-count-to-potato-been-a-meme-since-2010-mom-gives-a-shit-in-2012

Bell, C. M. (Ed.). (2011). *Blackness and disability: Critical examinations and cultural interventions.* Michigan State University Press.

Bell, T. (2020, July 1). Lawsuit over disability access policy decided in Disney's favor. *Disney Information Station.* https://www.wdwinfo.com/news-stories/lawsuit-over-disability-access-policy-decided-in-disneys-favor/

Belmonte, M. K. (2020). How individuals and institutions can learn to make room for human cognitive diversity. In H. Bertilsdotter Rosqvist, N. Chown, & A. Stenning (Eds.), *Neurodiversity studies: A new critical paradigm* (pp. 172–190). Routledge.

Benedet, J., & Grant, I. (2007). Hearing the sexual assault complaints of women with mental disabilities: Consent, capacity, and mistaken belief. *McGill Law Journal, 52*(2), 243–289. https://lawjournal.mcgill.ca/article/hearing-the-sexual-assault-complaints-of-women-with-mental-disabilities-consent-capacity-and-mistaken-belief/

Benjamin, W. (1982). The work of art in the age of mechanical reproduction. In *Modern art and modernism: A critical anthology* (1st ed., pp. 217–220). Harper & Row.

Bennett, C., & Keyes, O. (2020). What is the point of fairness?: Disability, AI and the complexity of justice. *ACM SIGACCESS: Accessibility and Computing, 125*(article 5), 1–5. https://doi.org/10.1145/3386296.3386301

Bennett, J. (2010). *Vibrant matter: A political ecology of things.* Duke University Press.

Bennett, J. A. (2018). Containing Sotomayor: Rhetorics of personal restraint, judicial prudence, and diabetes management. *Quarterly Journal of Speech, 104*(3), 257–278. https://doi.org/10.1080/00335630.2018.1486033

Bentley, S. (2017). The silencing invisibility cloak. In L. X. Z. Brown, E. Ashkenazy, & M. Giwa Onaiwu (Eds.), *All the weight of our dreams: On living racialized autism* (pp. 299–305). DragonBee Press.

Bergen, K. M., & Braithwaite, D. O. (2009). Identity as constituted in communication. In W. F. Eadie (Ed.), *21st century communication: A reference handbook* (pp. 165–173). Sage. http://www.credoreference.com.bianca.penlib.du.edu/entry/sagetfccomm/identity_as_constituted_in_communication

Bergmann, W. (2008). Anti-Semitic attitudes in Europe: A comparative perspective. *Journal of Social Issues, 64*(2), 343–362. https://doi.org/10.1111/j.1540-4560.2008.00565.x

Berne, P. (2015). Disability justice—A working draft by Patty Berne. Retrieved February 21, 2022, from http://sinsinvalid.org/blog/disability-justice-a-working-draft-by-patty-berne

Bertilsdotter Rosqvist, H., Brownlow, C., & O'Dell, L. (2013). Mapping the social geographies of autism—Online and off-line narratives of neuro-shared and separate spaces. *Disability & Society, 28*(3), 367–379. https://doi.org/10.1080/0968759 9.2012.714257

Bertilsdotter Rosqvist, H., Brownlow, C., & O'Dell, L. (2015). "What's the point of having friends?": Reformulating notions of the meaning of friends and friendship among autistic people. *Disability Studies Quarterly, 35*(4). https://doi.org/10.18061/dsq.v35i4.3254

Bertilsdotter Rosqvist, H., Chown, N., & Stenning, A. (Eds.). (2020a). *Neurodiversity studies: A new critical paradigm.* Routledge.

Bertilsdotter Rosqvist, H., Örulv, L., Hasselblad, S., Hansson, D., Nilsson, K., & Seng, H. (2020b). Designing an autistic space for research: Exploring the impact of context, space, and sociality in autistic writing processes. In H. Bertilsdotter Rosqvist, N. Chown, & A. Stenning (Eds.), *Neurodiversity studies: A new critical paradigm* (pp. 156–171). Routledge. https://doi.org/10.4324/9780429322297-15

Bielby, W. T., & Bielby, D. D. (1994). "All hits are flukes": Institutionalized decision making and the rhetoric of network prime-time program development. *American Journal of Sociology, 99*(5), 1287–1313. https://doi.org/10.1086/230412

biffcollins. (2015, December 31). *Where did the term "potato quality" come from?* [Social media]. Reddit. Retrieved June 1, 2021, from https://www.reddit.com/r/OutOfTheLoop/comments/3yzgku/where_did_the_term_potato_quality_come_from/

Billawalla, A., & Wolbring, G. (2014). Analyzing the discourse surrounding Autism in the *New York Times* using an ableism lens. *Disability Studies Quarterly, 34*(1), 1–25. https://doi.org/10.18061/dsq.v34i1.3348

REFERENCES 481

Birk, L. B. (2013). Erasure of the credible subject: An autoethnographic account of chronic pain. *Cultural Studies↔Critical Methodologies, 13*(5), 390–399. https://doi.org/10.1177/1532708613495799

Birt, L., Scott, S., Cavers, D., Campbell, C., & Walter, F. (2016). Member checking: A tool to enhance trustworthiness or merely a nod to validation? *Qualitative Health Research, 26*(13), 1802–1811. https://doi.org/10.1177/2F1049732316654870

Bivens, K. M., Cole, K., & Heilig, L. (2020). The activist syllabus as technical communication and the technical communicator as curator of public intellectualism. *Technical Communication Quarterly, 29*(1), 70–89. https://doi.org/10.108 0/10572252.2019.1635211

Blair, K. L., & Hoskin, R. A. (2019). Transgender exclusion from the world of dating: Patterns of acceptance and rejection of hypothetical trans dating partners as a function of sexual and gender identity. *Journal of Social & Personal Relationships, 36*(7), 2074–2095. https://doi.org/10.1177/0265407518779139

Blanck, P. (2021). On the importance of the *Americans with Disabilities Act* at 30. *Journal of Disability Policy Studies.* Advance online publication. https://doi.org/10.1177/10442073211036900

Blasius, M. (2015, October 19). Some fans ignore disability seating rules at Red Rocks. *Coloradoan.* https://www.coloradoan.com/story/news/local/colorado/2015/10/19/fans-ignore-disability-seating-rules-red-rocks/74208662/

Blaustein, B. W. (2005). *The Ringer* [Comedy; DVD]. 20th Century Fox Home Entertainment.

Blevins, J. L., Lee, J. J., McCabe, E. E., & Edgerton, E. (2019). Tweeting for social justice in #Ferguson: Affective discourse in Twitter hashtags. *New Media & Society, 21*(7), 1636–1653. https://doi.org/10.1177/1461444819827030

Blockmans, I. G. E. (2015). "Not wishing to be the white rhino in the crowd": Disability-disclosure at university. *Journal of Language & Social Psychology, 34*(2), 158–180. https://doi.org/10.1177/0261927X14548071

Blume, H. (1998). Neurodiversity. *The Atlantic.* http://www.theatlantic.com/magazine/archive/1998/09/neuro diversity/305909/

Bogaert, A. F. (2006). Toward a conceptual understanding of asexuality. *Review of General Psychology, 10*(3), 241–250. https://doi.org/10.1037/1089-2680.10.3.214

Bogage, J. (2019, March 28). *Esports continue TV push with ESPN and Turner, sparking enthusiasm, ire.* Retrieved May 18, 2021, from https://www.washingtonpost.com/sports/2019/03/28/esports-continue-tv-push-with-espn-turner-sparking-enthusiasm-ire/

Bogenschutz, M., Nord, D., & Hewitt, A. (2015). Competency-based training and worker turnover in community supports for people with IDD: Results from a group randomized controlled study. *Intellectual and Developmental Disabilities, 53*(3), 182–195. https://doi.org/10.1352/1934-9556-53.3.182

Borello, S. (2016, April 22). Sexual assault and domestic violence organizations debunk 'bathroom predator myth.' *ABC News.* Retrieved December 17, 2021, from https://abcnews.go.com/US/sexual-assault-domestic-violence-organizations-debunk-bathroom-predator/story?id=38604019

Bostad, I., & Hanisch, H. (2016). Freedom and disability rights: Dependence, independence, and interdependence. *Metaphilosophy, 47*(3), 71–384. https://doi.org/10.1111/meta.12192

482 REFERENCES

Botella, E. (2019, December 4). Tiktok admits it suppressed videos by disabled, queer, and fat creators. *Slate Magazine*. Retrieved November 15, 2021, from https://slate.com/technology/2019/12/tiktok-disabled-users-videos-suppressed.html

Boucher, E. M. (2015). Doubt begets doubt: Causal uncertainty as a predictor of relational uncertainty in romantic relationships. *Communication Reports, 28*(1), 12–23. https://doi.org/10.1080/08934215.2014.902487

Bower, W., & Sheppard-Jones, K. (2020). Advocacy: History of the Disability Rights Movement in the United States. In D. A. Harley & C. Flaherty (Eds.), *Disability studies for human services: An interdisciplinary and intersectionality approach* (pp. 75–90). Springer.

Bowers, J. S., & Pleydell-Pearce, C. W. (2011). Swearing, euphemisms, and linguistic relativity. *PLOSOne, 6*(7), e22341. https://doi.org/10.1371/journal.pone.0022341

Bowling, I (2019, February 1). Facebook. Retrieved December 10, 2019, from https://www.facebook.com/groups/theverybrexitproblemsclub/permalink/241068563484412/

Boylorn, R. M., & Orbe, M. P. (2014). *Critical autoethnography: Intersecting cultural identities in everyday life*. Left Coast Press.

Bradshaw, P., Pickett, C., van Driel, M. L., Brooker, K., & Urbanowicz, A. (2021). 'Autistic' or 'with autism'? Why the way general practitioners view autism matters. *Australian Journal of General Practice, 50*(3), 104–109. https://doi.org/10.31128/ajgp-11-20-5721

Braidotti, R. (1994). *Nomadic subjects: Embodiment and sexual difference in contemporary feminist theory*. Columbia University Press.

Braidotti, R. (2017). Posthuman critical theory. *Journal of Posthuman Studies, 1*(1), 9–25. https://doi.org/10.5325/jpoststud.1.1.0009

Braithwaite, D. O. (1991). "Just how much did that wheelchair cost?" Management of privacy boundaries by persons with disabilities. *Western Journal of Speech Communication, 55*(3), 245–274. https://doi.org/10.1080/10570319109374384

Braithwaite, D. O. (1990). From majority to minority: An analysis of cultural change from ablebodied to disabled. *International Journal of Intercultural Relations, 14*(4), 465–483. https://doi.org/10.1016/0147-1767(90)90031-Q

Braithwaite, D. O., & Braithwaite, C. A. (2011). "Which is my good leg?": Cultural communication of people with disabilities. In J. Stewart (Ed.), *Bridges not walls* (11th ed., pp. 470–483). McGraw Hill.

Braithwaite, D. O., & Eckstein, N. J. (2003). How people with disabilities communicatively manage assistance: Helping as instrumental social support. *Journal of Applied Communication Research, 31*(1), 1–26. https://doi.org/10.1080/00909880305374

Braithwaite, D. O., & Braithwaite, C. (1988). Viewing persons with disabilities as a culture. In L. A. Samovar & R. E. Porter (Eds.), *Intercultural communication: A reader* (pp. 147–153). Wadsworth.

Brandhorst, J. K. (2020). Combatting mental health stigma on college campuses. *Spectra, 56*(2), 24–27. https://www.natcom.org/Spectra

Braun, V., & Clarke, V. (2006). Using thematic analysis in psychology. *Qualitative Research in Psychology, 3*(2), 77–101. https://doi.org/10.1191/1478088706qp063oa

Brodwin, M. G., & Frederick, P. C. (2010). Sexuality and societal beliefs regarding persons living with disabilities. *Journal of Rehabilitation, 76*(4), 37–41.

Brody, L. R., & Hall, J. A. (2000). Gender, emotion, and expression. In M. Lewis & J. Haviland (Eds.), *Handbook of emotions* (2nd ed., pp. 447–460). Guilford Press.

Brown, L. X. Z. (2017a). Why the term "psychopath" is racist and ableist. In L. X. Z. Brown, E. Ashkenazy, & M. Giwa Onaiwu (Eds.), *All the weight of our dreams: On living racialized autism* (pp. 137–144). DragonBee Press.

Brown, L. X. Z. (2017b). Too dry to cry. In L. X. Z. Brown, E. Ashkenazy, & M. Giwa Onaiwu (Eds.), *All the weight of our dreams: On living racialized autism* (pp. 112–123). DragonBee Press.

Brown, L. X. Z. (2017c). Ableist shame and disruptive bodies: Survivorship at the intersection of queer, trans, and disabled existence. In A. Johnson, J. Nelson, & E. Lund (Eds.), *Religion, disability, and interpersonal violence* (pp. 163–178). Springer International Publishing. https://doi.org/10.1007/978-3-319-56901-7_10

Brown, L. X. Z., Ashkenazy, E., & Giwa Onaiwu, M. (Eds.). (2017). *All the weight of our dreams: On living racialized autism*. DragonBee Press.

Brown, M., & Anderson, S. L. (2020). Designing for disability: Evaluating the state of accessibility design in video games. *Games and Culture, 16*(6), 702–718. https://doi.org/10.1177/1555412020971500

Brown, R. L., & Moloney, M. E. (2019). Intersectionality, work, and well-being: The effects of gender and disability. *Gender & Society, 33*(1), 94–122. https://doi.org/10.1177/0891243218800636

Brown, T. (2017). The moon poem. In L. X. Z. Brown, E. Ashkenazy, & M. Giwa Onaiwu (Eds.), *All the weight of our dreams: On living racialized autism* (pp. 41–43). DragonBee Press.

Browning, E. R., & Cagle, L. E. (2017). Teaching a "critical accessibility case study": Developing disability studies curricula for the technical communication classroom. *Journal of Technical Writing and Communication, 47*(4), 440–463. https://doi.org/10.1177/2F0047281616646750

Brunkard, J., Namulanda, G., & Ratard, R. (2008). Hurricane Katrina deaths, Louisiana, 2005. *Disaster Medicine and Public Health Preparedness, 2*(4), 215–223. https://doi.org/10.1097/DMP.0b013e31818aaf55

Brynjolfsson, E., & McAfee, A. (2014). *The second machine age: Work, progress, and prosperity in a time of brilliant technologies*. Norton & Company.

Buchanan, N. T., & Settles, I. H. (2019). Managing (in)visibility and hypervisibility in the workplace. *Journal of Vocational Behavior, 113*, 1–5. https://doi.org/10.1016/j.jvb.2018.11.001

Bunch, M., Johnson, M., Moro, S.S., Adams, M.S., & Sergio, L. (2021). Virtual reality hope machines in a curative imaginary: Recommendations for neurorehabilitation research from a critical disability studies perspective. *Disability and Rehabilitation*. Advance online publication. https://doi.org/10.1080/09638288.2021.1982024

Burcaw, S. (2014). *Laughing at my nightmare*. Roaring Book Press.

Burcaw, S. (2019). *Strangers assume my girlfriend is my nurse*. Roaring Book Press.

Burgess, D. J., Bokhour, B. G., Cunningham, B. A., Do, T., Gordon, H. S., Jones, D. M., Pope, C., Saha, S., & Gollust, S. E. (2019). Healthcare providers' responses to narrative communication about racial healthcare disparities. *Health Communication, 34*(2), 149–161. https://doi.org/10.1080/10410236.2017.1389049

Burgess, J., & Green, J. (2009). *YouTube: Online video and participatory culture*. Policy Press.

Burke, J., Spence, P. R., & Lachlan, K. A. (2010). Crisis preparation, media use, and information seeking during Hurricane Ike: Lessons learned for emergency communication. *Journal of Emergency Management, 8*(5), 27–37. https://doi.org/10.5055/jem.2010.0030

484 REFERENCES

Burke, M. (2021, April 23). Father says son with autism was slammed to ground, punched by officer. *NBCNews.com*. Retrieved November 2, 2021, from https://www.nbcnews.com/news/us-news/father-says-son-autism-was-slammed-ground-punched-officer-n1265142

Butler, J. (1993). *Bodies that matter: On the discursive limits of sex*. Routledge.

Butler, J. (2006). *Gender trouble: Feminism and the subversion of identity* (2nd ed.). Routledge.

Butler, R. C., & Gillis, J. M. (2011). The impact of labels and behaviors on the stigmatization of adults with Asperger's disorder. *Journal of Autism Development Disorder, 41*(6), 741–749. https://doi.org/10.1007/s10803-010-1093-9

Byrd, G. A., Zhang, Y. B., Gist-Mackey, A. N., & Pitts, M. J. (2019). Interability contact and the reduction of interability prejudice: Communication accommodation, intergroup anxiety, and relational solidarity. *Journal of Language & Social Psychology, 38*(4), 441–458. https://doi.org/10.1177/0261927X19865578

Calder-Dawe, O., Witten, K., & Carroll, P. (2020). Being the body in question: Young people's accounts of everyday ableism, visibility, and disability. *Disability & Society, 35*(1), 132–155. https://doi.org/10.1080/09687599.2019.1621742

Calgaro, E., Craig, N., Craig, L., Dominey-Howes, D., & Allen, J. (2021). Silent no more: Identifying and breaking through the barriers that d/Deaf people face in responding to hazards and disasters. *International Journal of Disaster Risk Reduction, 57*. https://doi.org/10.1016/j.ijdrr.2021.102156

Calgaro, E., Villeneuve, M., & Roberts, G. (2020). Inclusion: Moving beyond resilience in the pursuit of transformative and just DRR practices for persons with disabilities. In A. Lukasiewicz & C. Baldwin (Eds.), *Natural hazards and disaster justice: Challenges for Australia and its neighbours* (pp. 319–348). Palgrave Macmillan. https://doi.org/10.1007/978-981-140466-2_17

Caliandro, A., & Anselmi, G. (2021). Affordances-based brand relations: An inquire on memetic brands on Instagram. *Social Media + Society, 7*(2), 1–18. https://doi.org/10.1177/20563051211021367

Cameron, C. (2014). *Disability studies: A student's guide*. Sage.

Cameron, D., & Stevenson, N. (2016). *Attitudes to potentially offensive language and gestures on TV and radio*. Research report. Retrieved January 16, 2020, from https://www.ofcom.org.uk/__data/assets/pdf_file/0022/91624/OfcomOffensiveLanguage.pdf

Cameron, L., Knezevic, I., & Hanes, R. (2021). Inspiring people or perpetuating stereotypes? The complicated case of disability as inspiration. In M. S. Jeffress (Ed.), *Disability representation in film, TV, and print media* (pp. 108–127). Routledge.

Cameron, N. O., Muldrow, A. F., & Stefani, W. (2018). The weight of things: Understanding African American women's perceptions of health, body image, and attractiveness. *Qualitative Health Research, 28*(8), 1242–1254. https://doi.org/10.1177/1049732317753588

Campbell, M. (2017). Disabilities and sexual expression: A review of the literature. *Sociology Compass, 11*(9), 1–19. https://doi.org/10.1111/soc4.12508

Canadian Working Group of Childhood Hearing. (2005). *Early hearing and communication development: Canadian working group of childhood hearing (CWGCH) Resource Document*. Minister of Public Works and Government Services Canada. Retrieved November 2015, from https://publications.gc.ca/collections/Collection/H124-10-2005E.pdf

Carey, J. (2009). *Communication as culture: Essays on media and society*. Routledge.

Carlson, L. (2016). Music, intellectual disability, and human flourishing. In N. Lerner, J. N. Straus, S. Jensen-Moulton, & B. Howe (Eds.), *The Oxford handbook of music and disability studies* (pp. 37–53). Oxford University Press.

Carmon, I. (2015, August 11). Donald Trump's worst offense? Mocking disabled reporter, poll finds. *NBC News*. https://www.nbcnews.com/politics/2016-election/trump-s-worst-offense-mocking-disabled-reporter-poll-finds-n627736

Carolin, R., & Tatum, C. (Directors). (2022). *Dog* [Film]. Metro-Goldwyn-Mayer.

CASLPA. (2006). *Position paper on cochlear implants in children*. SAC-OAC. Retrieved November 2016, from http://www.sac-oac.ca/sites/default/files/resources/Cochlear_implants_%20in_children_Oct_2006.pdf

Castruita, B. (2018, November 16). *Celeste interview with Matt Thorson of Matt Makes Games*. Retrieved May 18, 2021, from https://web.archive.org/web/20201108165429/; https://chargedshot.com/blog/2018/11/16/celeste-interview; Celeste. (n.d.). *Celeste*. Retrieved May 18, 2021, from http://www.celestegame.com

Center on Budget Policy and Priorities. (2000). *Policy basics: Introduction to Medicaid*. Retrieved December 21, 2021, from https://www.cbpp.org/research/health/policy-basics-introduction-to-medicaid

Center on the Developing Child at Harvard University. (2007). *A science-based framework for early childhood policy: Using evidence to improve outcomes for learning, behavior, and health for vulnerable children*. http://developingchild.harvard.edu/index.php/download_le/-/view/63

Centers for Disease Control and Prevention. (2020, September 16). *Disability impacts all of us*. National Center on Birth Defects and Developmental Disabilities. Retrieved January 2, 2022, from https://www.cdc.gov/ncbddd/disabilityandhealth/infographic-disability-impacts-all.html

Centers for Disease Control and Prevention. (2022). *What is early intervention*. Retrieved December 1, 2019, from https://www.cdc.gov/ncbddd/actearly/parents/states.html

Cerankowski, K. J., & Milks, M. (2010). New orientations: Asexuality and its implications for theory and practice. *Feminist Studies, 36*(3), 650–664, 699–700. https://www.jstor.org/stable/27919126

Chandler, E., Changfoot, N., Rice, C., LaMarre, A., & Mykitiuk, R. (2018). Cultivating disability arts in Ontario. *Review of Education, Pedagogy, and Cultural Studies, 40*(3), 249–264. https://doi.org/10.1080/10714413.2018.1472482

Chang, H., Ngunjiri, F. W., & Hernandez, K-A. C. (2013). *Collaborative ethnography*. Left Coast Press, Inc.

Charlton, J. (1998). *Nothing about us without us: Disability oppression and empowerment*. University of California Press.

Charmaz, K. (2014). *Constructing grounded theory*. Sage.

Charmaz, K., & Rosenfeld, D. (2006). Reflections of the body, images of the self: Visibility and invisibility in chronic illness and disability. In P. Vannini & D. Waskul (Eds.), *Body/embodiment: Symbolic interaction and the sociology of the body* (pp. 35–49). Taylor & Francis.

Charnin, M., & Strouse, E. (1977). "It's the hard knock life." [Song recorded by Annie and the Orphans]. On Columbia Records.

Chaudoir, S., & Quinn, D. (2010). Revealing concealable stigmatized identities: The impact of disclosure motivations and positive first-disclosure experiences on fear of

486 REFERENCES

disclosure and well-being. *Journal of Social Issues, 66*(3), 570–584. https://doi.org/10.1111/j.1540-4560.2010.01663.x

Chen, M. Y. (2012). *Animacies: Biopolitics, racial mattering, and queer affect.* Duke University Press.

Chennat, S. (Ed.). (2019). *Disability inclusion and inclusive education.* Springer.

Cherney, J. L. (1999). Deaf culture and the cochlear implant debate: Cyborg politics and the identity of people with disabilities. *Argumentation and Advocacy, 36*(1), 22–34. https://doi.org/10.1080/00028533.1999.11951635

Cherney, J. L. (2011). The rhetoric of ableism. *Disability Studies Quarterly, 31*(3). https://doi.org/10.18061/dsq.v31i3

Cherney, J. L. (2019). *Ableist rhetoric: How we know, value, and see disability.* Pennsylvania State University Press.

Chin, W. 2015. *Around 92% of people with impairments play games despite difficulties.* Retrieved May 18, 2021, from https://www.game-accessibility.com/documentation/around-92-of-people-with-impairments-play-games-despite-difficulties/

Cho, S. E., Jung, K., & Park, H. W. (2013). Social media use during Japan's 2011 earthquake: How Twitter transforms the locus of crisis communication. *Media International Australia, 141*(1), 28–40. https://doi.org/10.1177/1329878X1314900105

Chris, & and callmeshirley. (2012, February 13). *That really rustled my jimmies.* Know Your Meme. Retrieved June 1, 2021, from https://knowyourmeme.com/memes/that-really-rustled-my-jimmies

Christensen-Stryno, M. B., & Eriksen, C. B. (2020). Madeline Stuart as disability advocate and brand: Exploring the affective economies of social media. In J. Johanssen & D. Garrisi (Eds.), *Disability, media, and representations* (pp. 35–50). Routledge.

Christian, Y. (2017). They said I didn't act like a black. In L. X. Z. Brown, E. Ashkenazy, & M. Giwa Onaiwu (Eds.), *All the weight of our dreams: On living racialized autism* (pp. 195–198). DragonBee Press.

CICE (2020). Community Integration through Co-operative Education (CICE). Faculty of Health Sciences & Wellness. Humber College. Retrieved February 22, 2022, from https://healthsciences.humber.ca/programs/cice-ontario-college-certificate.html

Cirucci, A. M. (2017). Normative interfaces: Affordances, gender, and race in Facebook. *Social Media + Society, 3*(2), 1–10. https://doi.org/10.1177/2056305117717905

Cities slow to submit info on people in need of special evacuation assistance. (2015, March 10). *The Japan Times.* Retrieved November 30, 2019, from https://www.japantimes.co.jp/news/2015/03/10/national/cities-slow-to-submit-info-on-people-in-need-of-special-evacuation-assistance/

Clare, E. (1999). *Exile and pride: Disability, queerness, and liberation.* South End Press.

Clare, E. (2017). *Brilliant imperfection: Grappling with cure.* Duke University Press.

Clarke, L. (2015, August 27). Disabled Coventry woman thanks threatened employment support service for first job. *Coventry Observer.* Retrieved June 1, 2021, from https://coventryobserver.co.uk/news/disabled-coventry-woman-thanks-threatened-employment-support-service-for-first-job-9308/

Clinton "Halfcoordinated" Lexa [@Halfcoordinated]. (2019a, April 4). *I wrote up an alternate Celeste Assist Mode preamble and edited it with @Kathy_E_J to make sure key needs are covered, here's what we came up with. Pastebin with the same text.* https://pastebin.com/RDMJyqga. [Tweet]. Twitter. Retrieved May 18, 2021, from https://twitter.com/halfcoordinated/status/1113931964569071616?s=20

Clinton "Halfcoordinated" Lexa [@Halfcoordinated]. (2019b, April 4). *These are good suggestions and yes, Celeste overall handles it well! However, I feel obligated to mention that the Celeste assist mode preamble felt othering for many individuals when it mentioned "intended" gameplay, leaving folks feeling insulted for needing the assists at all.* [Tweet]. Twitter. Retrieved May 18, 2021, from https://twitter.com/halfcoordinated/status/1113880862121242624?s=20

Clogston, J. S. (1990). *Disability coverage in 16 newspapers.* Advocado Press.

CNN (2018). 16 insane things that happened in Trumpworld in just the last 48 hours, *The Point.* Retrieved January 16, 2020, from https://edition.cnn.com/2018/02/28/politics/48-hours-trump-analysis/index.html

COBRA—Confessions of a black rhapsodic aspie. (2017). You think I don't notice? In L. X. Z. Brown, E. Ashkenazy, & M. Giwa Onaiwu (Eds.), *All the weight of our dreams: On living racialized autism* (pp. 215–216). DragonBee Press.

Cohen, R., Fardouly, J., Newton-John, T., & Slater, A. (2019). #BoPo on Instagram: An experimental investigation of the effects of viewing body positive content on young women's mood and body image. *New Media & Society, 21*(7), 1546–1564. https://doi.org/10.1177/1461444819826530

Cole, S. (2020, August 7). Made to be broken [Audio podcast episode]. In *This American life.* WBEZ Chicago. Retrieved March 11, 2021, from https://www.thisamericanlife.org/713/made-to-be-broken/act-one-10

Coleman Brown, L. M. (2017). Stigma: An enigma demystified. In L. Davis (Ed.), *The disability studies reader* (5th ed., pp. 145–159). Routledge. https://doi.org/10.4324/9781315680668-18

Collier, M. J. (1997). Cultural identity and intercultural communication. In L. A. Samovar & R. E. Porter (Eds.), *Intercultural communication: A reader* (8th ed., pp. 36–44). Wadsworth Press.

Collins, B. & Zadrozny, B. (2020, April 17). In Trump's "LIBERATE" tweets, extremists see a call to arms. *NBC News.* https://www.nbcnews.com/tech/security/trump-s-liberate-tweets-extremists-see-call-arms-n1186561

Collisson, B., Edwards, J. M., Chakrian, L., Mendoza, J., Anduiza, A., & Corona, A. (2020). Perceived satisfaction and inequity: A survey of potential romantic partners of people with a disability. *Sexuality and Disability, 38*, 405–420. https://doi.org/10.1007/s11195-019-09601-7

Colorado Music Hall of Fame. (2019, March 22). History and future of Red Rocks Ampitheatre. https://cmhof.org/red-rocks-amphitheatre-kicks-off-another-season/

Complex Child Magazine. (2021). *Kentucky.* Retrieved January 17, 2022, from http://www.kidswaivers.org/ky

Connolly, W. (2005). *Pluralism.* Duke University Press.

Conrad, P. (1992). Medicalization and social control. *Annual Review of Sociology, 18*(1), 209–232. https://doi.org/10.1146/annurev.so.18.080192.001233

Constantino, C. (2016). *Stuttering gain* [Paper presentation]. International Stuttering Awareness Day Conference. Retrieved March 10, 2021, from http://isad.isastutter.org/isad-2016/papers-presented-by-2016/stories-and-experiences-with-stuttering-by-pws/stuttering-gain-christopher-constantino/

Corby, D., Taggart, L., & Cousins, W. (2020). The lived experience of people with intellectual disabilities in post-secondary or higher education. *Journal of Intellectual Disabilities, 24*(3), 339–357. https://doi.org/10.1177/1744629518805603

488 REFERENCES

Corrigan, P. W., Rafacz, J., & Rüsch (2011). Examining a progressive model of self-stigma and its impact on people with serious mental illness. *Psychiatry Research, 189*(3), 339–343. https://doi.org/10.1016/j.psychres.2011.05.024

Corrigan, P., Markowitz, F. E., Watson, A., Rowan, D., & Kubiak, M. A. (2003). An attribution model of public discrimination towards persons with mental illness. *Journal of Health and Social Behavior, 44*(2), 162–179. https://doi.org/10.2307/1519806

Costello, L., McDermott, M. L., & Wallace, R. (2017). Netnography: Range of practices, misperceptions, and missed opportunities. *International Journal of Qualitative Methods, 16*, 1–12. https://doi.org/10.1177/1609406917700647

Cotter, K. (2019). Playing the visibility game: How digital influencers and algorithms negotiate influence on Instagram. *New Media & Society, 21*(4), 895–913. https://doi.org/10.1177/1461444818815684

Couldry, N., Rodriguez, C., Bolin, G., Cohen, J., Volkmer, I., Goggin, G., Kraidy, M., Iwabuchi, K., Qiu, J. L., Wasserman, H., Zhao, Y., Rincón, O., Magallanes-Blanco, C., Thomas, P. N., Koltsova, O., Rakhmani, I., & Lee, K.-S. (2018). Media, communication and the struggle for social progress. *Global Media and Communication, 14*(2), 173–191. https://doi.org/10.1177/1742766518776679

Count to potato now 16. (n.d.). Me.Me. Retrieved June 1, 2021, from https://me.me/i/count-to-potato-now-16-girl-can-count-to-firetruck

Craig, M. (2002). *Ain't I a beauty Queen?: Culture, social movements, and the rearticulation of race.* Oxford University Press.

Craig, R. T. (2016). Metacommunication. In K. B. Jensen, R. T. Craig, J. D. Pooley, & E. W. Rothenbuhler (Eds.), *The international encyclopedia of communication theory and philosophy* (pp. 1–8). John Wiley & Sons. https://doi.org/10.1002/9781118766804.wbiect232

Crane, D. (2000). *Fashion and its social agendas: Class, gender, and identity in clothing.* University of Chicago Press.

Crawford, K. (2021). *The atlas of AI: Power, politics, and the planetary costs of artificial intelligence.* Yale University Press.

Crenshaw, K. (1991). Mapping the margins: Intersectionality, identity politics, and violence against women of color. *Stanford Law Review, 43*(6), 1241–1299. https://doi.org/10.2307/1229039

Cresswell, L., Hinch, R., & Cage, E. (2019). The experiences of peer relationships amongst autistic adolescents: A systematic review of the qualitative evidence. *Research in Autism Spectrum Disorders, 61*, 45–60. https://doi.org/10.1016/j.rasd.2019.01.003

Crompton, C. J., Hallett, S., Ropar, D., Flynn, E., & Fletcher-Watson, S. (2020). "I never realized everybody felt as happy as I do when I am around autistic people": A thematic analysis of autistic adults' relationships with autistic and neurotypical friends and family. *Autism: The International Journal of Research & Practice, 24*(6), 1438–1448. https://doi.org/10.1177/1362361320908976

Croom, A. M. (2013). How to do things with slurs: Studies in the way of derogatory words. *Language & Communication, 33*(3), 177–204. https://doi.org/10.1016/j.langcom.2013.03.008

Croom, A. M. (2015). An introduction to the special issue on Slurs. *Language Sciences, 52*, 1–2. https://doi.org/10.1016/j.langsci.2015.08.001

Csikszentmihalyi, M. (1990). *Flow: The psychology of optimal experience.* Harper & Row.

Csikszentmihalyi, M. (1997). *Finding flow: The psychology of engagement with everyday life*. Basic Books.

Csikszentmihalyi, M. (2008). *Flow: The psychology of optimal experience*. HarperCollins.

Culler, J. (2015). *Theory of the lyric*. Harvard University Press.

Cunningham, S., & Craig, D. R. (2019). *Social media entertainment: The new intersection of Hollywood and Silicon Valley*. New York University Press.

Daly, N., Holmes, J., Newton, J., & Stubbe, M. (2004). Expletives as signals in FTAs on the factory floor. *Journal of Pragmatics, 36*(5), 945–964. https://doi.org/10.1016/j.pragma.2003.12.004

Danforth, S., & Gabel, S. L. (Eds.). (2016). *Vital questions facing disability studies in education* (2nd ed.). Peter Lang.

Darling, R. B. (2013). *Disability and identity: Negotiating self in a changing society*. Lynne Rienner Publishers.

Daugherty, P. (2021, December 13). New California law cracks down on emotional support animal (ESA) fraud. *City Watch LA*. https://www.citywatchla.com/index.php/cw/animal-watch/23296-new-california-law-cracks-down-on-emotional-support-animal-esa-fraud

Daughter's wellbeing. (2019, May 10). esmemes.com. Retrieved June 4, 2021, from https://esmemes.com/i/isconcerned-for-her-daughters-wellbeing-draws-attention-to-her-on

Davidson, D., & La Monica, N. (2011). Disability definitions. In M. Z. Stange, C. K. Oyster, & J. E. Sloan (Eds.), *Encyclopedia of women in today's world* (Vol. 1, pp. 402–405). Sage.

davis halifax, n.v, Fancy, D., Rinaldi, J., Rossiter, K., & Tigchelaar, A. (2018). Recounting Huronia faithfully: Attenuating our methodology to the "fabulation" of truths-telling. *Cultural Studies, Critical Methodologies, 18*(3), 216–227. https://doi.org/10.1177/1532708617746421

Davis, A. C., & Lowery, W. (2015, October 7). FBI director calls lack of data on police shootings 'ridiculous,' 'embarrassing'. *The Washington Post*. Retrieved November 2, 2021, from https://www.washingtonpost.com/national/fbi-director-calls-lack-of-data-on-police-shootings-ridiculous-embarrassing/2015/10/07/c0ebaf7a-6d16-11e5-b31c-d80d62b53e28_story.html?utm_term=.30dae2e6b3a0

Davis, L. J. (1995). *Enforcing normalcy: Disability, deafness and the body*. Verso.

Davis, L. J. (2002). *Bending over backwards: Disability, dismodernism, and other difficult positions*. New York University Press.

Davis, L. J. (Ed.). (1997). *The disability studies reader*. Routledge.

Davis, L. J. (2021). In the time of pandemic, the deep structure of biopower is laid bare. *Critical Inquiry, 47*(S2), S138–S142. https://doi.org/10.1086/711458

Dawkins, R. (1989). *The selfish gene* (2nd ed.). Oxford Paperbacks.

De Hooge, A. N. (2019). Binary boys: Autism, aspie supremacy and post/humanist normativity. *Disability Studies Quarterly, 39*(1). https://doi.org/10.18061/dsq.v39i1.6461

De Jaegher, H. (2013). Embodiment and sense-making in autism. *Frontiers in Integrative Neuroscience, 7*, 1–19. https://doi.org/10.3389/fnint.2013.00015

DeGue, S., Fowler, K. A., & Calkins, C. (2016). Deaths due to use of lethal force by law enforcement. *American Journal of Preventive Medicine, 51*(5/S3), S173–S187. https://doi.org/10.1016/j.amepre.2016.08.027

Deitz, S., Lobben, A., & Alferez, A. (2021). Squeaky wheels: Missing data, disability, and power in the smart city. *Big Data & Society, 8*(2), 1–16. https://doi.org/10.1177/20539517211047735

490   REFERENCES

Dekker, M. (2020). From exclusion to acceptance: Independent living on the autistic spectrum. In S. K. Kapp (Ed.), *Autistic community and the neurodiversity movement: Stories from the frontline* (pp. 41–49). Palgrave Macmillan. https://doi.org/10.1007/978-981-13-8437-0

Deleuze, G. (1994). *Difference and repetition (P. Patton, Trans.).* Columbia University Press.

Delgado, M. R. (2019). Disability in the fourth industrial revolution. *Developmental Medicine and Child Neurology, 61*(9), 993. https://doi.org/10.1111/dmcn.14296

DeLuca, K. (1999). Articulation theory: A discursive grounding for rhetorical practice. *Philosophy and Rhetoric, 32*(4), 334–348. https://www.jstor.org/stable/40238046

Dengel, A., Devillers, L., & Schaal, L. M. (2021). Augmented human and human-machine co-evolution: Efficiency and ethics. In B. Braunschweig & M. Ghallab (Eds.), *Reflections on Artificial Intelligence for humanity* (pp. 203–227). Springer.

Denvir, D. (2013, December 16). A short history of the war on Christmas: How everyone from Bill O'Reilly to Jon Stewart became a co-conspirator in an annual farce. *Politico.* https://www.politico.com/magazine/story/2013/12/war-on-christmas-short-history-101222/

Denzin, N. (1997). *Interpreting ethnography: Ethnographic practices for the 21st century.* Sage.

Department of Work and Pensions. (2003). *Disabled for life*, DWP, London.

Dewaele, J.-M. (2010). The emotional force of swearwords and taboo words in the speech of multilinguals. *Journal of Multilingual and Multicultural Development, 25*(2-3), 204–222. https://doi.org/10.1080/01434630408666529

DeWelles, M. (2019). Just like but unlike: Sameness, difference, and disability in children's storybooks. *Journal of Teaching Disability Studies,* Issue 1. Retrieved April 7, 2020, from https://jtds.commons.gc.cuny.edu/just-like-but-unlike-sameness-difference-and-disability-in-childrens-storybooks/

Dhiman, S., Sahu, P. K., Reed, W. R., Ganesh, G. S., Goyal, R. K., & Jain, S. (2020). Impact of COVID-19 outbreak on mental health and perceived strain among caregivers tending children with special needs. *Research in Developmental Disabilities, 107*, 103790. https://doi.org/10.1016/j.ridd.2020.103790

Diamond, L. L., & Hogue, L. B. (2021). Preparing students with disabilities and police for successful interactions. *Intervention in School and Clinic, 57*(1), 3–14. https://doi.org/10.1177/1053451221994804

DiCicco-Bloom, B., & Crabtree, B. F. (2006). Making sense of qualitative research. *Medical Education, 40*(4), 314–321. https://doi.org/10.1111/j.1365-2929.2006.02418.x

Digital Asia Hub. (2017). *AI in Asia: AI for Social Good.* Conference, March 6–7, Waseda University. https://www.digitalasiahub.org/2017/02/27/ai-in-asia-ai-for-social-good/

Dionne, E. J. (2008, March 1). Culture wars? How 2004. *Real Clear Politics.* https://www.realclearpolitics.com/articles/2008/03/reclaiming_faith_and_politics.html

Doane, B., McCormick, K., & Sorce, G. (2017). Changing methods for feminist public scholarship: Lessons from Sarah Koenig's podcast serial. *Feminist Media Studies: Feminist Reception Studies in a Post-Audience Age: Returning to Audiences and Everyday Life, 17*(1), 119–121. https://doi.org/10.1080/14680777.2017.1261465

Dolmage, J. T. (2008). Mapping composition: Inviting disability in the front door. In C. Lewiecki-Wilson & B. J. Brueggemann (Eds.), *Disability and the teaching of writing: A critical sourcebook* (pp. 14–27). Bedford/St. Martin's.

Dolmage, J. T. (2014). *Disability rhetoric.* Syracuse University Press.

Dolmage, J. T. (2017). *Academic ableism: Disability and higher education*. University of Michigan Press.

Dolmage, J. T. (2018). *Disabled upon arrival: Eugenics, immigration, and the construction of race and disability*. Ohio State University Press.

Donner, J. (2015). *After access: Inclusion, development, and a more mobile Internet*. MIT Press.

Donovan, E. E., Thompson, C. M., LeFebvre, L., & Tollison, A. C. (2017). Emerging adult confidants' judgments of parental openness: Disclosure quality and post-disclosure relational closeness. *Communication Monographs, 84*(2), 179–199. https://doi.org/10.1080/03637751.2015.1119867

Doolittle, A. (2005, October 6). Katrina reveals lack of resources to evacuate deaf. *The Washington Times*, p. B01. Retrieved December 5, 2019, from https://www.washingtontimes.com/news/2005/oct/5/20051005-095340-4787r/

Dorwart, L. (2019, July 25). What a new report says about disability representation in children's TV shows. *Forbes*. Retrieved March 7, 2021, from https://www.forbes.com/sites/lauradorwart/2019/07/25/what-a-new-report-says-about-disability-representation-in-childrens-tv-shows/#4039adb173c7

Doyle, B. (2021, September 27). TikTok statistics—Everything you need to know. *Wallaroo Media*. Retrieved November 15, 2021, from https://wallaroomedia.com/blog/social-media/tiktok-statistics

Dufresne, A. (2021, December 13). Disney guests speak out on others abusing free disability service. *Inside the Magic*. https://insidethemagic.net/2021/12/disney-guests-speak-out-das-ad1/

Duggan, A., Bradshaw, Y., & Altman, W. (2010). How do I ask about your disability? An examination of interpersonal communication processes between medical students and patients with disabilities. *Journal of Health Communication, 15*(3), 334–350. https://doi.org/10.1080/10810731003686630

Duncan, M. C. (1994). The politics of women's body images and practices: Foucault, the panopticon, and Shape Magazine. *Journal of Sport and Social Issues, 18*(1), 48–65. https://doi.org/10.1177/019372394018001004

Durham, S. (1998). *Phantom communities: The simulacrum and the limits of postmodernism*. Stanford University Press.

Edelist, T. (2019). *Constructing parental choice in deaf diagnostic and intervention practices in Ontario*. (Publication No. 13421479) [Doctoral Dissertation, University of Toronto]. ProQuest Dissertations Publishing.

Edelman, A. (2018, May 5). *Collared: New laws crack down on fake service dogs*. NBCnews.com. Retrieved January 11, 2022, from https://www.nbcnews.com/politics/politics-news/collared-new-laws-crack-down-fake-service-dogs-n871541

Eilola, T. M., & Havelka, J. (2007). Emotional activation in the first and second language. *Cognition and Emotion, 21*(5), 1064–1076. https://doi.org/10.1080/02699930601054109

Eisenberg, E. M., & Riley, P. (2001). Organizational culture. In F. M. Jablin & L. L. Putnam (Eds.), *The new handbook of organizational communication* (pp. 291–322). Sage. https://doi.org/10.4135/9781412986243

Eisenberg, E. M., Trethewey, A., LeGreco, M., & Goodall, H. L., Jr. (2017). *Organizational communication: Balancing creativity and constraint* (8th ed.). Bedford/St. Martin's.

492 REFERENCES

Eisenmenger, A. (2019, December 12). Ableism 101: What it is, what it looks like, and what we can do to to [sic] fix it. *Access Living*. Retrieved December 21, 2019, from https://www.accessliving.org/newsroom/blog/ableism-101/

Elder, R. K. (2005, December 23). *'Ringer' endorsements don't patch its problems* [Newspaper]. *The Chicago Tribune*. Retrieved June 4, 2021, from https://www.chicagotribune.com/news/ct-xpm-2005-12-23-0512230148-story.html

Ellcessor, E. (2016). *Restricted access: Media, disability, and the politics of participation*. New York University Press.

Ellenkamp, J. J., Brouwers, E. P., Embregts, P. J., Joosen, M. C., & van Weeghel, J. (2016). Work environment-related factors in obtaining and maintaining work in a competitive employment setting for employees with intellectual disabilities: A systematic review. *Journal of Occupational Rehabilitation, 26*(1), 56–69. https://doi.org/10.1007/s10926-015-9586-1

Elliott, A. (2019). *The culture of AI: Everyday life and the digital revolution*. Routledge.

Elliott, D., & Hogle, P. S. (2013). Access rights and access wrongs: Ethical issues and ethical solutions for service dog use. *International Journal of Applied Philosophy, 27*(1), 1–14. https://doi.org/10.5840/ijap20132716

Ellis, C. (1999). Heartful autoethnography. *Qualitative Health Research, 9*(5), 669–683. https://doi.org/10.1177/104973299129122153

Ellis, C. (2007). Telling secrets, revealing lives: Relational ethics in research with intimate others. *Qualitative Inquiry, 13*(1), 3–29. https://doi.org/10.1170/780040947

Ellis, K., & Merchant, M. (2020). Disability media work. In K. Ellis, G. Goggin, B. Haller, & R. Curtis (Eds.), *The Routledge companion to disability and media* (pp. 387–399). Routledge.

Ellis, K., & Kao, K.-T. (2019). Who gets to play? Disability, open literacy, gaming. *Cultural Science Journal, 11*(1), 111–125. https://doi.org/10.5334/csci.128

Ellis, K., & Kent, M. (2011). *Disability and new media*. Routledge. https://doi.org/10.4324/9780203831915

Ellis, K., Goggin, G., Haller, B., Curtis, R., & (Eds.). (2020). *The Routledge companion to disability and media*. Routledge.

Ellis, P. E. (2017). Blood, sweat & tears: On assimilation. In L. X. Z. Brown, E. Ashkenazy, & M. Giwa Onaiwu (Eds.), *All the weight of our dreams: On living racialized autism* (pp. 23–29). DragonBee Press.

Ellison, R. (1952). *The invisible man*. Random House.

Elmore, K. (2013). Embracing interdependence: Technology developers, autistic users, and technical communicators. In L. Melonçon (Ed.), *Rhetorical accessability: At the intersection of technical communication and disability studies* (pp. 15–38). Routledge.

Emens, E. F. (2014). Compulsory sexuality. *Stanford Law Review, 66*(2), 303–386. https://doi.org/10.2139/ssrn.2218783

Emma. (2021, April 17). *Most remarkable service dog statistics in 2022*. Pawsome advice. Retrieved January 11, 2022, from https://pawsomeadvice.com/dog/service-dog-statistics/

Emry, R., & Wiseman, R. (1987). An intercultural understanding of nondisabled and disabled persons' communication. *International Journal of Intercultural Relations, 11*(1), 7–27. https://doi.org/10.1016/0147-1767(87)90029-0

Enger, J. E. (2019). "The disability rights community was never mine": Neuroqueer disidentification. *Gender & Society, 33*(1), 123–147. https://doi.org/10.1177/0891243218803284

Ensminger, J. J. (2010). *Service and therapy dogs in American society: Science, law and the evolution of canine caregivers*. Charles C. Thomas Publisher Ltd.

Entertainment Software Association [ESA]. (2018, April). *2018 essential facts about the computer and video game industry*. Retrieved May 18, 2021, from https://www.theesa.com/esa-research/2018-essential-facts-about-the-computer-and-video-game-industry/

Entertainment Software Association [ESA]. (2021, February). *2021 essential facts about the video game industry*. Retrieved January 2, 2022, from https://www.theesa.com/resource/2021-essential-facts-about-the-video-game-industry/

Entman, R. M. (2007). Framing bias: Media in the distribution of power. *Journal of Communication, 57*(1), 163–173. https://doi.org/10.1111/j.1460-2466.2006.00336.x

Epic Games. (2017). *Fortnite*. [Video game, PC, Nintendo Switch, PlayStation 4, PlayStation 5, Xbox One, Xbox Series X/S, iOS, Android]. Cary, North Carolina: Epic Games.

Erevelles, N., & Minear, A. (2010). Unspeakable offenses: Untangling race and disability in discourses of intersectionality. *Journal of Literary & Cultural Disability Studies, 4*(2), 127–145. https://doi.org/10.3828/jlcds.2010.11

Esposito, J. (2014). Pain is a social construction until it hurts: Living theory on my body. *Qualitative Inquiry, 20*(10), 1179–1190. https://doi.org/10.1177/1077800414545234

etan_causale. (2012, May 30). *When 4Chan attacks 9GAG* [Reddit Comment]. R/Funny. Retrieved June 4, 2021, from www.reddit.com/r/funny/comments/ucbx6/when_4chan_attacks_9gag/c4u8ugt/

Etikan, I., Musa, S. A., & Alkassim, R. S. (2016). Comparison of convenience sampling and purposive sampling. *American Journal of Theoretical and Applied Statistics, 5*(1), 1–4. https://doi.org/10.11648/j.ajtas.20160501.11

Evans, B. (2014). The foundations of autism: The law concerning psychotic, schizophrenic, and autistic children in 1950s and 1960s Britain. *Bulletin of the History of Medicine, 88*(2), 253–285. https://doi.org/10.1353/bhm.2014.0033

FAIR Health. (2020). *Risk Factors for COVID-19 Mortality among Privately Insured Patients: A Claims Data Analysis*. [White paper, in collaboration with the West Health Institute and Marty Makary, MD, MPH, from Johns Hopkins University School of Medicine]. https://s3.amazonaws.com/media2.fairhealth.org/whitepaper/asset/Risk%20Factors%20for%20COVID-19%20Mortality%20among%20Privately%20Insured%20Patients%20-%20A%20Claims%20Data%20Analysis%20-%20A%20FAIR%20Health%20White%20Paper.pdf

Fairman, S. K., & Huebner, R. H. (2001). Service dogs: A compensatory resource to improve function. *Occupational Therapy in Health Care, 13*(2), 41–52. https://doi.org/10.1080/J003v13n02_03

Family Policy Alliance (2021). *Transgenderism and gender dysphoria: God created mankind male and female, in his image and likeness, which cannot be changed*. Retrieved December 17, 2021, from https://familypolicyalliance.com/issues/sexuality/transgender/

Farman, J. (2012). *Mobile interface theory: Embodied space and locative media*. Routledge.

Farnall, O. F., & Lyons, K. (2012). Are we there yet? A content analysis of ability integrated advertising on prime-time TV. *Disability Studies Quarterly, 32*(1). https://doi.org/10.18061/dsq.v32i1.1625

Faulkner, S. (2016). *Poetry as method: Reporting research through verse.* Routledge.

Faulkner, S. (2017). Poetry is politics: An autoethnographic poetry manifesto. *International Review of Qualitative Research, 10*(1), 89–96. https://doi.org/10.1525/irqr.2017.10.1.89

Faulkner, S. (2020). *Poetic inquiry: Craft, method and practice* (2nd ed.). Routledge.

Favorite color of the alphabet. (n.d.). Memegenerator.Net. Retrieved June 4, 2021, from https://memegenerator.net/instance/25179076/i-can-count-to-potato-potato-is-my-favorite-color-of-the-alphabet

Fazel, S., Buxrud, P., Ruchkin, V., & Grann, M. (2010). Homicide in discharged patients with schizophrenia and other psychoses: A national case-control study. *Schizophrenia Research, 123*(2–3), 263–269. https://doi.org/10.1016/j.schres.2010.08.019

Fazelpour, S., & Danks, D. (2021). Algorithmic bias: Senses, sources, solutions. *Philosophy Compass, 16*(8), e12760. 1–16. https://doi.org/10.1111/phc3.12760

Ferguson, P. M., & Nusbaum, E. (2012). Disability studies: What is it and what difference does it make? *Research and Practice for Persons with Severe Disabilities, 37*(2), 70–80. https://doi.org/10.1177/154079691203700202

Ferris, J. (2004). The enjambed body: A step toward crippled poetics. *The Georgia Review, 58*(2), 219–233. https://www.jstor.org/stable/41402415

Ferris, J. (2008a). Just try having none. *Text and Performance Quarterly, 28*(1–2), 242–255. https://doi.org/10.1080/10462930701754499

Ferris, J. (2008b). Thirteen ways of looking at crip poetry. *Text and Performance Quarterly, 28*(1–2), 6–7. https://doi.org/10.1080/10462930701754275

Fielden, S. L., Moore, M. E., & Bend, G. L. (Eds.). (2020). *Palgrave handbook of disability at work.* Palgrave.

Filteau, A. (2017). Acting abled, acting white. In L. X. Z. Brown, E. Ashkenazy, & M. Giwa Onaiwu (Eds.), *All the weight of our dreams: On living racialized autism* (pp. 217–220). DragonBee Press.

Fine, A. H. (Ed.). (2019). *Handbook on animal-assisted therapy: Foundations and guidelines for animal-assisted interventions* (5th ed.). Elsevier.

Fistell, S. (2016, November 23). My life with Tourette's Syndrome. *New York Times.* https://www.nytimes.com/2016/11/23/opinion/my-life-with-tourettes-syndrome.html

Fjord, L. (2007). Disasters, race, and disability: [Un]seen through the political lens on Katrina. *The Journal of Race and Policy, 3*(1), 7–27. Retrieved March 1, 2022, from https://web.p.ebscohost.com/ehost/pdfviewer/pdfviewer?vid=0&sid=a0c62260-1d00-47f9-823c-a475236ff536%40redis

Fletcher, B., & Primack, A. J. (2017). Driving toward disability rhetorics: Narrative, crip theory, and eco-ability in *Mad Max: Fury Road. Critical Studies in Media Communication, 34*(4), 344–357. https://doi.org/10.1080/15295036.2017.1329540

Flores, N. (2014). Creating republican machines: Language governmentality in the United States. *Linguistics & Education, 25*, 1–11. https://doi.org/10.1016/j.linged.2013.11.001

Floridi, L., Cowls, J., King, T. C., & Taddeo, M. (2020). How to design AI for social good: Seven essential factors. *Science and Engineering Ethics, 26*, 1771–1796. https://doi.org/10.1007/s11948-020-00213-5

Flyvbjerg, B. (2006). Five misunderstandings about case-study research. *Qualitative Inquiry, 12*(2), 219–245. https://doi.org/10.1177/2F1077800405284363

Forrest, B. J. (2020). Crip feelings/feeling crip. *Journal of Literary & Cultural Disability Studies, 14*(1), 75–90. https://doi.org/10.3828/jlcds.2019.14

Foster, J. 2021. Framing disability in fashion. In R. L. Brown, M. Maroto, & D. Pettinicchio (Eds.), *The Oxford handbook of the sociology of disability* (online publication, n.p.). https://doi.org/10.1093/oxfordhb/9780190093167.013.15

Foster, J., & Pettinicchio, D. (2021). A model who looks like me: Communicating and consuming representations of disability. *Journal of Consumer Culture.* https://doi.org/10.1177/14695405211022074

Foster, P., Borgatti, S. P., & Jones, C. (2011). Gatekeeper search and selection strategies: Relational and network governance in a cultural market. *Poetics, 39*(4), 247–265. https://doi.org/10.1016/J.POETIC.2011.05.004

Foucault, M. (1972). *The archaeology of knowledge and the discourse on language* (A. Sheridan Smith, Trans.). Pantheon Books. (Original work published in 1969).

Foucault, M. (1975). *The birth of the clinic: An archaeology of medical perception.* (A. Sheridan Smith, Trans.). Vintage Books. (Original work published in 1973).

Foucault, M. (1978). *The history of sexuality. Volume 1, An introduction.* Penguin.

Foucault, M. (1980). Truth and power. In C. Gordon (Ed.), *Power/knowledge: Selected interviews & other writings by Michel Foucault, 1972–1977* (pp. 109–133). Vintage Books.

Foucault, M. (1994). *Birth of the clinic: An archaeology of medical perception.* (A. M. S. Smith, Trans.). Vintage Books. (Original work published 1973).

Foucault, M. (2003). The subject and power. In P. Rabinow & N. Rose (Eds.), *The essential Foucault: Selections from essential works of Foucault, 1954–1984* (pp. 126–144). The New Press.

Fram, S. M. (2013). The constant comparative analysis method outside of grounded theory. *The Qualitative Report, 18*(1), 1–25. http://www.nova.edu/ssss/QR/QR18/fram1.pdf

Frank, A. (2018, January 26). *Celeste is hard, but its creators are smart about difficulty.* Retrieved January 3, 2022, from https://www.polygon.com/2018/1/26/16935964/celeste-difficulty-assist-mode

French, S., & Corker, M. (Eds.). (1999). *Disability discourse.* Open University Press.

Freund, A. (2013). Toward an ethics of silence? Negotiating off-the-record events and identity in oral history. In A. Sheftel & S. Zembrzycki (Eds.), *Oral history off the record: Toward an ethnography of practice* (pp. 221–238). Palgrave Macmillan.

Friedlander, H. (1995). *The origins of Nazi genocide: From euthanasia to the Final Solution.* University of North Carolina Press.

Fuith, L., & Trombley, S. (2020). COVID-19 and the caregiving crisis: The rights of our nation's social safety net and a doorway to reform. *University of Miami Race & Social Justice Law Review, 11*(2), 159–184. Retrieved January 17, 2022, from https://repository.law.miami.edu/cgi/viewcontent.cgi?article=1132&context=umrsjlr

Fujii, K. (2012, October 31). The Great East Japan Earthquake and disabled persons—Background to their high mortality rate. *DINF.* Retrieved December 5, 2019, from https://www.ding.ne.jp/doc/english/twg/escap_121031/fujii.html

Gal, N., Shifman, L., & Kampf, Z. (2016). "It gets better": Internet memes and the construction of collective identity. *New Media & Society, 18*(8), 1698–1714. https://doi.org/10.1177/1461444814568784

Galinsky, A. D., Wang, C. S., Whitson, J. A., Anicich, E. M., Hugenberg, K., & Bodenhausen, G. V. (2013). The reappropriation of stigmatizing labels: The

496   REFERENCES

reciprocal relationship between power and self-labeling. *Psychological Science, 24*(10), 2020–2029. https://doi.org/10.1177/0956797613482943

Galloway, T. (2009). *Mean little deaf queer: A memoir.* Beacon Press.

Galloway, T. (2016). On being told "no": Keynote for *Celebrating disability through performance,* Georgia Southern's Patti Pace Performance Festival 2016. *Text and Performance Quarterly, 36*(2–3), 149–155. https://doi.org/10.1080/1046293 7.2016.1195507

Galloway, T., Nudd, D. M., & Sandahl, C. (2007). "Actual lives" and the Ethic of Accommodation. In P. Kuppers & G. Robertson (Eds.), *The community performance reader* (pp. 227–234). Routledge.

Galvin, K. M. (2014). Blood, law, and discourse: Constructing and managing family identity. In L. A. Baxter (Ed.), *Remaking 'family' communicatively* (pp. 17–32). Peter Lang.

Game Accessibility Guidelines. (n.d.). *Game accessibility guidelines: Full list.* Retrieved May 18, 2021, from http://gameaccessibilityguidelines.com/full-list/

Ganahl, D., & Arbuckle, M. (2001). The exclusion of persons with physical disabilities from prime time television advertising: A two-year quantitative analysis. *Disability Studies Quarterly, 21*(2), 1–8. https://doi.org/10.18061/DSQ.V21I2.278

Gardner, L., Campbell, J. M., & Westdal, J. (2018). Brief report: Descriptive analysis of law enforcement officers' experiences with and knowledge of autism. *Journal of Autism and Developmental Disorders, 49*(3), 1278–1283. https://doi.org/10.1007/s10803-018-3794-4

Garland-Thomson, R. (1997). *Extraordinary bodies: Figuring physical disability in American culture and literature.* Columbia University Press.

Garland-Thomson, R. (2002). The politics of staring: Visual representations of disabled people in popular culture. In S. L. Snyder, B. J. Brueggemann, & R. Garland-Thomson (Eds.), *Disability studies: Enabling the humanities* (pp. 56–75). Modern Language Association.

Garland-Thomson, R. (2009). *Staring: How we look.* Oxford University Press.

Garrisi, D., & Johanssen, J. (2020). Introduction. In J. Johanssen & D. Garrisi (Eds.), *Disability, media, and representations* (pp. 1–18). Routledge.

Gay & Lesbian Alliance Against Defamation. (2020). *Where we are on TV 2020-2021.* Retrieved November 15, 2021, from https://www.glaad.org/sites/default/files/GLAAD%20-%20202021%20WHERE%20WE%20ARE%20ON%20TV.pdf

Gelbar, N. W., Smith, I., & Reichow, B. (2014). Systematic review of articles describing experience and supports of individuals with autism enrolled in college and university programs. *Journal of Autism and Developmental Disorders, 44*(10), 2593–2601. https://doi.org/10.1007/s10803-014-2135-5

Genette, G. (1997). *Paratexts: Thresholds of interpretation.* Cambridge University Press.

George Washington University Online Public Health. (2020, November 5). *Equity vs. equality: What's the difference?* Retrieved May 18, 2021, from https://onlinepublichealth.gwu.edu/resources/equity-vs-equality/

George, A. M., Jacob, A. G., & Fogelfeld, L. (2015). Lean diabetes mellitus: An emerging entity in the era of obesity. *World Journal of Diabetes, 6*(4), 613–620. https://doi.org/10.4239/wjd.v6.i4.613

Gerber, E. (2009). Describing tragedy: The information access needs of blind people in emergency-related circumstances. *Human Organization, 68*(1), 73–81. https://doi.org/10.17730/humo.68.1.tm17684j7u301668

Gernsbacher, M. A., Raimond, A. R., Balinghasay, M. T., & Boston, J. S. (2016). "Special needs" is an ineffective euphemism. *Cognitive Research: Principles and Implications, 1*, 29. https://doi.org/10.1186/s41235-016-0025-4

Gibson, K. (2020, June 30). Face mask 'exemption' cards are fakes, feds warn. *CBS News*. https://www.cbsnews.com/news/face-mask-exemption-card-freedom-to-breathe-agency-fraudulent/

Gibson, M. J., Gregory, S. R., & Pandya, S. M. (2003). *Long-term care in developed nations: A brief overview*. Retrieved December 1, 2021, from http://research.aarp.org/health/2003

Giles, H., Linz, D., Bonilla, D., & Gomez, M. L. (2012). Police stops of and interactions with Latino and white (non-Latino) drivers: Extensive policing and communication accommodation. *Communication Monographs, 79*(4), 407–427. https://doi.org/10.1080/03637751.2012.723815

Gill, M. (2015). *Already doing it: Intellectual disability and sexual agency*. University of Minnesota Press.

Gilson, C., & andcallmeshirley. (2011, May 9). *Full retard*. Know Your Meme. Retrieved June 4, 2021, from https://knowyourmeme.com/memes/full-retard

Gingrich-Philbrook, C. (2007). Autoethnography's family values: Easy access to compulsory experiences. *Text and Performance Quarterly, 25*(4), 291–314. https://doi.org/10.1080/10462930500362445

Ginsburg, F. (2020). Foreword. In K. Ellis, G. Goggin, B. Haller & R. Curtis. (Eds.), *The Routledge companion to disability and media* (pp. xxii–xxvi). Routledge.

Ginsburg, F., & Rapp, R. (2019). "Not dead yet": Changing disability imaginaries in the twenty-first century. In V. Das & C. Han (Eds.), *Living and dying in the contemporary world* (pp. 525–541). University of California Press.

Giroux, H. (2017, March 22). The culture of cruelty in Trump's America. *Truthout*. https://truthout.org/articles/the-culture-of-cruelty-in-trump-s-america/

Glaser, B. G., & Strauss, A. L. (2017). *Discovery of grounded theory: Strategies for qualitative research*. Routledge.

Gleason, J., Ross, W., Fossi, A., Blonsky, H., Tobias, J., & Stephens, M. (2021). The devastating impact of Covid-19 on individuals with intellectual disabilities in the United States. *NEJM Catalyst*. https://catalyst.nejm.org/doi/full/10.1056/CAT.21.0051

Gleik, J. (2012). *The information: A history, a theory, a flood*. Pantheon Books.

Glenn, M. K., Foreman, A. M., Wirth, O., Shahan, K. M., Meade, B. J., & Thorne, K. L. (2017). Legislation and other legal issues relevant in choosing to partner with a service dog in the workplace. *Journal of Rehabilitation, 83*(2), 17–26. Retrieved January 11, 2022, from https://link.gale.com/apps/doc/A503309637/AONE?u=ucl_ttda&sid=bookmark-AONE&xid=613e0502

Gloviczki, P. J. (2015). *Journalism and memorialization in the age of social media*. Palgrave Macmillan.

Gloviczki, P. J. (2016). Leaving London: Three autoethnographic sketches. *Journal of Loss and Trauma, 21*(4), 286–289. https://doi.org/10.1080/1532502 4.2015.1067093

Gloviczki, P. J. (2021). *Mediated narration in the digital age: Storying the media world*. University of Nebraska Press.

Goad, K. (2018, November 2). What's race got to do with it? *AARP.* Retrieved May 20, 2021, from https://www.aarp.org/health/healthy-living/info-2018/role-of-race-in-diabetes.html

498 REFERENCES

Godart, F. C., & Mears, A. (2009). How do cultural producers make creative decisions? Lessons from the catwalk. *Social Forces, 88*(2), 671–692. https://doi.org/10.1353/sof.0.0266

Goffman, E. (1963). *Stigma: Notes on the management of spoiled identity.* Prentice-Hall.

Goffman, E. (1986). *Frame analysis: An essay on the organization of experience.* Northeastern University Press. (Original work published 1974).

Goggin, G. (2017). Communications rights, disability, and law: The Convention on the Rights of Persons with Disabilities in national perspective. *Law in Context, 35*(2), 129–149. https://doi.org/10.26826/law-in-context.v35i2.21

Goggin, G. (2021). *Apps: From mobile phones to digital lives.* Polity.

Goggin, G., & Newell, C. (2003). *Digital disability: The social construction of disability in new media.* Rowman & Littlefield.

Goggin, G., Yu, H., Fisher, K. R., & Li, B. (2019). Disability, technology innovation and social development in China and Australia. *Journal of Asian Public Policy, 12*(1), 34–50. https://doi.org/10.1080/17516234.2018.1492067

Goldsmith, D. J., & Domann-Scholz, K. (2013). The meanings of "open communication" among couples coping with a cardiac event. *Journal of Communication, 63*(2), 266–286. https://doi.org/10.1111/jcom.12021

Gonzales, L. (2018). Designing for intersectional, interdependent accessibility: A case study of multilingual technical content creation. *Communication Design Quarterly, 6*(4), 35–45. https://doi.org/10.1145/3309589.3309593

Good Morning America. (2022). *CDC director responds to criticisms on COVID-19 guidance* [Video]. YouTube. https://www.youtube.com/watch?v=gxZT7ra-oxs

Goodley, D. (2014). *Dis/ability studies: Theorising disablism and ableism.* Routledge.

Goodley, D. (2016). *Disability studies: An interdisciplinary introduction.* Sage.

Google. (n.d.-a). AI for Social Good. Retrieved February 25, 2022, from https://ai.google/social-good/

Google. (n.d.-b). Project Euphonia. Retrieved March 22, 2022, from https://sites.research.google/euphonia/about/.

Government accountability office: Report. (2017, February 9). *US Fed News (USA).* Retrieved December 5, 2019, from https://search-ebscohost-com.proxy.library.nyu.edu/login.aspx?direct=true&db=edsnbk&AN=1627092E3308BE38&site=eds-live

Government of Ontario. (2014a). *Newborn hearing screening: Parents are important partners* (Publication No. 018853) [Pamphlet]. Queen's Printer for Ontario. Retrieved February 2016, from http://www.children.gov.on.ca/htdocs/English/documents/earlychildhood/hearing/screening-parents/Screening-Parents-EN.pdf

Government of Ontario. (2014b). *Your baby needs a hearing assessment* (Publication No. 019573) [Pamphlet]. Queen's Printer for Ontario. Retrieved February 2016, from http://www.children.gov.on.ca/htdocs/English/documents/earlychildhood/hearing/assessment/Assessment-EN.pdf

Government of Ontario. (2014c). *Your baby has passed the screening but is at risk* (Publication #019609) [Pamphlet]. Queen's Printer for Ontario. Retrieved February 2016, from http://www.children.gov.on.ca/htdocs/English/documents/early-childhood/hearing/at-risk/At-Risk-EN.pdf

Government of Ontario. (2022a). *Your baby's hearing screen* [Pamphlet]. Infant Hearing Program. Retrieved January 12, 2022, from http://www.children.gov.on.ca/htdocs/English/documents/earlychildhood/hearing/screening/HearingScreen-EN.pdf

Government of Ontario. (2022b). *Infant Hearing Program*. Queen's Printer for Ontario. Retrieved January 11, 2022, from https://www.ontario.ca/page/infant-hearing-program#results

Grammenos, D., Savidis, A., & Stephanidis, C. (2009). Designing universally accessible games. *Computers in Entertainment, 7*(1), Article 8, 1–29. https://doi.org/10.1145/1486508.1486516

Green, S. J. (2021, February 16). Appeals Court rules Charleena Lyles wrongful-death suit against Seattle police can proceed. *The Seattle Times*. Retrieved October 31, 2021, from https://www.seattletimes.com/seattle-news/crime/appeals-court-rules-charleena-lyles-wrongful-death-suit-against-seattle-police-can-proceed/

Greene, K. L., & Serovich, J. M. (1996). Appropriateness of disclosure of HIV-testing information: The perspective of PWLAs. *Journal of Applied Communication Research, 24*(1), 50–65. https://doi.org/10.1080/00909889609365439

Greer, M., & Pierce, C. (2021). Examining the impact of the COVID-19 pandemic on caregivers of children with complex and chronic conditions. *Research, Advocacy, and Practice for Complex and Chronic Conditions, 40*(1), 1–26. https://doi.org/10.14434/rapcc.v40i1.33294

Grewe, B. (in press). On marking disability using language: A stain on the soul. *Listening: Journal of Communication Ethics, Religion, and Culture, 57*(2).

Grigoriadis, V. (2021, March 23). The beauty of 78.5 million followers. *The New York Times*. Retrieved November 15, 2021, from https://www.nytimes.com/2021/03/23/magazine/addison-rae-beauty-industry.html

Gross, Z. (2020, April 23). *Autism acceptance month and promoting neurodiversity in the workplace with ASAN*. [Webinar]. Partners for youth with disabilities. https://learn.pyd.org/webinars/#webinar-recordings-general

Grue, J. (2015). *Disability and discourse analysis*. Routledge.

Guest, C. M., Collis, G. M., & McNicholas, J. (2006). Hearing dogs: A longitudinal study of social and psychological effects of deaf and hard-of-hearing recipients. *Journal of Deaf Studies and Deaf Education, 11*(2), 252–261. https://doi.org/10.1093/deafed/enj028

Guidry-Grimes, L., Savin, K., Stramondo, J. A., Reynolds, J. M., Tsaplina, M., Burke, T. B., Ballantyne, A., Kittay, E. F., Stahl, D., Scully, J. L., Garland-Thomson, R., Tarzian, A., Doron, D., & Fins, J. J. (2020). Disability rights as a necessary framework for crisis standards of care and the future of health care. *Hastings Center Report, 50*(3), 28–32. https://doi.org/10.1002/hast.1128

Halberstam, J. (2005). *In a queer time and place*. New York University Press.

Hall, D. E. (2004). *Subjectivity*. Routledge.

Hall, G., & Kudsi, M. (2013, September 5). *Roar* [YouTube]. Retrieved June 4, 2021, from https://www.youtube.com/watch?v=CevxZvSJLk8

Hall, K. Q. (2011). *Feminist disability studies*. Indiana University Press.

Hall, S. (1973) *Encoding and Decoding in the television discourse*. Discussion Paper. University of Birmingham.

Hall, S. (1996). The problem of ideology: Marxism without guarantees. In D. Morley & K. H. Chen (Eds.), *Stuart Hall: Critical dialogues in cultural studies* (pp. 24–45). Routledge.

Hall, S. (1997). The work of representation. In S. Hall (Ed.), *Representation: Cultural representations and signifying practices* (2nd ed., pp. 13–74). Sage.

500 REFERENCES

Haller, B. (2000). How the news frames disability: Print media coverage of the Americans with Disabilities Act. *Social Science and Disability, 1*, 55–83. https://doi.org/10.1016/S1479-3547(00)80005-6

Haller, B., & Becker, A. B. (2014). Stepping backwards with disability humor? The case of NY Gov. David Paterson's representation on "Saturday Night Live." *Disability Studies Quarterly, 34*(1), 1-21. doi:https://doi.org/10.18061/dsq.v34i1.3459.

Haller, B., & Zhang, L. (2010). Survey of disabled people about media representations. *Media & Disability Resources.* Retrieved December 3, 2019, from https://mediadisability.wordpress.com/survey/

Hammer, G. (2016). "If they're going to stare, at least I'll give them a good reason to": Blind women's visibility, invisibility, and encounters with the gaze. *Signs: Journal of Women in Culture & Society, 41*(2), 409–432. https://doi.org/10.1086/682924

Hamraie, A. (2013). Designing collective access: A feminist disability theory of universal design. *Disability Studies Quarterly, 33*(4). https://doi.org/10.18061/dsq.v33i4.3871

Hamraie, A. (2017). *Building access: Universal design and the politics of disability.* University of Minnesota Press.

Hamraie, A., & Fritsch, K. (2019). Crip technoscience manifesto. *Catalyst, 5*(1), 1–33. https://doi.org/10.28968/cftt.v5i1.29607

Hansson, S., Orru, K., Siibak, A., Bäck, A., Krüger, M., Gabel, F., & Morsut, C. (2020). Communication-related vulnerability to disasters: A heuristic framework. *International Journal of Disaster Risk Reduction, 51*, 1–9. https://doi.org/10.1016/j.ijdrr.2020.101931

Hardin, M., & Hardin, B. (2004). Performance or participation...pluralism or hegemony? Images of disability & gender in Sports 'n Spokes Magazine. *Disability Studies Quarterly, 25*(4). https://doi.org/10.18061/dsq.v25i4.606

Hardy, O. T., Czech, M. P., & Corvera, S. (2012). What causes the insulin resistance underlying obesity? *Current Opinion in Endocrinology, Diabetes, and Obesity, 19*(2), 81–87. https://doi.org/10.1097/MED.0b013e3283514e13

Hargreaves, J., & Hardin, B. (2009). Women wheelchair athletes: Competing against media stereotypes. *Disability Studies Quarterly, 29*(2). https://doi.org/10.18061/dsq.v29i2.920

HarkenSlasher. (n.d.). 'Autistic' name calling: How and why it hurts an Autistic. In L. X. Z. Brown, E. Ashkenazy, & M. Giwa Onaiwu (Eds.), *All the weight of our dreams: On living racialized autism* (pp. 45–50). DragonBee Press.

Harper, M., & Cole, P. (2012). Member checking: Can benefits be gained similar to group therapy. *The Qualitative Report, 17*(2), 510–517. https://doi.org/10.46743/2160-3715/2012.2139

Harrington, E. (2018). Portable shame. In L. X. Z. Brown, E. Ashkenazy, & M. Giwa Onaiwu (Eds.), *All the weight of our dreams: On living racialized autism* (pp. 33–36). DragonBee Press.

Harris, C., Ayçiçeği, A., & Gleason, J. (2003). Taboo words and reprimands elicit greater autonomic reactivity in a first language than in a second language. *Applied Psycholinguistics, 24*(4), 561–579. https://doi.org/10.1017/S0142716403000286

Hart, L. A., Hart, B. L., & Bergin, B. (1987). Socializing effects of service dogs for people with disabilities. *Anthrozoos, 1*(1), 41–44. https://doi.org/10.2752/089279388787058696

Harter, L. M., Scott, J. A., Novak, D. R., Leeman, M., & Morris, J. F. (2006). Freedom through flight: Performing a counter-narrative of disability. *Journal of Applied Communication Research, 34*(1), 3–29. https://doi.org/10.1080/00909880500420192

Haw, M. H., & Leustek, J. (2015). Sharing the load: An exploratory analysis of the challenges experienced by parent caregivers of children with disabilities. *Southern Communication Journal, 80*(5), 404–415. https://doi.org/10.1080/1041794X.2015.108197

Hazlewood, J. (2019, September 25). New Guelph exhibit reveals history of eugenics education in Ontario. *CBC*. Retrieved February 22, 2022, from https://www.cbc.ca/news/canada/kitchener-waterloo/eugenics-ontario-guelph-museum-exhibit-1.5293653

Health Care Consent Act, Government of Ontario, S.O. 1996, c. 2, Sched. A (1996). https://www.ontario.ca/laws/statute/96h02

Healthwise Staff. (2021, July 28). Types of insulin. *The Children's Hospital of Montefiore*. Retrieved February 14, 2022, from https://www.cham.org/HealthwiseArticle.aspx?id=aa122570

HealthyPeople.gov. (2021). Disability health. Retrieved December 1, 2019, from https://www.healthypeople.gov/2020/law-and-health-policy/topic/disability-and-health

Heasley, S. (2020, July 7). Face mask exempt cards citing ADA are fake, Justice Department says. Disability Scoop. https://www.disabilityscoop.com/2020/07/07/face-mask-exempt-cards-ada-fake/28559/

Hebbeler, K., Barton, L. R., & Mallik, S. (2008). Assessment and accountability for programs serving young children with disabilities. *Exceptionality, 16*(1), 48–63. https://doi.org/10.1080/09362830701796792

Heilig, L. (2018). Silent maps as professional communication: Intersections of sociospatial considerations and information accessibility. *Business and Professional Communication Quarterly, 81*(4), 421–439. https://doi.org/10.1177/2F2329490618802446

Heilker, P. (2012). Autism, rhetoric, and whiteness. *Disability Studies Quarterly, 32*(4). https://doi.org/10.18061/dsq.v32i4.1756

Heiss, S. (2011). Locating the bodies of women and disability in definitions of beauty: An analysis of Dove's campaign for real beauty. *Disability Studies Quarterly, 31*(1). https://doi.org/10.18061/dsq.v31i1.1367

Hemingway, L., & Priestley, M. (2006). Natural hazards, human vulnerability and disabling societies: A disaster for disabled people? *Review of Disability Studies: An International Journal, 2*(3), 57–67. Retrieved March 2, 2022, from https://www.rdsjournal.org/index.php/journal/article/view/337/1037

Hendley, Y., Zhao, L., Coverson, D. L., Din-Dzietham, R., Morris, A., Quyyumi, A. A., Gibbons, G. H., & Vaccarino, V. (2011). Differences in weight perceptions among Blacks and whites. *Journal of Women's Health, 20*(12), 1805–1811. https://doi.org/10.1089/jwh.2010.2262

Hendren, S. (2020). *What can a body do?* Riverhead Books.

Henshaw, M., & Thomas, S. (2011). Police encounters with people with intellectual disability: Prevalence, characteristics and challenges. *Journal of Intellectual Disability Research, 56*(6), 620–631. https://doi.org/10.1111/j.1365-2788.2011.01502.x

Hernandez, J. (2021a, October 10). Police dragged a paraplegic man from his car after he told them he couldn't get out. *NPR*. Retrieved October 31, 2021, from https://www.npr.org/2021/10/10/1044884579/police-dragged-a-paraplegic-man-from-his-car-after-he-told-them-he-couldnt-get-o

502 REFERENCES

Hernandez, J. (2021b, September 29). A deaf man who couldn't hear police commands was tased and spent 4 months in jail. *NPR*. Retrieved October 31, 2021, from https://www.npr.org/2021/09/29/1041562502/deaf-man-tased-police-colorado-lawsuit

Heron, M. (2012). Inaccessible through oversight: The need for inclusive game design. *The Computer Games Journal, 1*(1), 29–38. https://doi.org/10.1007/BF03392326

Hill, D. R., King, S. A., & Mrachko, A. A. (2014). Students with autism, service dogs, and public schools: A review of state laws. *Journal of Disability Policy Studies, 25*(2), 106–116. https://doi.org/10.1177/1044207313477204

Hillary, A. (2020). Neurodiversity and cross-cultural communication. In H. Bertilsdotter Rosqvist, N. Chown, & A. Stenning (Eds.), *Neurodiversity studies: A new critical paradigm* (pp. 91–107). Routledge. https://doi.org/10.4324/9780429322297-10

Hinshaw, S. P. (2007). *The mark of shame: Stigma of mental illness and an agenda for change*. Oxford University Press.

Hipólito, I., Hutto, D. D., & Chown, N. (2020). Understanding autistic individuals: Cognitive diversity not theoretical deficit. In H. Bertilsdotter Rosqvist, N. Chown, & A. Stenning (Eds.), *Neurodiversity studies: A new critical paradigm* (pp. 193–209). Routledge. https://doi.org/10.4324/9780429322297-18

Hjorth, K., & Kim, K.-H. Y. (2011). The mourning after: A case study of social media in the 3.11 earthquake disaster in Japan. *Television & New Media, 12*(6), 552–559. https://doi.org/10.1177/1527476411418351

Hofmann, M., Kasnitz, D., Mankoff, J., & Bennett, C.L. (2020). Living disability theory: Reflections on access, research, and design. In T. Guerreiro, H. Nicolau, & K. Moffatt (Eds.), *22nd International ACM SIGACCESS Conference on Computers and Accessibility* (pp. 1-13). ACM. https://doi.org/10.1145/3373625.3416996

Holman Jones, S., Adams, T. E., & Ellis, C. (2013). Introduction: Coming to know autoethnography as more than a method. In S. Holman Jones, T. E. Adams, & C. Ellis (Eds.), *Handbook of autoethnography* (pp. 17–48). Left Coast Press.

Holmes, J. (2018, December 18). Trump Is milking the War on Christmas for every last penny. *Esquire*. https://www.esquire.com/news-politics/a25615175/donald-trump-war-on-christmas-fundraising-email/

Hoppe, A. D. (2019). License to tweak: Artistic license at first-tier Indian apparel suppliers. *Poetics, 76*. https://doi.org/10.1016/j.poetic.2019.05.001

Hoppe, A. D. (2020). Strategic balance or imperfect imitation? Style and legitimation challenges in a semi-peripheral city. In G. Cattani, S. Ferriani, F. Godart, & S. V. Sgourev (Eds.), *Aesthetics and style in strategy* (pp. 227–253). Emerald.

Hoppe, A. D. (2021). The microsociology of aesthetic evaluation: Selecting runway fashion models. *Qualitative Sociology*. https://doi.org/10.1007/s11133-021-09496-x

Horan, S., Martin, M., Smith, N., Schoo, M., Eidsness, M., & Johnson, A. (2009). Can we talk? How learning of an invisible illness impacts forecasted relational outcomes. *Communication Studies, 60*(1), 66–81. https://doi.org/10.1080/10510970802623625

Houghtalen, R. P., & Doody, J. (1995). After the ADA: Service dogs on inpatient psychiatric units. *The Bulletin of the American Academy of Psychiatry and the Law, 23*(2), 211–217. http://jaapl.org/content/jaapl/23/2/211.full.pdf

Houston, E. (2019). 'Risky' representation: The portrayal of women with mobility impairment in twenty-first-century advertising. *Disability & Society, 34*(5), 704–725. https://doi.org/10.1080/09687599.2019.1576505. https://www.cbpp.org/research/health/policy-basics-introduction-to-medicaid

REFERENCES   503

Hudson, A. (2009, August 12). Disaster plans leave disabled behind—Report. *The Washington Times*, p. A01. Retrieved December 5, 2019, from https://www.washingtontimes.com/news/2009/aug/12/disaster-plans-leave-disabled-behind/

Huell, J. C., & Erdely, J. L. (2020). Crafting empathy in *I got your back: A one(ish) person show exploring pain, empathy, and performance. Text and Performance Quarterly, 40*(4), 384–396. https://doi.org/10.1080/10462937.2020.1853213

Hughes, B. (2015). What can a Foucauldian analysis contribute to disability theory? In S. Tremain (Ed.), *Foucault and the government of disability* (pp. 78–92). University of Michigan Press.

Hughes, B., Russell, R., & Paterson, K. (2005). Nothing to be had 'off the peg': Consumption, identity and the immobilization of young disabled people. *Disability & Society, 20*(1), 3–17. https://doi.org/10.1080/0968759042000283601

Hughes, J. A. (2021). Does the heterogeneity of autism undermine the neurodiversity paradigm? *Bioethics, 35*(1), 47–60. https://doi.org/10.1111/bioe.12780

Humphries, T., Kushalnagar, P., Mathur, G., Napoli, D., Padden, C., Rathmann, C., & Smith, S. (2012). Language acquisition for deaf children: Reducing the harms of zero tolerance to the use of alternative approaches. *Harm Reduction Journal, 9*(16), 1–9. https://doi.org/10.1186/1477-7517-9-16

Hunter, M. L. (2006). *Race, gender, and the politics of skin tone*. Routledge.

Huntsman, S., Colton, J. S., & Phillips, C. (2018). Cultivating virtuous course designers: Using technical communication to reimagine accessibility in higher education. *Communication Design Quarterly, 6*(4), 12–23. https://doi.org/10.1145/3309589.3309591

Hurley, L. (2015, May 18). The Supreme Court just sided with 2 San Francisco cops who shot a mentally ill woman wielding a knife. *Business Insider*. Retrieved November 1, 2021, from http://www.businessinsider.com/r-us-top-court-backs-police-over-arrest-of-mentally-ill-woman-2015-5

Hurley, S. (2004). Imitation, media violence, and freedom of speech. *Philosophical Studies: An International Journal for Philosophy in the Analytic Tradition, 117*(1/2), 165–218. http://www.jstor.org/stable/4321442

Hurley, Z. (2019). Imagined affordances of Instagram and the fantastical authenticity of female Gulf-Arab social media influencers. *Social Media & Society, 5*(1), 1–16. https://doi.org/10.1177/2056305118819241

Huss, R. J. (2010). Why context matters: Defining service animals under federal law. *Pepperdine Law Review, 37*(4), 1163–1216. Retrieved June 17, 2022, from https://digitalcommons.pepperdine.edu/cgi/viewcontent.cgi?article=1054&context=plr

Huss, R. J. (2017a). Hounds at the hospital, cats at the clinic: Challenges associated with service animals and animal-assisted Interventions in healthcare facilities. *University of Hawaii Law Review, 40*(53), 53–113. Retrieved June 17, 2022, from https://papers.ssrn.com/sol3/papers.cfm?abstract_id=3249680

Huss, R. J. (2017b). Legal and policy issues for animal assisted interventions with special populations. *Applied Developmental Science, 21*(3), 217–222. https://doi.org/10.1080/10888691.2016.1231063

Huss, R. J., & Fine, A. H. (2017). Legal and policy issues for classrooms with animals. In N. R. Gee, A. H. Fine, & P. McCardle (Eds.), *How animals help students learn: Research and practice for educators and mental-health professionals* (pp. 27–38). Routledge.

Hutchings, L., & Archer, M. (2001). "Higher than Einstein": Constructions of going to university among working-class non-participants. *Research Papers in Education, 16*(1), 69–91. https://doi.org/10.1080/02671520010011879

Hyde, M. (2019, July 19). Held captive by his carers for four weeks, let's take a look at Boris Johnson's best bits. *The Guardian*. Retrieved December 10, 2019, from https://www.theguardian.com/commentisfree/2019/jul/19/held-captive-by-his-carers-for-four-weeks-lets-look-at-boris-johnsons-best-bits

Hyogo pref. to take steps to boost disaster assistance measures for elderly, disabled. (2017, January 16). *The Mainichi*. Retrieved November 30, 2019, from https://mainichi.jp/english/articles/ 20170116/p2a/00m/0na/010000c

I can count to potato. (n.d.). Funny Captions. Retrieved May 30, 2021, from http://www.funnycaptions.com/img/110633/i-can-count-to-potato/

I sued facebook. (2017). Meme Generator. Retrieved May 30, 2021, from http://memegenerator.net/instance/19446224/i-can-count-to-potato-i-sued-facebook-for-potato-dollars

Ibrahim, Y. (2021). *Digital icons: Memes, martyrs and avatars*. Routledge.

Illich, I. (1977). Disabling professions. In I. Illich, K. Zola, J. McKnight, J. Caplan, & H. Shaiken (Eds.), *Ideas in progress: Disabling professions* (pp. 11–39). Marion Boyars.

Image—128477. (2011, May 31). Know Your Meme. Retrieved May 30, 2021, from https://knowyourmeme.com/photos/128744-i-can-count-to-potato

Image—128745. (2011, May 31). Know Your Meme. Retrieved May 30, 2021, from https://knowyourmeme.com/photos/128745-i-can-count-to-potato

Image—128748. (2011, May 31). Know Your Meme. Retrieved May 30, 2021, from https://knowyourmeme.com/photos/128748-i-can-count-to-potato

Image—128749. (2011, May 31). Know Your Meme. Retrieved May 30, 2021, from https://knowyourmeme.com/photos/128749-i-can-count-to-potato

Image—251362. (2012, February 15). Know Your Meme. Retrieved May 30, 2021, from https://knowyourmeme.com/photos/251362-i-can-count-to-potato

Image—254453. (2012, February 19). Know Your Meme. Retrieved May 30, 2021, from https://knowyourmeme.com/photos/254453-i-can-count-to-potato

Inahara, M. (2009). This body which is not one: The body, femininity, and disability. *Body and Society, 15*(1), 47–62. https://doi.org/10.1177/1357034X08100146

InnerSloth. (2018). *Among Us.* [Video Game, PC, Nintendo Switch, PlayStation 4, PlayStation 5, Xbox One, Xbox Series X/S, iOS, Android]. InnerSloth.

Insomniac Games. (2020a). *Spider-Man: Miles Morales.* [Video game, PlayStation 4, PlayStation 5]. Sony Interactive Studio.

Insomniac Games. (2020b). *What Accessibility options does Marvel's Spider-Man: Miles Morales feature?* Retrieved May 18, 2021, from https://support.insomniac.games/hc/en-us/articles/360052412831-What-Accessibility-options-does-Marvel-s-Spider-Man-Miles-Morales-feature-

Institute for Health Metrics and Evaluation (2018). Findings from the Global Burden of Disease Study 2017. IHME.

Intel. (n.d.). AI for Good. Retrieved March 22, 2022, from https://www.intel.com/content/www/us/en/artificial-intelligence/ai4socialgood.html

Interaction Design Foundation. (2021). *What is usability?*. Retrieved May 14, 2021, from https://www.interaction-design.org/literature/topics/usability

Isbister, K. (2016). *How games move us: Emotion by design*. MIT Press. https://doi.org/10.7551/mitpress/9267.001.0001

Italiano, R., Ramirez, F., & Chattopadhyay, S. (2021). Perceptions of police use of force among U.S. adults and the role of communication accommodation in improving police–civilian interactions. *Journal of Applied Communication Research, 49*(6), 669–686. https://doi.org/10.1080/00909882.2021.1930103

ITU. (2021a). Artificial Intelligence for good. Retrieved March 22, 2022, from https://www.itu.int/en/mediacentre/backgrounders/Pages/artificial-intelligence-for-good.aspx

ITU. (2021b). Measuring digital development: Facts and figures 2021. Retrieved March 22, 2022, from https://www.itu.int/itu-d/reports/statistics/facts-figures-2021/

ITU. (2022, February 8). 100 ways AI will change our world. Keynote address. AI for Good 365 conference. Retrieved March 22, 2022, from https://aiforgood.itu.int/event/100-ways-ai-will-change-our-world/

Ivey, S. L., Tseng, W., Dahrouge, D., Engelman, A., Neuhauser, L., Huang, D., & Gurung, S. (2014). Assessment of state- and territorial-level preparedness capacity for serving deaf and hard-of-hearing populations in disasters. *Public Health Reports, 129*(2), 148–155. https://doi.org/10.1177/003335491412900208

Jaarsma, P., & Welin, S. (2012). Autism as a natural human variation: Reflections on the claims of the neurodiversity movement. *Health Care Analysis, 20*(1), 20–30. https://doi.org/10.1007/s10728-011-0169-9

Jackson, R., & Lyons, M. (2016). *Community care and inclusion for people with an intellectual disability.* Floris Books.

Jackson-Perry, D., Bertilsdotter Rosqvist, H., Layton Annable, J., & Kourti, M. (2020). Sensory strangers: Travels in normate sensory worlds. In H. Bertilsdotter Rosqvist, N. Chown, & A. Stenning (Eds.), *Neurodiversity studies: A new critical paradigm* (pp. 125–140). Routledge. https://doi.org/10.4324/9780429322297-12

Jacoby, T. A. (2015). A theory of victimhood: Politics, conflict and the construction of victim-based identity. *Millennium, 43*(2), 511–530. https://doi.org/10.1177/0305829814550258

James, W. (1996). *A pluralistic universe.* University of Nebraska Press.

Japan marks 8th anniversary of 3/11 disaster in Tohoku region. (2019, March 11). *The Asahi Shimbun.* Retrieved November 30, 2019, from http://www.asahi.com/ajw/articles/ AJ201903110021.html

Jardine, J. (2005, September 11). Being deaf means he can really help. *The Modesto Bee,* p. B1. Retrieved December 5, 2019, from https://search-ebscohost-com.proxy.library.nyu.edu/login.aspx?direct=true&db=edsnba&AN=10C9EBBAAF886948&site=eds-live

Jasanoff, S. (2015). Imagined and invented worlds. In S. Jasanoff & S.-H. Kim (Eds.), *Dreamscapes of modernity: Sociotechnical imaginaries and the fabrication of power* (pp. 321–341). University of Chicago Press.

Jaswal, V. K., & Akhtar, N. (2018). Being vs. appearing socially uninterested: Challenging assumptions about social motivation in autism. *Behavioral and Brain Sciences, 42*, 1–84. https://doi.org/10.1017/S0140525X18001826

Jay, K. L., & Jay, T. B. (2015). Taboo word fluency and knowledge of slurs and general pejoratives: Deconstructing the poverty-of-vocabulary myth. *Language Sciences, 52*, 251–259. https://doi.org/10.1016/j.langsci.2014.12.003

Jay, T. B. (2019). Taboo language awareness in early childhood. In K. Allan (Ed.), *The Oxford handbook of taboo words and language* (pp. 96–107). https://doi.org/10.1093/oxfordhb/9780198808190.013.6

506 REFERENCES

Jeffress, M. S. (2015). *Communication, sport and disability: The case of power soccer.* Routledge.

Jeffress, M. S. (Ed.). (2021). *Disability representation in film, TV, and print media.* Routledge.

Jeffress, M. S., & Brown, W. J. (2017). Opportunities and benefits for powerchair users through power soccer. *Adapted Physical Activity Quarterly, 34*(3), 235–255. https://doi.org/10.1123/apaq.2016-0022

Jennings, R. (2021, May 18). The blandness of TikTok's biggest stars. *Vox.* Retrieved November 15, 2021, from https://www.vox.com/the-goods/2021/5/18/22440937/tiktok-addison-rae-bella-poarch-build-a-bitch-charli-damelio-mediocrity

Jerslev, A. (2017). The elderly female face in beauty and fashion ads: Joan Didion for Céline. *European Journal of Cultural Studies, 21*(3), 349–362. https://doi.org/10.1177/1367549417708436

Johanssen, J., & Garrisi, D. (Eds.). (2020). *Disability, media, and representations: Other bodies.* Routledge.

Johnson, C. S. (2005, September 19). State donates 118 text phones to Louisiana to help deaf. *Independent Record.* Retrieved December 5, 2019, from https://search-ebscohost-com.proxy.library.nyu.edu/login.aspx?direct=true&db=edsnba&AN=12B5CE7895167BB8&site=eds-live

Johnson, M. L., & McRuer, R. (2014). Cripistemologies: Introduction. *Journal of Literary & Cultural Disability Studies, 8*(2), 127–147. https://doi.org/10.3828/jlcds.2014.12

Jones, C. T. (2016). *Writing intellectual disability: Glimpses into precarious processes of re/making a cultural phenomenon* (Unpublished doctoral dissertation). York University.

Jones, C. T., Collins, K., & Zbitnew, A. (2021). Accessibility as aesthetic in broadcast media: Critical access theory and disability justice as project-based learning. *Journalism & Mass Communication Educator, 77*(1), 24–42. https://doi.org/10.1177/10776958211000198

Jones, C. T., & Cheuk, F. (2020). Something is happening: Encountering silence in disability research. *Qualitative Research Journal, 21*(1), 1–14. https://doi.org/10.1108/QRJ-10-2019-0078

Jones, N. N. & Scott, J. B. (2017). *Call for proposals: Precarity and possibility: Engaging technical communication's politics.* Association of Teachers of Technical Writing. Retrieved May 14, 2021, from http://attw.org/attw-2018-conference-2/

Jones, N. N., Moore, K. R., & Walton, R. (2016). Disrupting the past to disrupt the future: An antenarrative of technical communication. *Technical Communication Quarterly, 25*(4), 211–229. https://doi.org/10.1080/10572252.2016.1224655

Jones, R. S. P., & Meldal, T. O. (2001). Social relationships and Asperger's syndrome. A qualitative analysis of first-hand accounts. *Journal of Intellectual Disabilities, 5*(1), 35–41. https://doi.org/10.1177/146900470100500104

Jones, S. (2020, June 19). 33–50 percent of police use-of-force incidents involve a person who is disabled. *WTHR.com.* Retrieved October 31, 2021, from https://www.wthr.com/article/news/33-50-percent-of-police-use-of-force-incidents-involve-a-person-who-is-disabled-has-disability/531-011bddff-a5f0-4d2a-9a-d2-6964623bc32d

Jung, E., & Hecht, M. L. (2004). Elaborating on the communication theory of identity: Identity gaps and communication outcomes. *Communication Quarterly, 52*(3), 265–283. https://doi.org/10.1080/03637759309376297

Jurgens, A. (2020). Neurodiversity in a neurotypical world: An enactive framework for investigating autism and social institutions. In H. Bertilsdotter Rosqvist, N. Chown, & A. Stenning (Eds.), *Neurodiversity studies: A new critical paradigm* (pp. 73–88). Routledge. https://doi.org/10.4324/9780429322297-8

k.johnson10. (2016). *Charlie Sheen DERP*. Imgflip. Retrieved May 30, 2021, from https://i.imgflip.com/11dvyf.jpg

Kafer, A. (2013). *Feminist, crip, queer*. Indiana University Press.

Kain, D. J. (2005). Constructing genre: A threefold typology. *Technical Communication Quarterly, 14*(4), 375–409. https://doi.org/10.1207/s15427625tcq1404_2

Kaiser Family Foundation. (2018). *Medicaid's future*. Retrieved January 12, 2020, from https://www.kff.org/tag/medicaids-future

Kalle69. (2013, October 21). *#Potato*. Know Your Meme. Retrieved May 30, 2021, from https://knowyourmeme.com/photos/627395-i-can-count-to-potato

Kanner, L. (1943). Autistic disturbances of affective contact. *Nervous Child, 2*(3), 217–250. http://simonsfoundation.s3.amazonaws.com/share/071207-leo-kanner-autistic-affective-contact.pdf

Kapp, S. K. (2013). Empathizing with sensory and movement differences: Moving toward sensitive understanding of autism. *Frontiers in Integrative Neuroscience, 7*(38), 1–6. https://doi.org/10.3389/fnint.2013.00038

Karetnick, J. (2019, September 24). *Service dogs 101—Everything you need to know*. American Kennel Club. Retrieved January 11, 2022, from https://www.akc.org/expert-advice/training/service-dog-training-101/

Kasnitz, D. (2020). The politics of disability performativity: An autoethnography. *Current Anthropology, 61*(21), S18–S25. https://doi.org/10.1086/705782

Kattari, S. K. (2019). The development and validation of the Ableist Microaggression Scale. *Journal of Social Service Research, 45*(3), 400–417. https://doi.org/10.108 0/01488376.2018.1480565

Katz, J., Floyd, J., & Schiepers, K. (Eds.). (2021). *Perceiving the future through new communication technologies: Robots, AI and everyday life*. Springer

Keller, R. M., & Galgay, C. E. (2010). Microaggressive experiences of people with disabilities. In D. W. Sue (Ed.), *Microaggressions and marginality: Manifestation, dynamics, and impact* (pp. 241–267). Wiley.

Kelly, B., Nevile, L., Sloan, D., Fanou, S., Ellison, R., & Herrod, L. (2009). From web accessibility to web adaptability. *Disability and Rehabilitation: Assistive Technology, 4*(4), 212–226. https://doi.org/10.1080/17483100902903408

Kelly, E. & Rice, C. (2020, January 16). Universities must open their archives and share their oppressive pasts. *The Conversation*. Retrieved February 11, 2022, from https://theconversation.com/universities-must-open-their-archives-and-share-their-oppressive-pasts-125539

Kelly, E., Manning, D. T., Boye, S., Rice, C., Owen, D., Stonefish, S., & Stonefish, M. (2021). Elements of a counter-exhibition: Excavating and countering a Canadian history and legacy of eugenics. *Journal of the History of the Behavioral Sciences, 57*(1), 12–33. https://doi.org/10.1002/jhbs.22081

Kelman, I., & Stough, L. M. (2014). (Dis)ability and (Dis)aster. In I. Kelman & L. M. Stough (Eds.), *Disability and disaster: Explorations and exchanges* (pp. 3–14). Palgrave Macmillan.

Kennedy, M. (2020). "If the rise of the TikTok dance and e-girl aesthetic has taught us anything, it's that teenage girls rule the internet right now": TikTok celebrity, girls and the Coronavirus crisis. *European Journal of Cultural Studies, 23*(6), 1069–1076. https://doi.org/10.1177/1367549420945341

Kenny, L., Hattersley, C., Molins, B., Buckley, C., Povey, C., & Pellicano, E. (2015). Which terms should be used to describe autism? Perspectives from the UK autism community. *Autism, 20*(4), 442–462. https://doi.org/10.1177/1362361315588200

Kent, M., & Ellis, K. (2015). People with disability and new disaster communications: Access and the social media mash-up. *Disability & Society, 30*(3), 319–431. https://doi.org/10.1080/09687599.2015.1021756

Kessler, G. (2016, August 2). Donald Trump's revisionist history of mocking a disabled reporter. *Washington Post.* https://www.washingtonpost.com/news/fact-checker/wp/2016/08/02/donald-trumps-revisionist-history-of-mocking-a-disabled-reporter/

Keyton, J. (2011). *Communication & organizational culture: A key to understanding work experiences* (2nd ed.). Sage.

Keyton, J. (2014). Organizational culture: Creating meaning and influence. In L. L. Putman & D. K. Mumby (Eds.), *The Sage handbook of organizational communication: Advances in theory, research, and methods* (3rd ed., pp. 549–568). Sage.

Kien, G. (2019). *Communicating with memes: Consequences in post-truth civilization.* Lexington Books.

Kim, E. (2011). Asexuality in disability narratives. *Sexualities, 14*(4), 479–493. https://doi.org/10.1177/1363460711406463

Kim, E. (2020, April). More trainings are not the answer to police violence against disabled people. Retrieved November 2, 2021, from https://www.criminallegal-news.org/news/2020/mar/18/more-trainings-are-not-answer-police-violence-against-disabled-people/

Kim, S.-H., Scheufele, D. A., & Shanahan, J. (2002). Think about it this way: Attribute agenda-setting function of the press and the public's evaluation of a local issue. *Journalism & Mass Communication Quarterly, 79*(1), 7–25. https://doi.org/10.1177/107769900207900102

Kim, Y. C., & Ball-Rokeach, S. J. (2006). Civic engagement from a communication infrastructure perspective. *Communication Theory, 16*(2), 173–197. https://doi.org/10.1111/j.1468-2885.2006.00267.x

Kim, Y. C., & Kang, J. (2010). Communication, neighborhood belonging and household hurricane preparedness. *Disasters, 34*(2), 470–488. https://doi.org/10.1111/j.1467-7717.2009.01138.x

Kim, Y. C., Moran, M. B., William, H. A., & Ball-Rokeach, S. J. (2011). Integrated connection to neighborhood storytelling network, education, and chronic disease knowledge among African Americans and Latinos in Los Angeles. *Journal of Health Communication, 16*(4), 393–415. https://doi.org/10.1080/1081073 0.2010.546483

Kinkaid, E., Emard, K., & Senanayake, N. (2020). The Podcast-as-method? Critical reflections on using podcasts to produce geographic knowledge. *Geographical Review, 110*(1–2), 78–91. https://doi.org/10.1111/gere.12354

Kirkpatrick, B. (2017). "A blessed boon": Radio, disability, governmentality and discourse of the "shut-in," 1920–1930. In E. Ellcessor & B. Kirkpatrick (Eds.), *Disability media studies.* New York University Press.

REFERENCES 509

Kitchin, R. (1998). 'Out of place,' 'knowing one's place': Space, power and the exclusion of disabled people. *Disability & Society, 13*(3), 343–356. https://doi.org/10.1080/09687599826678

Kittay, E. F. (2011). The ethics of care, dependence, and disability. *Ratio Juris, 24*(1), 49–58. https://doi.org/10.1111/j.1467-9337.2010.00473.x

Klepek, P. (2018, February 7). *Why the very hard 'Celeste' is perfectly fine with you breaking its rules.* Retrieved January 3, 2022, from https://www.vice.com/en/article/d3w887/celeste-difficulty-assist-mode

Klepek, P. (2019, September 16). *The small but important change 'Celeste' made to its celebrated assist mode.* Retrieved January 3, 2022, from https://www.vice.com/en/article/43kadm/celeste-assist-mode-change-and-accessibility

Klin, A., & Lemish, D. (2008). Mental disorders stigma in the media: Review of studies on production, content, and influences. *Journal of Health Communication, 13*(5), 434–449. https://doi.org/10.1080/10810730802198813

Knabb, R. D., Rhome, J. R., & Brown, D. P. (2005, December 20). *Tropical cyclone report: Hurricane Katrina, 23–30 August 2005.* National Hurricane Center. Retrieved January 10, 2022, from http://www.disastersrus.org/katrina/TCR-AL122005_Katrina.pdf

Knobel, M., & Lankshear, C. (2007). Online memes, affinities, and cultural production. In M. Knobel & C. Lankshear (Eds.), *A new literacies sampler* (pp. 199–227). Peter Lang.

Knoll, I. V., James, L., & Annas, G. D. (2016). Mass shootings and mental illness. In L. H. Gold & R. I. Simon (Eds.), *Gun violence and mental illness* (pp. 81–104). American Psychiatric Association Publishing.

Kögel, J., & Wolbring, G. (2020). What it takes to be a pioneer: Ability expectations from brain-computer interface users. *Nanoethics, 14*, 227–239. https://doi.org/10.1007/s11569-020-00378-0

Kozinets, R. (2015). *Netnography: Doing ethnographic research online.* Sage Press.

Krieger, N., Chen, J. T., Waterman, P. D., Kiang, M. V., & Feldman, J. (2015). Police killings and police deaths are public health data and can be counted. *PLOS Medicine, 12*(12). https://doi.org/10.1371/journal.pmed.1001915

kunoburesu. (2012, April 25). *4chan is putting all the blame on 9gag* [Social media]. Reddit. Retrieved May 30, 2021, from https://www.reddit.com/r/AdviceAnimals/comments/ssn0w/guess_who_just_found_out_she_was_a_meme/c4gpf9w/?utm_source=reddit&utm_medium=web2x&context=3

Kuppers, P. (2007). Performing determinism: Disability culture poetry. *Text and Performance Quarterly, 27*(2), 89–106. https://doi.org/10.1080/10462930701251066

Kuppers, P. (2017). *Theatre & disability.* Palgrave.

Kurzweil, R. (2003). The future of intelligent technology and its impact on disabilities. *Journal of Visual Impairment & Blindness., 97*(10), 582–584. https://doi.org/10.1177/0145482X0309701002

Kurzweil, R. (2005). *The singularity is near: When humans transcend biology.* Penguin.

Kuzma, C. (2018, November 16). *Everything you need to know before getting a service dog.* Vice.com. Retrieved January 11, 2022, from https://www.vice.com/en_us/article/j5zmak/everything-you-need-to-know-before-getting-a-service-dog

Lakin, K. C., Hill, B., & Bruininks, R. H. (1985). *An analysis of Medicaid's intermediate care facility for the mentally retarded (ICF-MR) program.* Retrieved December 1, 2019, from https://mn.gov/mnddc/parallels2/pdf/80s/85/85-AMI-UMN.pdf

REFERENCES

Lane, D. R., McNicholas, J., & Collis, G. M. (1998). Dogs for the disabled: Benefits to recipients and welfare of the dog. *Applied Animal Behaviour Science, 59*(1–3), 49–60. https://doi.org/10.1016/S0168-1591(98)00120-8

Langellier, K. M., & Peterson, E. E. (2004). *Storytelling in daily life: Performing narrative.* Temple University Press.

Lanzara, G. F. (2016). *Shifting practices: Reflections on technology, practices, and innovation.* MIT Press.

Latour, B. (2007). *Reassembling the social: An introduction to actor-network-theory.* Oxford University Press.

Lawson, M. (2021, January). How disabled creators on TikTok are going beyond "inspiration porn." *Allure.* Retrieved November 15, 2021, from https://www.allure.com/story/disabled-creators-on-tiktok

Lawson, R. (2019, July 4). Facebook. Retrieved December 10, 2019, from https://m.facebook.com/groups/theverybrexitproblemsclub/permalink/333412987583302/

Lawtoo, N. (2013). *The phantom of the ego: Modernism and the mimetic unconscious.* Michigan State University Press.

Lazar, J., & Stein, M.A. (Eds.) (2017). *Disability, human rights, and information technology.* University of Pennsylvania Press.

Lazar, J., Goldstein, D., & Taylor, A. (2015). *Ensuring digital accessibility through process and policy.* Morgan Kaufmann.

Lazzarato, M. (2014). *Signs and machines: Capitalism and the production of subjectivity.* Semiotext(e).

Leaver, T., Abidin, C., & Highfield, T. (2020). *Instagram: Visual social media cultures.* Polity Press.

LeBoeuf, M. (2007) The power of ridicule: An analysis of satire [Unpublished doctoral dissertation]. University of Rhode Island. Retrieved December 27, 2021, from https://digitalcommons.uri.edu/srhonorsprog/63/

Lee, E.-J., Ditchman, N., Thomas, J., & Tsen, J. (2019). Microaggressions experienced by people with multiple sclerosis in the workplace: An exploratory study using Sue's taxonomy. *Rehabilitation Psychology, 64*(2), 179–193. https://doi.org/10.1037/rep0000269

Lee, T. (2016). Criminalizing fake service dogs: Helping or hurting legitimate handlers? *Animal Law, 23*(325), 326–354.

Leneh Buckle, K. (2020). Autscape. In S. K. Kapp (Ed.), *Autistic community and the neurodiversity movement: Stories from the frontline* (pp. 109–122). Palgrave Macmillan. https://doi.org/10.1007/978-981-13-8437-0

Lett, K., Tamaian, A., & Klest, B. (2020). Impact of ableist microaggressions on university students with self-identified disabilities. *Disability & Society, 35*(9), 1441–1456. https://doi.org/10.1080/09687599.2019.1680344

Levin, S. (2017, June 19). Seattle woman killed by police while children were home after reporting theft. *The Guardian.* Retrieved October 31, 2021, from https://www.theguardian.com/us-news/2017/jun/19/seattle-police-shooting-charleena-lyles-mother

Lewis, J. (2021, February 2). 11 Black, body-positive influencers you should be following right now. *POPSUGAR Fitness.* Retrieved November 15, 2021, from https://www.popsugar.com/fitness/black-body-positive-influencers-to-follow-on-instagram-48140604

Lewis, T. A. (2015, April 26). Police brutality and deaf people. *American Civil Liberties Union*. Retrieved November 1, 2021, from https://www.aclu.org/blog/national-security/police-brutality-and-deaf-people

Lewthwaite, S., & Swan, H. (2013). Disability, web standards and the majority world. In L. Melonçon (Ed.), *Rhetorical accessability: At the intersection of technical communications and disability studies* (pp. 157–174). Routledge.

Li, D., & Ciechalski, S. (2021, October 9). Paraplegic man pulled from car, thrown to ground by police in Ohio. *NBCNews.com*. Retrieved October 21, 2021, from https://www.nbcnews.com/news/us-news/paraplegic-man-pulled-car-thrown-ground-police-ohio-n1281148

Li, N. P., Bailey, J. M., Kenrick, D. T., & Linsenmeier, J. A. (2002). The necessities and luxuries of mate preferences: Testing the tradeoffs. *Journal of Personality and Social Psychology, 82*(6), 947–955. https://doi.org/10.1037/0022-3514.82.6.947

Liddiard, K. (2014a). Liking for like's sake—The commodification of disability on Facebook. *Journal of Developmental Disabilities, 20*(3), 94–101. https://oadd.org/wp-content/uploads/2014/01/41019_JoDD_94-101_v13f_Liddiard.pdf

Liddiard, K. (2014b). The work of disabled identities in intimate relationships. *Disability and Society, 29*(1), 115–128. https://doi.org/10.1080/09687599.2013.776486

Lifted Team. (2018, September 19). Retrieved December 27, 2021, from https://www.liftedcare.com/dementia-disability-and-discrimination/

Lightfoot, E. B., & LaLiberte, T. L. (2006). Approaches to child protection case management for cases involving people with disabilities. *Child Abuse & Neglect, 30*(4), 381–391. https://doi.org/10.1016/j.chiabu.2005.10.013

Lillywhite, A., & Wolbring, G. (2020). Coverage of artificial intelligence and machine learning within academic literature, Canadian newspapers, and Twitter tweets: The case of disabled people. *Societies, 10*(1), 23. https://doi.org/10.3390/soc10010023

Lillywhite, A., & Wolbring, G. (2021). Coverage of ethics within the artificial intelligence and machine learning academic literature: The case of disabled people. *Assistive Technology, 33*(3), 129–135. https://doi.org/10.1080/10400435.2019.1593259

Lim, M. (2012). Clicks, cabs, and coffee houses: Social media and oppositional movements in Egypt, 2004–2011. *Journal of Communication, 62*(2), 231–248. https://doi.org/10.1111/j.1460-2466.2012.01628.x

Lincoln, Y. S., & Guba, E. G. (1985). *Naturalistic inquiry*. Sage.

Lindell, C. (2021, May 18). "My God makes no mistakes": Texas Senate oks ban on gender-affirming care for young Texans. *Austin American-Statesman*. Retrieved December 17, 2021, from https://www.statesman.com/story/news/2021/05/18/after-debating-theology-senate-oks-gender-care-ban-young-texans/5150720001/

Lindemann, K. (2010). Cleaning up my (father's) mess: Narrative containments of "leaky" masculinities. *Qualitative Inquiry, 16*(1), 29–38. https://doi.org/10.1177/1077800409350060

Lindlof, T. R., & Taylor, B. C. (2019). *Qualitative communication research methods* (4th ed.). Sage.

Lindsay, S., & Thiyagarajah, K. (2021). The impact of service dogs on children, youth and their families: A systematic review. *Disability and Health Journal, 14*(3), 101012. https://doi.org/10.1016/j.dhjo.2020.101012

Ling, R. S. (2012). *Taken for grantedness: The embedding of mobile communication into society*. MIT Press.

Linton, S. (1998). *Claiming disability: Knowledge and identity*. New York University Press.

512 REFERENCES

Lipari, L. (2014). *Listening, thinking, being: Toward an ethics of attunement.* Penn State University Press.

Lippincott, G. (2004). Gray matters: Where are the technical communicators in research and design for aging audiences? *IEEE Transactions on Professional Communication, 47*(3), 157–170. https://doi.org/10.1109/TPC.2004.833687

Livadas, G. (2005, September 11). Communication lines frayed for displaced deaf. *USA Today.* Retrieved December 5, 2019, from https://search-ebscohost-com.proxy.library.nyu.edu/login.aspx?direct=true&db=edsnba&AN=127C309259D098C8&site=eds-live

Llinares, D., Fox, N., & Berry, R. (Eds.) (2018). *Podcasting: New aural cultures and digital media.* Palgrave Macmillan. https://doi.org/10.1007/978-3-319-90056-8

Loebner, J. (2020). Advertising disability and the diversity directive. In K. Ellis, G. Goggin, B. Haller, & R. Curtis (Eds.), *The Routledge companion to disability and media* (pp. 341–355). Routledge.

Loeppky, J. (2021, October 26). When reporting on disability, advice about language is simple: Just ask. *Poynter.* Retrieved November 2, 2021, from https://www.poynter.org/reporting-editing/2021/when-reporting-on-disability-advice-about-language-is-simple-just-ask/

Loeser, C., Pini, B., & Crowley, V. (2018). Disability and sexuality: Desires and pleasures. *Sexualities, 21*(3), 255–270. https://doi.org/10.1177/1363460716688682

Lomax, A. (1980). Appeal for cultural equity. *African Music: Journal of the International Library of African Music, 6*(1), 22–31. https://doi.org/10.21504/amj.v6i1.1092

Longo, B. (1998). An approach for applying cultural study theory to technical writing research. *Technical Communication Quarterly, 7*(1), 53–73.

Longo, B. (2000). *Spurious coin: A history of science, management, and technical writing.* State University of New York Press.

Lorenz, T. (2020, December 11). The new influencer capital of America. *The New York Times.* Retrieved November 15, 2021, from https://www.nytimes.com/2020/12/11/style/atlanta-black-tiktok-creators.html

Low, R. (2021, October 9). Idaho Springs cops face another Taser lawsuit after using weapon on deaf man. *FOX3* Retrieved October 31, 2021, from https://kdvr.com/news/local/idaho-springs-cops-face-another-taser-lawsuit-after-using-weapon-on-deaf-man/

Lycan, W. G. (2015). Slurs and lexical presumption. *Language Sciences, 52,* 3–11. https://doi.org/10.1016/j.langsci.2015.05.001

M5000, & Y F. (2011, May 31). *I can count to potato.* Know Your Meme. Retrieved May 30, 2021, from https://knowyourmeme.com/memes/i-can-count-to-potato

Mackay, D. G., Shafto, M., Taylor, J. K., Marian, D. E., Abrams, L., & Dyer, J. R. (2004). Relations between emotion, memory, and attention: Evidence from taboo Stroop, lexical decision, and immediate memory tasks. *Memory & Cognition, 32,* 474–488. https://doi.org/10.3758/BF03195840

MacKinnon, C. (1989). *Toward a feminist theory of the state.* Harvard University Press.

MACPAC. Medicaid and CHIP Payment and Access Commission. (2017). *People with disabilities.* Retrieved December 12, 2019, from https://www.macpac.gov/subtopic/people-with-disabilities

Mader, B., Hart, L. A., & Bergin, B. (1989). Social acknowledgments for children with disabilities: Effects of service dogs. *Child Development, 60*(6), 1529–1534. https://doi.org/10.2307/1130941

Madison, D. S. (2020). *Critical ethnography: Methods, ethics, and performance* (3rd ed.). Sage.

Magee, S. K. (2018, November 6). Mayor of tsunami-hit city stresses resilience and inclusivity at U.N. *The Japan Times*. Retrieved November 30, 2019, from https://www.japantimes.co.jp/news/2018/11/06/national/mayor-tsunami-hit-city-stresses-resilience-inclusivity-u-n/

Making Space for Intimate Citizenship, (2016). "Let us show you"—Shona Casola. Retrieved February 21, 2022, from https://makingspaceforintimatecitizenship.wordpress.com/

Makkawy, A., & Moreman, S. T. (2019). Putting crip in the script: A critical communication pedagogical study of communication theory textbooks. *Communication Education, 68*(4), 401–416. https://doi.org/10.1080/03634523.2019.1643898

Mann, B. W. (2018). Rhetoric of online disability activism: #CripTheVote and civic participation. *Communication, Culture and Critique, 11*(4), 604–621. https://doi.org/10.1093/ccc/tcy030

Mann, B. W. (2019). Autism narratives in media coverage of the MMR vaccine-Autism controversy under a crip futurism framework. *Health Communication, 34*(9), 984–990. https://doi.org/10.1080/10410236.2018.1449071

Mann, B. W. (2020, November 11). *Theorizing intersectional stigma management communication at the crossroads: LGBTQIA+ and Autistic subjectivities* [Conference presentation]. National Communication Association.

Manos, M. M., Leyden, W. A., Resendez, C. I., Klein, E. G., Wilson, T. L., & Bauer, H. M. (2001). A community-based collaboration to assess and improve medical insurance status and access to health care of Latino children. *Public Health Reports, 116*(6), 575–584. https://doi.org/10.1093/phr/116.6.575

Mansell, R. (2015). Imaginaries, values, and trajectories: A critical reflection on the Internet. In G. Goggin & M. McLelland (Eds.), *Routledge companion to global Internet histories* (pp. 23–33). Routledge.

Mansell, R., & Raboy, M. (Eds.). (2011). *Handbook of global media policy*. Wiley-Blackwell.

Markwell, P., & Ratard, R. (2014). Deaths directly caused by Hurricane Katrina. *Louisiana Department of Health*. Retrieved December 5, 2019, from http://ldh.la.gov/assets/oph/Center-PHCH/Center-CH/stepi/specialstudies/2014Popwell Ratard_KatrinaDeath_PostedOnline.pdf

Maroto, M., Pettinicchio, D., & Patterson, A. C. (2019). Hierarchies of categorical disadvantage: Economic insecurity at the intersection of disability, gender, and race. *Gender & Society, 33*(1), 64–93. https://doi.org/10.1177/0891243218794648

Martino, A. S., & Schormans, A. F. (2018). When good intentions backfire: University research ethics review and the intimate lives of people labeled with intellectual disabilities. *Forum: Qualitative Social Research, 19*(3). https://doi.org/10.17169/fqs-19.3.3090

Masnick, M. (2005, January 5). *Since when is it illegal to just mention a trademark online?* Techdirt. Retrieved May 30, 2021, from https://www.techdirt.com/articles/20050105/0132239.shtml

Mass Shooting Tracker. (n.d.-a). About Mass Shooting Tracker. Retrieved September 2, 2019, from http://www.massshootingtracker.org/about

Mass Shooting Tracker. (n.d.-b). Data. Retrieved September 2, 2019, from http://www.massshootingtracker.org/data

Matsaganis, M. D., & Golden, A. G. (2015). Interventions to address reproductive health disparities among African-American women in a small urban community: The communicative construction of a "field of health action." *Journal of Applied*

Communication Research, 43(2), 163–184. https://doi.org/10.1080/0090988 2.2015.1019546

Matt Makes Games. (2018a). Celeste. [Video game, Windows, macOS, Linux, Nintendo Switch, PlayStation 4, Xbox One, Stadia]. Matt Makes Games.

Matt Makes Games. (2018b). Celeste press kit [Press release]. Retrieved May 18, 2021, from https://www.dropbox.com/sh/87lycjzncb0o9ns/AACcA3s5Uyzkeicn3-26qLBWa?dl=0

Matthewman, S. (2013). Accidentology: A critical assessment of Paul Virilio's "Political economy of speed." Cultural Politics, 9(3), 280–295. https://doi.org/10.121 5/17432197-2346982

Matthews, C. K., & Harrington, N. G. (2000). Invisible disability. In D. O. Braithwaite & T. L. Thompson (Eds.), Handbook of communication and people with disabilities: Research and application (pp. 405–422). Lawrence Erlbaum.

Matthews, M. (2019). Why Sheldon Cooper can't be black: The visual rhetoric of autism and ethnicity. Journal of Literary & Cultural Disability Studies, 13(1), 57–74. https://doi.org/10.3828/jlcds.2019.4

Mauldin, L. K. (2012). Parents of deaf children with cochlear implants: Disability, medicalization and neuroculture (Publication No. 3508706) [Doctoral dissertation, The City University of New York]. UMI Dissertation Publishing.

May, T. (2016, October 5). Full text: Theresa May's conference speech. The Spectator. Retrieved December 15, 2021, from https://www.spectator.co.uk/article/full-text-theresa-may-s-conservative-conference-speech/amp

Maybe she's born with it. (n.d.). Quickmeme. Retrieved June 1, 2021, from http://www.quickmeme.com/meme/3qrcpc

Mayer-Davis, E. J., Bell, R. A., Dabelea, D., D'Agostino, R., Imperatore, G., Lawrence, J. M., Liu, L., & Marcovina, S. (2009). The many faces of diabetes in American youth: Type 1 and type 2 diabetes in five race and ethnic populations: The search for diabetes in youth study. Diabetes Care, 32(2), S99–S101.

Mayo Clinic. (2020, October 16). Ehlers-Danlos syndrome. Retrieved January 11, 2022, from https://www.mayoclinic.org/diseases-conditions/ehlers-danlos-syndrome/symptoms-causes/syc-20362125

Mazzei, L. A. (2007). Inhabited silence in qualitative research: Putting poststructural theory to work (Vol. 318). Peter Lang.

McCann, D., Plummer, D., & Minichiello, V. (2010). Being the butt of the joke: Homophobic humor, male identity and its connection to emotional and physical violence for men. Health Sociology Review 19(4), 505-521). https://doi.org/10.5172/hesr.2010.1.9.4.505

McCormack, D. P. (2018). Atmospheric things: On the allure of elemental envelopment. Duke University Press.

McCoy, T. (2015, April 29). Freddie Gray's life a study on the effects of lead paint on poor Blacks. The Washington Post. Retrieved November 2, 2021, from https://www.washingtonpost.com/local/freddie-grays-life-a-study-in-the-sad-effects-of-lead-paint-on-poor-blacks/2015/04/29/0be898e6-eea8-11e4-8abc-d6aa3bad79dd_story.html.

McDonnell, A., & Milton, D. (2014). Going with the flow: Reconsidering "repetitive behaviour" through the concept of "flow states." In G. Jones & E. Hurley (Eds.), Good autism practice: Autism, happiness and wellbeing (pp. 38–47). BILD. https://doi.org/10.1080/00909882.2010.490841

McGrail, E., McGrail, J. P., & Rieger, A. (2020). Friday night disability: The portrayal of youthful social interactions in television's Friday Night Lights. *Disability Studies Quarterly, 40*(4). https://doi.org/10.18061/dsq.v40i4.6801

McKee, A. (2003). *Textual analysis: A beginner's guide.* Sage.

McKerrow, R. (1989). Critical rhetoric: Theory and praxis. *Communication Monographs, 56*, 91–111.

McMillan, C. T. (2019). *Thick: And other essays.* The New Press.

McRuer, R. (2006). *Crip theory: Cultural signs of queerness and disability.* New York University Press.

McRuer, R. (2018). *Crip times: Disability, globalization, and resistance.* New York University Press.

Mears, A. (2010). Size zero high-end ethnic: Cultural production and the reproduction of culture in fashion modeling. *Poetics, 38*(1), 21–46. https://doi.org/10.1016/j.poetic.2009.10.002

Mears, A. (2011). *Pricing beauty: The making of a fashion model.* University of California Press.

Medicaid.gov (2020). *Quality of care: Home and community based services (HCBS) waivers.* Retrieved January 5, 2022, from https://www.medicaid.gov/medicaid/quality-of-care/improvement-initiatives/hcbs/index.html

Meffert, E., Tillmanns, E., Heim, S., Jung, S., Huber, W., & Grande, M. (2011). Taboo: A novel paradigm to elicit aphasia-like trouble-indicating behavior in normally speaking individuals. *Journal of Psycholinguistic Research, 40*(307). https://doi.org/10.1007/s10936-011-9170-6

Meisenbach, R. (2010). Stigma management communication: A theory and agenda for applied research on how individuals manage moments of stigmatized identity. *Journal of Applied Communication Research, 38*(3), 268–292. https://doi.org/10.1080/00909882.2010.490841

Meisner, C., & Ledbetter, A. M. (2020). Participatory branding on social media: The affordances of live streaming for creative labor. *New Media & Society.* https://doi.org/10.1177/1461444820972392

Melonçon, L. (2013). Introduction. In L. Melonçon (Ed.), *Rhetorical accessability: At the intersection of technical communication and disability studies* (pp. 1–14). Routledge.

Meltzer, A. L., McNulty, J. K., Jackson, G., & Karney, B. R. (2014). Sex differences in the implications of partner physical attractiveness for the trajectory of marital satisfaction. *Journal of Personality and Social Psychology, 106*(3), 418–428. https://doi.org/10.1037/a0034424

Merleau-Ponty, M. (1962). *Phenomenology of perception.* Routledge.

Metzl, J., Piemonte, J., & McKay, T. (2021). Mental illness, mass shootings, and the future of psychiatric research into American gun violence. *Harvard Review of Psychiatry, 29*(1), 81–89. https://doi.org/10.1097/HRP.0000000000000280

Michalko, R. (2010). What's cool about blindness? *Disability Studies Quarterly, 30*(3/4). https://doi.org/10.18061/dsq.v30i3/4.1296

Microsoft. (n.d.). Seeing AI: An app for visually impaired people that narrates world around you. Retrieved March 22, 2022, from https://www.microsoft.com/en-us/garage/wall-of-fame/seeing-ai/

Miesenberger, K., Ossmann, R., Archambault, D., Searle, G., & Holzinger, A. (2008). More than just a game: Accessibility in computer games. In A. Holzinger (Ed.), *HCI and Usability for Education and Work* (pp. 247–260). Springer.

516   REFERENCES

Miles, A. L. (2019). "Strong black women": African American women with disabilities, intersecting identities, and inequality. *Gender & Society, 33*(1), 41–63. https://doi.org/10.1177/0891243218814820

Miles, P. (2010, May 13). *Service dog v. allergies—ADA accommodation conflict* [Web log post]. Law Office Space. Retrieved January 11, 2022, from https://www.lawfficespace.com/2010/05/service-dog-v-allergies-ada.html

Milford, P. (2019, July 29), Facebook. Retrieved December 10, 2019, from https://m.facebook.com/groups/theverybrexitproblemsclub/permalink/348750549382879/

Mills, M. (2022). *Hearing loss and the history of information theory*. Duke University Press.

Mills, M. L. (2017). Invisible disabilities, visible service dogs: The discrimination of service dog handlers. *Disability & Society, 32*(5), 635–656. https://doi.org/10.1080/09687599.2017.1307718

Milner, R. M. (2012). *The world made meme: Discourse and identity in participatory media* [Dissertation]. University of Kansas.

Milner, R. M. (2016). *The world made meme: Public conversations and participatory media*. The MIT Press.

Milton, D. E. M. (2012). On the ontological status of autism: The 'double empathy problem.' *Disability & Society, 27*(6), 883–887. https://doi.org/10.1080/09687599.2012.710008

Milton, D. E. M., Heasman, B., & Sheppard, E. (2018). Double empathy. In F. Volkmar (Ed.), *Encyclopedia of autism spectrum disorders* (pp. 1–8). Springer.

Milton, D., & Sims, T. (2016). How is a sense of well-being and belonging constructed in the accounts of autistic adults? *Disability and Society, 31*(4), 520–534. https://doi.org/10.1080/09687599.2016.1186529

Mingus, M. (2011, August 22). *Moving toward the ugly: A politic beyond desirability*. Femmes of Color Symposium keynote speech, Oakland, CA. Retrieved February 21, 2022, from http://leavingevidence.wordpress.com/2011/08/22/moving-toward-the-ugly-a-politic-beyond-desirability/

Ministry of Children and Youth Services. (2018). *Language development services guidelines: Ontario Infant Hearing Program* (Version 2018.02). Retrieved January 11, 2022, from https://www.uwo.ca/nca/pdfs/clinical_protocols/IHP%20Language%20Development%20Services%20Guidelines_2018.01.pdf

Ministry of Children, Community and Social Services. (2016). *Ontario Infant Hearing Program screening statistics* [Data set]. Government of Ontario. Retrieved February 2018, from https://data.ontario.ca/dataset/ontario-infant-hearing-program-ihp-screening-statisticsI

Ministry of Children, Community, and Social Services. (2019, July 15). *Protocol for universal newborn hearing screening in Ontario* (Version 2019.01). Retrieved January 11, 2022, from https://www.uwo.ca/nca/pdfs/clinical_protocols/IHP%20Screening%20Protocol%202019.01_Final_July_2019.pdf

Misawa, S. (2011, April 20). Petition for countermeasures against East Japan Great Earthquake and Tsunami disasters. *DPI-Japan*. Retrieved December 5, 2019, from http://dpi.cocolog-nifty.com

Mitchell, D. T., & Snyder, S. L. (2001). *Narrative prosthesis: Disability and the dependencies of discourse*. University of Michigan Press.

Mitchell, D. T., Snyder, S. L., & Ware, L. (2014). "[Every] child left behind": Curricular cripistemologies and the crip/queer art of failure. *Journal of Literary & Cultural Disability Studies, 8*(3), 295–314. https://doi.org/10.3828/jlcds.2014.24

Mitchell, D., & Snyder, S. (2013). Introduction: Disability studies and the double bind of representation. In D. T. Mitchell & S. Snyder (Eds.), *The body and physical difference: Discourses of disability* (pp. 1–31). University of Michigan.

Mizner, S. (2018, May 11). Police "command and control" culture is often lethal—especially for people with disabilities. *American Civil Liberties Union*. Retrieved November 3, from https://www.aclu.org/blog/criminal-law-reform/reforming-police/police-command-and-control-culture-often-lethal-especially

Moher, D., Liberati, A., Tetzlaff, J., & Altman, D. (2009). Preferred reporting items for systematic reviews and meta-analyses: The prisma statement. *Annals of Internal Medicine, 151*(4), 264–269. https://doi.org/10.1136/bmj.b2535

Mol, A. (2008). *The logic of care: Health and the problem of patient choice.* Routledge.

Mollow, A., & McRuer, R. (2012). Introduction. In R. McRuer & A. Mollow (Eds.), *Sex and disability* (pp. 1–36). Duke University Press.

Montgomerie, M. A. (2010). Visibility, empathy and derision. *Popular television representations of disability. Alter, 4*(2), 94–102. https://doi.org/10.1016/j.alter.2010.02.009

Moons, W. G., Chen, J. M., & Mackie, D. M. (2017). Stereotypes: A source of bias in affective and empathic forecasting. *Group Processes & Intergroup Relations, 20*(2), 139–152. https://doi.org/10.1177/1368430215603460

More barrier-free steps urged in disaster zone. (2012, June 27). *The Japan Times.* Retrieved November 30, 2019, from https://www.japantimes.co.jp/news/2012/06/27/national/more-barrier-free-steps-urged-in-disaster-zone/

Morella-Pozzi, D. (2014). The (dis)ability double life: Exploring legitimacy, illegitimacy, and the terrible dichotomy of (dis)ability in higher education. In R. M. Boylorn & M. P. Orbe (Eds.), *Critical autoethnography: Intersecting cultural identities in everyday life* (pp. 176–194). Left Coast Press.

Moreman, S. T. (2019). Accommodating desires of disability: A multi-modal approach to Terry Galloway and the Mickee Faust Club. *QED: A Journal of GLBTQ Worldmaking, 6*(3), 149–162. https://doi.org/10.14321/qed.6.3.0149

Morgan, J. M. (2021). Policing under disability law. *Stanford Law Review, 73*(6), 1401–1405. Retrieved November 1, 2021, from https://www.stanfordlawreview.org/print/article/policing-under-disability-law/

Morris, J., Thompson, N., Lippincott, B., & Lawrence, M. (2019). Accessibility User Research Collective: Engaging consumers in ongoing technology evaluation. *Assistive Technology Outcomes and Benefits, 13*(1), 38–56.

Morris, M. R. (2020). AI and accessibility. *Communications of the ACM, 63*(6), 35–37. https://doi.org/10.1145/3356727

Mortensen, C. D. (1997). *Miscommunication.* Sage.

Mortensen, T. E. (2018). Anger, fear, and games: The long event of #GamerGate. *Games and Culture, 13*(8), 787–806. https://doi.org/10.1177/1555412016640408

Moss, C. (2013). *The myth of persecution.* HarperCollins.

Mottron, L. (2017). Should we change targets and methods of early intervention in autism, in favor of a strengths-based education? *European Child & Adolescent Psychiatry, 26*(7), 815–825. https://doi.org/10.1007/s00787-017-0955-5

Mowatt, R. A., French, B. H., & Malebranche, D. A. (2013). Black/female/body *hypervisibility and invisibility.* A Black feminist augmentation of feminist leisure research. *Journal of Leisure Research, 45*(5), 644–660. https://doi.org/10.18666/jlr-2013-v45-i5-4367

Mulvey, A. (2020, December 9). Aha! An autoimmune disease. *Juvenile Diabetes Research Foundation*. Retrieved February 16, 2022, from https://www.jdrf.org/blog/2020/12/09/aha-autoimmune-disease/

Muñoz, J. E. (2006). Feeling brown, feeling down: Latina affect, the performativity of race, and the depressive position. *Signs: Journal of Women in Culture and Society, 31*(3), 675–688. https://doi.org/10.1086/499080

Muñoz, J. E. (2009). *Cruising utopia: The then and there of queer futurity*. New York University Press.

Muramatsu, R. S., Thomas, K. J., Leong, S. L., & Ragukonis, F. (2015). Service dogs, psychiatric hospitalization, and the ADA. *Psychiatric Services, 66*(1). Online publication. https://doi.org/10.1176/appi.ps.201400208

Murray, D., Lesser, M., & Lawson, W. (2005). Attention, monotropism and the diagnostic criteria for autism. *Autism, 9*(2), 139–156. https://doi.org/10.1177/1362361305051398

Murray, F. (2019, August). Me and monotropism. *Psychologist*, 44–48. https://thepsychologist.bps.org.uk/volume-32/august-2019/me-and-monotropism-unified-theory-autism

Murray, J. H. (1998). *Hamlet on the holodeck. The future of narrative in cyberspace*. MIT Press.

Nagle, A. (2017). *Kill all normies: The online culture wars from Tumblr and 4chan to the alt-right and Trump*. Zero Books.

Nakada, M., Kavathatzopoulos, I., & Asai, R. (2021). Robots and AI artifacts in plural perspective(s) of Japan and the West: The cultural–ethical traditions behind people's views on robots and AI artifacts in the information era. *Review of Socionetwork Strategies, 15*, 143–168. https://doi.org/10.1007/s12626-021-00067-8

Nakamura, K. (2009). Disability, destitution, and disaster: Surviving the 1995 Great Hanshin Earthquake in Japan. *Human Organization, 68*(1), 82–88. https://doi.org/10.17730/humo.68.1.bp20n6110341168x

Nakamura, K. (2019). My algorithms have determined you're not human: AI-ML, Reverse Turing Tests, and the disability experience. In J. P. Bigham (Ed.), *ASSETS '19: The 21st International ACM SIGACCESS Conference on Computers and Accessibility* (pp. 1–2). https://doi.org/10.1145/3308561.3353812

Naples, N. A., Mauldin, L., & Dillaway, H. (2019). From the guest editors: Gender, disability, and intersectionality. *Gender & Society, 33*(1), 5–18. https://doi.org/10.1177/0891243218813309

Nasim, R. (2010). Yahav's story: My way of living with Tourette's. *International Journal of Narrative Therapy & Community Work, 4*, 23–42.

Naslund, J. A., Aschbrenner, K. A., Marsch, L. A., & Bartels, S. J. (2016). The future of mental health care: Peer-to-peer support and social media. *Epidemiology and Psychiatric Sciences, 25*(2), 113–122. https://doi.org/10.1017/S2045796015001067

National Council on Disability. (2006). *The Impact of Hurricanes Katrina and Rita on people with disabilities: A look back and remaining challenges*. Retrieved December 5, 2019, from http://www.ncd.gov/publications/2006/Aug072006

National Institute of Justice. (2020, March). *Overview of police use of force*. Retrieved November 1, 2021, from https://nij.ojp.gov/topics/articles/overview-police-use-force

National Organization on Disability. (2006). *Report on Special Needs Assessment for Katrina Evacuees (SNAKE) Project*. Retrieved November 15, 2019, from https://www.preventionweb.net/files/9005_katrinasnakereport.pdf

Naughty Dog. (2016). *Uncharted 4: A Thief's End*. [Video game, PlayStation 4]. Sony Interactive Studio.

Naughty Dog. (2020). *The Last of Us 2*. [Video game, PlayStation 4]. Sony Interactive Studio.

Neely, E. L. (2017). No player is ideal: Why video game designers cannot ethically ignore players' real-world identities. *ACM SIGCAS Computers and Society, 47*(3), 98–111. https://doi.org/10.1145/3144592.3144602

Ne'eman, A., Stein, M. A., Berger, Z. D., & Dorfman, D. (2021). The treatment of disability under crisis standards of care: An empirical and normative analysis of change over time during COVID-19. *Journal of Health Political Policy Law, 46*(5), 831–860. https://doi.org/10.1215/03616878-9156005

Neilsen, L. (2008). Lyric inquiry. In J. G. Knowles & A. L. Cole (Eds.), *Handbook of the arts in qualitative research* (pp. 93–102). Sage Publications.

Nemeth, S. (2000). Society, sexuality, and disabled/ablebodied romantic relationships. In D. O. Braithwaite & T. L. Thompson (Eds.), *Handbook of communication and people with disabilities* (pp. 37–65). Lawrence Erlbaum.

Newman, J. (2021). Southern Ohio Police Department warns of fake handicap placards selling on marketplace. *SCIOTO Post.* (May 26). https://www.sciotopost.com/southern-ohio-police-department-warns-of-fake-handicap-placards-selling-on-marketplace/

Newzoo. (2021, July 1). *Newzoo Global Games Market Report 2021.* Retrieved January 2, 2022, from https://newzoo.com/insights/trend-reports/newzoo-global-games-market-report-2021-free-version/

Nichols, B. (1988). The work of culture in the age of cybernetic systems. *Screen (London), 29*(1), 22–47. https://doi.org/10.1093/screen/29.1.22

Nicolaidis, C., Raymaker, D. M., McDonald, K. E., Baggs, W. A. E. V., Dern, S., Kapp, S. K., Weiner, M., Boisclair, C., & Ashkenazy, E. (2015). "Respect the way I need to communicate with you": Healthcare experiences of adults on the autism spectrum. *Autism, 19*(7), 824–831. https://doi.org/10.1177/1362361315576221

Nissenbaum, A., & Shifman, L. (2017). Internet memes as contested cultural capital: The case of 4chan's /b/ board. *New Media & Society, 19*(4), 483–501. https://doi.org/10.1177/1461444815609313

Njelesani, J., Cleaver, S., & Tataryn, M. (2014). Practical strategies to meet the rights of persons with disabilities in disaster management initiatives. In D. Mitchell & V. Karr (Eds.), *Crises, conflict and disability: Ensuring equality* (pp. 84–89). Routledge. https://doi.org/10.4324/9780203069943

Norman, D. (2013). *The design of everyday things*. Basic Books.

O'Meara, V. (2019). Weapons of chic: Instagram influencer engagement pods as practices of resistance to Instagram platform labor. *Social Media & Society, 5*(4), 1–11. https://doi.org/10.1177/2056305119879671

O'Hara, K. (2004). "Curb cuts" on the information highway: Older adults and the internet. *Technical Communication Quarterly, 13*(4), 426–445. https://doi.org/10.1207/s15427625tcq1304_4

Oliver, M. (1983). *Social work with disabled people*. Macmillan Education.

Oliver, M. (1996). *Understanding disability: From theory to practice*. Macmillan Education.

Oliver, M. & Barnes, C. (2012). *The new politics of disablement*. Macmillan.

520 REFERENCES

Olkin, R., H'Sien, H., Schaff Abbene, M., & VanHeel, G. (2019). The experiences of microaggressions against women with visible and invisible disabilities. *Journal of Social Issues, 75*(3), 757–785. https://doi.org/10.1111/josi.12342

Onaiwu, M. G. (2017a). Don't let them be Autistic. In L. X. Z. Brown, E. Ashkenazy, & M. Giwa Onaiwu (Eds.), *All the weight of our dreams: On living racialized autism* (pp. 85–87). DragonBee Press.

Onaiwu, M. G. (2017b). Preface: Autistics of color: We exist....we matter. In L. X. Z. Brown, E. Ashkenazy, & M. Giwa Onaiwu (Eds.). *All the weight of our dreams: On living racialized autism* (pp. x–xxii). DragonBee Press.

Ontario Ministry of Health and Long-Term Care. (2001). Infant Hearing Program: Universal infant hearing screening assessment and communication development: Local implementation support document.

Ontario Ministry of Health and Long-Term Care. (2002). *Infant Hearing Program: Well-baby (DPOAE) screening protocol and training manual.* Retrieved June 2016, from www.mountsinai.on.ca/care/infant-hearing-program/documents/midwives-protocol.pdf

Orange, L. M. (2009). Sexuality and disability. In M.G. Brodwin, F.W. Siu, J. Howard, & E.R. Brodwin (Eds.). *Medical, psychosocial, and vocational aspects of disability* (3rd ed., pp. 263–272). Elliott & Fitzpatrick.

Osamu, N. (2014). The paradox of community-living and disaster. In D. Mitchell & V. Karr (Eds.), *Crises, conflict and disability: Ensuring equality* (pp. 142–146). Routledge. https://doi.org/10.4324/9780203069943

Ostiguy, B. J., Peters, M. L., & Shlasko, D. (2016). Ableism. In M. Adams, L. A. Bell, D. J. Goodman, & K. Y. Joshi (Eds.), *Teaching for diversity and social justice* (3rd ed., pp. 299–337). Routledge.

Oswal, S. K. (2014). Participatory design: Barriers and possibilities. *Communication Design Quarterly, 2*(3), 14–19. https://doi.org/10.1145/2644448.2644452

Oswal, S. K., & Hewett, B. L. (2013). Accessibility challenges for visually impaired students and their online writing instructors. In L. Melonçon (Ed.), *Rhetorical accessability: At the intersection of technical communication and disability studies* (pp. 135–156). Routledge.

Oswal, S. K., & Melonçon, L. (2014). Paying attention to accessibility when designing online courses in technical and professional communication. *Journal of Business and Technical Communication, 28*(3), 271–300. https://doi.org/10.117 7/2F1050651914524780

Oswal, S. K., & Melonçon, L. (2017). *Saying no to the checklist: Shifting from an ideology of normalcy to an ideology of inclusion in online writing instruction.* WPA: *Writing Program Administration-Journal of the Council of Writing Program Administrators, 40*(3) https://wpacouncil.org/aws/CWPA/asset_manager/get_file/400647?ver=526

Oswald, A. G., Avory, S., & Fine, M. (2021, March 2). Intersectional expansiveness born at the neuroqueer nexus. *Psychology & Sexuality.* Advance online publication. https://doi.org/10.1080/19419899.2021.1900347

Otake, T. (2013, March 10). Filmmaker captures the 3/11 stress of Tohoku's deaf. *The Japan Times.* Retrieved November 30, 2019, from https://www.japantimes.co.jp/culture/2013/03/10/films/.filmmaker-captures-the-311-stress-of-tohokus-deaf/

Owen, P. R. (2012). Portrayals of schizophrenia by entertainment media: A content analysis of contemporary movies. *Psychiatric Services, 63*(7), 655–659. https://doi.org/10.1176/appi.ps.201100371

Owens, D. C. (2021). Listening to Black women saves Black lives. *The Lancet, 397*(10276), 788–789. https://doi.org/10.1016/S0140-6736(21)00367-6

Pacanowsky, M. E., & O'Donnell-Trujillo, N. (1982). Communication and organizational cultures. *Western Journal of Speech Communication, 46*(2), 115–130. https://doi.org/10.1080/10570318209374072

Pacanowsky, M. E., & O'Donnell-Trujillo, N. (1983). Organizational communication as cultural performance. *Communication Monographs, 50*(2), 126–147. https://doi.org/10.1080/03637758309390158

Pacanowsky, M. E., & O'Donnell-Trujillo, N. (1990). Communication and organizational cultures. In S. R. Corman, S. P. Banks, C. R. Bantz, & M. E. Mayer (Eds.), *Foundations of organizational communication* (pp. 142–153). Longman.

Padden, C. (2015). Communication. In R. Adams, B. Reiss, & D. Serlin (Eds.), *Keywords for disability studies* (pp. 43–45). New York University Press.

Palmeri, J. (2006). Disability studies, cultural analysis, and the critical practice of technical communication pedagogy. *Technical Communication Quarterly, 15*(1), 49–65. https://doi.org/10.1207/s15427625tcq1501_5

Park, S., & Humphry, J. (2019). Exclusion by design: Intersections of social, digital and data exclusion. *Information, Communication & Society, 22*(7), 934–953. https://doi.org/10.1080/1369118X.2019.1606266

Parker, R. (2009). Sexuality, culture and society: Shifting paradigms in sexuality research. *Culture, Health & Sexuality, 11*(3), 251–266. https://doi.org/10.1080/13691050701606941

Parsons, A. L., Reichl, A. J., & Pedersen, C. L. (2017). Gendered ableism: Media representations and gender role beliefs' effect on perceptions of disability and sexuality. *Sexuality and Disability, 35*(2), 207–225. https://doi.org/10.1007/s11195-016-9464-6

Partlow, K. (2019, August). *12 misconceptions about service dogs and those who use them.* Animal Health Foundation. Retrieved January 11, 2022, from https://www.animalhealthfoundation.org/blog/2019/08/12-misconceptions-about-service-dogs-and-those-who-use-them/?sfw=pass1640721218

Pasquale, F. (2015). *The black box society: The secret algorithms that control money and information.* Harvard University Press.

Pasquale, F. (2020). *New laws of robotics.* Harvard University Press.

Pass, E. (2013). Accessibility and the web design student. In L. Melonçon (Ed.), *Rhetorical accessability: At the intersection of technical communication and disability studies* (pp. 115–134). Routledge.

Pate, E. (2017). The middle, or—The Mestiza and the coffee shop. In L. X. Z. Brown, E. Ashkenazy, & M. Giwa Onaiwu (Eds.), *All the weight of our dreams: On living racialized autism* (pp. 221–240). DragonBee Press.

Paterson, K. (2012). It's about time! Understanding the experience of speech impairment. In A. Roulstone, C. Thomas, & N. Watson (Eds.), *Routledge handbook of disability studies* (pp. 165–177). Routledge.

Pathakji, N. (2018). *Corporations and disability rights: Bridging the digital divide.* Oxford University Press.

Paul, C. A. (2018). *The toxic meritocracy of video games: Why gaming culture is the worst.* University of Minnesota Press. https://doi.org/10.5749/j.ctt2204rbz

Payne, B. M. (2010). Your art is gay and retarded: Eliminating discriminating speech against homosexual and intellectually disabled students in the secondary arts education classroom. *Art Education, 63*(5), 52–55. https://doi.org/10.1080/0004312 5.2010.11519088

Payne, D. A., Hickey, H., Nelson, A., Rees, K., Bollinger, H., & Hartley, S. (2016). Physically disabled women and sexual identity: A photovoice study. *Disability & Society, 31*(8), 1030–1049. https://doi.org/10.1080/09687599.2016.1230044

Pelias, R. J. (2021). *Lessons on aging and dying: A poetic autoethnography.* Routledge.

Pelisek, C. (2021, September 30). Deaf Colorado man says he was arrested after not obeying police commands he couldn't hear: Lawsuit. *People.com.* Retrieved October 30, 2021, from. https://people.com/crime/deaf-colorado-man-arrested-not-obeying-police-commands-could-not-hear-lawsuit/

Pérez-Latorre, Ó., Oliva, M., & Besalú, R. (2017). Videogame analysis: A social-semiotic approach. *Social Semiotics, 27*(5), 586–603. https://doi.org/10.108 0/10350330.2016.1191146

Perlin, M. L., & Lynch, A. J. (2016). *Sexuality, disability, and the law: Beyond the last frontier?* Palgrave Macmillan.

Pernick, M. S. (1996). *The black stork: Eugenics and the death of "defective" babies in American medicine and motion pictures since 1915.* Oxford University Press.

Perrow, C. (1999). *Normal accidents: Living with high-risk technologies.* Princeton University Press.

Perry, D. M. (2017, September 25). 4 disabled people dead in another week of police brutality. *The Nation.* Retrieved November 1, 2021, from https://www.thenation.com/article/four-disabled-dead-in-another-week-of-police-brutality/

Perry, D. M., & Carter-Long, L. (2014, May 6). How misunderstanding disability leads to police violence. *The Atlantic.* Retrieved November 21, 2021, from https://www.theatlantic.com/health/archive/2014/05/misunderstanding-disability-leads-to-police-violence/361786/

Perry, D. M., & Carter-Long, L. (2016). *The Ruderman White paper on media coverage of law enforcement use of force and disability.* Retrieved October 31, 2021, from https://rudermanfoundation.org/wp-content/uploads/2017/08/MediaStudy-PoliceDisability_final-final.pdf

Petri, G., Beadle-Brown, J., & Bradshaw, J. (2017). "More Honoured in the Breach than in the Observance"—Self-advocacy and human rights. *Laws, 6*(4), 26. https://doi.org/10.3390/laws6040026

Petri, G., Beadle-Brown, J., & Bradshaw, J. (2020). Redefining self-advocacy: A practice theory-based approach. *Journal of Policy and Practice in Intellectual Disabilities, 17*(3), 207–218. https://doi.org/10.1111/jppi.12343

Petronio, S. S. (2002). *Boundaries of privacy: Dialectics of disclosure.* State University of New York Press.

Pettinicchio, D. (2019). *Politics of empowerment: Disability rights and the cycle of American policy reform.* Stanford University Press.

Phair, D. (2017). Unpacking the diagnostic TARDIS. In L. X. Z. Brown, E. Ashkenazy, & M. Giwa Onaiwu (Eds.), *All the weight of our dreams: On living racialized autism* (pp. 336–344). DragonBee Press.

Phạm, M. T. (2015). *Asians wear clothes on the internet: Race, gender, and the work of personal style blogging.* Duke University Press.

Philaretou, A. G., & Allen, K. R. (2001). Reconstructing masculinity and sexuality. *The Journal of Men's Studies, 9*(3), 301–321. https://doi.org/10.3149/jms.0903.301

Phillips, M. (2016). Service and emotional support animals on campus: The relevance and controversy. *Research and Teaching in Developmental Education, 33*(1), 96–99. Retrieved January 11, 2022, from http://www.jstor.org/stable/44290251

Phillips, M. J. (1990). Damaged goods: Oral narratives of the experience of disability in American culture. *Social Science & Medicine, 30*(8), 849–857.

Pickens, T. A. (2019). *Black madness: Mad blackness.* Duke University Press.

Piepzna-Samarasinha, L. L. (2018). *Care work: Dreaming disability justice.* Arsenal Pulp Press.

Pierce, C. (1970). Offensive mechanisms. In F. Barbour (Ed.), *The black seventies* (pp. 265–282). Porter Sargent.

Pierce, K. L. (2018, October 8). *Understanding and working with service dog handlers.* Counseling Today. Retrieved January 11, 2022, from https://ct.counseling.org/2018/10/understanding-and-working-with-service-dog-handlers/

Pitaru, A. (2008). E is for everyone: The case for inclusive game design. In K. Salen (Ed.), *The Ecology of Games: Connecting Youth, Games, and Learning* (pp. 67–86). MIT Press. https://doi.org/10.1162/dmal.9780262693646.06

PlayStation. (2020). *The Last of Us Part II.* Retrieved May 18, 2021, from https://www.playstation.com/en-ca/games/the-last-of-us-part-ii/

Polkinghorne, D. E. (1995). Narrative configuration in qualitative analysis. *International Journal of Qualitative Studies in Education, 8*(1), 5–23. https://doi.org/10.1080/0951839950080103

Porter, G. L., & Richler, D. (1991). *Changing Canadian schools: Perspectives on disability and inclusion.* The Roeher Institute.

Porter, J. R., & Kientz, J. A. (2013). An empirical study of issues and barriers to mainstream video game accessibility. *Proceedings of the 15th International ACM SIGACCESS Conference on Computers and Accessibility—ASSETS '13*, 1–8. https://doi.org/10.1145/2513383.2513444

Potato girl—Quickmeme. (n.d.). Me.Me. Retrieved June 1, 2021, from https://me.me/i/all-these-memes-ace-got-me-feeling-downs-quickmeme-com-all

Potts, L., & Salvo, M. (Eds.). (2017). *Rhetoric and experience architecture.* Parlor Press.

Powell, A., Overington, C., & Hamilton, G. (2018). Following #JillMeagher: Collective meaning-making in response to crime events via social media. *Crime, Media, Culture, 14*(3), 409–428. https://doi.org/10.1177/1741659017721276

Prendergast, M., Leggo, C., & Sameshima, P. (2009). *Poetic inquiry: Vibrant voices in the social sciences.* Sense.

Price, M. (2011). *Mad at school: Rhetorics of mental disability and academic life.* University of Michigan Press.

Price, M., & Kerschbaum, S. L. (2016). Stories of methodology: Interviewing sideways, crooked and crip. *Canadian Journal of Disability Studies, 5*(3), 18–56. https://doi.org/10.15353/cjds.v5i3.295

Primrose v. The Western Union Telegraph Co., 154 U.S. 1 (1894). Retrieved March 11, 2021, from https://supreme.justia.com/cases/federal/us/154/1/

Pritchard, E. (2017). Cultural representations of dwarfs and their disabling effects on dwarfs in society. *Considering Disability, 1*, 1–31, file:///C:/Users/M706A~1.JEF/AppData/Local/Temp/1985-cultural-representations-of-dwarfs-and-their-disabling-affects-on-dwarfs-in-society-1.pdf

Protevi, J. (2009). *Political affect: Connecting the social and the somatic.* University of Minnesota Press.

524 REFERENCES

Prouty, R. W., Smith, G., & Lakin, K. C. (2003). *Residential services for persons with developmental disabilities: Status and trends through 2002.* Retrieved December 1, 2019, from https://rtc.umn.edu/docs/RISP2007.pdf

Przybylo, E. (2011). Crisis and safety: The asexual in sexusociety. *Sexualities, 14*(4), 444. https://doi.org/10.1177/1363460711406461

Przybylo, E. (2016). Asexuals against the Cis-tem! *Transgender Studies Quarterly, 3*(3-4), 653–660. https://doi.org/10.1215/23289252-3545347

Puar, J. K. (2009). Prognosis time: Towards a geopolitics of affect, debility and capacity. *Women & Performance: A Journal of Feminist Theory, 19*(2), 161–172. https://doi.org/10.1080/07407700903034147

Puar, J. K. (2017). *The right to maim: Debility, capacity, disability.* Duke University Press.

Pucket, J., Tregde, D., & Spry Jr., T. (2020, June 25). VERIFY: Face mask exemption cards are fake. *9 news.* https://www.9news.com/article/news/verify/verify-fraudulent-face-mask-exempt-card-doesnt-actually-do-anything/

Pullin, G. (2009). *Design meets disability.* MIT.

Putnam, M. (2005). Conceptualizing disability: Developing a framework for political disability identity. *Journal of Disability Policy Studies, 16*(3), 188–198.

Putnam, R. (1993). The prosperous community: Social capital and public life. *The American Prospect, 13*(4), 249–263. Retrieved January 5, 2022, from http://www.prospect.org/print/vol/13

Rains, S. A. (2018). *Coping with illness digitally.* MIT Press.

Rambo, C. (2007). Sketching as autoethnographic practice. *Symbolic Interaction, 30*(4), 531–542. https://doi.org/10.1525/si.2007.30.4.531

Rasmussen, M. L. (2004). "That's so gay!": A study of the deployment of signifiers of sexual and gender identity in secondary school settings in Australia and the United States. *Social Semiotics, 14*(3), 289–308. https://doi.org/10.1080/10350330408629681

Raw video released of Rob Ford smoking crack. (2016, August 11). [Newspaper]. *The Globe and Mail.* Retrieved May 30, 2021, from https://www.theglobeandmail.com/canada/toronto/video-video-raw-video-released-of-rob-ford-smoking-crack/

Ray, D. S., & Ray, E. J. (1998). Adaptive technologies for the visually impaired: The role of technical communicators. *Technical Communication, 45*(4), 573–579. https://www.jstor.org/stable/43088583

Raymaker, D. M. (2020). Shifting the system: AASPIRE and the loom of science and activism. In S. K. Kapp (Ed.), *Autistic community and the neurodiversity movement: Stories from the frontline* (pp. 133–144). Palgrave Macmillan. https://doi.org/10.1007/978-981-13-8437-0

Reagan, T. (2011). Ideological barriers to American Sign Language: Unpacking linguistic resistance. *Sign Language Studies, 11*(4), 606–636. https://doi.org/10.1353/sls.2011.0006

redhatGizmo. (2019, April 12). *Video game difficulty is an accessibility issue.* [Online forum post]. Reddit. Retrieved May 18, 2021, from https://www.reddit.com/r/gaming/comments/bcbg1g/video_game_difficulty_is_an_accessibility_issue/

Redmon Bray. (2012, April 25). *Round 2.* Know Your Meme. Retrieved May 30, 2021, from https://knowyourmeme.com/photos/291683-i-can-count-to-potato

Reed-Danahay, D. (1997). *Auto/ethnography: Rewriting the self and the social.* Berg.

Resene, M. (2017). From evil queen to disabled teen: Frozen introduces Disney's first disabled princess. *Disability Studies Quarterly, 37*(2). https://doi.org/10.18061/dsq.v37i2.5310

Retznik, L., Wienholz, S., Seidel, A., Pantenburg, B., Conrad, I., Michel, M., & Riedel-Heller, S. (2017). Relationship status: Single? Young adults with visual, hearing, or physical disability and their experiences with partnership and sexuality. *Sexuality & Disability, 35*(4), 415–432. https://doi.org/10.1007/s11195-017-9497-5

Reynolds, J. M. (2017). "I'd rather be dead than disabled"—The ableist conflation and the meanings of disability. *Review of Communication, 17*(3), 149–163. https://doi.org/10.1080/15358593.2017.133125

Rice, C., Chandler, E., Liddiard, K., Rinaldi, J., & Harrison, E. (2018). Pedagogical possibilities for unruly bodies. *Gender and Education, 30*(5), 663–682. https://doi.org/10.1080/09540253.2016.1247947

Rich, A. (1980). Compulsory heterosexuality and lesbian existence. *Signs, 5*(4), 631–660.

Richards, D., Miodrag, N., & Watson, S. L. (2006). Sexuality and developmental disability: Obstacles to healthy sexuality throughout the lifespan. *Developmental Disabilities Bulletin, 34*(1-2), 137–155.

Richards, M.-L. (2018). Hyper-visible invisibility: Tracing the politics, poetics and affects of the unseen. *Field Journal, 7*(1), 39–52. Retrieved January 11, 2022, from http://field-journal.org/wp-content/uploads/2018/01/3-Hyper-visible-Invisibility.pdf

Richards, R. (2008). Writing the othered self: Autoethnography and the problem of objectification in writing about illness and disability. *Qualitative Health Research, 18*(12), 1717–1728. https://doi.org/10.1177/1049732308325866

Richardson, L. (1994). Writing as a method of inquiry. In N. K. Denzin & Y. S. Lincoln (Eds.), *Handbook of Qualitative Research* (pp. 516–529). Sage.

Richardson, L. (2003). Writing: A method of inquiry. In Y. S. Lincoln & N. K. Denzin (Eds.), *Turning points in qualitative research: Tying knots in a handkerchief* (pp. 379–396). AltaMira Press.

Riessman, C. K. (2008). *Narrative methods for the human sciences.* Sage.

Rintala, D. H., Matamoros, R., & Seitz, L. L. (2008). Effects of assistance dogs on persons with mobility or hearing impairments: A pilot study. *Journal of Rehabilitation Research and Development, 45*(4), 489–504. https://doi.org/10.1682/JRRD.2007.06.0094

Rivera, G. N., Smith, C. M., & Schlegel, R. J. (2019). A window to the true self: The importance of I-sharing in romantic relationships. *Journal of Social & Personal Relationships, 36*(6), 1640–1650. https://doi.org/10.1177/0265407518769435

Roberge, J., & Castelle, M. (Eds.) (2021). *The cultural life of machine learning: An incursion into critical AI studies.* Springer.

Rodriguez, K. E., Bibbo, J., & O'Haire, M. E. (2020a). The effects of service dogs on psychosocial health and wellbeing for individuals with physical disabilities or chronic conditions. *Disability and Rehabilitation, 42*(10), 1350–1358. https://doi.org/10.1080/09638288.2018.1524520

Rodriguez, K. E., Greer, J., Yatcilla, J. K., Beck, A. M., & O'Haire, M. E. (2020b). The effects of assistance dogs on psychosocial health and wellbeing: A systematic literature review. *PloS ONE, 15*(12), e0243302. https://doi.org/10.1371/journal.pone.0243302

Roffee, J., & Wailing, A. (2016). Rethinking microaggressions and anti-social behavior against LGBTIQ+ youth. *Safer Communities, 15*(4), 190–201. https://doi.org/10.1108/SC-02-2016-0004

Romaniuk, O., & Terán, L. (2022). First impression sexual scripts of romantic encounters: Effect of gender on verbal and non verbal immediacy behaviors in American media dating culture. *Journal of Social and Personal Relationships, 39*(2), 107–131. https://doi.org/10.1177/02654075211033036

Ronai, C. R. (1995). Multiple reflections of child sex abuse: An argument for a layered account. *Journal of Contemporary Ethnography, 23*(4), 395–426. https://doi.org/10.1177/089124195023004001

Rosa, H. (2003). Social acceleration: Ethical and political consequences of a desynchronized high-speed society. *Constellations, 10*(1), 3–33. https://doi.org/10.1111/1467-8675.00309

Rose, E. J. (2016). Design as advocacy: Using a human-centered approach to investigate the needs of vulnerable populations. *Journal of Technical Writing and Communication, 46*(4), 427–445. https://doi.org/10.1177/2F0047281616653494

Rose, H., & Conama, J. B. (2018). Linguistic imperialism: Still a valid construct in relation to language policy for Irish Sign Language. *Language Policy, 17*(3), 385–404. https://doi.org/10.1007/s10993-017-9446-2

Roth, W. D. (2016). The multiple dimensions of race. *Ethnic and Racial Studies, 39*(8), 1310–1338. https://doi.org/10.1080/01419870.2016.1140793

Rouhban, B. (2014). Natural hazards: Enhancing disaster preparedness and resilience of people with disabilities. In D. Mitchell & V. Karr (Eds.), *Crises, conflict and disability: Ensuring equality* (pp. 75–83). Routledge. https://doi.org/10.4324/9780203069943

Roulstone, A. (2016). *Disability and technology: An interdisciplinary and international approach*. Palgrave Macmillan.

Rubin, S., Biklen, D., Kasa-Hendrickson, C., Kluth, P., Cardinal, D. N., & Broderick, A. (2001). Independence, participation, and the meaning of intellectual ability. *Disability & Society, 16*(3), 415–429. https://doi.org/10.1080/09687590120045969

Rupar, A. (2019, August 5). "Mental illness and hatred pulls (*sic.*) the trigger": Trump's speech about shootings ignored the real problem. *Vox*. http://www.vox.com/2019/8/5/20754770/trump-el-paso-dayton-speech-white-house-mental-illness-video-games-guns

Russell, G. (2020). Critiques of the neurodiversity movement. In S. K. Kapp (Ed.), *Autistic community and the neurodiversity movement: Stories from the frontline* (pp. 287–303). Palgrave Macmillan. https://doi.org/10.1007/978-981-13-8437-0

Ryan, E. B., Anas, A. P., & Gruneir, A. J. S. (2006). Evaluations of overhelping and underhelping communication: Do old age and physical disability matter? *Journal of Language & Social Psychology, 25*(1), 97–107. https://doi.org/10.1177/0261927X05284485

Ryan, E. B., Bajorek, S., Beaman, A., & Anas, A. P. (2005). "I just want you to know that 'them' is me": Intergroup perspectives on communication and disability. In J. Harwood & H. Giles (Eds.), *Intergroup communication: Multiple perspectives* (pp. 117–140). Peter Lang. https://doi.org/10.1177/0261927X05284485

Ryan, S., & Räisänena, U. (2008). "It's like you are just a spectator in this thing": Experiencing social life the "aspie" way. *Emotion, Space and Society, 1*(2), 135–143. https://doi.org/10.1016/j.emospa.2009.02.001

SAC. (2010). *SAC Position paper on universal newborn hearing screening in Canada*. Retrieved January 10, 2022, from https://www.sac-oac.ca/professional-resources/resource-library/sac-position-paper-universal-newborn-hearing-screening-2010?_ga=2.220293402.382556165.1641852772-1275366536.1641852772

SAC. (2018a). *About SAC*. Retrieved April 2018, from https://www.sac-oac.ca/about-sac/about-sac

SAC. (2018b). *SAC position paper on cochlear implants in children.* Retrieved January 11, 2022, from https://www.sac-oac.ca/sites/default/files/resources/SAC-OAC-Cochlear_Implants_PP_EN.pdf

Sætra, H. S. (2021). AI in context and the Sustainable Development Goals: Factoring in the unsustainability of the sociotechnical system. *Sustainability, 13*(4), 1738. https://doi.org/10.3390/su13041738

Saldaña, J. (2009). *The coding manual for qualitative researchers.* Sage.

Saldaña, J. (2016). *The coding manual for qualitative research* (3rd ed.). Sage.

Salen, K., & Zimmerman, E. (2004). *Rules of play: Game design fundamentals.* MIT Press.

Salter, M. (2018). From geek masculinity to gamergate: The technological rationality of online abuse. *Crime, Media, Culture, 14*(2), 247–264. https://doi.org/10.1177/1741659017690893

Samsung. (2021). Accessibility for everyone. Retrieved March 22, 2022, from https://www.design.samsung.com/global/contents/accessibility_design/

Samuels, E. (2014). *Fantasies of identification: Disability, gender, race.* New York University Press.

Samuels, E. (2017). Six ways of looking at crip time. *Disability Studies Quarterly, 37*(3) https://dsq-sds.org/article/view/5824/4684

San Pedro, T. J. (2015). Silence as shields: Agency and resistances among Native American students in the urban Southwest. *Research in the Teaching of English, 50*(2), 132–153. https://www.jstor.org/stable/24890030

Sandahl, C. (2003). Queering the crip or cripping the queer? Intersections of queer and crip identities in solo autobiographical performance. *GLQ: A Journal of Lesbian and Gay Studies, 9*(1-2), 25–56. https://muse.jhu.edu/article/40804

Sandahl, C. (2006). More than just funny: Reading Galloway from a disability perspective. *Liminalities: A Journal of Performance Studies, 2*(3), 1–7. http://liminalities.net/2-3/san.htm

Sandahl, C. (2008). Why disability identity matters: From dramaturgy to casting in John Belluso's *Pyretown. Text and Performance Quarterly, 28*(1–2), 225–241. https://doi.org/10.1080/10462930701754481

Sandahl, C. (2018). Using our words: Exploring representational conundrums in disability drama and performance. *Journal of Literary & Cultural Disability Studies, 12*(2), 129–144. https://doi.org/10.3828/jlcds.2018.11

Sandry, E. (2020). Interdependence in collaboration with robots. In K. Ellis, G. Goggin, B. Haller, & R. Curtis (Eds.), *Routledge companion to disability and media* (pp. 316–326). Routledge.

Sarrett, J. C. (2018). Autism and accommodations in higher education: Insights from the autism community. *Journal of Autism & Developmental Disorders, 48*(3), 679–693. https://doi.org/10.1007/s10803-017-3353-4

Sass, J. S. (2000). Emotional labor as cultural performance: The communication of caregiving in a nonprofit nursing home. *Western Journal of Communication, 64*(3), 330–358. https://doi.org/10.1080/10570310009374679

Saul, R. (2010). KevJumba and the adolescence of YouTube. *Educational Studies, 46*(5), 457–477. https://doi.org/10.1080/00131946.2010.510404

Schoenfeld-Tacher, R., Hellyer, P., Cheung, L., & Kogan, L. (2017). Public perceptions of service dogs, emotional support dogs, and therapy dogs. *International Journal of Environmental Research and Public Health, 14*(6), 642. https://doi.org/10.3390/ijerph14060642

Schreiner, N., Pick, D., & Kenning, P. (2018). To share or not to share? Explaining willingness to share in the context of social distance. *Journal of Consumer Behaviour, 17*(4), 366–378. https://doi.org/10.1002/cb.1717

Scott, J. B. (2003). *Risky rhetoric: AIDS and the cultural practices of HIV testing.* Southern Illinois University Press.

Scott, J.-A. (2012). "Cripped" heroes: An analysis of physically disabled professionals' narratives of performance of identity. *Southern Communication Journal, 77*(4), 307–328. https://doi.org/10.1080/1041794X.2012.673852

Scott, J.-A. (2013). Problematizing a researcher's performance of "insider status": An autoethnography of "designer disabled" identity. *Qualitative Inquiry, 19*(2), 101–115. https://doi.org/10.1177/1077800412462990

Scott, J.-A. (2018). *Embodied performance as applied research, art and pedagogy.* Palgrave Macmillan.

Scott, J.-A. (2020). Disrupting compulsory performances: Snapshots and stories of masculinity, disability, and parenthood in cultural currents of daily life. In A. L. Johnson & B. LeMaster (Eds.), *Gender futurity, intersectional autoethnography: Embodied theorizing from the margins* (pp. 24–36). Routledge.

scwizard, & Sophie. (2010, September 27). *Limes guy / Why can't I hold all these limes?* Know Your Meme. Retrieved May 30, 2021, from https://knowyourmeme.com/memes/limes-guy-why-cant-i-hold-all-these-limes

Segev, E., Nissenbaum, A., Stolero, N., & Shifman, L. (2015). Families and networks of Internet memes: The relationship between cohesiveness, uniqueness, and quiddity concreteness. *Journal of Computer-Mediated Communication, 20*(4), 417–433. https://doi.org/10.1111/jcc4.12120

Seidel, K. (2020). Neurodiversity.com: A decade of advocacy. In S. K. Kapp (Ed.), *Autistic community and the neurodiversity movement: Stories from the frontline* (pp. 89–107). Palgrave Macmillan. https://doi.org/10.1007/978-981-13-8437-0

Semprini, A. (1995). *L'objet comme procès et comme action: De la nature et de l'usage des objets dans la vie quotidienne* [The Object as Process and as Action: On the Nature and Use of Objects in Everyday Life]. L'Harmattan.

Servaes, J., & Malikhao, P. (2010). Advocacy strategies for health communication. *Public Relations Review, 36*(1), 42–49. https://doi.org/10.1016/j.pubrev.2009.08.017

Settles, I. H., Buchanan, N. T., & Dotson, K. (2019). Scrutinized but not recognized: (In)visibility and hypervisibility experiences of faculty of color. *Journal of Vocational Behavior, 113*, 62–74. https://doi.org/10.1016/j.jvb.2018.06.003

Shaffer, A. (2007, September 27). Pas de deux: Why are there only two sexes? *Slate.* https://slate.com/human-interest/2007/09/why-are-there-only-two-sexes.html

Shah, S., Wallis, M., Conor, F., & Kiszely, P. (2015). Bringing disability history alive in schools: Promoting a new understanding of disability through performance methods. *Research Papers in Education, 30*(3), 267–286. https://doi.org/10.108 0/02671522.2014.891255

Shakespeare, T. (1993). Disabled people's self-organisation: A new social movement? *Disability, Handicap and Society, 8*(3), 249–264. https://doi.org/10.1080/02674649366780261

Shakespeare, T. (1994). Cultural representation of disabled people: Dustbins for disavowal? *Disability and Society, 9*(3), 283–299. https://doi.org/10.1080/09687599466780341

Shakespeare, T. (1999). Joking a part. *Body and Society, 5*(4), 47–52. https://doi.org/10.1177/1357034x99005004004

Shakespeare, T. (2006). The social model of disability. In L. J. Davis (Ed.), *The disability studies reader* (2nd ed., pp. 197–204). Routledge.

Shakespeare, T. (2010). The social model of disability. In L. Davis (Ed.), *The disability studies reader* (3rd ed., pp. 266–273). Routledge. https://doi.org/10.432 4/9780203077887-25

Shakespeare, T. (2017). *Disability: The basics.* Routledge.

Shakespeare, T., Ndagire, F., & Seketi, Q. E. (2021). Triple jeopardy: Disabled people and the COVID-19 pandemic. *The Lancet, 397*(10282), 1331–1333. https://doi.org/10.1016/S0140-6736(21)00625-5

Shakespeare, T., Thompson, S., & Wright, M. J. (2009). No laughing matter: Medical and social factors in restricted growth. *Scandinavian Journal of Disability Research, 12*(1), 19–31. https://doi.org/10.1080/15017410902909118

Shanouda, F. (2019). *The Politics of passing: Disabled and mad students' experiences of disclosure in higher education.* (Unpublished doctoral dissertation). University of Toronto.

Shapira, S., & Granek, L. (2019). Negotiating psychiatric cisgenderism-ableism in the transgender-autism nexus. *Feminism & Psychology, 29*(4), 494–513. https://doi.org/10.1177/0959353519850843

Shapiro, J. P. (1994). *No pity: People with disabilities forging a new civil rights movement.* Three Rivers Press.

Shaw, A. (2010). What is video game culture? Cultural studies and game studies. *Games and Culture, 5*(4), 403–424. https://doi.org/10.1177/1555412009360414

Sheldon, J. (2017). Problematizing reflexivity, validity, and disclosure: Research by people with disabilities about disability. *The Qualitative Report, 22*(4), 984–1000. https://doi.org/10.46743/2160-3715/2017.2713

Shelton, S. S., & Waddell, T. F. (2021). Does 'inspiration porn' inspire? How disability and challenge impact attitudinal evaluations of advertising. *Journal of Current Issues and Research in Advertising, 42*(3), 258–276. https://doi.org/10.1080/1064173 4.2020.1808125

Sheppard, E. (2020). Performing normal but becoming crip: Living with chronic pain. *Scandinavian Journal of Disability Research, 22*(1), 39–47. https://doi.org/10.16993/sjdr.619

Shew, A. (2018). Different ways of moving through the world. *Logic, 5.* Retrieved February 21, 2022, from https://logicmag.io/failure/different-ways-of-moving-through-the-world/

Shifman, L. (2013). *Memes in digital culture.* The MIT Press.

Show and tell tomorrow? Potato. (n.d.). Quickmeme. Retrieved June 1, 2021, from http://www.quickmeme.com/meme/3p931v

Showalter Salas, H. (2011). Cochlear implants and deaf children. In D. Diekema, M. Mercurio, & M. Adam (Eds.), *Clinical ethics in pediatrics: A case-based textbook* (pp. 154–159). Cambridge University Press.

Shrayber, M. (2019, July 9). *Exclusive: Spencer Pratt opened up about Heidi Montag's plastic surgery and it's actually heartbreaking.* Cosmopolitan. Retrieved June 1, 2021, from https://www.cosmopolitan.com/entertainment/tv/a28339096/the-hills-new-beginnings-episode-2-recap-spencer-pratt-heidi-plastic-surgery/

Shriver, T. (2008, August 12). *Special Olympics chairman Timothy Shriver's remarks at "Tropic Thunder" protest.* Special Olympics. Retrieved June 4, 2021, from http://www.specialolympics.org/Special+Olympics+Public+Website/English/Press_Room/Global_news/Tropic+Thunder/Shriver+Protest+Remarks.htm

530 REFERENCES

Shuttleworth, R., & Meekosha, H. (2013). The sociological imaginary and disability enquiry in late modernity. *Critical Sociology, 39*(3), 349–367. https://doi.org/10.1177/0896920511435709

Sidhu, D. (2008). Cujo goes to college: On the use of animals by individuals with disabilities in postsecondary institutions. *University of Baltimore Law Review, 38*(2), 276–303. https://scholarworks.law.ubalt.edu/ublr/vol38/iss2/3

Siebers, T. (2001). Disability in theory: From social constructionism to the new realism of the body. *American Literary History, 13*(4), 737–754. https://doi.org/10.1093/alh/13.4.737

Siebers, T. (2004). *Disability as masquerade. Literature and medicine, 23*(1), 1–22. https://doi.org/10.1353/lm.2004.0010

Siebers, T. (2008). *Disability theory.* University of Michigan Press.

Siegal, A. (2011, August 13). The education of Ashif Jaffer. *BBC* [The Documentary Podcast BBC World Service]. Retrieved February 21, 2022, from https://www.bbc.co.uk/programmes/p02rth23

Silverman, R., & Rowe, D. (2020). Introduction. Blurring the body and the page: The theory, style, and practice of autoethnography. *Cultural Studies↔Critical Methodologies, 20*(2), 91–94. https://doi.org/10.1177/1532708619878762

Sinai Health System. (2012). *Communicating with parents: Sample scripts for each pamphlet.* [Video File]. Retrieved October 2017, from https://vimeo.com/61719338

Sinclair, J. (2010). Being autistic together. *Disability Studies Quarterly, 30*(1). https://doi.org/10.18061/dsq.v30i1.1075

Singer, J. (1999). "Why can't you be normal for once in your life?" From a "problem with no name" to the emergence of a new category of difference. In M. Corker & S. French (Eds.), *Disability discourse* (pp. 59–67). Open University Press.

Singer, P. W. (2006, June 2). DHS seeks to better serve disaster victims with disabilities. *Government Executive: Web Edition.* Retrieved March 2, 2022, from https://www.govexec.com/defense/2006/06/dhs-seeks-to-better-serve-disaster-victims-with-disabilities/21956/

Siperstein, G. N., Pociask, S. E., & Collins, M. A. (2010). Sticks, stones, and stigma: A study of students' use of the derogatory term retard. *Intellectual and Developmental Disabilities, 48*(2), 126–134. https://doi.org/10.1352/1934-9556-48.2.126

Small, A., & Cripps, J. (2012). On becoming: Developing an empowering cultural identity framework for deaf youth and adults. In A. Small, J. Cripps, & J. Côté (Eds.), *Cultural space and self/identity development among deaf youth* (pp. 29–41). Canadian Cultural Society of the Deaf.

Small, M. L. (2009). 'How many cases do I need?' On science and the logic of case selection in field-based research. *Ethnography, 10*(1), 5–38. https://doi.org/10.1177/2F1466138108099586

Smith, A. (2020a, April 16). Tea party-style protests break out across the country against stay-at-home orders. *NBC News.* https://nbcnews.com/politics/donald-trump/tea-party-style-protests-break-out-across-country-against-stay-n1185611

Smith, A. (2020b, July 20). Trump gives masks his strongest endorsement yet after having downplayed them for months. *NBC News.* https://nbcnews.com/politics/donald-trump/trump-gives-masks-his-strongest-endorsement-yet-after-downplaying-them-n1234388

Smith, B. (2018, May 7). Using AI to empower people with disabilities. *Microsoft on the Issues.* https://blogs.microsoft.com/on-theissues/2018/05/07/using-ai-to-empower-people-with-disabilities/

Smith, R. A. (2007). Language of the lost: An explication of stigma communication. *Communication Theory, 17*(4), 462–485. https://doi.org/10.1111/j.1468-2885.2007.00307.x

Smith, S. (2020c, August 9). Unmasked: How Trump's mixed messaging on face-coverings hurt U.S. coronavirus response. *NBC News.* https://www.nbcnews.com/politics/donald-trump/calendar-confusion-february-august-trump-s-mixed-messages-masks-n1236088

Smith-Frigerio, S. (2019). Coping, community and fighting stereotypes: An exploration of multidimensional social capital in personal blogs discussing mental illness. *Health Communication, 35*(4), 410–418. https://doi.org/10.1080/1041023 6.2018.1564959

Smith-Frigerio, S. (2020). Grassroots mental health groups' use of advocacy strategies in social media messaging. *Qualitative Health Research, 30*(14), 2205–2216. https://doi.org/10.1177/1049732320951532

Smith-Frigerio, S., & Houston, J. B. (2018). Crazy, insane, nut job, wacko, basket case, and psycho: Donald Trump's tweets surrounding mental health issues and attacks on media personalities. In M. Lockhart (Ed.), *President Donald Trump and his political discourse* (pp. 114–130). Routledge.

Snoddon, K. (2009). *American sign language and early literacy: Research as praxis* (Publication No. NR61098) [Doctoral Dissertation, University of Toronto]. ProQuest Dissertations Publishing.

Snyder, S. L., & Mitchell, D. T. (2006). *Cultural locations of disability.* University of Chicago Press.

Social Blade. (2022, March 7). *Top 100 most followed TikTok accounts (sorted by followers count).* Retrieved March 7, 2022, from https://socialblade.com/tiktok/top/100

Spanakis, E. K., & Golden, S. H. (2013). Race/ethnic difference in diabetes and diabetic complications. *Current Diabetes Reports, 13*(6), 1–18. https://doi.org/10.1007/s11892-013-0421-9

Special Olympics. (2008, August 14). *Special Olympics and coalition of disability organizations protest DreamWorks' "Tropic Thunder."* Special Olympics. Retrieved February 10, 2022, from https://www.specialolympics.org/Special+Olympics+Public+Website/English/Press_Room/Global_news/R-Word-Tropic+Thunder.htm

Speedy, J. (2015). *Staring at the park: A poetic autoethnographic inquiry.* Routledge.

Spocchia, G. (2022, January 9). *"My disabled life is worthy": CDC prompts backlash for comments on Omicron deaths.* The Independent. Retrieved January 10, 2022, from: https://www.independent.co.uk/news/world/americas/cdc-omicron-covid-disabilities-deaths-b1989524.html

Spinuzzi, C. (2007). Accessibility scans and institutional activity: An activity theory analysis. *College English, 70*(2), 189–201. https://doi.org/10.2307/25472260

Spitzberg, B. H., & Cupach, W. R. (1984). *Interpersonal communication competence.* Sage.

Sports Night. (2012a). Dear Louise. *Sports Night Youtube Channel.* 11 June. (Original air date: November 11, 1998). https://www.youtube.com/watch?v=hJPENIO-G2M

Sports Night. (2012b). Kyle Whitaker's got two sacks. *Sports Night Youtube Channel.* 12 June. (Original air date: December 14, 1999). https://www.youtube.com/watch?v=ActOViNAbJw

Squirmy and Grubs. (2020a, January 11). *Conspiracy theories about our relationship.* [Video]. YouTube. Retrieved April 7, 2020, from https://www.youtube.com/watch?v=7OxYV7liwso

532 REFERENCES

Squirmy and Grubs. (2020b, June 22). *Does Shane's disease affect his sex drive? Intimacy and disability Q&A part 3*. [Video]. YouTube. Retrieved April 7, 2020, from https://www.youtube.com/watch?v=3LJJnULUyFY

Squirmy and Grubs. (2020c, May 20). *Intimacy & disability—How we make it work—Q&A part 1*. [Video]. YouTube. Retrieved April 7, 2020, from https://www.youtube.com/watch?v=8iBROcohmxk

Squirmy and Grubs. (2020d, May 10). *Physical affection and intimacy in our relationship*. [Video]. YouTube. Retrieved April 7, 2020, from https://www.youtube.com/watch?v=5tq83yqreU0

Squirmy and Grubs. (2020e, June 9). *Sexual function and Shane's disease—intimacy and disability Q&A part 2*. [Video]. YouTube. Retrieved April 7, 2020, from https://www.youtube.com/watch?v=P_CbYrTTUdo

Srikanth, A. (2021, March 17). National Database on police killings tracked 1,127 deaths last year. *The Hill*. Retrieved November 1, 2021, from https://thehill.com/changing-america/respect/equality/543712-national-database-on-police-killings-tracked-1127-police

St. Lawrence, J. S., Husfeldt, B. A., Kelly, J. A., Hood, H. V., & Smith, S. (1990). The stigma of AIDS: Fear of disease and prejudice toward gay men. *Journal of Homosexuality, 19*(3), 85–99. https://doi.org/10.1300/J082v19n03_05

St. Pierre, J. (2012). The construction of the disabled speaker: Locating stuttering in disability studies. *The Canadian Journal of Disability Studies, 1*(3), 1–21.

St. Pierre, J. (2015a). Cripping communication: Speech, disability, and exclusion in liberal humanist and posthumanist discourse. *Communication Theory, 25*(3), 330–348. https://doi.org/10.1111/comt.12054

St. Pierre, J. (2015b). Distending straight-masculine time: A phenomenology of the disabled speaking body. *Hypatia, 30*(1), 49–65. https://doi.org/10.1111/hypa.12128

St. Pierre, J., & Peers, D. (2016). Telling ourselves sideways, crooked and crip: An introduction. *Canadian Journal of Disability Studies, 5*(3), 1–11. https://doi.org/10.15353/cjds.v5i3.293

Stake, R. E. (1995). *The art of case study research*. Sage.

Stanley-Becker, I. (2020, May 12). Mask or no mask? Face coverings become tool in partisan combat. *Washington Post*. https://www.washingtonpost.com/politics/in-virus-response-riven-by-politics-masks-are-latest-rorschach-test/2020/05/12/698477d4-93e6-11ea-91d7-cf4423d47683_story.html

Steinkuehler, C. A., & Williams, D. (2006). Where everybody knows your (screen) name: Online games as "third places." *Journal of Computer-Mediated Communication, 11*(4), 885-909. https://doi.org/10.1111/j.1083-6101.2006.00300.x

Stenning, A. (2020). Understanding empathy through a study of autistic life writing. In H. Bertilsdotter Rosqvist, N. Chown, & A. Stenning (Eds.), *Neurodiversity studies: A new critical paradigm* (pp. 108–124). Routledge. https://doi.org/10.4324/9780429322297-11

Stephens, R., Atkins, J., & Kingston, A. (2009). Swearing as a response to pain. *Neuroreport, 20*(12), 1056–1060. https://doi.org/10.1097/WNR.0b013e32832e64b1

Sterne, J. (2021). *Diminished faculties: A political phenomenology of impairment*. Duke University Press.

Stiller, B. (2008, August 13). *Tropic thunder*. [Film] Dreamworks Pictures.

Stone, J., (2017, August 7). Brexit caused by low levels of education, study finds. *The Independent*. Retrieved December 10, 2019, from https://www.independent.co.

uk/news/uk/politics/brexit-education-higher-university-study-university-leave-eu-remain-voters-educated-a7881441.html?amp

Stough, L. M., & Kelman, I. (2017). People with disabilities and disasters. Retrieved January 3, 2022, from https://oaktrust.library.tamu.edu/bitstream/handle/1969.1/165520/Stough%20%26%20Kelman-FINAL%20CLEAN%20COPY%206-19.pdf?sequence=1&isAllowed=y

Strauss, J. (2017). Passing – and passing. In L. X. Z. Brown, E. Ashkenazy, & M. Giwa Onaiwu (Eds.), *All the weight of our dreams: On living racialized autism* (pp. 187–191). DragonBee Press.

Stubblefield, A. (2007). "Beyond the pale": Tainted whiteness, cognitive disability, and eugenic sterilization. *Hypatia, 22*(2), 162–181. https://doi.org/10.1111/j.1527-2001.2007.tb00987.x

Student Disability Services. (2021, December 30). *The myth of the unfair advantage.* University of Mississippi. https://sds.olemiss.edu/the-myth-of-the-unfair-advantage/

Sturgeon, J. (2017). Sometimes I wonder if I'm being masochistic. In L. X. Z. Brown, E. Ashkenazy, & M. Giwa Onaiwu (Eds.), *All the weight of our dreams: On living racialized autism* (pp. 72–75). DragonBee Press.

Suárez-Orozco, C., Casanova, S., Martin, M., Katsiaficas, D., Cuellar, V., Smith, N. A., & Dias, S. I. (2015). Toxic rain in class: Classroom interpersonal micro-aggressions. *Educational Researcher, 44*(3), 151–160. https://doi.org/10.3102/0013189X15580314

Sue, D. W. (2010a). *Microaggressions and marginality: Manifestation, dynamics, and impact.* Wiley and Sons.

Sue, D. W. (2010b). Microaggressions, marginality, and oppression. In D. W. Sue (Ed.), *Microaggressions and marginality: Manifestation, dynamics, and impact* (pp. 3–24). Wiley & Sons.

Sue, D. W., Capodilupo, C. M., Torino, G. C., Bucceri, J. M., Holder, A. M. B., Nadal, K. L., & Esquilin, M. (2007). Racial microaggressions in everyday life: Implications for clinical practice. *American Psychologist, 62*(4), 271–286. https://doi.org/10.1037/0003-066X.62.4.271

Sullivan, M. (2015). Subjected bodies: Paraplegia, rehabilitation, and the politics of movement. In S. Tremain (Ed.), *Foucault and the government of disability* (pp. 27–44). University of Michigan Press.

Summer, S., & Waddell, F. (2021). Does 'inspiration porn' inspire? How disability and challenge impact attitudinal evaluations of advertising. *Journal of Current Issues & Research in Advertising, 42*(3), 258–276. https://doi.org/10.1080/10641734.2020.1808125

Syndrome of a down. (n.d.). Memegenerator.Net. Retrieved June 4, 2021, from https://memegenerator.net/instance/25176266/i-can-count-to-potato-my-favorite-band-is-syndrome-of-a-down

Takahashi, R. (2019, October 14). Japan criticized for lack of foreign-language information during Typhoon Hagibis. Retrieved November 30, 2019, from https://www.japantimes.co.jp/news/2019/10/14/national/japan-criticized-lack-foreign-language-information-typhoon-hagibis/#.XdtnEuj7TIU

Takayama, K. (2017). Disaster relief and crisis intervention with deaf communities: Lessons learned from the Japanese deaf community. *Journal of Social Work in Disability & Rehabilitation, 16*(3-4), 247–260. https://doi.org/10.1080/1536710X.2017.1372241

534 REFERENCES

Taters gonna tate. (n.d.). Quickmeme. Retrieved June 1, 2021, from http://www.quickmeme.com/meme/3p1llv

Taylor, C. (2003). *Modern social imaginaries.* Duke University Press.

Tesser, A. (1988). Towards a self-evaluation maintenance model of social behavior. In L. Berkowitz (Ed.), *Advances in experimental social psychology* (pp. 181–227). Academic.

The Guardian. (n.d.). Culture: Games. Retrieved May 18, 2021, from https://www.theguardian.com/games

The Japan Times. (n.d.). *120-year history of* The Japan Times. Retrieved December 11, 2019, from https://cdn-japantimes.com/wp-ontent/uploads/2017/03/JT_NYT_Media_Guide_v.4.0e.pdf

The Mainichi Shimbun. (n.d.). *The History of the Mainichi Shimbun.* Retrieved January 18, 2022, from https://www.mainichi.co.jp/company/history-e.html

The Minnesota Governor's Council on Developmental Disabilities. (2022). *Parallels in time. A history of developmental disabilities.* Retrieved June 15, 2023 from https://mn.gov/mnddc/parallels/five/5a/6.html

The Washington Post (2020, January 22). Fatal force: Police shootings database. *The Washington Post.* https://www.washingtonpost.com/graphics/investigations/police-shootings-database/

Theofanos, M. F., & Redish, J. (2003). Bridging the gap: Between accessibility and usability. *Interactions, 10*(6), 36–51. https://doi.org/10.1145/947226.947227

Theofanos, M. F., & Redish, J. G. (2005). Helping low-vision and other users with web sites that meet their needs: Is one site for all feasible? *Technical Communication, 52*(1), 9–20. https://www.ingentaconnect.com/content/stc/tc/2005/00000052/00000001/art00002

Thomas, C. (2007). *Sociologies of disability and illness: Contested ideas in disability studies and medical sociology.* Macmillan International Higher Education.

Thomas, K. (2021, July 19). *Hyper-invisibility: What it's like to be Black in engineering: Biomedical-optics researcher Audrey Bowden discusses systemic racism, implicit bias, and five guiding principles for implement change.* SPIE: The International Society for Optics and Photonics. Retrieved January 11, 2022, from https://spie.org/news/hyper-invisibility-what-its-like-to-be-black-in-engineering-

Thompson, R. (2012). Screwed up, but working on it: (Dis)ordering the self through E-stories. *Narrative Inquiry, 22*(1), 86–104. https://doi.org/10.1075/ni.22.1.06tho

Thompson, V. (2021, February 10). Understanding the policing of Black, disabled bodies. *Center for American Progress.* Retrieved October 31, 2021, from https://www.americanprogress.org/issues/disability/news/2021/02/10/495668/understanding-policing-black-disabled-bodies/

Thomson, R. G. (2014). The story of my work: How I became disabled. *Disability Studies Quarterly, 34*(2). http://dsq-sds.org/article/view/4254/3594

Tigert, M. K., & Miller, J. H. (2021). Ableism in the classroom: Teaching accessibility and ethos by analyzing rubrics. *Communication Teacher.* https://doi.org/10.1080/17404622.2021.2006254

Tilbury, K. (2018, May 16). Fake service dogs, real problems. Associated Press. https://apnews.com/article/1a28f8e528424fdca2040ea8139e3014

Timke, E. (2019). Disability and advertising. *Advertising & Society Quarterly, 20*(3). https://doi.org/10.1353/asr.2019.0024

Ting-Toomey, S. (1993). Communicative resourcefulness: An identity negotiation theory. In R. L. Wiseman & J. Koester (Eds.), *Intercultural communication competence* (pp. 72–111). Sage.

Ting-Toomey, S. (1998). Intercultural conflict competence. In J. N. Martin, T. K. Nakayama, & L. A. Flores (Eds.), *Readings in cultural contexts* (pp. 401–413). Mayfield Publishing.

Tisoncik, L. A. (2020). Austistics.org and finding our voices as an activist movement. In S. K. Kapp (Ed.), *Autistic community and the neurodiversity movement: Stories from the frontline* (pp. 65–76). Palgrave Macmillan. https://doi.org/10.1007/978-981-13-8437-0

Titchkosky, T. (2003). *Disability, self, and society.* University of Toronto Press.

Titchkosky, T. (2007). *Reading & writing disability differently: The textured life of embodiment.* University of Toronto Press.

Titchkosky, T. (2019). Disability imaginaries in the news. In K. Ellis, G. Goggin, B. Haller, & R. Curtis (Eds.), *Routledge companion to disability and media* (pp. 13–22). Routledge.

Titchkosky, T., & Michalko, R. (2009). Introduction. In T. Titchkosky & R. Michalko (Eds.), *Rethinking normalcy: A disability studies reader* (pp. 1–15). Canadian Scholars' Press.

Tkaczyk, V., Mills, M., & Hui, A. (Eds.). (2020). *Testing hearing: The making of modern aurality.* Oxford University Press.

Tokyo's Sumida ward spearheads project to assist disabled residents in times of disaster. (2016, February 21). *The Mainichi.* Retrieved November 30, 2019, from https://mainichi.jp/english/articles/20160221/p2a/00m/0na/004000c

Tomašev, C. J., Hutter, F., Mohamed, S., Picciariello, A., Connelly, B., Belgrave, D. C. M., Ezer, D., van der Haert, F. C., Mugisha, F., Abila, G., Arai, H., Almiraat, H., Proskurnia, J., Snyder, K., Otake-Matsuura, M., Othman, M., Glasmachers, T., de Wever, W., et al. (2020). AI for social good: Unlocking the opportunity for positive impact. *Nature Communications, 11*(1), 2468. https://doi.org/10.1038/s41467-020-15871-z

Tomberry, & Don. (2009, August 19). *The Internet is serious business.* Know Your Meme. Retrieved June 1, 2021, from https://knowyourmeme.com/memes/the-internet-is-serious-business

Toshimabousai. (2019, November 10). Tweet. Retrieved November 10, 2019, from https://twitter.com/toshimabousai/status/1182808626605506560

Toyosaki, S., & Pensoneau-Conway, S. L. (2013). Autoethnography as a praxis of social justice: Three ontological contexts. In S. H. Jones, T. E. Adams, & C. Ellis (Eds.), *Handbook of autoethnography* (pp. 557–575). Left Coast Press.

Tracy, S. J. (2020). *Qualitative research methods: Collecting evidence, crafting analysis, communicating impact* (2nd ed.). Wiley Blackwell.

Treviranus, J. (2016). The future challenge of the ADA: Shaping humanity's transformation. *Inclusion, 4*(1), 30–38. https://doi.org/10.1352/2326-6988-4.1.30

Treviranus, J. (2019). The value of being different. In A. Hurst & C. Duartes (Eds.), *W4A '19: Proceedings of the 16th International Web for All Conference* (pp. 1–7). https://doi.org/10.1145/3315002.3332429

Trieschmann, R. B. (1988). *Spinal cord injuries: Psychological, social, and vocational rehabilitation.* Demos Medical Publishing.

536 REFERENCES

Trippity, F. (2013, December 15). Toronto mayor Rob Ford can't count to potato. *Funny Meme-Mories.* Retrieved June 1, 2021, from http://funnymeme-mories.blogspot.com/2013/12/toronto-mayor-rob-ford-cant-count-to.html

Trujillo, N. (1985). Organizational communication as cultural performance: Some managerial considerations. *Southern Speech Communication Journal, 50*(3), 201–224. https://doi.org/10.1080/10417948509372632

Truong-Vu, K.-P. (2022). On the margins of hyperinvisibility and hypervisibility: The paradox of being an Asian-American during the COVID-19 pandemic. In M. Heath, A. K. Darkwah, J. Beoku-Betts, & B. Purkayastha (Eds.), *Global feminist autoethnographies during COVID-19: Displacements and disruptions* (pp. 199–210). Routledge.

Tucker, E. C., Jones, J. L., Gallus, K. L., Emerson, S. R., & Manning-Ouellette, A. L. (2020). Let's take a walk: Exploring intellectual disability as diversity in higher education. *Journal of College and Character, 21*(3), 157–170. https://doi.org/10.1080/2194587X.2020.1781659

Tufekci, Z., & Wilson, C. (2012). Social media and the decision to participate in political protest: Observations from Tahrir Square. *Journal of Communication, 62*(2), 363–379. https://doi.org/10.1111/j.1460-2466.2012.01629.x

Turner, D. M., Bohata, K., & Thompson, S. (2017). Introduction. Special issue. Disability, work and representation: New perspectives. *Disability Studies Quarterly, 37*(4). https://doi.org/10.18061/dsq.v37i4.6101

Twigg, J., Kett, M., & Lovell, E. (2018, July). Disability inclusion and disaster risk reduction: Overcoming barriers to progress. Briefing note. *ODI.* Retrieved January 5, 2022, from https://www.odi.org/sites/ odi.org.uk/files/resource-documents/12324.pdf

Tyler, I. (2008). Chav mum chav scum. *Feminist Media Studies, 8*(1), 17–34. https://doi.org/10.1080/14680770701824779

U mad bro? (n.d.). Quickmeme. Retrieved June 1, 2021, from http://www.quick-meme.com/meme/3qcfzx

U.S. Census Bureau. (2015, July 29). *Facts for features: Hurricane Katrina 10th anniversary: Aug. 29, 2015.* Retrieved December 5, 2019, from https://www.census.gov/newsroom/facts-for-features/2015/cb15-ff16.html

U.S. Department of Health and Human Services. (2010). *Understanding Medicaid home and community services.* Retrieved December 1, 2019, from https://aspe.hhs.gov/system/files/pdf/76201/primer10.pdf

U.S. Department of Justice. (2011). *Service animals.* Retrieved January 11, 2022, from https://www.ada.gov/service_animals_2010.htm

U.S. Department of Justice. (2015) *Frequently asked questions about service animals and the ADA.* Retrieved January 11, 2022, from https://www.ada.gov/regs2010/service_animal_qa.html

U.S. Department of Justice, Civil Rights Division. (2010). Americans with Disabilities Act ADA Compliance BRIEF: Restriping Parking Spaces. https://www.denvergov.org/content/dam/denvergov/Portals/643/documents/Offices/Disability/DPEP/ADA%20Parking%20Lot%20Requirements.pdf

U.S. Department of Justice, Civil Rights Division. (2015). Frequently asked questions about service animals and the ADA. https://www.ada.gov/regs2010/service_animal_qa.html

U.S. Department of Justice, Office of Public Affairs. (2020, June 30). *The Department of Justice warns of inaccurate flyers and postings regarding the use of face masks and the*

Americans with Disabilities Act. [Press Release]. https://www.justice.gov/opa/pr/department-justice-warns-inaccurate-flyers-and-postings-regarding-use-face-masks-and

UN Office for Disaster Risk Reduction (UNDRR). (n.d.). *UN global survey explains why so many people living with disabilities die in disasters.* Retrieved January 10, 2022, from https://www.unisdr.org/archive/35032

UNESCO. (2021). *Recommendation on the Ethics of Artificial Intelligence.* UNESCO. Document code: SHS/BIO/REC-AIETHICS/2021. UNESCO. Retrieved March 22, 2022, from https://unesdoc.unesco.org/ark:/48223/pf0000380455

United Nations, General Assembly. (n.d.). *Addressing the Vulnerability and Exclusion of Persons with Disabilities: The Situation of Women and Girls, Children's Right to Education, Disasters and Humanitarian Crises,* Item 5(D) (June 9–11, 2015). Retrieved December 2019, from https://www.un.org/disabilities/documents/COP/crpd_csp_2015_4.doc

Upgrading anti-disaster measures. (2016, March 11). *The Japan Times.* Retrieved November 30, 2019, from https://www.japantimes.co.jp/opinion/2016/03/11/editorials/upgrading-anti-disaster-measures-2/

Uthappa, N. R. (2017). Moving closer: Speakers with mental disabilities, deep disclosure, and agency through vulnerability. *Rhetoric Review, 36*(2), 164–175. https://doi.org/10.1080/07350198.2017.1282225

Valencia, D. (2017). Passing without trying. In L. X. Z. Brown, E. Ashkenazy, & M. Giwa Onaiwu (Eds.), *All the weight of our dreams: On living racialized autism* (pp. 246–253). DragonBee Press.

Van Lancker, D., & Cummings, J. L. (1999). Expletives: Neurolinguistic and neurobehavioral perspectives on swearing. *Brain Research Reviews, 31*(1), 83–104. https://doi.org/10.1016/S0165-0173(99)00060-0

Vandenbosch, L., Vervloessem, D., & Eggermont, S. (2013). "I might get your heart racing in my skin-tight jeans": Sexualization on music entertainment television. *Communication Studies, 64*(2), 178–194. https://doi.org/10.1080/1051097 4.2012.755640

Vargas, T. (2018, April 24). Settlement reached in police-custody death of man with Down Syndrome. *The Washington Post.* Retrieved October 31, 2021, from https://www.washingtonpost.com/local/settlement-reached-in-police-custody-death-of-man-with-down-syndrome/2018/04/24/7d53c0ca-47fe-11e8-827e-190efaf1f1ee_story.html

Vaz, P., & Bruno, F. (2003). Types of self-surveillance: From abnormality to individuals 'at risk'. *Surveillance & Society, 1*(3), 272–291. https://doi.org/10.24908/ss.v1i3.3341

Venom123. (2012, April 25). *"I can count to potato" girl finally realizes she's a meme!—Off-Topic.* Comic Vine. Retrieved June 1, 2021, from https://comicvine.gamespot.com/forums/off-topic-5/i-can-count-to-potato-girl-finally-realizes-shes-a-664306/

Véron. E. (1987). *La sémiosis sociale: Fragments d'une théorie de la discursivité* [Social Semiosis: Fragments of a Theory of Discursivity]. Presses Universitaires de Vincennes.

Villanueva, G., Broad, G. M., Gonzalez, C., & Ball-Rokeach, S. (2016). Communication asset mapping: An ecological field application toward building healthy communities. *International Journal of Communication, 10,* 2704–2724. https://ijoc.org/index.php/ijoc/article/viewFile/5335/1674

Villepoux, A., Vermeulen, N., Niedenthal, P., & Mermillod, M. (2015). Evidence of fast and automatic gender bias in affective priming. *Journal of Cognitive Psychology*, *27*(3), 301–309. https://doi.org/10.1080/20445911.2014.1000919

Virilio, P. (2007). *The original accident* (J. Rose, Trans.). Polity.

Voorhees, J. (2014, August 27). "Suicide by cop" is a horrible, misleading phrase. We need to stop saying it. *Slate Magazine*. Retrieved November 3, 2021, from https://slate.com/news-and-politics/2014/08/suicide-by-cop-the-dangerous-term-that-stops-us-from-asking-hard-questions-about-police-shootings.html

Wahl, O. F. (1992). Mass media images of mental illness: A review of the literature. *Journal of Community Psychology*, *20*(4), 343–352. https://doi.org/10.1002/1520-6629(199210)20:4%3C343::AID-JCOP2290200408%3E3.0.CO;2-2

Wald, M. (2020). AI data-driven personalisation and disability inclusion. *Frontiers in Artificial Intelligence*, *5*(571955), 1–7. https://doi.org/10.3389/frai.2020.571955

Walker, C. (2017, November 16). Following lawsuit, Red Rocks trying new ticketing system for accessible seats. *Westword*. https://www.westword.com/music/red-rocks-to-implement-new-ticketing-system-following-disability-lawsuit-9700315

Walker, N. (2012). Throw away the master's tools: Liberating ourselves from the pathology paradigm. In J. Bascom (Ed.), *Loud hands: Autistic people, speaking* (pp. 154–162). The Autistic Press.

Walker, N. (2021). Neuroqueer: An introduction. *Neuroqueer: The writings of Dr. Nick Walker*. Retrieved December 17, 2021, from https://neuroqueer.com/neuroqueer-an-introduction/

Walsh-Warder, M. (2016). The disproportionate impact of Hurricane Katrina on people with disabilities. *Verge*, *13*, 2–20. Retrieved January 4, 2022, from https://mdsoar.org/bitstream/handle/11603/3744/Verge13_Walsh-WarderMolly.pdf?sequence=1&isAllowed=y

Walters, S. (2010). Toward an accessible pedagogy: Dis/ability, multimodality, and universal design in the technical communication classroom. *Technical Communication Quarterly*, *19*(4), 427–454. https://doi.org/10.1080/10572252.2010.502090

Walther, S., Yamamoto, M., Thigpen, A. P., Garcia, A., Willits, N. H., & Hart, L. A. (2017). Assistance dogs: Historic patterns and roles of dogs placed by ADI or IGDF accredited facilities and by non-accredited U.S. facilities. *Frontiers in Veterinary Science*, *4*, 1–14. https://doi.org/10.3389/fvets.2017.00001

Walton, R. (2016). Supporting human dignity and human rights: A call to adopt the first principle of human-centered design. *Journal of Technical Writing and Communication*, *46*(4), 402–426. https://doi.org/10.1177/2F0047281616653496

Walton, R., Moore, K. R., & Jones, N. N. (2019). *Technical communication after the social justice turn: Building coalitions for action*. Routledge.

Warner, M. (1999). Normal and normaller: Beyond gay marriage. *GLQ: A Journal of Lesbian & Gay Studies*, *2*, 119–171. https://doi.org/10.1215/10642684-5-2-119

We ride the same bus. (n.d.). Memegenerator.Net. Retrieved June 4, 2021, from https://memegenerator.net/instance/25176748/i-can-count-to-potato-hey-i-know-you-we-ride-the-same-bus

Weaver, S. (2022). *The rhetoric of Brexit humour: comedy, populism and the EU referendum*. Routledge.

Web Accessibility Initiative. (2016). Web Accessibility Initiative (WAI) Highlights. World Wide Web Consortium. Retrieved May 14, 2021, from http://www.w3.org/WAI/highlights/archive#x20131220a

Web trolls: Mum's horror over abuse of down's syndrome daughter. (2012, April 12). *BBC News.* Retrieved June 4, 2021, from. https://www.bbc.com/news/uk-england-coventry-warwickshire-17676553

Webster, A. (2020, June 1). *The Last of Us Part II isn't just Naughty Dog's most ambitious game—it's the most accessible, too.* Retrieved May 18, 2021, from https://www.theverge.com/21274923/the-last-of-us-part-2-accessibility-features-naughty-dog-interview-ps4

Wee, L. (2015). Mobilizing affect in the linguistic cyberlandscape: The R-word campaign. In R. Rubdy & S. Ben Said (Eds.), *Conflict, exclusion and dissent in the linguistic landscape* (pp. 185–203). Palgrave Macmillan UK. https://doi.org/10.1057/9781137426284

Weeden, J., & Sabini, J. (2005). Physical attractiveness and health in Western societies: A review. *Psychological Bulletin, 131*(5), 635–653. https://doi.org/10.1037/0033-2909.131.5.635

Weedon, C. (1987). *Feminist practice and poststructuralist theory.* Blackwell.

Weeks Schroer, J., & Bain, Z. (2020). The message in the microaggression: Epistemic oppression at the intersection of disability and race. In L. Freeman & J. Weeks Schroer (Eds.), *Microaggressions and philosophy* (pp. 226–250). Routledge.

Wemigwans, J. (2018). *A digital bundle: Protecting and promoting Indigenous knowledge online.* University of Regina Press.

What is vulnerability? (n.d.). *The International Federation of Red Cross and Red Crescent Societies.* Retrieved December 10, 2019, from https://www.ifrc.org/en/what-we-do/disaster-management/about-disasters/what-is-a-disaster/what-is-vulnerability/

Whelan, D., Askey, C. J., & Mann, C. P. (2020). Disability awareness training: A train the trainer program for first responders. *The National Center on Criminal Justice & Disability.* Retrieved February 1, 2022, from https://thearc.org/policy-advocacy/legal-advocacy/#what_arc_doing

White, B. (2006). Disaster relief for Deaf persons: Lessons for Hurricanes Katrina and Rita. *Review of Disability Studies: An International Journal, 2*(3) Retrieved December 10, 2019, from https://www.rdsjournal.org/index.php/journal/article/view/336

White, G., Fox, M. H., Rooney, C., & Cahill, A. (2006, April 20). *Assessing the impact of Hurricane Katrina on Persons with Disabilities: Interim Report.* Law, Health Policy and Disability Center. Retrieved January 20, 2022, from https://disability.law.uiowa.edu/dpn_hi/345.pdf

White, M., & Dorman, S. M. (2001). Receiving social support online: Implications for health education. *Health Education Research, 16*(6), 693–707. https://doi.org/10.1093/her/16.6.693

Whittaker, M., Alper, M., Bennett, C.L., Hendren, S., Kaziunas, L., Mills, M., Morris, M. R., Rankin, J., Rogers, E., Salas, M., & West, S. M. (2019). *Disability, bias, and AI.* AI Now Institute, New York University. Retrieved March 22, 2022, from https://ainowinstitute.org/disabilitybiasai-2019.pdf

Whittington-Walks, F. (2018). "One of us" or two? Conjoined twins and the paradoxical relationships of identity in American Horror Story: Freak Show. In J.L. Schatz & A.E. George (Eds.), *The image of disability: Essays on media representations* (pp. 11-27). McFarland & Company, Inc.

WHY CANT I HOLD ALL THESE POTATOES. (n.d.). Me.Me. Retrieved June 1, 2021, from https://me.me/i/why-cant-i-hold-all-these-potatoes-none

540 REFERENCES

Wick, K. G. (2017). Love letter to my autism. In L. X. Z. Brown, E. Ashkenazy, & M. Giwa Onaiwu (Eds.), *All the weight of our dreams: On living racialized autism* (pp. 124–127). DragonBee Press.

Widdows, H. (2019). *Perfect me: Beauty as an ethical ideal*. Princeton University Press.

Wiemann, J. M. (1977). Explication and test of a model of communicative competence. *Human Communication Research, 3*(3), 195–213. https://doi.org/10.1111/j.1468-2958.1977.tb00518.x

Wiggins, B. E., & Bowers, G. B. (2015). Memes as genre: A structurational analysis of the memescape. *New Media & Society, 17*(11), 1886–1906. https://doi.org/10.1177/1461444814535194

Wilkin, H. A., & Ball-Rokeach, S. J. (2006). Reaching at risk groups: The importance of health storytelling in Los Angeles Latino media. *Journalism, 7*(3), 299–320. https://doi.org/10.1177/2F1464884906065513

Wilkin, H. A., & Ball-Rokeach, S. J. (2011). Hard-to-reach? Using health access status as a way to more effectively target segments of the Latino audience. *Health Education Research, 26*(2), 239–253. https://doi.org/10.1093/her/cyq090

Wilkin, H. A., Stringer, K. A., O'Quin, K., Montgomery, S. A., & Hunt, K. (2011). Using communication infrastructure theory to formulate a strategy to locate "hard-to-reach" research participants. *Journal of Applied Communication Research, 39*(2), 201–221. https://doi.org/10.1080/00909882.2011.556140

Williams, E. & Musumeci, M. (2021). *Children with special health care needs: Coverage, affordability, and HCBS access* (Issue Brief). Kaiser family Foundation. Retrieved June 15, 2022 from https://www.kff.org/medicaid/issue-brief/children-with-special-health-care-needs-coverage-affordability-and-hcbs-access/

Williamson, B. (2019). *Accessible America: A history of disability and design*. New York University Press.

Wilson, J. C. (2000). Making disability visible: How disability studies might transform the medical and science writing classroom. *Technical Communication Quarterly, 9*(2), 149–161. https://doi.org/10.1080/10572250009364691

Wilson, J. C., & Lewiecki-Wilson, C. (2001). *Embodied rhetorics: Disability in language and culture*. Southern Illinois University Press.

Wilson, S. R., & Sabee, C. M. (2003). Explicating communicative competence as a theoretical term. In J. O. Greene & B. R. Burleson (Eds.), *Handbook of communication and social interaction skills* (pp. 3–50). Lawrence Erlbaum Associates. https://doi.org/10.4324/9781410607133-7

Wilson, Z. (2019, August 10). Facebook. Retrieved December 10, 2019, from https://www.facebook.com/groups/theverybrexitproblemsclub/search/?query=BENNY&epa=SEARCH_BOX

Winkle, M., Crowe, T. K., & Hendrix, I. (2012). Service dogs and people with physical disabilities partnerships: A systematic review. *Occupational Therapy International, 19*(2012), 54–66. https://doi.org/10.1002/oti.323

Wisner, B. (2002). Disability and disaster: Victimhood and agency in earthquake risk reduction. *Radix—Radical Interpretations of Disaster*. Retrieved December 5, 2019, from http://www.radixonline.org/ disability2.html

Wissinger, E. (2015). *This year's model: Fashion, media, and the making of glamour*. New York University Press.

Wodak, R. (2001). What CDA is about: A summary of its history, important concepts and its developments. In R. Wodak & M. Meyer (Eds.), *Methods of critical discourse analysis* (pp. 1–13). Sage Publications.

REFERENCES 541

Wolbring, G. (2016). Employment, disabled people and robots: What is the narrative in the academic literature and Canadian newspapers? *Societies, 6*(15), 1–16. https://doi.org/10.3390/soc6020015

Wolbring, G., & Yumakulov, S. (2014). Social robots: Views of staff of a disability service organization. *International Journal of Social Robotics, 6*, 457–468. https://doi.org/10.1007/s12369-014-0229-z

Wolfdash94. (2010). *Arguing on the internet is like running in the Special Olympics* [Photo]. https://www.flickr.com/photos/57149147@N08/5264741674/

Woman Alive. (2020, December 15). There's more to me than just having down's syndrome. *Woman Alive.* https://www.womanalive.co.uk/stories/view?articleid=3335

Wong, A. (2016). #CripTheVote: Our voices, our vote. Retrieved January 16, 2020, from https://disabilityvisibilityproject.com/2016/01/27/cripthevote-our-voices-our-vote/

Woods, R. (2021, May 16). Down's syndrome campaigner Heidi Crowter on marriage and loving life. *BBC News.* https://www.bbc.com/news/uk-england-coventry-warwickshire-57089602

Woods, R., Milton, D., Arnold, L., & Graby, S. (2018). Redefining critical autism studies: A more inclusive interpretation. *Disability & Society, 33*(6), 974–979. https://doi.org/10.1080/09687599.2018.1454380

World CP Day (n.d.). Retrieved December 28, 2021, from https://worldcpday.org

World Health Organization. (2017). 'Depression: let's talk' says WHO, as depression tops list of causes of ill health. http://www.who.int/en/news-room/detail/30-03-2017%2D%2Ddepression-let-s-talk-says-who-as-depression-tops-list-of-causes-of-ill-health

Yin, R. K. (2013). *Case study research: Design and methods* (5th ed.). Sage.

Worldometer. (2022). COVID-19 Coronavirus pandemic. https://www.worldometers.info/coronavirus/

Xurd, N. S. Raceabelism. (n.d.). In L. X. Z. Brown, E. Ashkenazy, & M. Giwa Onaiwu (Eds.), *All the weight of our dreams: On living racialized autism* (pp. 148–149). DragonBee Press.

Yamaguchi, M. (2020, March 5). Japan opens part of last town off-limits since nuclear leaks. *ABC News.* Retrieved January 10, 2022, from https://abcnews.go.com/International/wireStory/japan-opens-part-town-off-limits-nuclear-leaks-69377729

Yamamoto, M., & Hart, L. A. (2019). Professionally- and self-trained service dogs: Benefits and challenges for partners with disabilities. *Frontiers in Veterinary Science, 6*, 1–15. https://doi.org/10.3389/fvets.2019.00179

Yan, K. (2021, January 25). Diabetes stigma is everywhere, but you can do something about it. *diaTribe.* Retrieved February 14, 2022, from https://diatribe.org/diabetes-stigma-everywhere-you-can-do-something-about-it

Yanagihara, H. (2021, May 10). Who gets to be beautiful now? *The New York Times.* Retrieved November 15, 2021, from https://www.nytimes.com/2021/05/10/t-magazine/beauty-transforming-self.html

Yep, G. A. (2013). Queering/quaring/kauering/crippin'/transing "other bodies" in intercultural communication. *Journal of International and Intercultural Communication, 6*(2), 118–126. https://doi.org/10.1080/17513057.2013.777087

Yep, G. A. (2016). Toward thick(er) intersectionalities: Theorizing, researching, and activating the complexities of communication and identities. In K. Sorrells & S. Sekimoto (Eds.), *Globalizing intercultural communication: A reader* (pp. 85–93). Sage.

542 REFERENCES

Yep, G. A., & Lescure, R. (2019). A thick intersectional approach to microaggressions. *Southern Communication Journal, 84*(2), 113–126. https://doi.org/10.108 0/1041794X.2018.1511749

Yergeau, M. (2010). Circle wars: Reshaping the typical Autism essay. *Disability Studies Quarterly, 30*(1). https://doi.org/10.18061/dsq.v30i1.1063

Yergeau, M. (2013, January 7). But I never think of you as disabled! Accessing paternalism, erasure, and other happy feel-good theories. *Autistext.* http://autistext. com/2012/01/07/but-i-never-think-of-you-as-disabled-accessing-paternalism-erasure-and-other-happy-feel-good-theories/

Yergeau, M. R. (2018). *Authoring autism: On rhetoric and neurological queerness.* Duke University Press.

Yin, R. K. (2003). *Case study research design and methods* (3rd ed.). Sage.

Yoshizaki-Gibbons, H. H., & O'Leary, M. E. (2018). Deviant sexuality: The hypersexualization of women with bipolar disorder in film and television. In J. L. Schatz & A. E. George (Eds.), *The image of disability: Essays on media representations* (pp. 93–106). McFarland & Company.

You can count to potato? (n.d.). Quickmeme. Retrieved June 1, 2021, from http:// www.quickmeme.com/meme/3ozguz

YOU RUSTLED MY DAUGHTERS JIMMIES. (n.d.). Me.Me. Retrieved June 1, 2021, from https://me.me/i/yourustled-mydaughters-jimmies-o-myonerator-ne-none

Young, A., Carr, G., Hunt, R., McCracken, W., Skipp, A., & Tattersall, H. (2006). Informed choice and deaf children: Underpinning concepts and enduring challenges. *Journal of Deaf Studies and Deaf Education, 11*(3), 322–336. https://doi. org/10.1093/deafed/enj041

Young, N. A. (2021). Childhood disability in the United States: 2019. (Issue Brief ACSBR-006), U.S. Department of Commerce, U.S. Census Bureau. Retrieved January 1, 2022, from https://www.census.gov/content/dam/Census/library/ publications/2021/acs/acsbr-006.pdf

Youngblood, S. A. (2013). Communicating web accessibility to the novice developer from user experience to application. *Journal of Business and Technical Communication, 27*(2), 209–232. https://doi.org/10.1177/2F1050651912458924

Yu, H., & Moeller, M. (2018). *Accountability in technical communication.* Association for Teachers of Technical Writing. Retrieved May 4, 2020, from http://attw. org/2019-conference-cfp/

Yuan, B., Folmer, E., & Harris, F. C. (2011). Game accessibility: A survey. *Universal Access in the Information Society, 10*(1), 81–100. https://doi.org/10.1007/ s10209-010-0189-5

Yumakulov, S., Yergens, D., & Wolbring, G. (2012). Imagery of disabled people within social robotics research. In S. S. Ge, O. Khatib, J.-J. Cabibihan, R. Simmons, & M.-A. Williams (Eds.), *Social robotics. Proceedings of the 4th International Conference, ICSR 2012, Chengdu, China, October 29–31, 2012* (pp. 168–177). Springer.

Zahara, A. (2016, March 21). Refusal as research method in discard studies. Retrieved February 21, 2022, from https://discardstudies.com/2016/03/21/refusal-as-research-method-in-discard-studies/

Zajko, M. (2021). Conservative AI and social inequality: Conceptualizing alternatives to bias through social theory. *AI & Society, 36*, 1047–1056. https://doi. org/10.1007/s00146-021-01153-9

Zappa, A. (2017). Beyond erasure: The ethics of art therapy research with trans and gender-independent people. *Art Therapy, 34*(3), 129–134. https://doi.org/10.1080/ 07421656.2017.1343074

Zbitnew, A. (2015). Visualizing absence: Memorializing the histories of the former Lakeshore Psychiatric Hospital. Retrieved February 21, 2022, from https://visualizingabsence.wixsite.com/visualizing-absence1-space-gallery

Zdenek, S. (2009). Accessible podcasting: College students on the margins in the new media classroom. *Computers and Composition Online*, 1–21. http://www.cconlinejournal.org/Zdenek_Word_version_CConline.pdf

Zdenek, S. (2011). Which sounds are significant? Towards a rhetoric of closed captioning. *Disability Studies Quarterly, 31*(3). https://doi.org/10.18061/dsq.v31i3.1667

Zdenek, S. (2015). *Reading sounds: Closed-captioned media and popular culture*. University of Chicago Press.

Zdenek, S. (2017). Call for proposals: Reimagining accessibility and disability in technical and professional communication. *Communication Design Quarterly*. Retrieved May 14, 2021, from http://readingsounds.net/wp-content/uploads/CFP-CDQ-2017/CFP-ReimaginingAccessibility-CDQSpecial-Issue.html

Zdenek, S. (2018). Guest editor's introduction: Reimagining disability and accessibility in technical and professional communication. *Communication Design Quarterly, 6*(4), 4–11. https://doi.org/10.1145/3309589.3309590

Zhang, L., & Haller, B. (2013). Consuming image: How mass media impact the identity of people with disabilities. *Communication Quarterly, 61*(3), 319–334. https://doi.org/10.1080/01463373.2013.776988

Zhu, X., Smith, R. A., & Parrott, R. L. (2017). Living with a rare health condition: The influence of a support community and public stigma on communication, stress, and available support. *Journal of Applied Communication Research, 45*(2), 179–198. https://doi.org/10.1080/00909882.2017.1288292

Zimmerman, N. (2012, April 26). *Girl with down's is unwitting subject of mean internet meme*. Gawker. http://gawker.com/5905373/girl-with-downs-is-unwitting-subject-of-mean-internet-meme

Zitzelsberger, H. (2005). (In)visibility: Accounts of embodiment of women with physical disabilities and differences. *Disability and Society, 20*(4), 389–403. https://doi.org/10.1080/09687590500086492

Zoller, H. M. (2005). Health activism: Communication theory and action for social change. *Communication Theory, 15*(4), 341–364. https://doi.org/10.1111/j.1468-2885.2005.tb00339.x

Zoller, H. M., & Kline, K. N. (2008). Theoretical contributions of interpretive and critical research in health communication. *Annals of the International Communication Association, 32*(1), 89–135. https://doi.org/10.1080/23808985.2008.11679076

Zulli, D., & Zulli, D. J. (2020). Extending the internet meme: Conceptualizing technological mimesis and imitation publics on the TikTok platform. *New Media & Society*. https://doi.org/10.1177/1461444820983603

INDEX[1]

NUMBERS AND SYMBOLS
#CripTheVote, 9, 17, 26, 468, 469
#Disability, 273, 277, 279
#DisabilityTikTok, 273–286

A
Abbott, D., 297, 300, 302, 303
Able-bodied, 6, 70, 75, 88, 90, 93n1,
  101, 104, 105, 107, 108, 115, 117,
  123, 130, 164, 166, 175, 179, 186,
  193, 196, 197, 235, 298, 300, 302,
  309, 346, 402
Ableism, 10, 40, 48, 70, 74, 79, 90,
  99–109, 113, 115, 117, 127, 141,
  142, 190, 191, 198, 253–268, 283,
  300, 311n2, 352, 357, 374
  See also Ableist
Ableist, 6, 11, 33, 39, 71, 73, 75, 76, 78,
  79, 100–109, 113, 115, 130, 131,
  148, 253, 254, 263, 274, 280, 297,
  300, 305, 311, 351, 394
  language, 394
  rhetoric, 11, 100, 102–105
Accessibility as Aesthetic, 352, 354,
  357, 365

Accessibility measures, 226, 228, 230,
  231, 234, 235, 237
  See also Accessibility settings
Accessibility settings, 229–231, 233,
  236, 238
Accessibility/accessible design,
  401–412
ADA, *see* Americans with Disabilities Act
Adaptive technologies, 403, 405, 410
ADHD, *see* Attention deficit hyperactivity
  disorder
Advocacy fatigue, 331–346
Advocacy strategies, 462–466, 468–472
Affordance, 223, 224, 227, 229, 232,
  235, 236, 238, 274, 277, 278
Agency, 12, 36–38, 82, 85, 87, 89,
  91–93, 195, 211, 223, 224, 227,
  230–232, 235, 236, 238, 279, 299,
  305, 308, 332, 371, 376, 387, 425,
  429, 455, 464, 470, 471
Aggrievement politics, 185–198
AI, *see* Artifical intelligence
AI for Good, 210–212
Alper, M., 206, 210
American Sign Language (ASL), 70, 71,
  76, 309, 385, 395, 449

[1] Note: Page numbers followed by 'n' refer to notes.

© The Author(s), under exclusive license to Springer Nature
Switzerland AG 2023
M. S. Jeffress et al. (eds.), *The Palgrave Handbook of Disability and
Communication*, https://doi.org/10.1007/978-3-031-14447-9

545

546 INDEX

Americans with Disabilities Act (ADA), 191–195, 197, 198, 211, 331–336, 339, 340, 345, 346, 370, 386, 387, 389–392, 395, 404
Annamma, S. A., 149, 159
  See also Connor, D.; Ferri, B.
Artificial intelligence (AI), 10, 205–215
  See also Machine learning
Ascribed disabled identity, 196
Ashcraft, K. L., 369, 373–375, 378
ASL, *see* American Sign Language
Assist Mode, 226–228, 234, 235, 239n2
Assistive device, 306, 340, 342, 343
Attention deficit hyperactivity disorder (ADHD), 8, 24, 46, 54, 71, 75, 196, 409
Autism, 21, 22, 45, 46, 50, 284, 335, 388, 391, 393, 394, 409, 462
  See also Autistic
Autistic, 21, 24, 45, 47, 48, 50–52, 54, 58, 284, 388, 429
Autoethnography, 116, 129–142, 243, 244
Avowed disabled identity, 196

B
Ball-Rokeach, S. J., 421–423, 425, 426, 434
Barnes, C., 280
Basas, C. G., 332, 337, 344–346
Baudrillard, J., 254, 257, 258, 263, 267
Becker, A. B., 276, 281, 282
Bertilsdotter Rosqvist, H., 45, 46, 48, 50, 51, 53, 54, 57
Biocertification, 105
Bio-power, 443, 447
BIPOC, 48, 59, 125, 387
Birk, L. B., 133
Black, 9, 10, 99, 104, 120–122, 124, 145–160, 249, 253, 279, 283, 301, 317–329, 357, 359–361, 386, 390, 391
Blockmans, I. G. E., 164, 165, 178
Braidotti, R., 38, 39, 42, 243–245
Braithwaite, D. O., 6, 46, 50, 78, 163, 186, 196
Brexit, 11, 24, 317–329
  See also Leavers; Remainers
Burcaw, S., 83–91, 93n1

C
CAC, *see* Communication action context
Cameron, C., 321, 322, 324–327
Carey, J., 31, 33, 36, 39, 40
Carter-Long, L., 386, 387, 390–394
Celeste, 225–228, 234, 235, 238
Cerebral palsy (CP), 7, 22, 71, 72, 75, 108, 114, 120, 123, 125, 169, 244, 245, 273, 277, 279, 281, 283, 391
Chang, H., 336, 337
Children with disabilities, 12, 206, 418–420, 425, 434–436
Cho, S. E., 299, 300
Chronic pain, 2, 8, 10, 73, 115, 129–142, 279, 340
The CICE Team, 351–355, 357, 359, 363–365
CIT, *see* Communication infrastructure theory
Class, 4, 6–8, 10, 38, 99, 107, 115, 116, 118–120, 122, 123, 125, 126, 142, 147, 149, 150, 159, 160, 309, 333, 338–342, 358, 360, 387
Clogston, J.S., 306
Cochlear implant (CI), 208, 442, 449–455
Cognitive impairment, 253, 254, 260, 261, 263–267
Collaborative autoethnography, 332, 336–337, 345
Collier, M. J., 196
Communication accidents, 9, 32, 33, 39, 40
Communication action context (CAC), 421–423, 426–432, 435
Communication as ritual, 33
Communication competence, 9, 45–59
Communication infrastructure theory (CIT), 421–423, 425, 426, 434
Communication training, 386, 387, 392–394
Compulsory able-bodiedness, 9, 87, 117, 126, 254, 264, 372
Confidence, 141, 169, 176–177, 429
Connor, D., 149, 159
Constantino, C., 41
Content analysis, 11, 296, 297, 306, 311
Co-opting disabled identity, 189, 191, 192, 197

COVID pandemic, 2, 102, 126, 141, 167, 186, 195, 197, 198, 355, 420
Craig, D. R., 274, 277, 278, 285
Craig, M., 275
Crip, 26, 108, 128n2, 261, 375–378
  poetics, 134–135, 142
  theory, 108, 371–374
  time, 40, 130–135, 141, 142
Cripistemology, 11, 369, 373–376
Critical autoethnography, 113–127
  See also Autoethnography
Critical disability studies (CDS), 82, 258, 355, 357, 401–412
Critical humanism, 244
Critical posthuman, 245–251
Critical race theory, 149
Cross-neurotype communication, 9, 45–59
Crowter, Heidi, 253, 254, 262–268
Csikszentmihalyi, M., 54, 224
Cultural categories, 46, 47, 52–58
Cultural equity, 221–239
Cunningham, S., 274, 277, 278, 285
Custodial caregiver, 418, 420, 421, 423–427, 430–436

D
D/deaf hard of hearing (DHH), 298, 299, 303, 304, 307–310, 455
Dating, 163, 164, 167, 170–174, 176, 177, 179, 226, 281, 282
Davis, L. J., 7, 92, 99, 100, 102, 105, 106, 234, 238, 265, 404, 448
Deaf, 20–23, 68, 70, 71, 108, 208, 246, 251, 282, 298, 304, 305, 307, 309, 357, 385, 388, 391, 395, 441–457
Deaf culture, 442, 450–452, 456
Deafness/hard of hearing, 245, 246, 248, 250, 251, 388, 391, 441–457
"Defective" norm *vs.* ideal, 105, 106
Deleuze, G., 257, 258, 264
Delgado, M. R., 209
Dementia, 22, 23, 46, 320–325, 328, 329
Denzin, N., 116
DHH, *see* D/deaf hard of hearing

Diabetes
  type one diabetes, 146–151, 153, 155, 159
  type two diabetes, 147–149, 155, 159
Disability
  definition, 81–83
  justice, 8, 11, 12, 79, 208, 351, 353, 357–358, 364, 365
  as metaphor, 23, 268
  networks, 425–427, 431–432, 434
  studies, 1, 4–9, 11, 38, 79, 82, 99, 105, 108, 130, 133, 134, 149, 207, 212, 244, 258, 259, 275, 280, 297, 298, 318, 344, 402, 404, 405, 408, 409, 433, 441, 443, 463
  and technology, 207, 208, 215
Disability-first terminology, 21
Disability Issues Caucus (DIC), 6–9
Disaster communication, 296–304
  See also Disaster information
Disaster information, 295–297
Disaster preparation, 301
Disaster Risk Reduction (DRR), 297, 298, 300, 301, 304, 311
Disaster studies, 298
Disclosure, 71, 78, 164–166, 178, 466, 471
Discourse analysis, 83, 225, 254, 443
DisCRT, 149
Dolmage, J. T., 100, 356, 357, 402, 403
Down syndrome, 10, 22, 46, 253, 254, 260–267, 386, 396
DRR, *see* Disaster Risk Reduction
Duggan, A., 164, 165, 178
Durham, S., 257, 258
Dwarfism, 19, 20
Dysfluent speaker, 32, 37
Dyslexia, 46, 196, 409
Dysphemistic, 23

E
Ecosystems of activity, 407
Educational strategies, 466, 472
Ellis, C., 132, 243, 244
Ellis, K., 222, 236, 274, 275, 299
  See also Kent, M.

548 INDEX

Embodiment, 2, 3, 7, 8, 11n2, 23, 39, 115–117, 127, 134, 142, 186, 245, 371, 372, 408
Emotional support and therapy animals, 333
Erasure, 378, 387, 392–393
Erdely, J.L., 133
Esposito, J., 133, 134
Ethic of Accommodation, 375
Ethnography, 7, 8, 116, 371, 372
Eugenics, 100–102, 106, 141, 268, 319, 356
Euphemisms, 18, 23

F
Family, 5, 12, 17, 19, 21, 31, 48, 69, 70, 76, 103, 146, 147, 149, 150, 154–156, 170, 196, 246, 248, 257, 263, 265, 268, 307–309, 329, 342, 344, 387, 418–422, 427–436, 442, 444, 446, 449, 451, 453–455
Ferri, B., 149, 159
Ferris, J., 129, 134, 135, 137, 138, 140, 372
Fibromyalgia, 73, 74, 77, 135
FitCrip, 10, 113–127
Fitness, 115–119, 121–126, 280
Fjord, L., 297, 300, 309
Flores, N., 443
Flow, 9, 34, 37, 38, 41, 54, 187, 224, 226, 230–232, 236, 246, 308, 341, 373, 375, 377, 378, 430
Foster, J., 10, 11, 274, 276, 277, 281, 285
Foucault, M., 7, 83, 85, 92, 108, 140, 225, 259, 443, 447
Fourth Industrial Revolution, 209
Framing/Framing theory, 196, 207, 211, 232, 280–284, 305–311, 387, 392–396, 407
Fritsch, K., 208, 215, 352, 354, 357, 360, 362–365

G
Galgay, C. E., 67–69, 71, 73, 76–78, 332, 337, 338, 346
Galloway, T., 375

Game Accessibility Guidelines, 223, 229, 231
Game design, 222, 223, 225–233, 236, 238
Game mechanics, 221–239
Game studies, 223, 224
Garland Thomson, R., 2, 7, 8, 99, 103, 104, 106, 117, 166, 167, 186, 195, 259, 280, 402, 404
Gender, 4, 6, 7, 10, 27, 56, 67, 68, 79, 90, 99–101, 103–106, 117, 127, 142, 145–160, 164, 166, 174, 196, 213, 266, 274, 275, 279, 281, 326, 329, 342, 373, 376, 387, 402, 468
Genette, G., 225, 226
Gingrich-Philbrook, C., 132
Goffman, E., 87, 92, 178, 306, 321
Goggin, G., 10, 206, 210, 211, 214, 299
Goodley, D., 234, 235, 259
Google, 206, 211
Governmentality, 443, 444

H
Hall, S., 107, 223
Haller, B., 5, 186, 244, 276, 281, 282, 297, 306
Hammer, G., 166, 167, 179
Hamraie, A., 208, 215, 352, 354, 357, 360, 362–365, 408
Hashtag, 9, 12, 17, 26, 273, 277–279, 282, 300, 462–472
HCBS, *see* Home and community based waivers
Hearing screening, 441, 442, 444, 448
Hearing technologies, 442, 447–454
Helpless, 70, 73–75, 79, 167, 235, 300
Helplessness, 68, 73, 328
See also Helpless
Hemingway, L., 297, 302, 306
Heterosexual, 10, 105, 164, 166, 167
High affect display, 56, 57
Higher education, 191, 356–358, 365
Holman Jones, S., 132
Holocaust, 101, 102
Home and community based waivers (HCBS), 417–419, 433, 434, 436
Horan, S., 163, 166, 178
Huell, J.C., 133

Human dignity, 12, 402, 405, 407, 409–411
Humanizing, 463, 465, 466
Humor, 26, 180, 256, 264, 317–329
Hurricane Katrina, 11, 295–311
Huss, R. J., 334, 335
Hyper-invisibility, 331–346

I

Ibrahim, Y., 254, 255, 257, 258
I Can Count to Potato, 10, 253–268
  See also Potato meme
Identity, 1–10, 20–22, 26, 27, 45, 52, 68, 70, 71, 79, 82, 85, 86, 89, 91, 99, 100, 103, 104, 106, 108, 109, 115, 116, 120, 124, 126, 127n1, 128n2, 132, 147, 159, 160, 163–180, 185–199, 214, 254, 256–258, 260, 264, 266, 267, 318, 321, 322, 328, 337, 338, 341, 343, 345, 346, 370, 371, 373, 387, 388
Ideology, 83, 102, 107, 189, 258, 264, 442, 450
IHP, *see* Ontario Infant Hearing Program
Imaginaries, 187, 209–210, 212–215, 320
Improvisations, 355, 375–378
Inahara, M., 88, 92
Inclusion, 10, 11, 19, 23, 26, 58, 59, 119, 127, 158, 206, 207, 211–213, 215, 231, 238, 239, 252, 274–277, 279, 286, 300, 305, 307, 311, 356–358, 360, 361, 365, 377, 406, 463, 465, 469, 471
Indigenous communities, 21
Infantilization, 68, 76, 83, 85, 92
Intellectual disabilities, 102, 195, 197, 260, 261, 263, 264, 266–268, 320, 351–365, 392, 393
Interable/interabled, 84, 93n1, 163–180
Interest system, 46, 52–54, 58
  See also Monotropism; Polytropism
Interface, 37, 212, 225, 404, 405, 407–409, 472
Internalization, 179
Internet archeology, 254
Intersectional/intersectionality, 7–10, 13, 47, 48, 56, 59, 79, 99–109,

159, 186, 352, 353, 356, 357, 363, 365, 369, 371–373
Invisible disability, 71, 73, 154–160, 163, 164, 189, 191, 193, 196, 331, 334–338, 340, 341, 343, 346

J

Jacoby, T. A., 188, 189, 197
Jasanoff, S., 209
Johnson, Boris, 319, 324–327
Jurgens, A., 53

K

Kanner, L., 50
Kapp, S. K., 46, 48–50, 54
Keller, R. M., 67–69, 71, 73, 76–78, 332, 337, 338, 346
Kent, M., 299
  See also Ellis, K.
Kerschbaum, S. L., 355
Kim, Y. C., 421–423
Knowing-making, 352, 354, 357, 358, 360, 363–365
Kuppers, P., 134, 375
Kurzweil, R., 208

L

Langellier, K. M., 116
The Last Of Us Part II (TLOU2), 225, 230–233, 236–238
Leavers, 273, 318, 319, 324, 325
Lebensunwerten Lebens, 101, 102
Lillywhite, A., 212
Linton, S., 100, 108, 402, 404
Lipari, L., 34, 39, 40
Little Britain, 326–327
Loebner, J., 275–277
Low affect display, 56, 57
Lyric autoenthography, 129–142
  See also Autoethnography

M

Machine learning, 205, 206, 210, 215
Machinic enslavement, 36
MacKinnon, C., 452

550 INDEX

Malikhao, P., 464, 468, 471, 472
Mansell, R., 210, 211
Marvel's Spider-Man: Miles Morales, 225,
    229–230, 236, 238
    See also Miles Morales
Mass shooting, 12, 189, 461, 462,
    464, 466–472
May, T., 318
McRuer, R., 42, 87, 93, 108, 117, 131,
    264, 372–374, 378
Media representation, 187, 189, 194,
    274–276, 279, 361
Medicaid, 152, 417–436
Medical model, 4, 6, 48, 196–198, 393
    of disabilities, 4, 77, 82, 105, 190,
    191, 195–196, 234
    See also Pathology paradigm
Medical racism, 155, 157–159
Meme, 10, 253–268, 465
Mental health concerns, 462–472
    See also Mental illness
Mental illness, 12, 20, 22, 24, 25, 189,
    318, 324, 325, 328, 392, 393, 409,
    462, 465–468, 470
Michalko, R., 82, 376
Michelle P. Waiver (MPW),
    419–421, 423–436
Microaggressions, 5, 8, 9,
    67–79, 331–346
Miles Morales, 229, 230, 236, 238
Mills, M. L., 331, 332, 336, 337, 339,
    342, 345, 346
Monotropism, 53, 54
Moral model of disability, 4
Morgan, J. M., 390
MPW, *see* Michelle P. Waiver
Murray, D., 53, 54
Murray, F., 53–55, 57

N
Nazi genocide, 101
Neely, E. L., 224, 228
Neilsen, L., 134
Neoliberal, 357, 378, 454
Neurodivergent/neurodivergence/
    neurodiversity, 4, 9, 21, 45–59, 108,
    109, 373, 375, 401, 407, 409, 411
    See also Neuro-variation
Neuroqueer, 108, 109

Neuro-separate spaces, 47, 51–52
Neuro-shared spaces, 47, 51–52
Neuro-variation, 47, 48, 51–52
Newell, C., 210, 299
Njelesani, J., 300
Normalcy, 7, 11, 45, 48, 82, 83, 87, 92,
    93n1, 103–105, 107, 189, 198,
    214, 234, 235, 408, 448, 452, 453
Normal is natural (Aristotle),
    103–106, 109
Normative, 2–4, 37, 48, 56, 75, 85, 87,
    88, 90, 92, 93, 106, 123, 127, 131,
    188, 278, 283, 298, 373, 376,
    408, 454–456
    See also Normalcy

O
O'Donnell-Trujillo, N., 370
Oliver, M., 82, 280
Ontario Infant Hearing Program (IHP),
    441–450, 452–457
Organizational communication,
    11, 369–378
Organizational culture,
    370–372, 374–378
Osteogenesis imperfecta (OI), 69, 74, 75

P
Pacanowsky, M. E., 370
Padden, C., 40
Participant observation, 355, 372
Paterson, K., 39
Pathology paradigm, 46
Patronization, 68, 70, 76
People of color, 56, 132, 147–149,
    159, 357
Performance, 5–7, 19, 39, 40, 42, 56,
    102, 108, 115–127, 128n2, 133,
    134, 149, 186, 192, 209, 236, 250,
    337, 370–372, 375, 376, 408
    See also Performativity
Performativity, 116, 118, 127
Perrow, C., 34–36, 38
Perry, D. M., 386, 387, 390–394
Person-first terminology, 21
Peterson, E. E., 116
Pity, 74, 139, 164, 190, 276, 280,
    341, 343

INDEX   551

Plain language translation, 352
Platforms, 11, 58, 85, 86, 211, 221,
    226, 228, 255, 267, 274, 277, 278,
    285, 286, 299, 300, 466, 467,
    470, 472
Podcast, 11, 58, 351–365
Police brutality, 11, 56, 385–396
    See also Police violence
Police violence, 387, 392
Political correctness, 20
Polytropism, 53, 54
Popular culture, 10, 86, 221, 222,
    243–245, 251, 267
Porter, S., 297, 300, 302, 303
Posthuman critical theory, 10, 243–252
    See also Critical posthuman
Potato meme, 253, 254, 259–266, 268
Priestley, M., 297, 302, 306
Pritchard, E., 328
Productivity, 12, 53, 131
Progeria, 67, 69
Project Euphonia, 211
Psychiatric disabilities, 132,
    390–393, 407

R

Race, 4, 6, 7, 10, 56, 67, 68, 78, 79, 90,
    99–101, 104–107, 117, 127, 142,
    145–160, 196, 213, 248–250, 274,
    275, 279, 326, 329, 342, 376, 377,
    387, 392
Race and disability, 100, 105, 147–150
    See also DisCRT
Remainers, 318–321, 325–327
Retarded, 253, 259, 260
    See also R-word
Retznik, L., 164, 179
Rhetoric, 11, 12, 48, 76, 100–109, 166,
    186–191, 317–329, 359, 402, 409,
    446, 447, 469
Rich, A., 117
Richards, R., 133
Riessman, C. K., 425, 426
The Ringer, 253, 259, 260, 262, 265, 268
Ritual, 33, 39–42, 128n2, 376
Romantic relationship, 49, 163–180
    See also Dating
Rouhban, B., 297, 299
Roulstone, A., 207, 208

Rowe, D., 132
R-word, 17–19, 253, 259–263, 268

S

Samuels, E., 100, 104, 105, 131, 142
Sandahl, C., 108, 372
Satire, 260, 318, 327–328
Scott, J.-A., 116, 117, 133, 166, 186,
    371, 372
Self-worth, 176–177, 179, 345
    See also Confidence
Sense-sharing, 369–378
Sensory-defensive behavior, 55
Sensory-seeking behavior, 55
Servaes, J., 464, 468, 471, 472
Service dog, 78, 331–346
Service dog handler, 11, 331, 332, 334,
    336, 338, 345
Sexism, 10, 48, 79, 100, 103, 104, 109,
    222, 253–268, 394
Sexuality, 4, 6, 7, 9, 10, 27, 67, 81–93,
    99, 103, 127, 142, 179, 275, 280,
    281, 376, 377
Sexual subjectivity, 82, 86–88, 91
Shakespeare, T., 5, 9, 19, 20, 22, 23, 26,
    48, 197, 235, 237, 318, 321, 322
Shifman, L., 255, 256, 259, 261,
    262, 265
Short stature, 19, 20
Sign language, 20, 305, 391, 442,
    443, 449–456
Silence, 341, 355, 362, 364, 365
Silverman, R., 132
Simulacra, 253–260, 263–267
Sinclair, J., 47, 49, 51, 52, 54, 55, 57, 58
Smith-Frigerio, S., 12, 462–464,
    470, 471
SNAKE Project, 302, 308, 309, 311
Social construction model, 305
Social control, 5, 426, 427, 430
Social justice, 8, 248, 249, 277, 336,
    337, 356, 372, 396, 401, 405–406,
    410, 411
Social media, 11, 12, 19, 25, 58, 126,
    167, 172, 193, 206, 254, 255, 261,
    267, 273, 274, 277–278, 284–286,
    299, 300, 319, 326, 328, 425, 431,
    434, 462, 464, 467–470
    See also Platforms

552 INDEX

Social model of disability, 4, 21, 47, 82, 87, 264
Sociosemiotics, 223, 225, 226, 238
Sociospatial model of disability, 408
Special Olympics, 260, 268
Spoken language approach, 443, 445, 447, 449, 451, 453, 455
Sport, 8, 10, 103, 124, 127, 128n2, 245, 248, 250, 251, 421
Sports Night, 10, 243–252
Spread the Word to End the Word, 259–261, 268
Squirmy and Grubs, 84–86, 89, 90
Stammer, 32
Stereotype, 11, 24, 49, 85, 87, 92, 164, 165, 179, 253, 267, 274, 276, 280–283, 285, 319, 320, 324–328, 342
Stigma, 2, 5, 6, 9, 10, 19, 25, 47, 49–51, 57, 81, 84, 85, 87, 117, 166, 177, 179, 186, 231, 239, 267, 268, 280, 342, 343, 392, 393, 422, 465, 466
Storytelling network (STN), 421–422, 435
Structured sociality, 57, 58
Stutter, 32, 41, 42
    See also Stammer
Syllogism, 103
Systems theory, 34, 37, 38

T
Taboo words, 9, 17–27
Takayama, K., 302, 303, 307, 308
Technical communication, 11, 12, 401–412
T4 program, 101
TikTok, 11, 273, 274, 277–286
Titchkosky, T., 82, 93, 209, 447, 448
TLOU2, *see The Last Of Us Part II*
Tōhoku, 11, 295–311
Toxic positivity, 71, 78
Transgress, 89
Transmission model, 32–34, 38, 39
Trope of victimhood, 186
Tropic Thunder, 259–261
Trump, Donald (President), 23, 24, 185, 190, 191, 198, 462–465, 467, 469, 471
Tweets, 212, 320, 463, 465–472

Twigg, J., 297–299
Twitter, 17, 24, 26, 230, 296, 299, 300, 320, 461–472
    See also Tweets
Tyranny of normality, 234–235

U
UN, *see* United Nations
UNESCO, *see* United Nations Educational, Scientific and Cultural Organization
United Nations (UN), 211, 212, 214, 297, 309, 311
United Nations Educational, Scientific and Cultural Organization (UNESCO), 214, 215
Unstructured sociality, 57
U.S. Department of Justice, 192, 194, 195, 332, 333, 388, 393
Utilitarian, 404
Utilitarianism, 24

V
Very Brexit Problems Club, 317–323, 325, 326
Video games, 10, 221–239
View of self, 173–175, 179
    See also Identity

W
Weaponized disability, 192, 194, 195
Weaver, S., 318, 322, 324
Web Content Accessibility Guidelines (WCAG 2.1), 401, 407–409
Western Union Telegraph, 34, 36, 37
Wolbring, G., 212, 282, 285
Women with disabilities, 164, 166, 178, 179

Y
YouTube, 83, 84, 86, 89, 244, 274, 278

Z
Zhang, L., 186, 244, 306
Zitzelsberger, H., 163, 165, 167, 179

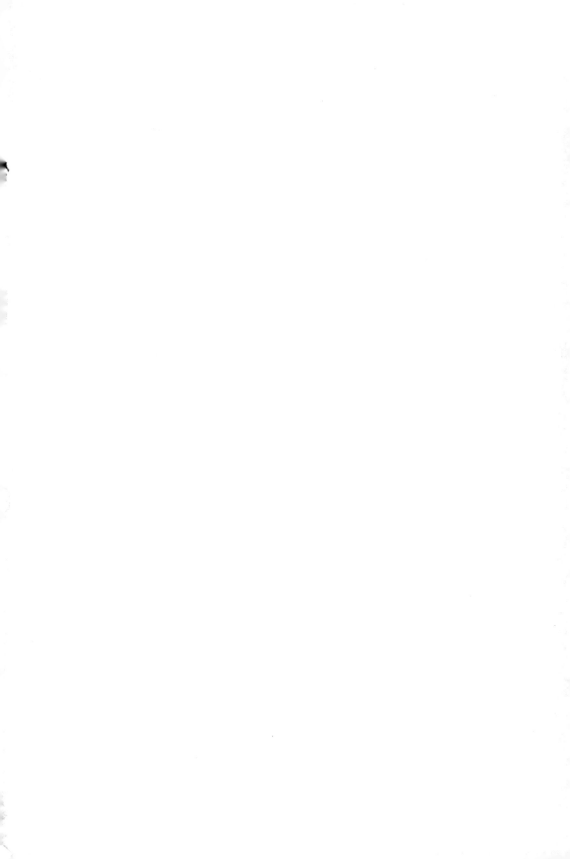

Printed in the United States
by Baker & Taylor Publisher Services